Maureen Friel

A Practical Approach
to Angiography

A Practical Approach to Angiography

Second Edition

Irwin S. Johnsrude, M.D.

Clinical Professor of Radiology, East Carolina University School of Medicine, Greenville, North Carolina; Chief of Special Procedures in Radiology, Pitt County Memorial Hospital, Greenville, North Carolina

Donald C. Jackson, M.D., F.R.C.R., F.R.C.P.(C)

Clinical Professor of Radiology, Duke University School of Medicine, Durham, North Carolina; Staff Radiologist, Craven County Hospital, New Bern, North Carolina

N. Reed Dunnick, M.D.

Professor of Radiology, and Chief of Vascular and Interventional Radiology, Duke University Medical Center, Durham, North Carolina

Little, Brown and Company
Boston/Toronto

Competence, without compassion,
is labor lost.
Compassion, without competence,
is perilous.

Confucius

Contents

Preface

The radiologist has an increasing variety of diagnostic methods with which to work, and the role of each is constantly changing in importance. Although angiography is one of the most dynamic and exciting of these methods, it is invasive and should be undertaken only when noninvasive techniques fail. The excellent anatomic detail provided by ultrasound, computed tomography, and magnetic resonance imaging serve to limit and make more precise the indications for angiography. Advances in angiography itself, in both technology and techniques of performance, allow us to employ a full range of selective catheterizations together with magnification and pharmacoangiography. Technologic advances in digital angiography (intravenous and intraarterial) have broadened the base of patient selection, allowing some studies to be performed on an outpatient basis with saving in cost and with fewer complications for the patient. Therapeutic catheter techniques have rapidly developed and their scope greatly broadened.

Technological advances of the past decade require more than simple diagnostic studies of the vascular system. Often a lesion amenable to intravascular therapeutic methods is uncovered during a procedure. The decision to treat must be addressed at the time of the study. This requires technical skill, a mind open to sudden changes in goals of the procedure, a close rapport with the attending clinicians and surgeons, and an armamentarium of immediately available catheterization equipment of increasing complexity and cost.

The primary purpose of A *Practical Approach to Angiography* is to lessen the danger to patients by familiarizing the angiographer with available equipment and the latest angiographic and therapeutic techniques. This book also attempts to provide the angiographer with an understanding of indications and contraindications thus preventing complications.

We have outlined a practical approach—a technical manual—to management of the patient once he or she has been selected for an angiographic or intravascular therapeutic procedure. In the early chapters, the text guides the inexperienced angiographer, making him aware of the tools with which he must work, familiarizing him with good working habits, and warning him of traps. Discussion of anatomy and physiology are purposefully kept brief. This section also includes an introduction in general terms to therapeutic techniques.

Later in the text, more precise details of angiographic techniques, together with indications and contraindications, and a general approach to solving a problem in specific body and organ areas by angiographic methods are discussed. In addition, a brief section on therapeutic maneuvers is included in each chapter. These chapters may also act as reminders for the angiographer who needs a quick reference before undertaking an unfamiliar procedure.

Because technique of performance naturally evolves while a study is in progress and varies according to the specific pathologic process under study, abnormal angiographic patterns of a wide variety of conditions have been summarized and illustrated. References are provided for more in-depth understanding of many of these diseases.

The final chapter is devoted to cardiopulmonary resuscitation.

This new edition of A *Practical Approach to Angiography* renews the position of angiography as it relates to improving noninvasive imaging technology. Areas from the first edition that are now less pertinent or seem obsolete have been deleted. The second edition also incorporates the impact made by digital subtraction angiography and the newer (but more expensive) contrast agents. It includes manufacturer's improvements in angiographic equipment which further enhance angiographic capabilities. The role of intravascular interventional radiology has been expanded substantially.

The angiographer should at all times carefully evaluate expected information and benefit versus the risks of the angiographic study or therapeutic endeavors as they apply to the particular patient. Once decided upon, the procedure should be skillfully performed and the findings correctly interpreted and managed. In these sometimes difficult tasks, we hope A *Practical Approach to Angiography* will benefit our readers and their patients.

I. S. J.
D. C. J.
N. R. D.

Contributing Authors

Simon D. Braun, M.D.

Assistant Professor of Radiology, Duke University Medical Center, Durham, North Carolina

N. Reed Dunnick, M.D.

Professor of Radiology, and Chief of Vascular and Interventional Radiology, Duke University Medical Center, Durham, North Carolina

Donald C. Jackson, M.D., F.R.C.R., F.R.C.P.(C)

Clinical Professor of Radiology, Duke University Medical Center, Durham, North Carolina; Staff Radiologist, Craven County Hospital, New Bern, North Carolina

Curtis B. Johnsrude, M.D.

Fellow in Cardiothoracic Anesthesia, Cleveland Clinic Foundation, Cleveland, Ohio

Irwin S. Johnsrude, M.D.

Clinical Professor of Radiology, East Carolina University School of Medicine, Greenville, North Carolina; Chief of Special Procedures in Radiology, Pitt County Memorial Hospital, Greenville, North Carolina

Glenn E. Newman, M.D.

Assistant Professor of Radiology, Duke University Medical Center, Durham, North Carolina

Preliminary Considerations

Because of their numerous and expanding capabilities, the catheter techniques of diagnostic and interventional angiography are some of the most exciting endeavors in radiology. The potential for doing good, however, is sometimes offset by the capacity to cause harm. For this reason the diagnostic possibilities of an angiographic study must be carefully weighed against its potential complications, and other techniques that are noninvasive should be considered first. If the diagnostic information that will be obtained is greater than the anticipated danger, the angiographer should proceed with the study. On the other hand, if the danger outweighs the potential information, the angiographer should think again. He should consider noninvasive techniques or wait until conditions are more favorable.

If intravascular therapeutic techniques are to be accepted and performed, surgery is considered the gold standard against which they must be compared. Percutaneous intervention should prove to be of at least equal therapeutic value, with equal or smaller complication rates. The procedure should be more expeditious and cost effective. Intravascular therapy should be performed with the cooperation of the attending surgeon.

All of the following factors are important in both angiographic and interventional procedures. Optimal results can only be obtained by the suitable interaction of these factors: the patient, the clinical indications for the study, the radiologist, and the angiographic equipment.

The Patient

The angiographic procedure should be discussed with the patient with particular reference to the benefits that may be obtained. If a therapeutic procedure is to be performed, the advantages and disadvantages of the procedure, together with alternative methods of therapy must be carefully spelled out. Possible complications should be explained. The patient should be carefully evaluated at every stage of the procedure.

1. Before the procedure. The clinical history should be obtained and an examination done especially of the cardiovascular and neurologic symptoms. Increased risk occurs with the following conditions:

   advanced age
   low cardiac output
   congestive heart failure
   recent or impending myocardial infarction
   hypertension
   wide pulse pressure (over 100 mm Hg)
   dehydration
   immunosuppression
   impaired renal function
   severe arteriosclerosis
   previous severe reaction to contrast medium

2. During the procedure. The patient has a right to expect communication, compassion, and competence from the radiologist.
3. After the procedure. The radiologist should look for possible complications such as hematoma formation, occluded vessels, or delayed reactions to contrast agents.

Follow-up care is very important in the therapeutic studies, particularly with indwelling catheters and ongoing therapy.

Clinical Indications

The angiographic study should be clearly indicated. The worst disaster that can befall a physician and his patient is the occurrence of a serious complication when the study was not indicated in the first place. Factors increasing the risks of the study should be considered and corrected if possible.

The Cardiovascular Radiologist

The cardiovascular interventional radiologist should be convinced that he is the proper person to perform and interpret the angiographic procedure by reason of his interest, attitudes, training, and dexterity, both in the performance of the procedure and the management of complications. He should have well-trained technical personnel, suitable equipment, and impeccable technique. He should also be skilled in the interpretation of films, because superb films are of little value if they are not correctly interpreted.

Informed Consent

Because radiologists often perform hazardous cardiovascular procedures on patients, they are morally and legally obligated to obtain informed consent. Since the beginning of this century, the courts have decreed that "every human being of adult years and sound mind has the right to determine what shall be done with his own body" [4]. The patient must have at his disposal, in easily understood terms, "complete current information available concerning diagnosis, treatment, and prognosis" [2]. As physicians, therefore, it is our legal and moral duty to inform patients fully of the nature, risks, possible complications, benefits, and alternatives to any diagnostic or therapeutic procedure that we may perform on them [1, 4, 5]. Moreover, the courts have stated that the details of such information must be documented in writing [3]. Because lack of communication is probably the most important antecedent of medical malpractice suits, it is imperative that those directly involved in performing the procedures communicate personally with the patient. This communication may be augmented by some form of written information, designed primarily to increase the patient's understanding and will serve as a permanent record that the patient has been informed.

References

1. Goldie, R. R. The requirements of informed consent: Hospitals. *J.A.H.A.* 46:58, 126, 1972.
2. Grants Administration Manual (TN. 71.6). Washington, D.C.: Department of Health, Education, and Welfare, April 15, 1971. Part I, Chapter 40.
3. *Irving Trust Co. (as Executors of Ross V. Rosomott et al.)*, N.Y.S. 2d (Superior Court, Westchester County) Index # 9499/67, April 8, 1971.
4. *Schloendorff v. New York Hospital*, 105 N.E. 92 (1940).
5. Toole, J. F. Informed consent (editorial). *Circulation* 43:1, 1973.

I

Equipment
and General
Techniques

Notice

The indications and dosages of all drugs in this book have been recommended in the medical literature and conform to the practices of the general medical community. The medications described do not necessarily have specific approval by the Food and Drug Administration for use in the diseases and dosages for which they are recommended. The package insert for each drug should be consulted for use and dosage as approved by the FDA. Because standards for usage change, it is advisable to keep abreast of revised recommendations, particularly those concerning new drugs.

Conventional Angiographic and Digital Angiographic Equipment

Angiographic equipment falls into two major categories. The larger equipment—radiographic equipment, high-pressure injectors, physiologic monitoring equipment, and resuscitative apparatus—is discussed in this chapter. The second category consists of the disposable items used for invasive intravascular procedures, contrast agents, and other required drugs. These are considered in Chapter 2.

Radiographic Equipment

Proper hemodynamic and morphologic assessment of the rapidly moving, pulsatile cardiovascular system requires multiple rapid radiographic exposures of vessels or cardiac chambers, both as they fill with contrast medium and when they empty. Multiple projections add additional information. The major radiographic equipment necessary to do this includes the following:

x-ray generators
x-ray tubes and collimators
x-ray image recorders (film changers; 70-, 90-, or 105-mm cameras; cineradiographic apparatus; videotape; digital subtraction methods)
image intensification fluoroscopy (with television tube and monitor and, preferably, with digital subtraction capabilities)
x-ray table

The type of equipment chosen varies, depending on available funds and on the volume, type, and level of sophistication of the special cardiovascular procedures anticipated at the hospital or institution.

Before selecting equipment, one should keep in mind the basic tenets of good radiography. Because the primary goal is multiple film recordings of superior image quality, each component part in the general system of information transfer must be carefully selected. Geometric distortion, motion blurring, scattered radiation, and background noise must be minimized. One should also consider the following factors: minimum patient radiation dose, optimum radiographic exposure factors, rapid repetitive x-ray exposure requirements, and films that can be easily and rapidly developed.

Obtaining consistently good arteriograms involves a series of compromises. The tube of the smallest focal spot produces the least distortion; however, its heat storage capacity limits its use to the shorter radiographic "runs" on smaller body parts [14]. Moreover, the smaller anode angles required for these focal spots produce a smaller field. The higher the milliamperage used, the shorter is the required exposure time, resulting in less motion blurring; the results are the added expense of a shorter tube life and an increase in effective focal-spot size. High-ratio grids help to clean up scattered radiation; this in turn demands more radiation. High-speed screens are crucial in angiography because they increase film darkening and thus reduce radiation demands; the larger crystals increase distortion. Increased focal spot–film distance improves geometry but greatly increases radiation requirements.

The angiographer must continually reassess the equipment available to him and must be closely attuned to advances in radiographic technology that may pertain to his field. An adequate angiographic room should meet several basic requirements [2, 5, 11], as detailed in the following sections.

THE ANGIOGRAPHIC ROOM

An area of at least 400 square feet is required, with additional space for storage of equipment (Fig. 1-1). The height of the ceiling should be 10 ft to allow for high-placed tubes for large-field angiography. Covered floor troughs hide unsightly cable attachments to the x-ray units. There should be a wide access door to receive stretchers and beds. An electrical supply of 480 volts is required.

4

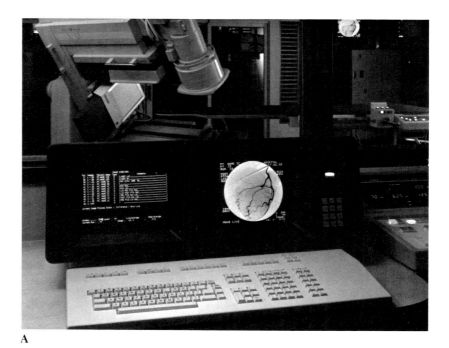

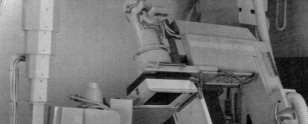

A

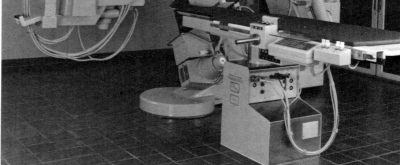

B

Fig. 1-1. Angiographic room. Biplane angiographic room with U arm, attached Puck film changers, a 100-mm photofluorographic camera, and digital subtraction capabilities.

A. The controls panels are located in a shielded area with a good view of the entire angiographic suite. This contains the controls for the biplane serio-graphs, the digital subtraction units, the photo-fluorographic camera, remote tabletop movement with U-arm manipulation, generator controls, and the console for the automatic high-pressure injector.

B. Angiographic table with biplane seriographic unit in position. The image amplifier has been replaced with the anteroposterior Puck changer in Towne position. The lateral Puck changer is in position for biplane study.

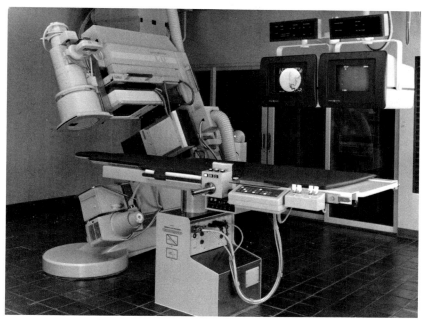

C

C. U-arm configuration with image amplifier rotated 30 degrees from the vertical axis, permitting a Towne projection of the head.

GENERATORS

The units should be three-phase 12-pulse generators with a minimum output of 100 kW. Constant potential generators with a range of up to 2000 mA are available but not necessary. For simultaneous biplane studies, a single 2000-mA constant potential generator or two 1000-mA three-phase generators may be used [21].

TUBES, FLEXIBLE TUBE HANGERS, AND COLLIMATORS

For heavy-duty nonmagnification angiography, tubes with high-speed rotating anodes (up to 10,000 rpm) with dual effective focal spots of 1.2 (large) and 0.3 to 0.6 mm (small) are currently available [13]. For 2× linear magnification angiography, 0.3-mm focal-spot tubes are available, and 0.1-mm, 0.15-mm, and 0.2-mm grid biased focal-spot tubes are available for up to 3× or 4× linear magnification. The latter tubes have a target angle of 7 degrees, which produces a limited field coverage on the film. A 10- to 12-degree target angle is required to cover a 14 × 14-in. field at a 40-in. source image distance.

Tube Distance

For most angiography the distance from the tube focal spot to the film—called *focal-film distance* (FFD)—is 40 in. Exceptions are found in magnification angiography, large-field angiography, and sometimes in biplane simultaneous or alternate firing studies of the head. In magnification studies the small focal-spot tube (0.3 mm or less) is placed closer to the patient while the film is placed farther away from him (Figs. 1-2, 1-3). In large-field studies the tube must hang closer to the ceiling in order to give the greater FFD required to cover the entire radiographic field (Fig. 1-4) [21]. During biplane nonmagnification studies the basic roentgenographic rule of close object-film distance may be thwarted. In order to accommodate the object in the center of the field on one projection (e.g., head on anteroposterior film changer), the same object may be as much as 6 to 10 in. away from the center of the remaining changer. To reduce the resulting distortion, the FFD of the appropriate tube must be increased up to 60 in. or more (Fig. 1-5). These geometric requirements must be kept in mind when an angiographic room is being planned.

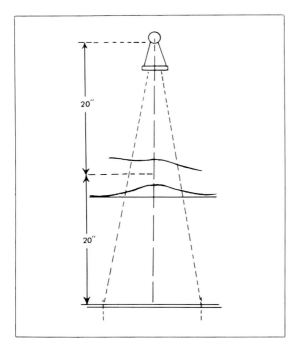

Fig. 1-2. Magnification arteriography. With a focal spot–film distance of 40 in. and a focal spot–object distance of 20 in., the linear magnification achieved is 2×. The field size covered is halved. A small focal spot is required to obtain a sharp image. Scatter is absorbed by the air gap, often making a grid unnecessary.

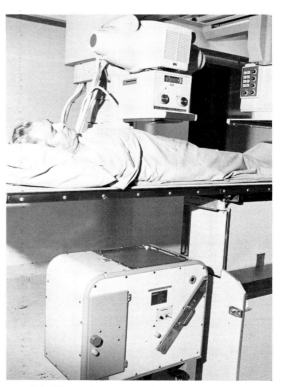

Fig. 1-3. The tabletop raises the patient and permits a long object-film distance, which is necessary for magnification arteriography.

GRIDS

During an x-ray exposure, useless scatter and secondary emission produce film background fog. Coning, particularly in areas with much overlying soft tissue structure, helps to curtail this effect. Grids also decrease scatter and must be chosen carefully. Stationary grids used for 40-in. FFDs are focused (30 to 42 in.) and have a 10:1 or 12:1 ratio. For biplane studies an 8:1 cross-hatched parallel grid is desirable for the lateral projection. If FFDs greater than 42 in. are being used (to curtail distortion), or if an angled tube direction is frequently used, grid "cutoff" may occur, and par-

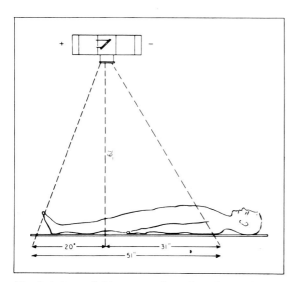

Fig. 1-4. Large-field angiography. This schema shows 51-in. coverage of the lower abdomen, pelvis, and lower extremities, which requires a 79-in. distance from the focal spot to the film. Either a cone or a collimator may be used; somewhat greater distance may be required if a collimator is used. A gradient x-ray screen

should be used, with high speed at the top end and detail speed toward the feet. A 12:1 grid is inserted over the abdomen and an 8:1 grid over the thigh and lower extremity areas. If the anode is nearer the feet, the heel effect decreases radiation to the feet and increases it to the rest of the body. A wedge-shaped aluminum filter (1 cm thick toward the feet, 0.5 cm at the midportion, and 0 at the abdomen) may still be necessary to equalize radiation.

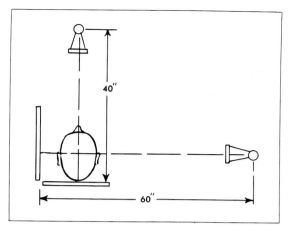

Fig. 1-5. Biplane angiography. The lateral changer should be applied to the side being investigated to decrease distortion. A small focal spot (0.6 mm) should be used. The focal spot–film distance of the lateral tube should be increased.

allel grids are necessary. Grids are often not necessary in magnification angiography because the scattered radiation is dissipated in the air gap between the patient and the film. An air gap of 20 in. is equivalent to attenuation of scatter provided by an 8:1 grid [4].

FILTERS

Filters are used to equalize radiographic density in fields with nonuniform thickness. They are usually made of aluminum and are of various shapes and thicknesses (Fig. 1-6).

Fig. 1-6. Aluminum filters help to equalize radiographic density. A biwedged filter (right) is used for evaluating both mediastinal and pulmonary vascular structures. A single-wedge filter (left) for brachiocephalic and peripheral angiography.

SCREENS AND FILMS

High-speed screens are necessary to accommodate the rapid exposures required in angiography [17]. The choice of screen must be closely matched to the speed of the film. The speed of the intensifying screen is influenced by the size of the crystals used, the thickness of the phosphor layer, and the efficiency of x-ray absorption and light conversion of the phosphor. Although increasing the thickness of the phosphor and the size of the crystals increases x-ray absorption, there is a trade-off in decreased resolution. Thus with x-ray film that is sensitive to the blue-violet light spectrum, extra-high-speed screens produce poor resolution and graininess when matched with high-speed film. Currently available rare-earth screens are much more rapid (up to 12 times) than par-speed screens, with no change in resolution but with some increase in mottling [6]. In addition, low-absorption carbon fiber has been incorporated into angiographic tabletops and face plates of serial film changers. This combination allows considerably more transmission of the x-ray beam than was previously possible, more rapid exposures with lower radiation requirements, longer tube life, and use of tubes with smaller focal spots. These factors are distinct advantages in magnification angiography, in which the small focal spot limits tube output.

IMAGING

Fluoroscopy

Cesium iodide phosphor image intensifiers allow optimum resolution. Television monitors permit frequent checking of catheter positions under good lighting conditions. Tubes with a dual effective

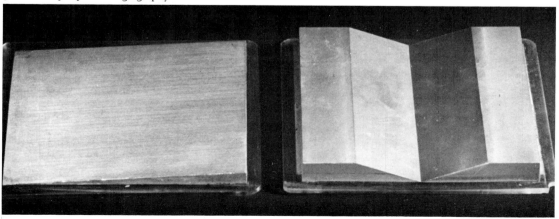

focal spot, with a smallest size of 0.3 mm, provide optimum detail.

Seriography

Seriography requires a mechanical rapid film changer [3]. A variety of such devices are available. Roll film changers permitting exposures up to 12 frames per second may be obtained. These film changers allow for exposure areas of 14 × 12 in. or less. Examples of this type of changer are the Franklin and the Elema Schonander. The CGR changer is loaded as a roll film changer, but the film is cut to individual 14 × 14-in. pieces after each exposure. This changer delivers up to 8 films per second. Cut film changers deliver individual films of 10 × 12 in. or 14 × 14 in. at variable rates of up to 6 films per second; examples of these are the Schonander (AOT) and the Memco. The Puck is a light-weight model with easy loading and occasionally with a fluoroscopic "see-through" capability. A maximum rate of 4 films per second and a total of 20 films are available in the Puck changer. Vacuum methods to enhance film screen contact (and fluoroscopic see-through capabilities) have been used by Amplatz in his changer design. The Picker changer uses individually vacuum-packed cassettes, which can be exposed at variable rates of up to 4 per second. Exposure rates and the relation of radiation exposures to contrast injections are computer controlled in the Picker, Schonander AOT, and Puck changers. The Sanchez-Perez changer is a chain-driven unit that changes 12 individual 10 × 12-in. cassettes at rates up to 2 per second. Limitations of field size and total number and rate of exposures detract from its value, however, and this unit is now considered obsolete.

These rapid film changers are used for angiographic evaluation of the aorta, pulmonary arteries, selective visceral arteries, brain, and brachiocephalic and brachial arteries and for evaluation of the aortoiliac region. They are occasionally used for study of limited areas of the lower and upper extremities in the evaluation of conditions such as tumors and arteriovenous fistulas. They can be used for complete coverage of the lower extremities by programming x-ray tabletop movements to correspond with vascular opacification. In most of the changers at least three different exposure rates of varying length can be programmed during a single series of exposures, thus allowing evaluation of the arterial, capillary, and venous phases of angiography. Simultaneous biplane studies can be performed, but two individual changers are required. Scatter radiation often detracts from the study; this effect can be partially counteracted by tight coning to the immediate area of interest. Alternate firing of the exposures also reduces scatter. Alternate firing may be accomplished (with the Schonander AOT) from the programmer controls, with the films loaded in the normal sequence. A certain amount of scatter still occurs on the film being advanced into position in the one changer by the exposure on the other changer with the film in place. Another method of reducing scatter is alternate loading of film magazines (e.g., spaces 1, 3, 5, 7, . . . on the anteroposterior changer; spaces 2, 4, 6, 8, . . . on the lateral). Because the film must be in place between the screens before there can be an exposure, when the frontal exposure is triggered, the film in the lateral changer has not yet been advanced. Obviously the maximum exposure rate is halved when this approach is used; it is two exposures per second when the programmer is set at four per second.

Large-field Seriography

Large-field seriographs, up to 51 in. in length, capture the arteriographic pattern of large areas (see Fig. 1-4) [20]. They are used primarily in the investigation of the lower abdominal aorta and the lower extremities. An automatic timer is usually available, which permits a total of five or six exposures at varying intervals ranging from one every second to one every 10 seconds or longer. The great length of the exposure field requires a high-placed tube (72-in. FFD for a 36-in. long exposure field, 79-in. FFD for a 51-in. field length). The radiographic density over this wide area of exposure can be made uniform by directing the anode position toward the feet (heel effect) and by using appropriate wedge filters with the thick part directed toward the feet, graduated screens, and varied grids.

Cineradiography

Cineradiography is a helpful adjunct in the study of the dynamics of the circulatory system [1]. Resolution, contrast, and image sharpness, however, are degraded in the cine system by photon noise inherent in the image amplifier. The geometry of focal spot to object and film is not as satisfactory as that obtained by serial roentgenographic techniques. Modern, large three-phase generators, high-speed fractional focal-spot tubes, grid pulse x-ray production, and 35-mm over-framed high-speed cameras produce satisfactory images in select areas of interest in which the study of motion and evaluation of small changes in contrast are critical. Examples of such areas are in coronary arteriograms and in angiocardiography for determining the competence of valves and the presence of shunts. The limitations of cineradiography in other areas of angiographic interest lie in the small field size and also somewhat poorer detail in the visualization of fine structures.

Photofluorography

Photofluorography is spot-film photography of the output phosphor of a fluoroscopic image intensifier. Roll films of 70-mm, 90-mm, 100-mm, and 105-mm width can be used with seriographic rates of up to 12 exposures per second. Advantages of this technique include lower patient radiation dose, low film cost, and a convenient, rapid manner of imaging precisely what is seen on the fluoroscopic screen. Smaller field size, reduced image (minification), and slightly less resolution, however, limit the use of this modality to small selective and superselective vessel studies (e.g., coronary arteriography, carotid and renal artery bifurcations in multiple projections, documentation of venous effluent collections).

Video Tape and Disc Recordings

Video tape and disc recordings allow replay of fleeting fluoroscopic pictures, such as test injections of contrast and catheter positions. They are often used in conjunction with cine recordings and can be reviewed until the more permanent cine film is processed. The resolution with current video tape and disc units, however, is not adequate as the final recorded image of angiographic information.

DIGITAL SUBTRACTION ANGIOGRAPHY

Subtraction angiography is a simple technique in which the first contrast-free image in an angiographic series is reversed and converted into a negative "mask," which, when superimposed on a subsequent image of a contrast-filled vessel, eliminates the background material and makes the vessels more conspicuous (Fig. 1-7). Digital subtraction angiography (DSA) is the computerized

version of this simple concept. It provides angiographic studies that can be reviewed in "real time" with intraarterial injections of greatly diluted (and, therefore, lesser quantities of) contrast material. The arteries can also be imaged by injecting larger quantities of contrast media into the venous system and subtracting out the arterial phase of the examination. This has the advantages of being less invasive and causing less patient discomfort. Because an arterial puncture is not required, the risks are limited to those of a venous injection. This also broadens the scope of the procedure to a wider population, for whom it can be used as a screening procedure on an outpatient basis.

DSA requires the acquisition of quality images, the conversion of the x-ray image to one that is digitized, a computerized manipulation of the digitized image by means of subtraction and enhancement, and finally the storage and archiving of the finished product [8, 12, 13, 15, 18].

Newer advances in video technologies and roentgenographic densitometry in DSA are promising not only for improved imaging of the vascular system but also for a broad understanding of some of the functional information that can be obtained by the dynamics of the circulatory system [7].

High-quality images are necessary. They require a powerful computer controlled generator, a high heat capacity x-ray tube, a high-resolution image intensifier, an automatic gain controlled amplifier, a logarithmic video amplifier, and, perhaps most important, a high-quality plumbicon television system with a signal-to-noise ratio of 1000:1 or better [10]. A high-speed analog to digital (A-D) converter then transforms the analog electronic signals received from the television fluoroscopic image point by point into digital information. A speed of 10 million conversions per second may digitize a 512 × 512 matrix in 1/30th of a second (one video frame time). Information is stored in two different digital memory banks. The original contrast-free digital images are placed in one of them and reversed to make a mask (Fig. 1-8). The contrast-filled digital images are placed in the second memory bank. The images from the two banks are subsequently subtracted and enhanced by digital manipulation in the digital processor. The subtraction studies are performed and can be reviewed almost simultaneously with the injection (real time). They can be stored on a digital hard or floppy disk for later review and interpretation; se-

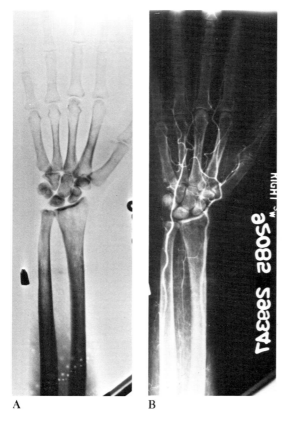
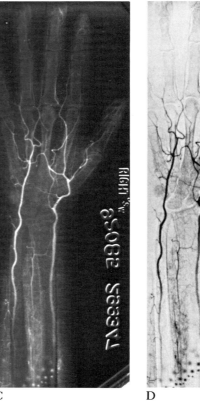
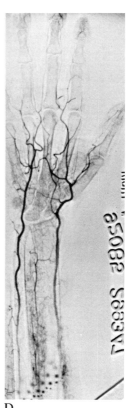

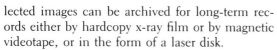

A   B   C   D

Fig. 1-7. Subtraction angiography.
A. A negative image of a "mask" film (without angiographic contrast medium).
B. Single film with contrast medium.
C. Superimposition of A on B.
D. Exposed and developed subtraction angiogram.

lected images can be archived for long-term records either by hardcopy x-ray film or by magnetic videotape, or in the form of a laser disk.

The subtracted images may be acquired by one of two methods. They may be obtained serially, using short pulsed x-ray exposures at a rate varying from 1 to 30 frames per second, depending on body size (using a 512 × 512 matrix). By this technique, the images are of higher resolution due to increased available photon flux (technical factors: 0.9 to 1.0 mm focal spot [FS]; 80–90 peak kilovoltage [kVp]; 20–80 milliamperes times time in seconds [mAS] depending on body part). Alternatively, they can be acquired in a dynamic, continuous mode of 30 frames or more per second (technical factors: continuous exposure on 0.6 mm FS of 75–85 kVp; 4–25 mAS; images obtained continuously for approximately 12–15 seconds). In that case, shorter x-ray exposure times result in decreased photon flux and, therefore, less resolution. While the serial, sometimes slower frame rate is useful in studying pathologic anatomy seen in the systemic vessels, the dynamic mode is more

useful in studying rapidly moving structures such as the left ventricle. Another helpful technique, using the dynamic mode, is "time interval difference," in which the subtraction is performed between each successive image, or adjacent temporal image sums, rather than from a single first image (Fig. 1-9). With this method, during diastole, the cardiac chamber outer dimension may register as white, but in systole it may register as black. This feature can be useful in evaluating cardiac function.

The resolution of the digital image is directly related to the number of picture elements (pixels) in the image (matrix) and to the size of the field over which it is spread. For example, a matrix size of 1024 × 1024 pixels allows an image that is considerably improved over one with 256 × 256 pixels; it requires memory banks and a central pro-

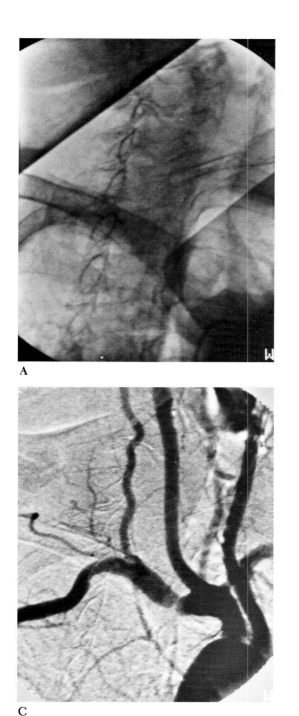

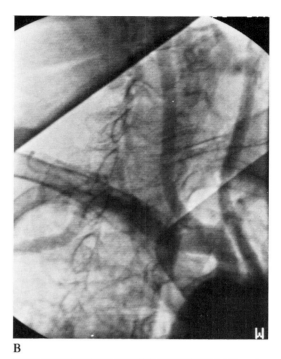

A

B

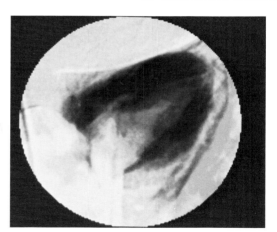

Fig. 1-9. Time interval difference. Note diastole (registered as black) and systole (registered as white).

C

Fig. 1-8. Digital subtraction angiogram.
A. Image collected immediately prior to arrival of contrast agent is reversed by the computer. Note linear dense shadows cast by copper plates inserted to equalize densities.
B. Image following injection of contrast prior to subtraction and enhancement.
C. Image following subtraction and enhancement.

cessing unit with a considerably larger (24 times) and more expensive capacity, and, consequently, much more time for transferring and storage of the information; fewer frames per second (between 7 and 8) may be obtained. It is important to understand that if a given number of pixels is spread too thinly over an overly large image intensifier field size, a loss of spatial resolution results. Digital image quality is also directly related to the shades of

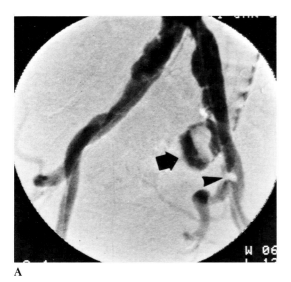

A

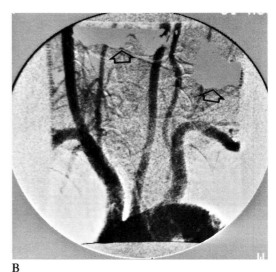

B

Fig. 1-10. Artifacts of digital subtraction angiography.
A. Misregistration due to peristalsis of gas (*large arrow*). Catheter in subatheromatous space (*small arrow*).
B. Artifact due to overpenetration in an area with unequal densities (*open arrow*).

gray that are allotted by the A-D converter to each discrete pixel in the image. Most current digital systems provide 1024 (10 bits, or 2^{10}) gray levels.

A number of artifacts that occur during the study can degrade the image (Fig. 1-10). A study of the arterial system obtained by intravenous injection of contrast agent (IV-DSA) may be compromised in patients with a low cardiac output due to delayed flow of diluted contrast material. Motion by the patient following registration of the mask prevents accurate superimposition. Involuntary motion, such as swallowing, peristalsis of gas, pulsating movement of calcium plaques, and excursions of the cardiac cycle, causes misregistration. There are a number of video processing methods that can be used to overcome these artifacts in order to produce high-quality images. There may be real-time processing, occurring during the time that the angiogram is being displayed (bandpass filters [16] and moving mask high-pass filters [9]). Postprocessing subtraction techniques can remove motion artifacts in a number of ways.

1. The image chosen for a mask may be changed to one closer in sequence to that of the opacified vessel, i.e., remasking. With some equipment, a mask can be chosen from images at the end of the run, after the contrast has left the area of interest. This is particularly helpful when the patient has moved at the beginning of the contrast injection but then remained relatively still.

2. The sequence of images obtained prior to arrival of the contrast may be "averaged" before being made into a mask, allowing for less misregistration on the subtracted image, i.e., integrated masking.

3. The misregistrated contrast-filled image may be physically shifted from a fraction of a pixel to a number of pixels in horizontal, vertical, or rotational directions to fit the masked mode, i.e., reregistration. This shift is performed by means of an array processor, a specialized component of the computer that rapidly performs computations on large arrays of numbers.

4. Another method is matched filtration. By use of continuous low-intensity video frame rates (30/second), a set of images of contrast-filled vessels is acquired, and the information on all of these frames is combined throughout the full length of the bolus injection. This technique contrasts with the conventional one of obtaining a sequence of 10 to 20 short but intense x-ray exposures following the injection of which only one or two are ultimately used. The combined images, weighted proportionally to the amount of contrast agent present in the individual video frame, produces a single DSA image of comparable or better quality than

those obtained in routine fashion. There is also a considerable reduction in radiation exposure [19].

5. Misregistration due to motion elicited from the different phases of the cardiac cycle can be overcome in part by electrocardiograph (ECG) "gated" studies. The mask and each subtracted image are registered during the same phase of the cardiac cycle, the process being triggered by an accompanying ECG.

6. Another concept requiring specially constructed generators may resolve the problem of motion artifact by using energy subtraction rather than temporal subtraction. The concept is based on the subtraction of differences obtained in images by exposing them at different kilovoltages within milliseconds of each other so that motion no longer introduces an artifact. The severe filtration of the x-ray beam required for this maneuver decreases its efficiency and limits its use to small body parts or infants. A combination of energy subtraction with temporal subtraction (hybrid subtraction) may obviate this problem and is currently available from certain manufacturers.[1]

CATHETERIZATION TABLE

A floating tabletop permits adequate multidirectional tabletop movement (10 in. laterally on each side and 51 in. longitudinally). With this flexibility the operator can easily position the patient over the film changer without disturbing catheter positions. The tabletop should allow for minimal patient film distance in the desired exposure projection. It should be constructed with material of low x-ray absorption (carbon fiber). If magnification capabilities are required, the tabletop or the seriographic changer should provide increased object-film distance. Oxygen and suction attachments, attachments for physiologic monitoring, a high-intensity light, and push-button finger control under sterile conditions are necessary. Some tables have added attachments to mechanically rotate patients into varying degrees of obliquity. Special programmers may be installed to move the tabletop sequentially at preset intervals in order to follow vascular opacification of the extremities. Still others (usually in

combination with a C- or U-arm fluoroscopic-radiographic unit) can be swung up to 180 degrees on either side of an isocenter.

C- OR U-ARM UNITS

These are rotation units, either floor or ceiling mounted, which have an x-ray tube mounted on one side and an image intensifier on the other [11]. In addition to attached digital equipment, other imaging devices, such as serial film changer, cineradiographic equipment, or photofluorographic equipment, may also be mounted on the same side as the image intensifier (see Fig. 1-1). The film changer is interchangeable with the image intensifier when fluoroscopy is completed and serial films need to be taken. The patient on the pedestal x-ray table described above is positioned stationary within the circle of the arm, while the unit can be rotated to provide any degree of angulation in the transverse plane and up to 35 to 45 degrees in the cranial or caudal direction. Both single and biplane units are available. Another biplane option is a single rotational unit with the additional installation of a ceiling mounted tube and a floor mounted film changer. The capacity to fluoroscope at variable angles makes a C- or U-arm configuration helpful in interventional procedures other than angiography and intraarterial therapeutic maneuvers. It helps to simplify and make more accurate needle punctures deep within the body for purposes of biopsy, abscess drainage, nephrostomy, cholangiography, and biliary drainage procedures.

The many capabilities of a rotational multiangulation mounting unit makes it ideal for a comprehensive special procedures room. Disadvantages include a limitation of the type of film changer that can be used to a smaller, lighter version (Puck, CGR Maximax) with filming capabilities of only 20 films (Puck) or 25 films (Maximax) and a maximum exposure rate of 4 films per second. In addition, although femoral approaches may be easily accessible, certain designs make axillary approaches difficult. Also, with the familiar configuration of the image intensifier located above the patient and the x-ray tube below during fluoroscopy, there are two options once filming is contemplated. One can retain the same configuration, thus not allowing the localizer light to outline the projected collimated radiographic field. Here also a certain lack of geometric sharpness of

[1] Manufactured by General Electric Medical Systems Group, 3000 N. Grandview Blvd., P.O. Box 414, Milwaukee, WI 53201.

posterior structures (aorta, kidneys) is created. The other option is to invert the unit, obviating these problems, but this is both cumbersome and time consuming. With most available units one can fluoroscope with the x-ray tube above the patient and the image intensifier and interchangeable film changer below; this method causes more radiation for the operator unless the x-ray tube is adequately shielded. In addition, the increased bulk of the intensifier and changer machinery below the x-ray table often necessitates an inconveniently high table location. The considerable advantages of these units outweigh the disadvantages, and improved designs are continually being developed.

FILM PROCESSOR

A compact 90-second automatic film processor gives good quality film processing, takes up a minimum of space, and may be conveniently located in a darkroom immediately adjacent to the special procedures room.

INJECTORS

Specially designed injectors are available for angiography. Most units automatically trigger the x-ray exposure and the seriograph to coincide with the onset of the injection moments before or after the injection has commenced. The injectors are programmed to deliver a predetermined amount of contrast agent (up to 100 or 200 ml) at a preset rate. The desired amount and rate of contrast agent injection may be preset via the unit controls for delivery any time before or after the exposure is triggered. Some units have an additional feature that can trigger one or multiple serial injections, together with the x-ray exposures, in relation to the phase of the cardiac cycle. This feature is helpful in cardiac chamber injections. Also, if injections of contrast agent are started early in diastole during midstream aortic or pulmonary arteriograms, the thrust of systole more adequately opacifies the takeoff vessels and branches, thereby reducing the required amount of contrast agent. During digital intravenous injections, with the catheter located in the superior vena cava or the right atrium, rapid injections during atrial diastole may prove beneficial.

The rate of injection of contrast media into the vascular system may vary considerably. Thirty to forty milliliters per second may be injected midstream into large vessels such as the aorta, while only 2 ml per second may be required in small, selected venous radicles. Because too large a bolus or too rapid a rate of injection can cause an organ infarction, and because a bolus that is too small or injected too slowly may produce an inadequate result, accurate control of these factors is critical.

The pressure applied at the origin of the catheter rapidly diminishes due to resistance by the catheter and the viscosity of the material that passes through it. The resistance offered by the catheter depends on the length of the tube through which the contrast agent has to travel, the inside diameter of the tube, and the number and size of side holes present near its tip. Obviously a long, narrow tube with high-viscosity contrast medium requires considerably more pressure than a short, wide-diameter tube with low-viscosity medium (see Fig. 2-9). The resistance encountered by the contrast medium as it passes through the tube is decreased by adding numerous large side holes at the tip of the catheter.

Earlier constant-pressure models of some injectors (Gidlund, Amplatz) use compressed gas to activate a hydraulic system, which in turn operates the injector syringe. These injectors require the pressure in pounds per square inch (psi) needed for the injection rate of a given volume of contrast agent. Calibrated charts, using catheters of standard diameter and length, and contrast media of varying viscosity, are required for accurate control of delivery rate. More modern and efficient computer controlled constant-flow injectors usually take more of these factors into consideration.[2] These injectors are generally driven by an electromechanical system, and the volume of contrast is given at the required rate, regardless of the resistance derived from the catheter and the viscosity of the contrast agent. A slow rise time in pressure during the early part of the delivery of contrast medium will prevent the catheter from recoiling out of a selected vessel. This timing feature is built into the modern models.

If the rate of injection is too high for a catheter,

[2] Such constant-flow injectors (and their manufacturers) include Cordis injector (Cordis Corp., P.O. Box 428, Miami, FL 33237); Viamonte-Hobbs (Liebel-Flarsheim Co., 11 E. Amity Rd., Cincinnati, OH 45215); Medrad injector (Technology for People, 566 Alpha Dr., Pittsburgh, PA 15238); Contract III E 3X (Siemens Corp., 186 Wood Ave. S., Iselin, NJ 08830); MRI Digital injection system (Medical Research International, 55991 Penn Circ. S., Pittsburgh, PA 15206).

it ruptures. The point of rupture occurs where the pressure is the highest, at the most proximal portion of the catheter, where it is connected to the injector. Transparent Teflon connecting tubes with high tensile strength are, therefore, interposed between the catheter and the injector.

An injector can be a lethal machine. Care should be taken to make sure that all connections are airtight, that all air is out of the system, and that the proper factors for a given injection are applied. The syringe head should be turned down so that any small collections of air are trapped high in the syringe, and the final 10 to 20 ml of contrast agent should not be injected in order to prevent injection of air emboli. A good rule to consider is insisting that two sets of eyes check all the injection factors before an injection is made.

The injectors have safety features to prevent inadvertent injection of larger than desired volumes. Adequate grounding and electrical insulation of the syringe (which communicates directly with the patient) from the injector motor prevent fatal arrhythmias. Indeed, all electrical circuits in the angiographic room must be carefully designed and adequately grounded. They should be rechecked frequently to prevent high voltage and current shock as well as small current-induced ventricular fibrillation.

Physiologic Monitoring Equipment

Physiologic monitoring equipment is necessary for safe intracardiac catheter manipulation. Constant electrocardiographic and intravascular pressure recordings during these procedures are minimal requirements. Intravascular pressure recordings may also be used during catheterization of vessels supplying vital structures such as the heart or brain. This monitoring permits early detection of dampening of the pressure at the catheter tip, which signifies occlusion of the catheter tip (by thrombus, wedge position, or plaque). Pressure measurements are important in determining the presence of gradients across valves or areas of vascular stenosis. They monitor the success or failure of an angioplastic procedure. An oscilloscope must be available for ongoing display of these hemodynamic functions in full view of all personnel in the special procedures room. In addition, the measurements of these functions should be permanently recorded for later calculations. One must become familiar with these monitoring units and know how to balance and calibrate them.

Resuscitative Equipment

Resuscitative equipment includes the following (see also Chap. 25):

direct current (DC) defibrillator
oxygen
suction equipment
endotracheal tubes and other airways
laryngoscope
bag and mask for assisted forced breathing

References

1. Abrams, H. *Abrams Angiography* (3rd ed.), Vol. 1. Boston: Little, Brown, 1983. Pp. 105–185.
2. Abrams, H., et al. Optimal radiologic facilities for examination of the chest and cardiovascular system. *Circulation* 43:A135, 1971.
3. Amplatz, K. Rapid Film Changers. In H. Abrams (ed.), *Abrams Angiography* (3rd ed.), Vol. 1. Boston: Little, Brown, 1983. Pp. 105–124.
4. Bookstein, J., and Voegel, E. A critical analysis of magnification radiography: Laboratory investigation. *Radiology* 98:23, 1971.
5. Brinker, R., and Skukas, J. *Radiology Special Procedures Room.* Baltimore: University Park, 1973.
6. Brodeur, A. E., et al. Three tier rare earth imaging system. *A.J.R.* 136:755, 1981.
7. Bwisch, J., and Heintzer, P. Parametric imaging. *Radiol. Clin. North Am.* 23(3):321, 1985.
8. Crummy, A. B., et al. Digital video subtraction angiography for evaluation of peripheral vascular disease. *Radiology* 141:33, 1981.
9. Hardin, C., et al. Realtime digital angiocardiography using a temporal high pass filter. *Radiology* 151:517, 1984.
10. Harrington, D. P., Boxt, L. M., and Murray, P. D. Digital subtraction angiography: Overview of technical principles. *A.J.R.* 139:781, 1982.
11. Levin, D., and Dunhom, L. New equipment considerations for angiographic laboratories. *A.J.R.* 139:755, 1982.
12. Levin, D., et al. Review: Digital subtraction angiography: Principles and pitfalls of image improvement techniques. *A.J.R.* 134:447, 1984.
13. Meaney, T. F., et al. Digital subtraction angiography of the human cardiovascular system. *A.J.R.* 135:1153, 1980.
14. Milne, E. The role and performance of minute focal spots in roentgenology, with special reference to magnification. *C.R.C. Crit. Rev. Radiol. Sci.* 2:269, 1971.

15. Mistretta, C. A., et al. (eds.). *Digital Subtraction Arteriography*. Chicago: Year Book, 1982.
16. Nelson, J., et al. Digital subtraction angiography using a bandpass filter. *Radiology* 145:309, 1982.
17. Ovitt, T., Moore, R., and Amplatz, K. The evaluation of high speed screen film combinations in angiography. *Radiology* 114:449, 1975.
18. Ovitt, T., and Newell, J. Digital subtraction angiography: Technology equipment and techniques. *Radiol. Clin. North Am.* 23:177, 1985.

19. Reiderer, S. J., et al. The application of matched filtering to x-ray exposure reduction in digital subtraction angiography: Clinical results. *Radiology* 146:349, 1983.
20. Roy, P. Peripheral angiography in ischemic arterial diseases of the limbs. *Radiol. Clin. North Am.* 5:467, 1967.
21. Thompson, T. T. *A Practical Approach to Modern X-ray Equipment*. Boston: Little, Brown, 1978. Pp. 17–50.

Equipment for Intravascular Invasive Techniques

Intravascular invasive techniques require a wide variety of needles, guidewires, and catheters. Catheter introducers, catheter sheaths, connecting tubes, adapters, and stopcocks are also necessary. A number of injectables must always be on hand. These include local anesthetics, drugs (see Appendix 1), and contrast agents. Finally, a growing array of materials used for intravascular therapeutic endeavors, together with their delivery systems, must be stocked (see Chap. 5–7).

Needles

A variety of needle assemblies are available for arterial punctures (Fig. 2-1); the simplest is a 2- or 3-in. long, 18-gauge, thin-walled, sharply beveled metal needle, which easily transmits a 0.035- or 0.038-in. guidewire. With this needle assembly, only the anterior wall of the vessel need be punctured. Patients with severe atherosclerosis or those who are obese may present problems in arterial puncture with this technique. There are also needle assemblies with overlying Teflon sleeves, which help to reduce the complications of hematoma, dissection, and other causes of failure. One such needle has component parts that include a hollow steel shaft, a sharply beveled, diamond-shaped steel obturator, and an overlying Teflon sleeve. These special needle assemblies are of varying lengths and diameters; the one we usually use is 18 gauge and 3 in. long. As the vessel is punctured and pulsatile blood is encountered, the sleeve alone is advanced into the artery. Once the Teflon sleeve is well within the artery, catheter exchange may be more easily performed. Other needles are available, both with and without overlying Teflon sleeves.

Catheters

Catheter material is chosen for ease of manipulation or torque. It must also be capable of maintaining its shape during catheterization; this property is termed its *memory*. A smooth outer surface decreases arterial trauma. In catheters having equal outside diameters, a thin-wall catheter provides a higher flow capability than one with a thick wall due to the greater inside diameter of the former. Radiopaque catheters (made by adding lead, bismuth, or barium salts) are easily seen under the fluoroscope. The tensile strength of the catheter and its capacity for being formed to the angiographer's need are important considerations in the choice of catheter material. The diameter should be the smallest size that allows adequate delivery of a given dose of contrast material. The outside diameter of a 1 French catheter measures $\frac{1}{3}$ mm; therefore, a catheter with an outside diameter of 3 French measures 1 mm, 6 French measures 2 mm, and 30 French measures 10 mm. The inside diameter, or the diameter of the inner passage, which transports the contrast medium, is obviously less and depends on the thickness of the catheter wall. Catheter size is particularly important when the angiographer is dealing with infants and children. Sizes 3, 4, 5, and 6 French catheters are available for use with children. In adults, sizes 4 through 7 French catheters are commonly used. Generally, those catheters with larger inside diameters are used for large-dose, rapid, midstream injections, while the smaller ones are sufficient for the lower dose, slower delivery required for selective studies. Coaxial systems have been developed in which small (2 to 3 French) catheters may be introduced through larger (6.5 to 7 French) catheters. At the other extreme, 30 French catheters may be used to introduce special filters or other intravascular manipulative devices. The smaller, more dilute contrast requirements of intraarterial digital subtraction angiography allows use of smaller catheters. The general trend is toward using smaller diameter, thin-walled catheters.

A tapered catheter tip is necessary for an atraumatic entrance through the vessel wall, but this same taper tends to diminish the flow rate. Special thin-walled catheter sheaths are necessary (see

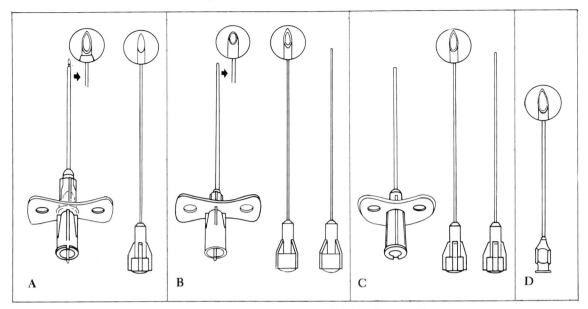

Fig. 2-1. Needles used for percutaneous puncture.
A. Standard Amplatz needle with overlying Teflon
    catheter sleeve.
B. Potts needle with both sharp and blunt obturator.
C. UMI needle with both sharp and blunt obturator.
D. Thin-walled needle for single wall puncture.

Chaps. 5 and 7) to introduce the nontapered catheters used for injecting certain emboli or for introducing coaxial systems. A high-pressure injection through an end-hole catheter creates a dangerous jet effect, which may cause laceration and perforation of the arterial wall or endocardium. High-pressure injections may cause circumferential negative pressure, which is transmitted to the vessel wall and may cause a transient localized narrowing just distal to the catheter tip. Side holes in the catheter tip minimize the trauma by diminishing the jet effect out the end hole, enhance mixing of the contrast agent in the bloodstream, and decrease catheter recoil. These same side holes may prove dangerous, however, unless they are flushed forcefully and frequently. Clots may form within the holes and may embolize into the target organ during the ensuing high-pressure injection.

Catheters with side holes but without an end hole are particularly useful for intracardiac right heart and pulmonary artery injections. There is no jet effect and little recoil with the use of such catheters. Because there is no end hole, these catheters cannot be introduced percutaneously except through a paper-thin Mylar or Teflon sheath. The sheath must first be introduced over a short end-hole catheter. The use of these non-end-hole catheters is almost entirely limited to the venous system, the right side of the heart, and the pulmo-

nary arteries in adults; they may also be used in the smooth-walled arteries of children. Such a catheter is undesirable for manipulation through diseased arteries, because, without an end hole, it cannot be led by a protective guidewire.

The introduction of foreign materials such as catheters and guidewires into the vascular system initiates thrombus formation, which can cause serious complications of thromboembolism [22]. Formation of clots occurs by adhesion of platelet aggregates to the foreign surface, resulting in a white thrombus. This process accelerates the formation of thromboplastin, thrombin, and eventually a fibrin network, which incorporates red cells to form the red thrombus. The thrombus can be dislodged and travel into vessels supplying vital structures, or it can be stripped off at the site of entry as the catheter is withdrawn, and thrombosis of the vessel may result. Clots rarely form if tests are done expeditiously and careful attention is directed to flushing catheters, avoiding arterial trauma, spasm, and wedged position of the catheter tip. In prolonged procedures, or in high-risk, hypercoagulable patients, there are two approaches to prevent clot formation. First, the patient may be systemically anticoagulated during the study if there is no contraindication. Usually a dosage of 45 international units (IU) per kilogram (given as an initial dose at the start of the examination) suffices for a study of approximately 1 to 1½ hours' duration. The second approach is to treat the catheter surface with thromboresistant material. A benzylkonium heparin precipitate may be applied to the outer surface of the catheter in a very thin layer. It should not be applied to the luminal surface, because it may be dislodged by the guidewire and embolized to unwanted areas. This coating prevents clot formation for approximately 1 to 1½ hours, the usual length of an angiographic procedure. A means for heparinizing surfaces of polymeric materials has been devised with the use of a substance that does not deteriorate on exposure to blood and has negligible local and systemic effects [11, 25]. This approach may be helpful in limited circumstances such as when one is considering the long-term use of catheters during intraluminal therapeutic techniques.

There are a variety of different commonly used catheter materials.

1. Catheters made from Teflon are useful for midstream injections, in which high pressures are required for rapid delivery of contrast medium. Teflon has a low coefficient of friction, is strong, and can withstand autoclaving and high-pressure injections. Its memory is good, but temperatures as high as 350°F are required to form a curve. The catheter tip is sharp, and it must be used with caution.

2. Catheters made from polyurethane have a softer tip and are, therefore, safer for selective placement into aortic branches. Because this rubbery material is rather soft, the catheters are manufactured with a wire mesh within the walls of the catheter shaft. This mesh gives body and good torque control, which is particularly useful in selective work. The wire mesh takes up space within the wall of the catheter, giving it a somewhat thicker wall and smaller inside diameter than other catheters. The catheter's distal 5 cm, bonded firmly to the catheter shaft, contains no wire mesh. This permits extrusion of the tip to smaller diameters and molding of various tip shapes. In order to mold a polyurethane catheter for a specific need, the desired shape must be formed. Next,

it is boiled for approximately 3 minutes in water, or for a shorter time in hot glycerine. Because polyurethane is a rubbery material, steel guidewires often become stuck within the catheters. Specially prepared Teflon-coated guidewires (with a low coefficient of friction) must, therefore, be used to introduce these catheters percutaneously. Polyurethane catheters have preformed shapes and curves produced by the manufacturer for a given selective procedure. They must be cold- or gas-sterilized.

3. Polyethylene catheters are easily molded to suit one's requirements. The attenuated catheter tip can be easily formed by pulling the catheter over an old guidewire and cutting the distal pulled tip with a sharp blade. A few seconds of immersion in boiling water produces a curve with good memory. Side holes are easily placed, and the proximal end of the catheter can be "funneled" by slowly rotating it in a flame (Fig. 2-2), which permits attachment of the catheter to an adapter. Virgin polyethylene is clear and radiolucent; impregnation with lead salts add radiopacity to the catheters. Some of these are also manufactured with an inner wire mesh for added torque control. Polyethylene catheters must be cold- or gas-sterilized.

4. The woven Dacron catheters commonly used include the NIH catheter (side holes but no end hole), Gensini catheter (side holes and end hole), Lehman catheter (end hole but no side hole), and Sones catheter (distal 2.5 cm tapered to 5.5 French with four side holes at the tip),[1] among others. These catheters are useful in pulmonary angiography, in cardiac work, for obtaining pressures within the cardiac system, and in coronary arteriography, respectively. Woven Dacron catheters must be cold- or gas-sterilized.

5. A newer polyurethane catheter coextruded with an inner nylon wall has been developed which provides a thin wall with high tensile strength.[2] This provides high flow rates of contrast medium with lower delivery pressures than that required for singly extruded catheters.

---

[1]Manufactured by USCI, A Division of C. R. Bard, Inc., Box 566, Billerica, MA 01821.
[2]Manufactured by Mallinckrodt, Diagnostic Products Division, St. Louis, MO 63134.

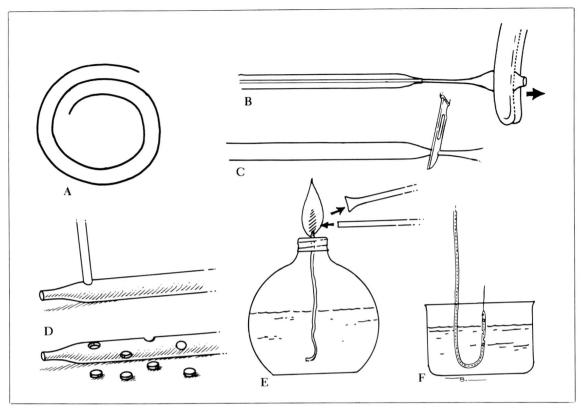

Fig. 2-2. How to make your own catheter.
A. Coiled polyethylene catheter material commercially available in 10-ft or longer sections. Straighten the material by injecting warm water intraluminally and cut to desired length.
B. Introduce guidewire to just proximal to tip, grasp the tip with forceps, quickly immerse in hot water, and "pull" the tip. This procedure ensures a taper that fits snugly to the chosen guidewire.
C. Cut tapered end with a sharp blade.
D. Punch side holes with sharp cannula, and then count the plugs, because they must not be lost in the catheter.
E. Funnel the proximal end by rapid, transient, repetitive application to the base of the flame of an alcohol burner. An adapter can now be applied.
F. Insert a wire to form a catheter shape. Momentarily, insert the curve (but not the tip, which deforms with heat) into boiling water and then into cold water.

Polyurethane, Dacron, and sometimes polyethylene catheters require prior dilatation of the arterial wall at the point of entry to prevent damage to the catheter tip and to the artery. This procedure is performed with a smoothly tapered dilator made of a more durable Teflon material of similar or slightly smaller diameter than the catheter to be used.

Advances in angiography and expansion of angiographic techniques to allow treatment of certain diseases have resulted in a growing interest in developing newer catheter techniques and materials, which has occurred in both the experimental and the clinical laboratory. Coaxial catheter systems [10], balloon-tipped catheters [9, 13, 24, 37, 43, 45], Silastic catheters [10], catheters with detachable balloons [6, 45], catheters that sheath electrodes, and catheters capable of guidance by magnets [20] are only some of the systems that are in various stages of development or are currently available. They will be described in later chapters.

Guidewires

Guidewires are used to guide the catheter percutaneously into the artery and to advance it safely to its final location within the arterial system. A general rule is that the catheter should not be advanced in the arteries without a guidewire; however, this is not true in the venous system, in the right side of the heart, and in the smooth vessels of children. Guidewires are composed of an external metal spring and a tapered inner steel core that runs throughout the entire length of the wire for added strength. Some guidewires have a fixed hyperflexible tip, which may vary in length from 3 to 9 in. Others have a movable inner core that can be withdrawn from the tip to permit flexibility of varying lengths in the same wire. Some wires have an inner tapered mandrel, which provides a gradual transition of variable length from the flexible tip to the more rigid shaft. These wires are helpful in selective angiography, since, once advanced into the vessels, they permit the catheter to follow its course more easily. This feature is particularly important in positioning catheters accurately in peripheral locations for therapeutic embolization or vessel dilatation. A particular stiff steel-wire shaft with a flexible tip (the Lunderquist exchange wire, Amplatz heavy-duty wire) is invaluable in advancing catheters through resistant areas, such as through markedly tortuous vessels, across the aortic bifurcation, or in percutaneous biliary and urinary interventional procedures. Limited torque control of the guidewire tip can be obtained by soldering the inner mandrel to the external metal spring at regular intervals along its length.

A special small-gauge (0.014 in., 0.016 in.), externally steerable, platinum-tipped guidewire is available for manipulation through coronary arteries, second- or third-order renal branches, lower extremity vessels distal to the trifurcation, or very tight areas of stenosis (Figs. 2-3 and 2-4). The platinum alloy improves visibility despite its small caliber [30].

Guidewire tips may be straight, or they may be J-shaped with a gentle or tight radius. Straight guidewires are used in young patients in whom tortuosity and atherosclerosis are not a problem; J-shaped guidewires allow better maneuverability through tortuous vessels and added safety as they brush over plaques of diseased arteries. A special type of variable stiffness wire is available that, when flexible, can be safely advanced through diseased vessels. When rigidity is required for advancing an overlying catheter, this can be imposed on the guidewire by an external manipulator (Fig. 2-5C).

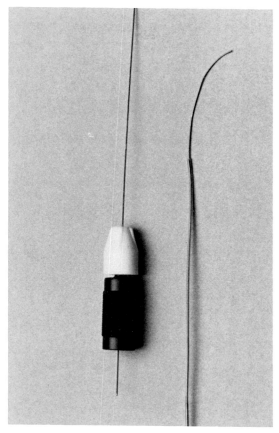

Fig. 2-3. Steerable 0.016-in. platinum alloy guidewire tip introduced coaxially through an "injectable guidewire." Removable manipulator on the hub of the 0.6-in. guidewire allows good control.

Still another guidewire (see Fig. 2-3) has a removable inner core (an open-ended guidewire catheter) allowing injection of contrast media and therapeutic agents, transportation of inner steerable guidewires, and measurement of pressures in otherwise inaccessible locations [42].

Some guidewires may be specially coated with benzylkonium heparin precipitate, which prevents clots from forming [1]. Standard guidewire lengths vary from 50 to 145 cm. Extra long guidewires ranging up to 260 cm may be obtained. These are useful in exchanging long catheters positioned selectively in a peripheral location, where one does not wish to lose the advantage of the selective catheter placement. Guidewire diameters range

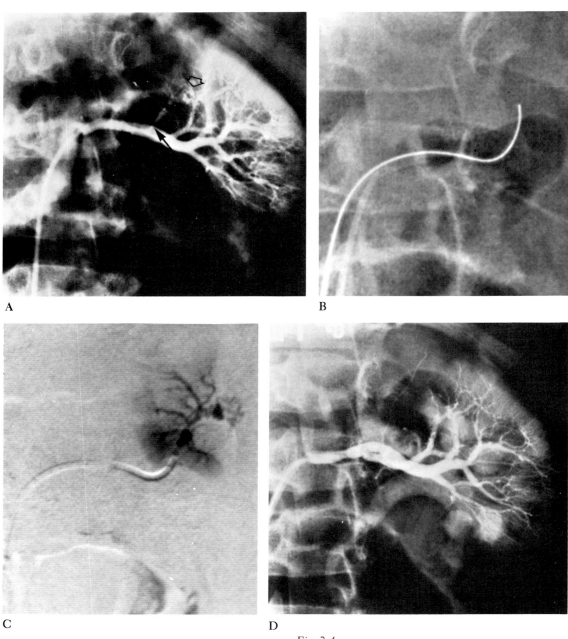

A

B

C

D

Fig. 2-4.

A. Stenosed left renal interlobar branch (*arrow*) causing hypertension in a 6-year-old boy. Note collaterals (*open arrow*).

B. 0.016-in. steerable guidewire advanced through stenosis.

C. 5 French catheter proximal to stenosis used for embolization with Ivalon microparticles.

D. Sequential branch occluded. Hypertension disappeared in 2 days but recurred 6 months later (required heminephrectomy).

from 0.014 to 0.052 in.; the guidewires most frequently used in adults are 0.035 and 0.038 in. in diameter. A guidewire can be used to assist catheter placement selectively in maneuvers that are sometimes difficult. The flexible wire should be carefully advanced well into the target artery, where it acts as an anchor or "lead" for advancement of the overlying catheter.

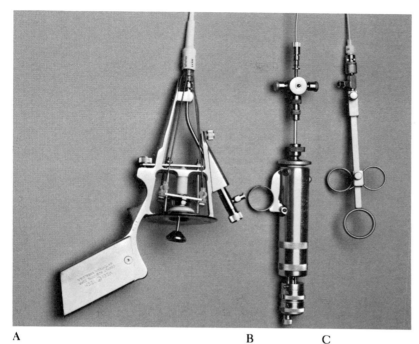

A   B   C

Fig. 2-5. External catheter manipulators.
A. Meditech.
B. Muller.
C. Cook, Inc.

There are certain precautions to consider in the use of guidewires.

1. The correct guidewire should be chosen to match the catheter that is being used. The two should be well fitted. If the fit is too loose, a punch biopsy of an arterial wall can occur as the catheter is introduced over the wire. If the fit is too tight, the flexible tip can be pulled off the guidewire as it is being withdrawn from the catheter (this is more likely to occur if the steel core within the guidewire breaks). The guidewire must be at least 20 cm longer than the catheter.
2. The Teflon coating of the guidewire may be stripped or flaked off and embolized within the vascular tree. This is more likely to occur if the guidewire is used more than once.
3. The guidewire must be checked closely before use and discarded after the procedure has been terminated.

Sterile Tray Assembly

Items on the sterile tray include the following:

1. Sterile gloves and gown (mask and cap not sterile).
2. Povidone-iodine (Betadine), Kelly forceps, 4 × 4-in. gauze pads, and drapes for preparing and draping the patient.
3. Local anesthetic—20-ml vial of 1 or 2% lidocaine (without epinephrine), 25 and 21-gauge disposable needles.
4. For angiographic procedures, a 500-ml container of sterile 5% dextrose for intravascular injection (add 1000 IU of heparin if not contraindicated, and if systemic heparinization is not anticipated) (a closed system is advantageous); basin with heparinized sterile 5% dextrose for catheter, guidewire, and needle cleaning; 50-ml container of low-density contrast agent (see Appendix 3) for test injection (tabulate amount used); sterile drapes, both large and small; sterile covering for control mechanisms for fluoroscopy and tabletop movement; four 10-ml syringes; four 20-ml syringes; one 2-way stopcock; translucent Teflon connecting tube (between catheter and injector); catheters; and guidewires.

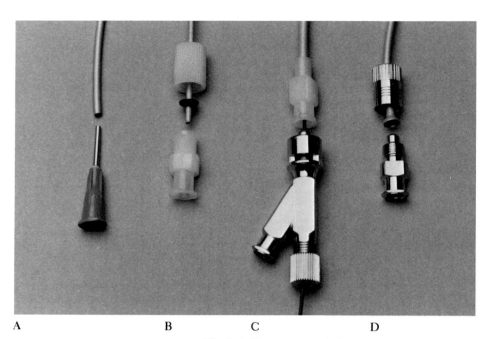

A   B   C   D

Fig. 2-6. Various types of adapters for catheter hubs.
A. Simple adapter (for hand injection only).
B. O-ring adapter for straight catheter hub. Accepts high-pressure injections.
C. Touhy-Borst adapter with sidearm. Accepts small coaxial catheter or guidewire.
D. Standard adapter for funnel-shaped hub.

5. Heparin (45 IU/kg, 3000 IU for a 70-kg adult) is used only if not contraindicated (do not use in patients with bleeding diathesis, internal or external bleeding, dissecting aneurysm, or trauma, or if anticipated length of angiographic study is shorter than 20 minutes). Protamine sulfate is an antidote for heparin and can be given if the procedure is shorter than anticipated. The usual dose is 1 ml (10 mg) per 1000 IU of heparin given.

Other Helpful Accessories

1. A variety of catheter hubs that fit catheters from 3 to 9 French (Fig. 2-6). These are made to accept catheters with flared ends or with straight ends. The latter require a Touhy-Borst adapter with rubber O-ring and screw to clamp over and secure the catheter end. Catheter hubs may also be obtained in the form of blunt needle hubs of varying gauges.

2. Adapters (preferably Luer-Lok). Male to male, female to female, with and without rotating capabilities, with and without sidearms to be used for flushing (Fig. 2-7), with and without proximal O-ring; one-way valves to prevent reflux and close flow around the guidewire or coaxial catheter; also Luer plugs to occlude male and female adapters.

3. Dependable stopcocks—two-way, three-way.

4. Manifolds with one, two, or more sidearms, with and without rotating adapters.

5. Thin-walled introducer sheaths of varying diameters and lengths, with and without sidearms for flushing; and one-way rubber valves to prevent reflux or bleeding around the hub (hemostasis valves). Currently, there are three common types of introducer sheaths available. In one[3] there is a self-sealing hemostasis valve at its proximal end, which is successful in preventing back-bleeding when a catheter diameter of similar caliber or 1 French size smaller is used. Detachable balloons may be dislodged when drawn through this type of valve. In another[4] any size catheter of similar or smaller diameter may be introduced without fear of leaking, and detachable balloons

[3] Manufactured by Cordis Corp., 125 NE 40th St., Miami, FL 33137.
[4] Manufactured by Cook, Inc., P.O. Box 489, Bloomington, IN 47401.

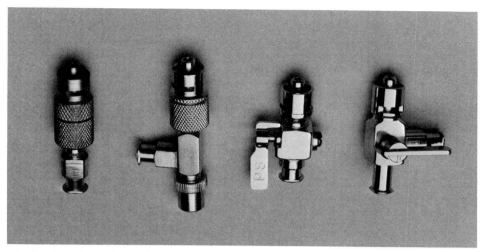

Fig. 2-7. Rotating and straight connectors with and without side ports.

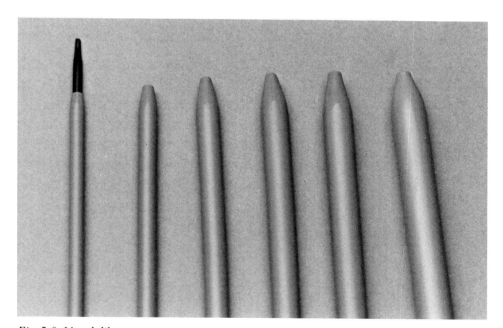

Fig. 2-8. Vessel dilators.

will not be dislodged. In a third type[5] the sheath has no valve at its proximal end. Back-bleeding is prevented by attaching a Y-shaped Touhy-Borst adapter to the hub. "Peel-away" sheaths, which can be easily removed once the catheter has been introduced, are also available.

[5]Manufactured by Ingenor Medical Systems, 70 rue Orfila, 75020 Paris, France.

6. Dilators of varying diameters, 5 French (1.67 mm outside diameter) through 30 French (10 mm outside diameter) (Fig. 2-8).
7. Accessory polyethylene catheter material from 3 French to 9 or 10 French (for making your own catheters).
8. Translucent connecting tubes of varying lengths, of high tensile strength, and malleable, with leak-proof adapters.
9. At least two different types of external catheter manipulating devices (see Fig. 2-5).

10. Positive pressure pumps for continuous flushing of coaxial catheter systems (for high-pressure arterial circulation).
11. A portable Doppler ultrasonography unit for detecting pulses.
12. Hot water, steam (preferably under pressure), or hot glycerine to mold catheter tips to your needs; an alcohol flame to flare the proximal catheter end to accommodate the adapter; flat-tipped but sharpened needles of varying diameters to make side holes of varying diameters in the catheter tips.
13. Various accessories for interventional work, including catheter retrieval sets, embolic material, balloon occlusive catheters, balloon dilating catheters (see Chaps. 5, 6, and 7).
14. A variety of drugs (listed in Appendix 1).

Contrast Media

POSITIVE (RADIODENSE) CONTRAST AGENTS

The ideal contrast agent for intravascular use would be radiopaque, of low viscosity, and easily miscible with blood; it would remain within the vascular system; it would be inert, easily excreted, and free of toxic effect on the body. Such an agent is not available at the present time. However, two broad groups of radiopaque contrast agents are currently available: (1) ionic—the standard organic ionic salts of triiodobenzoic acid (Table 2-1), and (2) nonionic—the more recently developed nonionic iodinated organic compounds with three iodine atoms per benzene ring (Table 2-2).

The organic ionic salts of triiodobenzoic acid have a high iodine content and have enjoyed wide use as angiographic contrast agents over the past 3 decades [27]. The three main ionic triiodobenzoic angiographic contrast agents used have a common triiodo-, 2-, 4-, 6-benzene ring structure with minor variation in the 3-, 5-acetylamine component. They are either sodium or methylglucamine salts of diatrizoates, iothalamates, or metrizoates, and come in low, medium, and high concentrations.

The nonionic agents are fully substituted organic compounds with three iodine atoms per benzene ring. They are not charged and do not dissociate into ionic components. They include Metrizamide (Sterling Winthrop), Iopamidol (Squibb), Iopromide (Berlex), and Iohexol (Sterling Winthrop) [4]. Metrizamide is known to be unstable in solution, is difficult and expensive to manufacture, and is used primarily in myelography. Dimers of benzene rings are also being tested. One such is a dimer of two benzene rings (with six iodine atoms) attached to a single cation. When dissociated, the dimer provides only half as many ions as do standard ionic contrast agents of similar iodine content.

Density of contrast medium on an angiogram is a reflection of the concentration of iodine present and the rate at which it is delivered. Osmolarity is a measure of the number of ions or molecules dissolved in a liter of solution. Because a diagnostic angiographic study requires many of these iodine-containing ions, the osmolarity of the standard agents is high (estimated to be 5 to 10 times as high as the osmolarity of blood). This high osmolarity may account for most of the chemotoxic effects of injected ionic contrast agents. The vasodilation, sensation of heat and pain, and fall in hematocrit that may occur with high-dose studies may be explained by this hypertonicity [16, 46]. It is not surprising, and indeed is gratifying, to find markedly lesser systemic and vascular effects when the newer, nonionic agents (with subsequent lower osmolarity) are used [19].

As stated in Poiseuille's law, the rate of delivery of the contrast agent is related not only to the diameter and length of the catheter through which it is injected but also to its viscosity (Fig. 2-9). Viscosity in turn is determined by the size of molecules injected: the larger the molecules, the greater the viscosity. Because sodium is a much smaller cation than methylglucamine, any ionic agent containing more sodium is less viscous. The sodium, however, is more toxic. Although the methylglucamine is less toxic, in the pure form it has a greatly increased viscosity, making rapid injection of a large bolus more difficult. A compromise in these standard agents is a combination of the two.

Reactions to Contrast Media

A number of reactions can occur when contrast medium is injected into the vascular system [38, 39, 40]. These include antigen-antibody reactions, histamine release, complement activation and coagulation changes; a small number of reactions may be attributed to psychogenic factors. The largest number of reactions can be attributed to the

Table 2-1. Physical characteristics of ionic contrast media in common use[*]

Product	Anion	Cation(s)	Concentration (%)	Iodine (mg/ml)	Viscosity (cP) (37°C)	Osmolarity (mOsm/kg)
Hypaque 30% (Winthrop)	Diatrizoate	Meglumine	30	141	1.43	633
Conray-30 (Mallinckrodt)	Iothalamate	Meglumine	30	141	1.5	600
Conray-43 (Mallinckrodt)	Iothalamate	Meglumine	43	202	2.0	1000
Hypaque 50% (Winthrop)	Diatrizoate	Sodium	50	300	2.5	1550
Hypaque 60% (Winthrop)	Diatrizoate	Meglumine	60	282	4.2	1415
Reno-M-60 (Squibb)	Diatrizoate	Meglumine	60	282	4.0	1500
Angiovist 292 (Berlex)	Diatrizoate	Meglumine 52% Sodium 8%	60	292	4.0	1500
Conray-60 (Mallinckrodt)	Iothalamate	Meglumine	60	282	4.1	1400
Renografin-60 (Squibb)	Diatrizoate	Meglumine 52% Sodium 8%	60	288	3.9	1420
Hypaque-M 76% (Winthrop)	Diatrizoate	Meglumine 66% Sodium 10%	76	370	8.3	2016
Renografin-76 (Squibb)	Diatrizoate	Meglumine 66% Sodium 10%	76	370	9.1	1940
Angiovist 370 (Berlex)	Diatrizoate	Meglumine 66% Sodium 10%	76	370	8.4	2100
MD-76 (Mallinckrodt)	Diatrizoate	Meglumine 66% Sodium 10%	76	370	9.1	2140
Renovist (Squibb)	Diatrizoate	Meglumine 34.3% Sodium 35%	70	372	6.0	1900
Hypaque M-75 (Winthrop)	Diatrizoate	Meglumine 50% Sodium 25%	75	385	8.0	2108
Conray-400 (Mallinckrodt)	Iothalamate	Sodium	67	400	4.5	2300
Vascoray (Mallinckrodt)	Iothalamate	Meglumine 52% Sodium 26%	78	400	9.0	2400

[*]For a more comprehensive review, see Fischer H. W. Catalog of intravascular contrast media. *Radiology* 159:561, 1986.

Table 2-2. Physical characteristics of low-osmolarity angiographic contrast media in common use

Product	Generic name	Concentrations (%)	Iodine (mg/ml)	Viscosity (cP) (37°C)	Osmolarity (mOsm/kg)
Isovue	Iopamidol	61.0	300	4.7	616
Isovue	Iopamidol	76.0	370	9.4	796
Omipaque	Iohexol	64.7	300	6.8	709
Omipaque	Iohexol	75.5	350	11.2	862
Hexabrix	Ioxaglate Meglumine 39.3% Sodium 19.6%	58.9	320	7.5	600

Source: Data from Fischer, H. W. Catalog of intravascular contrast media. *Radiology* 159:561, 1986.

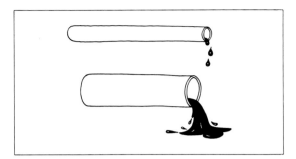

Fig. 2-9. Poiseuille's law: Flow $\propto \Delta Pr^4/L\eta$. The longer and narrower the catheter and the more viscous the material, the slower is the flow. ΔP = pressure gradient; r = radius of tube; L = length of tube; η = viscosity of fluid.

complement system, which can be activated by contrast media to cause histamine release from basophils and mast cells, alter capillary permeability, mobilize leukocytes, and interact with the coagulation, kinin, and fibrinolytic systems [28]. In special circumstances, breakdown products of the complement system can produce anaphylatoxins which can alter capillary permeability and contract smooth muscles. Other breakdown products can attack and destroy membranes, causing hemolysis.

Chemotoxicity of Contrast Agents

In high concentrations, ionic agents have a chemotoxic but usually rapidly reversible effect on blood vessels and on their contents. Damage to arterial endothelium and red blood cells with hemolysis, red blood cell crenation, and intravascular sludging of red blood cells occurs in varying degrees with different agents. Locally increased serum potassium and vasodilatation are known to occur. The high protein-binding capabilities of the older, more toxic agents have been shown to be almost negligible with more modern contrast media. Although the effect of nonionic agents on red-blood-cell aggregation is essentially the same as with standard contrast agents, there is no deformity of the erythrocytes. There are markedly decreased adverse effects on blood flow and endothelial damage, and there is no binding of plasma proteins with the nonionic agents [1].

Chemotoxicity is also related to the amount of contrast agent that escapes from the endothelial membrane to make contact with parenchymal cells. The manner of escape of contrast agent across endothelial capillary lining cells is explained in part by the activation of endothelial cellular pinocytotic vesicles. Under normal conditions these vesicles do not permit transport of macromolecules across the capillary walls. However, hypertonicity of the contrast agent adversely permits these vesicles to transport contrast molecules across the membrane into the perivascular spaces.

Adverse Effects on the Central Nervous System

There is an additional factor at work, in the brain, which is not thought to be due to contrast agent hypertonicity. Normally the central nervous system (CNS) is protected by the blood-brain barrier, and the contrast medium does not pass into the brain tissue. Tight junctions (closely apposed cellular surfaces in the capillary endothelium of the brain) do open, however, with repeated injections of standard contrast medium [36]. This process violates the interface between the capillary and the glial cell and is thought by some to permit direct contact of the cell with macromolecules of contrast agent. Once across the membrane, the contrast agent does have an adverse effect on parenchymal cells, shifting the oxygen dissociation curve to the left and causing an increased affinity of hemoglobin for oxygen at the expense of the surrounding tissue, with resulting tissue hypoxia. Convulsions and other neurologic sequelae may follow the intracerebral injection of contrast agent [12, 21], particularly in patients with underlying cerebral ischemia and brain tumors. There is only minimal alteration of the blood-brain barrier and brain cellular toxicity, with much greater tolerance, when nonionic contrast agents are used [15].

Medullary shock has occurred when large amounts of contrast medium reach the spinal vessels [5, 8]. This condition consists of transient episodes, varying in severity, of spastic and/or myoclonic contractions of the lower extremities; it can occur during selective injections into lumbar or intercostal arteries in patients with spinal arteriovenous malformations, or during an inadvertently large-dose injection in patients with normal spines. Medullary shock has been seen in midstream aortic injections during Valsalva maneuver or other low-flow states in which large quantities of contrast medium may remain stagnant within these vessels. Transverse myelitis resulting in permanent cord damage is extremely rare with the newer contrast agents.

Adverse Effects on the Cardiovascular System

Contrast agents cause a number of electrophysiologic and hemodynamic effects, on both the central (cardiac) and the peripheral circulation [19]. In the heart, standard hyperosmolar ionic agents have a direct inhibitory effect on smooth muscle, myocardial cells, and the conduction system. Secondary effects occur as a consequence of activating compensatory circulatory reflexes [19]. Thus, following an injection into the root of the aorta or into the main pulmonary artery, there is an initial elevation of the blood pressure for the first 5 seconds, followed by a blood pressure depression for the next 30 seconds. A peripheral injection of contrast medium can lower the blood pressure due to vasodilatation. Bradycardia mediated via the vasomotor centers may lower the blood pressure further. This may be particularly dangerous in patients with cerebral or coronary vascular insufficiency. Standard contrast agents contain chelators that bind free calcium; this increases the potential for fibrillation and has a negative inotropic effect on the myocardium. Decreased contractility and increased left ventricular end-diastolic pressure (LVEDP) and decreased rate of development of ventricular pressure (dp/dt) can prove dangerous in patients with impending heart failure.

The nonionic agents have less severe cardiac effect, have fewer arrhythmogenic effects, fewer ECG changes, and little adverse effect on contractility. They have no change on LVEDP with coronary or left ventricular injections [4]. Thus, patients with pulmonary hypertension, patients with impending or real heart failure, and patients with significant coronary artery disease or conduction defects who are to have pulmonary, ventricular, or coronary contrast studies should be examined with the less toxic nonionic agents whenever possible.

Adverse Effects on the Kidneys

Contrast agents are excreted by glomerular filtration, which in turn induces a prompt diuresis. Both direct chemical toxicity and hypertonicity can play a role in nephrotoxicity. The effect of contrast agents on normal kidneys is transient, with increased renal flow due to vasodilatation, increased glomerular filtration, and reactive vasoconstriction [14]. There may be subsequent decreased renal tubular function. Renal function rapidly returns to normal under most circumstances. However, in patients with prior renal failure, diabetes mellitus, proteinuria due to multiple myeloma, or other causes [34, 35], and in patients who are dehydrated or are in congestive heart failure, renal function can be further impaired by contrast agents [26, 32]. This effect is not necessarily dose-related and occurs in a larger number of patients than formerly suspected. Acute tubular necrosis can occur and presents clinically as oliguria soon after the angiographic study is completed. This condition can progress to complete anuria, which is often refractory to treatment with mannitol and other diuretics. Recovery usually occurs spontaneously and is complete within a week. Surgery should be avoided until there is a clinical recovery from renal failure. It is wise to obtain measurements of the serum creatinine level, both before and after angiography, on all susceptible patients; this is particularly important in all surgical candidates. In these patients the possible benefits of angiography should be carefully weighed against the risks involved. They should be well hydrated before and during the study, and very careful attention should be paid to the amount of contrast agent used. A radiographic observation signaling impending problems is a persistent nephrogram on a radiograph of the abdomen taken the day following an angiogram. Experimental findings indicate that the lower osmolarity of nonionic agents decreases the adverse effects on renal function [44], and their use should be considered in all patients with azotemia who require angiographic studies.

Contrast Agents in Children

Ionic contrast media are acidic. For this reason, particularly in children in whom pH balance may be critical, doses of contrast media must be closely watched [29]. Although these pH changes are usually rapidly reversible, it is wise to wait 20 minutes between injections in the pediatric patient. For these patients the less toxic, nonionic contrast media may prove most helpful.

Allergic Reactions to Contrast Agents

Finally, allergic reactions, initiated by an inherent histamine releasing capacity of the contrast agents, can occur. This type of reaction, which is less common, produces angioneurotic edema, laryngoedema, bronchospasm, and anaphylactic reactions. Susceptible, atopic patients can have these reactions despite no previous contrast injections, for they may have been exposed to and developed antibodies to halogenated benzene ring derivatives in other forms (e.g., food additives, pesticides, herbicides). These can then cross-react with the contrast medium molecules when they are injected. Thus, allergic reaction is not limited to patients with prior exposure to a contrast medium, for the antibody induction is initiated by a variety of similar chemical agents. Because there is less activation of the complement system by the nonionic agents, we should expect fewer reactions with their use.

A prior history of contrast reactions is only a relative contraindication to angiography. If the angiographic procedure is essential, the study may be performed but with extra caution [17, 23, 47].

A definite decrease in the rate and severity of reactions to repeat contrast injections has been found by pretreating the patient with corticosteroids. Although many regimens exist, they all include the use of pharmacologic doses of corticosteroids. Some authors favor pretreatment for as long as 3 or 4 days before the examination, while others allow one dose the night before and a second dose the morning of the study. We routinely use prednisone, 20 mg PO every 6 hours for 24 hours, before contrast medium injection.

There is also wide variation in the use of antihistamines to prevent allergic reactions to contrast media. Benadryl is recommended for blocking the H1 receptors and is often given in a single dose prior to contrast injections. More recently it has been shown that the use of both an H2 and an H1 antagonist was more effective than an H1 blocker alone. Thus, cimetidine (Tagamet), which is a very benign drug over a short course, may be useful [31]. We occasionally add Benadryl, 50 mg IM, and cimetidine, 300 mg IV, the morning of the study in patients with a history of a severe contrast medium reaction.

Many physicians make a distinction between major and minor contrast media reactions when deciding whether or not to give contrast material. Major reactions are those resulting in cardiovascular collapse, severe arrhythmia, or pulmonary edema, while minor reactions include a rash or urticaria. Edema involving the airway and bronchospasm may also be considered major reactions, since impairment of gas exchange may lead to cardiovascular collapse. Contrast studies can usually be safely performed after minor contrast reactions, but such tests should be done with caution if the previous reaction was severe.

During the examination, an anesthesiologist should be on stand-by call, and an open intravenous line and an emergency cart should be ready as added precautions. Epinephrine must be immediately available to treat those patients who demonstrate cardiovascular collapse (hypotension and tachycardia) [3]; 0.3 to 0.5 mg may be given in an intravenous bolus with repeated injections following close monitoring of the blood pressure and heart rate. These patients must be differentiated from those with hypotension and bradycardia caused by vasovagal attacks. The latter may or may not be associated with contrast media injections, and respond to intravenous injection of 0.5 to 1.0 mg of atropine.

Which Contrast Agents to Use and When

Certain organs tolerate one contrast agent better than another, and higher concentrations of one contrast agent over another. From both experimental and clinical reports, all organs appear to tolerate the nonionic better than the ionic contrast agents. Nonionic agents cause less pain, have fewer effects on the kidney, myocardium, brain, vessel walls, and coagulation system, and, if preliminary results are verified, may have fewer allergic manifestations [33]. Their cost relative to ionic agents is, however, significantly higher. The angiographer must be familiar with the characteristics of the available agents (Table 2-1 and Table 2-2) as well as their cost. Of the ionic contrast agents, those with high concentrations, including Hypaque 90% and Angio-Conray, are rarely required. Indeed, we have never had occasion to use them. Medium-concentration contrast agents, which include those with iodine content from 350 to 400 mg per milliliter are generally satisfactory for midstream aortic and pulmonary artery injections, for selective injections into the mesenteric arteries and celiac axis, and sometimes for iliac and femoral arteriography and for caval angiography. The low-concentration ionic contrast agents used in angiography include those containing primarily methylglucamine salts with iodine contents ranging from 282 to 300 mg per milliliter. These agents are preferred for selective organ injection and can be satisfactory in femoral arteriography provided they are given in large doses and are rapidly injected. By this means, the amount of iodine injected per second is comparable to that of a smaller dose of the more concentrated (of higher osmolarity and, therefore, more toxic) contrast agents. Low-concentration iothalamates and pure methylglucamine salts appear to be better tolerated in the brain than other contrast agents [7]. In coronary arteriography it is necessary that a certain amount of sodium be included with the contrast agent because complete absence of salt results in ventricular fibrillation [41]. Calcium added to the standard agents has been shown to decrease adverse effects of the ionic agents on the myocardium. Electrocardiographic changes indicating transient conduction defects are usually seen following the introduction of any ionic contrast agent during coronary arteriography [2, 41], but these are significantly reduced with the nonionic agents.

It appears that there are many advantages to using the more recently developed nonionic agents; chemotoxic and allergic reactions are fewer and less intense; patient and organ tolerance is better than with the standard agents [33, 35, 44]. Their price is a major drawback and their use may have to be reserved for the pediatric patient, those with severe cardiac disease or pulmonary hypertension, and those with renal disease or previous history of severe contrast media reactions. They may be considered for more routine use when patient discomfort and safety and motion are significant considerations (i.e., coronary, spinal, external carotid, peripheral extremity arteriography, and digital subtraction angiography).

NEGATIVE (RADIOLUCENT) CONTRAST AGENTS

Negative contrast agents include air, carbon dioxide, and nitrous oxide. These agents may be used to delineate retroperitoneal, intraperitoneal, and intrathoracic structures. Only carbon dioxide may be used intravascularly.

Capnoangiography is the use of carbon dioxide as an intravascular contrast agent. Carbon dioxide is 20 times more miscible in blood than air and is absorbed within 1 to 3 minutes. Up to 100 cc of gas may be used in a single rapid injection. Most experience with this agent to date has been in the venous system, and few if any complications occur with this route of injection. Carbon dioxide can be used very effectively when injected directly into the arterial system, subtracted out, and enhanced by digital subtraction. This technique should be considered a viable alternative to standard contrast agents in patients with contraindications to their use [18].

A rare contraindication to capnoangiography is severe respiratory disease, in which the patient might have difficulty excreting the carbon dioxide. It should not be used in the region of the head, because carbon dioxide can decrease the sensitivity of respiratory and cardiac centers.

Indications for the use of radiolucent contrast agents include

1. Allergy to radiopaque contrast media; intraarterial digital subtraction studies below the diaphragm
2. Evaluation of the hepatic veins, inferior vena cava, or renal venous obstruction
3. Evaluation of tricuspid insufficiency (the hepatic veins in tricuspid insufficiency would be larger during systole)
4. Evaluation of the superior vena cava syndrome
5. Evaluation of thickness of pericardium (rarely performed if adequate ultrasonography facilities are available)

References

1. Aspelin, P. Effect of ionic and non-ionic contrast media on morphology of human erythrocytes. *Acta Radiol. [Diagn.] (Stockh.)* 19:675, 1978.
2. Banks, D., Raftery, E., and Oram, S. Evaluation of contrast media used in coronary arteriography. *Br. Heart J.* 31:645, 1969.
3. Barach, E. M., et al. Epinephrine for treatment of anaphylactic shock. *J.A.M.A.* 21:2118, 1984.
4. Bettmann, M. Angiographic contrast agents: Conventional and new media compared. *A.J.R.* 139:787, 1982.
5. Cornell, S. Spasticity of the lower extremities following abdominal angiography. *Radiology* 93:377, 1969.
6. Debrun, G., et al. Detachable balloon and calibrated-leak balloon techniques in the treatment of cerebrovascular lesions. *J. Neurosurg.* 49:635, 1978.
7. Dempsey, P., et al. The effect of contrast media on patient motion during cerebral angiography. *Radiology* 115:207, 1975.
8. DiChiro, G. Unintentional spinal cord arteriography: A warning. *Radiology* 112:231, 1974.
9. Dotter, C., et al. Transluminal iliac artery dilatation: Nonsurgical catheter treatment of atheromatous narrowing. *J.A.M.A.* 117:230, 1974.
10. Dotter, C., et al. Injectable flow guided co-axial

catheters for selective angiography and controlled vascular occlusion. *Radiology* 104:421, 1972.

11. Eldh, P., and Jacobson, B. Heparinized vascular catheters: A clinical trial. *Radiology* 111:289, 1974.

12. Fischer, H. W. Occurrence of seizure during cranial computed tomography. *Radiology* 137:563, 1980.

13. Fogarty, T., Cranley, J., and Krause, R. A method of extraction of arterial emboli and thrombi. *Surg. Gynecol. Obstet.* 116:241, 1963.

14. Forrest, J. B., Howards, S. S., and Gillenwater, J. Y. Osmotic effects of intravenous contrast agents on renal function. *J. Urol.* 125:147, 1981.

15. Goldman, K. The blood brain barrier: Effects of non-ionic contrast media with and without addition of calcium ions and magnesium ions. *Invest. Radiol.* 14:305, 1979.

16. Grainger, R. G. Osmolality of intravascular radiological contrast media. *Br. J. Radiol.* 53:739, 1980.

17. Greenberger, P. A., et al. Pretreatment of high-risk patients requiring radiographic contrast media studies. *J. Allergy Clin. Immunol.* 67:185, 1981.

18. Hawkins, I. F., Jr. Carbon dioxide digital subtraction arteriography. *A.J.R.* 139:19, 1982.

19. Higgins, C. B. Overview and methods used for the study of the cardiovascular actions of contrast materials. *Invest. Radiol.* 15(Suppl.):S188, 1980.

20. Hilal, S., et al. Magnetically guided devices for vascular exploration and treatment. *Radiology* 113:529, 1974.

21. Howitz, N., and Weiner, L. Temporary cortical blindness following angiography. *Neurosurgery* 40:583, 1974.

22. Jacobsson, B., and Schlossman, D. Thrombogenic properties of vascular catheter materials in vitro. *Acta Radiol. [Diagn.] (Stockh.)* 14:385, 1973.

23. Kelly, J. F., et al. Radiographic contrast media studies in high-risk patients. *J. Allergy Clin. Immunol.* 62:181, 1978.

24. Kerber, C. Balloon catheter with a calibrated leak: A new system for superselective angiography and occlusive catheter therapy. *Radiology* 120:547, 1976.

25. Lagergren, H., Olsson, P., and Swendenborg, J. Inhibited platelet adhesion: A nonthrombogenic characteristic of a heparin coated surface. *Surgery* 75:643, 1974.

26. Lang, E. K., et al. The incidence of contrast medium induced acute tubular necrosis following arteriography. *Radiology* 138:203, 1981.

27. Lasser, E. C. Contrast material symposium. *Invest. Radiol.* 15(Suppl.):S1, 1980.

28. Lasser, E. C., et al. Activation system in contrast idiosyncrasy. *Invest. Radiol.* 15(Suppl.):S2, 1980.

29. Levin, A., Effect of angiocardiography on fluid and electrolyte balance. *A.J.R.* 105:777, 1969.

30. Meyerovitz, M., Levin, D., and Boxt, L. Superselective catheterization of small caliber arteries with a new high visibility steerable guidewire. *A.J.R.* 144:785, 1985.

31. Meyers, G. E., and Bloom, F. L. Cimetidine (Tagamet) combined with steroids and H1 antihistamines for the prevention of serious radiographic contrast material reactions. *Cathet. Cardiovasc. Diagn.* 7:65, 1981.

32. Older, R. A., et al. Contrast-induced acute renal failure: Persistent nephrogram as clue to early detection. *A.J.R.* 134:339, 1980.

33. Pfister, R. C., et al. Contrast-medium-induced electrocardiographic abnormalities: Comparison of bolus and infusion of methylglucamine iodamine and methylglucamine/sodium diatrizoate. *A.J.R.* 140:149, 1983.

34. Pillay, V., et al. Acute renal failure following intravenous urography in patients with long-standing diabetes mellitus and azotemia. *Radiology* 95:633, 1970.

35. Port, F., Wagoner, R., and Fulton, R. Acute renal failure after angiography. *A.J.R.* 121:544, 1974.

36. Rapoport, S. Reversible Opening of the Blood-Brain Barrier by Osmotic Shrinkage of the Cerebro-Vascular Endothelium: Opening up the Tight Junctions as Related to Carotid Arteriography. In S. Hilal (ed.), *Small Vessel Angiography: Imaging, Morphology, Physiology, and Clinical Applications* St. Louis: Mosby, 1973.

37. Rapoport, S., et al. Experience with metrizamide in patients with previous severe anaphylactoid reactions to ionic contrast agents. *Radiology* 143:321, 1982.

38. Shehadi, W. H. Contrast media adverse reactions: Occurrence, recurrence, and distribution patterns. *Radiology* 143:11, 1982.

39. Shehadi, W. H., and Toniolo, G. Adverse reactions to contrast media. *Radiology* 137:299, 1983.

40. Siegle, R. L., and Lieberman, P. A review of untoward reactions to iodinated contrast material. *J. Urol.* 119:581, 1978.

41. Snyder, C., Cramer, R., and Amplatz, K. Isolation of sodium as a cause of ventricular fibrillation. *Invest. Radiol.* 6:245, 1971.

42. Sos, T., et al. A new open ended guidewire catheter. *Radiology* 154:817, 1985.

43. Swan, H., et al. Catheterization of the heart in man with use of a flow-directed balloon-tipped catheter. *N. Engl. J. Med.* 283:447, 1970.

44. Tornquist, C., et al. Proteinuria following nephroangiography. VII. Comparison between ionic, monomeric, monoacidic, dimeric, and non-ionic contrast media in the dog. *Acta Radiol. [Suppl.] (Stockh.)* 362:49, 1980.

45. White, R. I., Jr. et al. Therapeutic embolization with detachable balloons. *Cardiovasc. Intervent. Radiol.* 14:35, 1979.

46. Widrich, W. C., et al. Iopamidol: A non-ionic contrast agent for peripheral arteriography. *Radiology* 145:53, 1982.

47. Zweiman, B., Mishkin, M. M., and Hildreth, E. A. An approach to the performance of contrast studies in contrast material-reactive persons. *Ann. Intern. Med.* 83:159, 1975.

Catheterization Techniques

Although they are widely accepted, angiographic procedures are not without danger, discomfort, and expense to the patient and should not be recklessly initiated. When they are requested, the clinician has often exhausted all other means for obtaining a definitive diagnosis, and no room remains for equivocation because of an inadequate study. With this in mind, one should give due consideration, prior to undertaking a procedure, to the finer details of the technique to be employed and should evaluate the films and images carefully prior to completion of the procedure.

Preangiographic Evaluation

PATIENT CHART REVIEW

The patient's cardiovascular, hematologic, renal, and neurologic status should be reviewed prior to the study. There are no absolute contraindications to angiography; however, anuria, heart failure, impending or recent myocardial infarction, impending cerebral vascular accident, the presence of blood dyscrasias, and a previous severe reaction to contrast agents represent high-risk situations.

At this point, consider those who may be studied by less invasive techniques of intravenous digital subtraction angiography (IV-DSA). Although the intravenous route would be helpful in high-risk patients with poor pulses, not all of these patients are candidates for this procedure. This method generally requires an alert, cooperative patient with a reasonably good cardiac output and renal function. It should be reserved primarily for those vessels or organs that can be regionally isolated from other superimposed structures, such as the vessels in the neck (cervical portions of the carotid and vertebral arteries) or in the extremities. Major vessels of the abdomen or pelvis may also be evaluated. Occasionally the pulmonary arteries may be studied. Patients in heart failure, with poor contractility of the left ventricle, or with aortic insufficiency will not provide optimal levels of vascular opacification by IV-DSA. Patients at risk for the high doses of contrast media required for IV-DSA should be screened out. Those with diabetes mellitus, pulmonary hypertension, multiple myeloma, coronary artery disease, and poor renal function may be better studied by intraarterial DSA (IA-DSA), for which considerably smaller doses of contrast are required than with conventional angiography. Here also, nonionic contrast materials should be strongly considered. IA-DSA with nonionic agents or carbon dioxide may also be used in those with a history of severe reaction to contrast material.

The scope of angiography has clearly broadened with the addition of the less toxic nonionic agents and digital imaging techniques. The drawbacks and indications for using these techniques in favor of conventional angiography must be considered during the preangiographic evaluation, but in all cases, the physician should weigh the benefit of the study against the possible complications that may arise.

PREANGIOGRAPHIC ORDERS

The following regimen is a guide for adults. The physician should use his own judgment and should adjust the regimen to suit the needs of individual patients. The first three items should be considered for both conventional as well as digital subtraction angiographic studies.

1. The patient should sign the operative permit following appropriate discussion with the physician. Informed consent is an important consideration [1].
2. The patient should abstain from solid food for 6 to 8 hours before the study, but not from clear liquids. Fasting is indicated if general anesthesia is being considered.
3. The patient should be well hydrated, with intravenous administration of physiologic solutions (e.g., 5% dextrose) if necessary. The physician should beware of the patient having undergone 2 or 3 days of repeated fasting to accommodate numerous diagnostic proce-

dures; renal failure has been encountered following angiography in such cases.

4. The following preangiographic medications should be given when the patient is called to the radiology department for conventional angiography or IA-DSA: atropine, 0.6 to 1.0 mg intramuscularly (to reduce vasovagal reactions); meperidine hydrochloride (Demerol), 50 to 100 mg intramuscularly; and diazepam (Valium), 5 to 10 mg, or sodium secobarbital, 50 to 100 mg, orally.

5. Aspirin, 325 mg, may be given the night (but preferably for 2 or 3 days) before the study to prevent platelet adhesiveness.

6. The groin or axilla should be shaved and prepared.

7. All anticoagulants should be discontinued if the consulting physician agrees. This is not entirely necessary if an intravenous route is being considered.

Approaches to Angiographic Procedures

GENERAL PRINCIPLES

Physical Evaluation

Before deciding on an approach to a vascular study, the angiographer must study the possible target vessels. Evaluation of a vessel prior to a puncture includes comparing the strength of the pulse of the artery to that on the opposing limb. A decreased pulse pressure at the site of the intended puncture indicates disease at or proximal to the area, and this vessel should be approached with caution. If available, the noninvasive cardiovascular laboratory findings should be reviewed. Arteries in the periphery of the limb must also be checked and marked for postangiographic reference.

The findings on physical examination influence the details of the technique to be used (i.e., the amount and concentration of contrast agent, the timing and number of films, and the pressure to be used for the injection). Thus in a patient with an arteriovenous communication, the rapid flow, strong pulse with high pulse pressure requires a large dose of concentrated contrast agent with a fast injection and rapid timing of films. In contrast, the poor pulses and cold, shiny, hairless skin in the limb with arterial obliterative disease require

slower delivery, a smaller dose and concentration of contrast agent, and sometimes surprisingly slow timing of the films. The film timing and the dosages and rates of contrast media mentioned in this text are therefore subject to considerable variation, and the angiographer must use judgment in each study.

It is always possible to obtain an angiographic study, regardless of the extent of disease that is present. Familiarity with the percutaneous approach to the femoral arteries, axillary arteries, brachial arteries, and the major veins, as well as the translumbar approach, will preclude failure (Fig. 3-1).

The Percutaneous Arterial Approach

In the percutaneous approach, the arterial wall is punctured and the needle is advanced into the artery. The guidewire is fed through the needle into the artery, the needle is withdrawn, and a catheter is inserted into the vessel over the guidewire. This method is known as the Seldinger technique [15] of catheter placement within the vascular system (see Figs. 3-3, 3-4). The general principles of this technique will be discussed in the following sections; individual variations for selected approaches will be mentioned separately.

THE PUNCTURE. Prepare the skin over a wide area around the puncture site and drape the chosen site with sterile towels and sheets. Use a local anesthetic (lidocaine 1%) to infiltrate widely the perivascular tissues of the puncture site. Use of the anesthetic not only provides anesthesia but prevents vasospasm. The next step is to make a 2-mm nick in the skin approximately 1 to 2 cm beyond the intended site of arterial entry and gently loosen the subcutaneous tissues with a small curved forceps. This allows a port of escape for blood and may prevent formation of a hematoma. Choose your needle carefully (Fig. 3-2). Its outside diameter should not exceed that of the subsequently used catheter; otherwise, an annoying leak can occur at the site of puncture. Introduce the needle, making sure that the component parts of the needle assembly are properly fitted. Localize the pulsating artery with gentle pressure applied on the needle. The pulsations should be transmitted through the needle in a to-and-fro motion. If the motion is localized to one side or the other, the pulsations transmitted to the needle indicate that the needle is either medial or lateral to the artery.

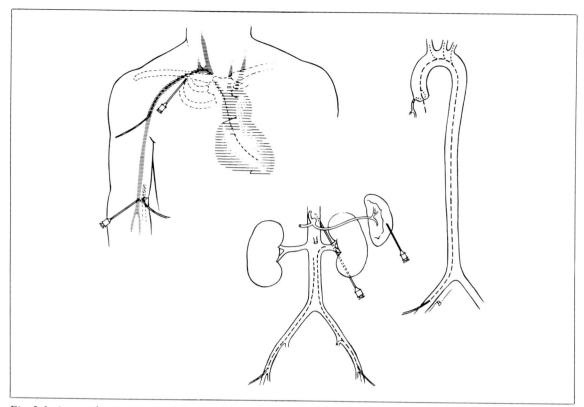

Fig. 3-1. Approaches to angiographic procedures. The femoral artery is the most common approach for studying the arteries of the lower extremities, pelvis, abdominal aorta and its branches, thoracic aorta and its branches, brachiocephalic vessels, coronary arteries, and left ventricle. If the femoral artery is occluded, the other approaches are available. The translumbar approach outlines the abdominal aorta and the vessels peripheral to it, but it does not allow selective catheterization of branches. The axillary approach allows angiography of the left ventricle and the entire aorta and selective catheterization of the brachiocephalic vessels, coronary arteries, and vessels below the diaphragm. When all peripheral arteries are occluded, IV-DSA usually provides adequate studies of the arterial system.

The optimal method uses a sharply beveled needle without an internal stylet; it may have an overlying Teflon sleeve. The needle is slowly advanced through the anterior wall of the artery until pulsatile flow is seen (Fig. 3-3). The flow at this point must be a round, well-pulsating flow of blood. Advance the needle into the artery and, if good flow remains, replace the metal shaft of the needle with the guidewire. As an alternate, sometimes easier method, puncture both walls of the artery (Fig. 3-4), withdraw the sharp stylet, and bend the

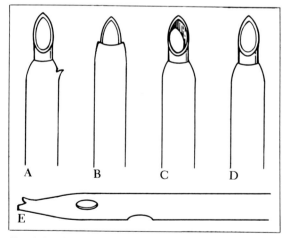

Fig. 3-2. The angiographer should be aware of improper needle and catheter assemblies.
A. Teflon sleeve is frayed.
B. More friable Teflon sleeve is too long.
C. Sharp obturator is too short.
D. Component parts of the needle assembly are properly fitted. The sharp obturator is presenting, followed by the metal sleeve and subsequently by the well-tapered Teflon sleeve. This assembly permits atraumatic arterial puncture.
E. Catheter tip is frayed.

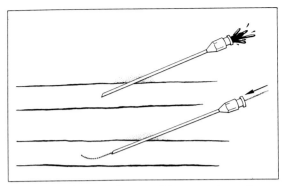

Fig. 3-3. Seldinger technique. Direct anterior wall puncture. (See text.)

needle with its Teflon sleeve almost parallel to the skin. Slowly withdraw the needle. Pulsatile flow indicates when the needle is within the arterial lumen. Again advance the Teflon sleeve, remove the needle shaft, and replace it with a guidewire. Occasionally the femoral nerve lies behind the artery and may be injured with the latter technique (Fig. 3-5).

Poor flow patterns demand caution. A forceful but irregular spraying flow may indicate arterial stenosis in the vicinity of the needle. A dripping or barely pulsatile flow may indicate several things. First, it can be caused by severe hypotension, such

Fig. 3-4. The Seldinger technique of percutaneous catheter placement within a vessel. (See text for details.)

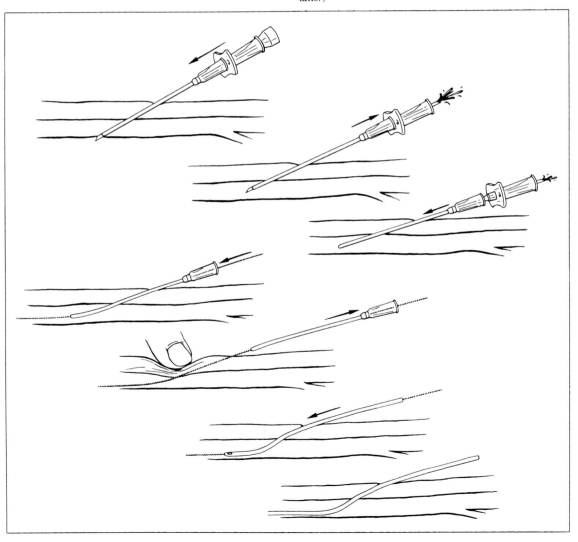

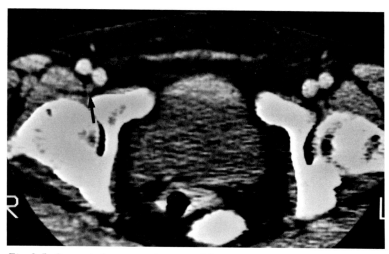

Fig. 3-5. Computed tomography scan of the inguinal region demonstrating a femoral nerve lying immediately posterior to the femoral artery (*arrow*).

as that seen in a vasovagal attack. Second, polycythemia may sometimes produce an almost pulseless, dark flow of blood, suggesting that the needle may be in a vein. Finally, the poor flow is often due to occlusive disease, a subintimal location of the needle, or drainage of a hematoma. Under these circumstances, think carefully before continuing.

Once the vessel is entered, the guidewire should be advanced at least 15 to 20 cm into the vessel, to a point well beyond the junction of the flexible tip with its more firm shaft. Failure at this point will result in the flexible portion of the guidewire being insufficiently stable to permit passage of the catheter through the tissues (Fig. 3-6), which will cause inadvertent withdrawal of the guidewire and trauma to the artery. Do not force the needle assembly or the guidewire as you are advancing up the artery, since arterial walls can be injured or dissected and atherosclerotic plaques undermined. If a large plaque presents an obstruction to the advancing needle and wire assembly, it may sometimes be circumvented by twisting the guidewire tip. If this maneuver is unsuccessful, it is necessary to repuncture at a slightly higher or lower level. Another approach may have to be attempted. Be sure to secure hemostasis prior to your second attempt at puncture.

CATHETER PLACEMENT (see Fig. 3-4). With the guidewire well within the artery, pressure must be applied over the puncture site to prevent hema-

toma formation after the needle is removed. The next step is to pass the appropriate catheter into the artery. By bringing the catheter tip through the skin as close to the artery as possible, with a rotary movement, the smoothly tapered tip of the catheter may be gently inserted over the immobilized

Fig. 3-6. A complication of catheter insertion: The guidewire is insufficiently rigid for the catheter to follow through the arterial wall into the arterial lumen. As the catheter tip traumatizes the arterial wall, the guidewire is inadvertently removed and successful catheter placement is aborted.

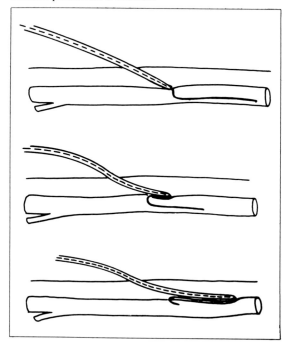

guidewire into the vessel. Under fluoroscopic control, the catheter may now be advanced into the artery, with the protective tip of the flexible guidewire always preceding the catheter tip.

It is important to keep the following points in mind: Do not introduce the guidewire unless there is a good flow from the needle or catheter. Do not force the introduction of the guidewire. Do not leave the guidewire within the catheter or blood vessel for more than a few seconds, because a clot will form over the guidewire and will be stripped off as the wire is withdrawn. Be sure that the stiff portion of the guidewire is well into the vessel.

When the intravascular catheter is at the appropriate level, promptly remove the guidewire and attach the connecting tube and syringe. Aspirate and flush the catheter with sterile 5% dextrose. This procedure should be repeated at 1- to 2-minute intervals.

Certain catheters (polyurethane, woven Dacron) have blunt or friable tips that may injure the arterial wall during the percutaneous insertion. Introduction of these catheters must be preceded by the prior insertion of a smoothly tapered, smooth-walled catheter of more durable material (usually Teflon). The diameter of this "persuader" or dilator must be no greater than, and usually 1 French size smaller than, the diameter of the proposed catheter. These blunt-tipped catheters may also be introduced through a previously placed sheath at the puncture site.

All injections through the catheter should be preceded by a slight aspiration to remove air bubbles present in the catheter hub. A small test injection of contrast material serves to check the catheter position and to exclude subintimal injection or otherwise improper catheter position. Never fail to perform this. If the catheter tip is in a ventricular cavity, a major pulmonary artery, or the root of the aorta, it must move freely with the pulsations of vascular flow. If the catheter tip is fixed, injection into the myocardium or the intima or a wedged position may ensue. Check the catheter position following any change in position of the patient or his extremities, since the tip may advance into an undesirable position with motion.

PREVENTION OF THROMBUS FORMATION. Special measures must be taken to prevent thrombus formation. All flushing solutions should contain heparin (1000 IU/500 ml of 5% dextrose). Alternatively, catheters treated with heparin coating on both inner and outer surfaces can be used [2]. The advantages of these catheters are (1) the very high concentration of heparin at the blood-catheter interface, which prevents clot formation, and (2) the lack of danger from systemic administration of anticoagulants. If the procedure is going to be long and arduous, and multiple small vessels must be catheterized, the patient may be systemically heparinized at the start of the procedure; this is accomplished by administering 45 IU of heparin per kilogram body weight directly into the artery through the catheter [17]. If the angiographic procedure takes approximately 1 hour, the major effects of the heparin will have worn off by its termination, and few extra precautions to secure hemostasis are necessary. Ten milligrams of protamine sulfate per 1000 IU of heparin administration may be administered intravenously if prolonged bleeding at the puncture site is a problem. Patients should not be heparinized routinely; contraindications include bleeding diathesis, the translumbar approach, intraabdominal, intrathoracic, or intracranial bleeding or a lesion predisposing to bleeding, severe hypertension or aortic insufficiency, follow-up needle aspiration of intraabdominal or thoracic structures, or immediately postoperative patients.

CATHETERIZATION IN CHILDREN. Special considerations must be given to the techniques used in children, since their arteries are especially prone to spasm and thrombosis. A sharp 18- or 20-gauge thin-walled needle (without an obturator) is used with the bevel facing anteriorly. A "butterfly" needle (after the attached plastic tubing is removed) is a helpful instrument. As soon as the anterior wall of the artery is punctured and pulsatile flow is obtained, a small diameter guidewire is introduced through the needle up to the distal aorta. The needle is removed, and dilators of gradually increasing sizes are introduced prior to placement of the catheter over the guidewire. Avoid using large-diameter catheters.

OCCLUDED CATHETER REPLACEMENT. During the course of a study, an intravascularly placed catheter may become occluded. It may be replaced by one of two methods:

1. *Use of a paper-thin Mylar or Teflon sheath.* Introduce the sheath into the vessel over the hub of the catheter, after removing the adapter

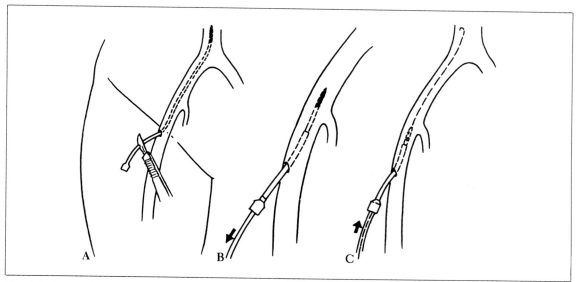

Fig. 3-7. Removal of an occluded catheter and insertion of a replacement catheter through a paper-thin Mylar or Teflon sheath.
A. Remove hub of catheter.
B. Insert a paper-thin, well-fitted Mylar sheath over the catheter through the skin incision and into the artery at the puncture site. Withdraw the occluded catheter. Be sure to have the replacement catheter with inserted guidewire ready for rapid insertion at this point.
C. Introduce the new catheter with presenting guidewire through the Mylar or Teflon sheath.

(Fig. 3-7). Remove the occluded catheter. Place a guidewire (with flexible tip presenting) through a fresh catheter and replace the occluded catheter with this assembly.

2. *Guidewire placement.* Withdraw the catheter tip to near the point of puncture and drill a small hole into one side of the catheter (Fig. 3-8). Anchor 2 or 3 mm of guidewire into this hole, advance the catheter with its clotted tip into the lower aorta, pulling the guidewire with the catheter along its outside surface into the vessel lumen. Withdraw the 2- or 3-mm embedded portion of the guidewire from the catheter. The guidewire is now free within the vessel lumen and a new catheter may be introduced over the guidewire once the occluded catheter has been removed.

CATHETER REMOVAL. At the conclusion of the study, withdraw the catheter close to the site of entry and check the peripheral pulses. If they are decreased, perform a "pull-out" angiogram to exclude clot formation or arterial spasm (Fig. 3-9). To relieve arterial spasm, 10 ml of 1% lidocaine may be injected into the tissues surrounding the puncture site and nitroglycerin 100 to 300 μg injected into the spastic artery. A milking action of the femoral artery immediately following pull-out of the catheter and the release of a short spurt of blood with catheter removal may extrude a small intraarterial clot (Fig. 3-10). Adequate hemostasis at the arterial puncture site (not the site of the skin incision) must be secured by compression hard enough to prevent bleeding. After the first 2 or 3 minutes, compression should be sufficiently relaxed to permit intermittent pulsation of peripheral vessels. Arteries that were patent at the termination of an angiographic procedure have been known to occlude with a clot as a result of overzealous compression. Compression should be maintained for approximately 10 minutes, but the duration varies depending on the catheter size, heparinization, the length of the procedure, and the age and blood pressure of the patient.

POSTANGIOGRAPHIC EVALUATION. Postangiographic evaluation for signs of possible complications is essential and includes checking for changes in pulse pressure, temperature, color, and motor function in the extremity chosen for puncture. Both retroperitoneal and external hematoma formation are possible. Fluoroscopy of the contrast-filled bladder following each arterial study may forewarn of possible problems by revealing bladder

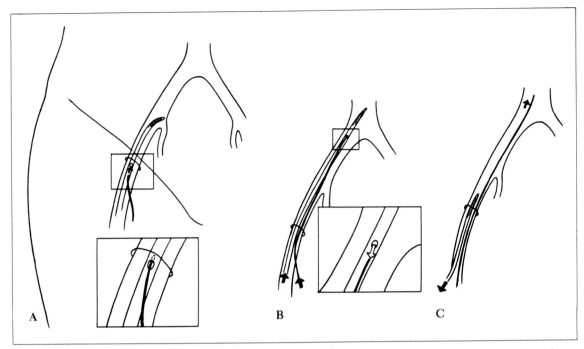

Fig. 3-8. Occluded catheter replacement with guide-wire alone. (See text for details.)

displacement (see Fig. 3-34). Following return to the ward, the patient is placed on "vital signs status," with frequent checks made of the puncture site and also of the peripheral extremity. The patient is encouraged to drink fluids and is kept at complete bed rest for approximately 12 hours. If renal failure is suspected, the serum creatinine level is monitored. Immediate surgical and medical consultation must be sought in the event of complications.

THE FEMORAL ARTERY APPROACH

Indications
The femoral artery approach is the single most important commonly used approach to study and sometimes to treat diseases of vessels of

1. The lower extremities
2. The pelvic area
3. The abdominal aorta and its numerous branches
4. The thoracic aorta and the bronchial and intercostal arteries
5. The brachiocephalic vessels
6. The coronary arteries and the left ventricle

Contraindications
Contraindications to the use of the femoral artery approach include

1. Severe aortic, iliac, or common femoral arterial occlusive disease
2. Marked tortuosity of the iliac arteries, precluding accurate catheter placement or manipulation
3. Severe blood dyscrasias
4. Dacron grafts extending to the femoral artery (this is only a relative contraindication)
5. Femoral artery aneurysm

Technique
The femoral artery passes lateral to the femoral vein under the inguinal ligament and overlies the most medial aspect of the femoral head (Fig. 3-11). It arches in a dorsal medial direction to become the external iliac artery when it enters the pelvis. This arching of the femoral artery over the pectineus muscle is an important consideration to be kept in mind during the catheterization procedure. If one attempts to enter the artery at a point

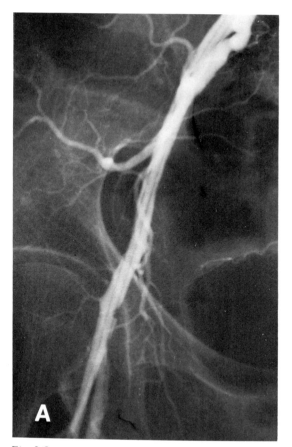

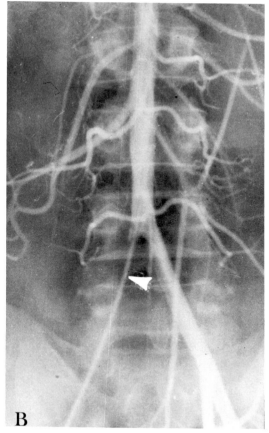

Fig. 3-9.

A. "Pull-out" angiogram. Note the fibrin collections along the course of the catheter; they cause a radiolucent line.

B. Pull-out angiogram performed on another patient with absent peripheral pulse recognized prior to withdrawal of the catheter. There is a spasm of the right iliac vessels around the catheter (*arrowhead*) as well as thrombus in the left common iliac artery. Mild paresthesias but no pallor or pain were experienced by the patient. Symptoms disappeared and pulses returned 2 hours after the catheter was removed. Prior to withdrawal of the catheter, 3000 IU of intraarterial heparin and 15 ml of periarterial lidocaine were introduced.

just cephalad to this arch, the needle may travel deep into the pelvis without reaching the artery, and it may enter the bladder. If the puncture is made considerably below this point, advancement of the needle is more difficult; in addition, the deep femoral artery (arteria profunda femoris) may be entered instead. If the artery is entered at the apex of the arch and the needle is adequately angled (approximately 45 degrees to the skin surface), the approach is facilitated and success is ensured. In obese persons, the crease between the abdominal panniculus and the thigh in the region of the groin is lower than the inguinal ligament. The unwary angiographer will mistake this landmark for that of the ligament, making a puncture that is too low. Even in obese patients, do not puncture above the inguinal crease. In patients who are slim, on the other hand, one tends to make an approach that is too high for successful puncture. If indeed puncture is successful with this too-cephalad approach (into the external iliac artery), hemostasis is more difficult to secure following removal of the needle or catheter, and retroperitoneal hemorrhage may ensue. Remember that occasionally the femoral nerve lies immediately posterior, rather than lateral, to the femoral artery, and it may be inadvertently damaged.

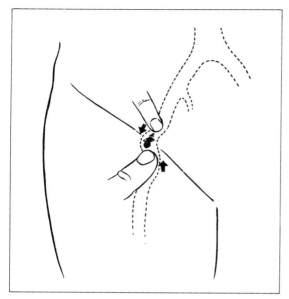

Fig. 3-10. Extrusion of a clot formed close to the puncture site. If a pull-out angiogram demonstrates a clot, a milking action of the femoral artery immediately following catheter removal may extrude a small intraarterial clot.

The technique for puncture is as described earlier, in the section General Principles. The angiographer should be sure to mark peripheral pulses before the study as a reference point for possible occlusive complications. The direction of needle placement in Figure 3-11 is retrograde (upstream) to the flow of blood.

An antegrade direction may be used if catheter placement for therapy (e.g., chemotherapy, selective occlusion of feeding branches to an arteriovenous malformation, transluminal angioplasty) is anticipated (Fig. 3-12). In order to enter the common femoral artery, the skin puncture site must be at least 2 cm above the inguinal ligament, a procedure that is sometimes difficult in obese patients. The point at which the needle enters the artery must, however, be below the inguinal ligament to avoid retroperitoneal hemorrhage following withdrawal of the catheter. The guidewire-catheter assembly is more likely to descend down the superficial femoral artery rather than the profunda femoris artery if a more lateromedial and superficial approach is used, if the foot is internally rotated (thus throwing the posteriorly located profunda laterally), or if the patient's leg is placed in a "frogleg" position. Placing a pillow under the hip

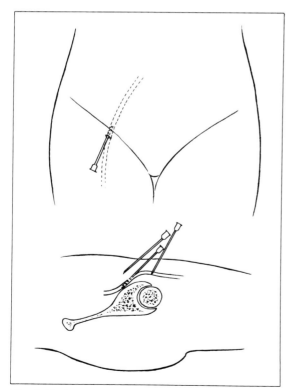

Fig. 3-11. Anatomy of the femoral artery pertinent to puncture. (See text for details.)

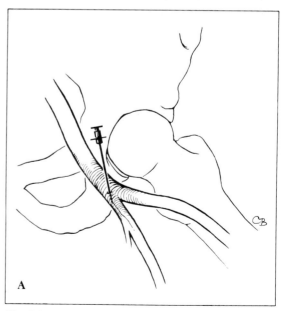

Fig. 3-12. Anterograde puncture of the femoral artery. (See text.)
A. Frogleg position facilitates entry into the common femoral artery.

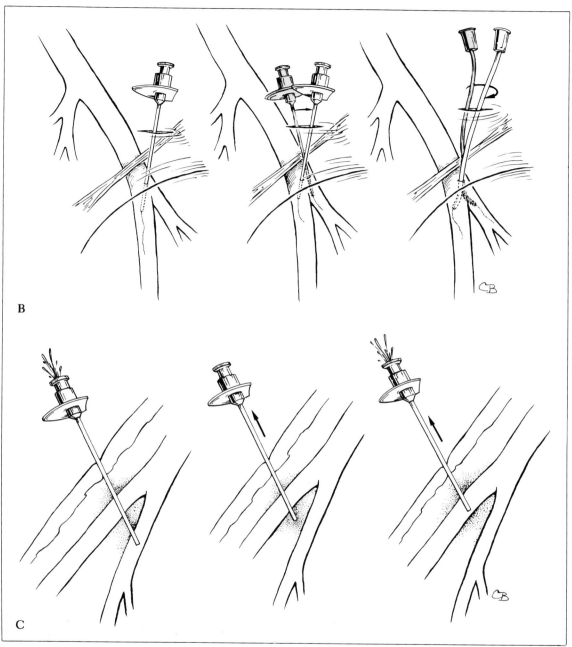

B

C

B. Skin incision is 2 cm above the inguinal ligament; common femoral arterial puncture is below the inguinal ligament. A lateromedial approach directs entry into the superficial femoral rather than into the profunda femoris branch. If the profunda is entered, redirect the needle hub; alternatively, manipulate an introducer with a curved distal tip that has been exchanged for the needle.

C. The superficial femoral artery has been traversed to enter the profunda femoris artery. Substantiate with contrast injection, withdraw the needle, and advance the guidewire into the superficial femoral artery.

of the groin being approached is helpful with an obese patient. If the profunda is instead cannulated, there are a number of methods available to redirect the guidewire and catheter into the superficial femoral artery. The simplest is to direct the needle cannula so as to advance the guidewire in the more ventral and medial direction of the superficial femoral artery. Occasionally, a curved vascular torque wire or a short 5 French polyethylene introducer with a sharply angled tip may help direct the entry into the superficial femoral artery. Sometimes the needle has traversed through the superficial femoral artery to enter the profunda femoris. After first checking with a contrast injection, careful withdrawal of the needle will result in absent flow as it leaves the profunda, to actively spurt again as the needle tip withdraws into the superficial femoral artery.

Sometimes the femoral pulse is barely palpable or imperceptible due to an upstream obstruction. Catheter placement may be desired to view peripheral run-off distal to the point of obstruction, or to attempt angioplasty of the compromised artery. This may be accomplished by blindly puncturing with the standard angulation and approach over the medial femoral head. The position of the vessel may also be localized by IV-DSA "road mapping." A contrast filled mask obtained by IV-DSA is displayed on the monitor which provides a static image of the vessel, through which the position of the needle, guidewire or catheter can be monitored. Obviously the patient must not move once the road map has been made. Doppler ultrasonography may be invaluable in finding the precise location of the vessel.

THE TRANSLUMBAR APPROACH
Indications
The translumbar approach is used

1. When the femoral artery cannot be used to evaluate the abdominal aorta and peripheral vessels due to occlusive disease, marked vascular tortuosity, or presence of compromised vascular grafts
2. When adequate detail cannot be provided by IV-DSA

Contraindications
Contraindications to the translumbar approach include

1. Blood dyscrasia (be sure the patient is not taking dicumarol, heparin, or thrombolytic agents)
2. Abdominal aneurysm or dissecting aneurysm at the site of the proposed abdominal aortic puncture
3. Aortic graft in the region of the puncture site, particularly if it is complicated by infection or fistulas
4. Severe systemic hypertension or aortic insufficiency

Technique
The angiographer should study preliminary films of the abdomen in anteroposterior and lateral projections for signs of vascular calcification.

The patient is prone. The left side may be slightly elevated right anterior oblique (RAO); this position brings the aorta to the left, lateral to the vertebral bodies, making it more accessible. The point of needle entry in the back is 1 to 2 cm below the left twelfth rib, approximately four fingerbreadths lateral to the spinous processes (Fig. 3-13A). The twelfth rib should be recognized either on a preliminary film or by fluoroscopy prior to needle insertion. To mistake the eleventh rib for the twelfth would place the needle too high and result in pneumothorax or hemothorax.

Local anesthetic is used for the skin wheal and is also introduced through the long needle on its way down to the aorta. An 8-inch, 18-gauge, Teflon-sheathed needle is used in combination with a sharp obturator. It is directed obliquely, ventrad and cephalad, until the vertebral body of T12 is identified with the needle tip (Fig. 3-13B). The needle is then withdrawn at least 5 cm and directed more laterally and ventrally to bypass the vertebral body. It is again advanced slowly until the pulsations of the abdominal aorta are transferred to the needle, being identified both visually and tactilely. The aortic wall is penetrated with a short, controlled forward motion by passing the needle 1 cm into the aortic lumen. *Only the proximal wall is punctured.* Removing the sharp obturator should result in pulsatile flow. This flow is usually not as pulsatile as that seen with puncture of other arteries through shorter needles.

The special guidewire with its flexible distal curve is then inserted into the inner steel needle shaft and advanced cephalad into the low thoracic aorta (Fig. 3-13C). If the guidewire cannot be introduced easily into the aortic lumen, the needle

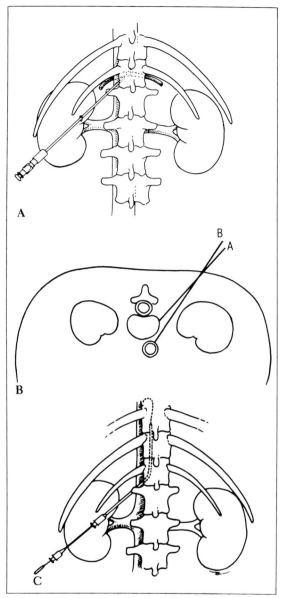

Fig. 3-13. Three stages of translumbar puncture. (See text for details.)

this approach. Occasionally guidewire manipulation descending into the abdominal aorta is possible (Fig. 3-14); an anterograde injection can thus be made and is more desirable in evaluating the distal aorta and peripheral vessels. Following guidewire removal, the position of the Teflon catheter should be checked with fluoroscopy. A high-pressure connecting tube is applied to the catheter. In an adult, if the Teflon catheter has advanced into a descending thoracic aorta, the angiographer should use 85 to 100 ml of Renografin-76 (delivered at 17 to 20 ml per second for 5 seconds) if one wishes to see the femoral arterial run-off [16]. Sixty milliliters at the same rate is required to see the abdominal aorta. If the Teflon sleeve descends into the abdominal aorta, much less contrast agent is required for an adequate study (50 ml at 10 ml per second). A nonionic contrast agent can be used to reduce the heat sensation and provide a more comfortable examination.

An alternative approach uses a modification in the shape of the 5 French catheter sleeve overlying the needle shaft. By applying a 90-degree curve on the distal 1.5 cm of this sleeve and adding a number of side holes near the distal tip, the catheter can be manipulated into an anterograde position down the abdominal aorta [6]. The needle with overlying modified sleeve is introduced in routine fashion at the T12 level. When pulsatile flow is obtained, the needle is withdrawn, and the catheter tip assumes its curve, frequently pointing directly downstream. If not, it can be rotated appropriately and the catheter sheath is advanced downstream over a J-shaped guidewire. A tip-occluding wire introduced immediately prior to the contrast injection not only straightens out the curve (precluding inadvertent injection into side branches) but also forces the contrast agent out through the side holes.

There is still another approach by which to enter the lower abdominal aorta. This may be used if obstructive disease is suspected below the aortic bifurcation and the visceral vessels are not required as part of the study. The needle is advanced transversely and anteriorly (Fig. 3-15) to enter the aorta at the lower border of L2. This approach misses the kidney and renal artery. The overlying sleeve may then be easily advanced downstream.

The translumbar approach can be used for evaluating the aortic arch and selecting brachiocephalic vessels [12]. Once the routine translumbar

should be withdrawn minimally, since resistance is usually caused by the proximity of the catheter needle tip to the opposite aortic wall. Once the guidewire is properly placed, the angiographer should slowly advance the Teflon sleeve into the aorta over the guidewire, simultaneously withdrawing the steel needle assembly and guidewire from the aorta. The Teflon sleeve and guidewire usually enter the descending thoracic aorta with

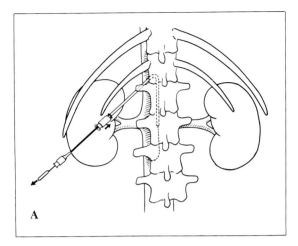

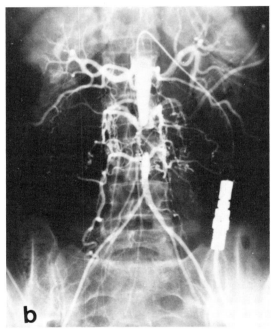

Fig. 3-14. Guidewire manipulation in a descending anterograde fashion into the abdominal aorta.
A. Line drawing showing patient in prone position.
B. Abdominal aortogram viewed in anteroposterior projection showing complete segmental occlusion below the level of the renal arteries. Fifty milliliters of Conray-60 (15 ml per second) provides an adequate study.

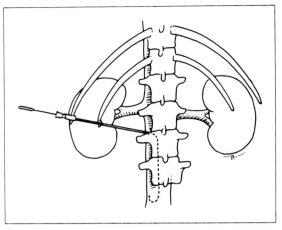

Fig. 3-15. Low translumbar approach. The Teflon sleeve is advanced anterograde down the abdominal aorta.

approach has been accomplished, an Amplatz heavy-duty exchange guidewire is introduced through the needle sleeve into the low thoracic aorta. The needle sleeve is replaced over this guidewire with a 5 French introducer over which lies a 20-cm long 5.5 French Desilets Hoffman catheter exchange sheath[1] fitted with a hemostasis valve. No. 5 French high-flow "pigtail" catheters can be introduced through this sheath for aortic arch studies. Selective catheterization of the brachiocephalic vessels can be accomplished with 65-cm 5 French end-hole catheters with appropriate curves.

Comments and Precautions

Improper needle placement can lead to various problems. If the initial skin nick is too medial, the direction of the needle is not sufficiently oblique and only the lateral wall of the aorta may be reached; the needle may completely miss the aorta. If the approach is too lateral, the direction of the needle may be too shallow and the needle may pass between the aorta and vertebral body, thus once again bypassing the aorta (Fig. 3-16). If no pulsations have been felt or seen and the needle has been introduced to approximately 7 in. or more, the latter situation is the most likely cause and a more medial approach should be considered. If the needle passes more cephalad than the body of T12, the left pleural space may be entered,

[1] Manufactured by Cook, Inc., P.O. Box 489, Bloomington, IN 47401.

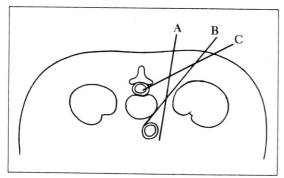

Fig. 3-16. Improper needle placement in the translumbar approach.
A. If the approach is too medial, only the lateral wall of the aorta is reached. The aorta may be completely missed.
B. If the approach is too lateral, the needle passes between the vertebral body and the aorta.
C. If the direction of the needle is too shallow, it may even enter the spinal canal. The needle may be inserted too high with intrathoracic placement.
      The Teflon sleeve may be advanced selectively into visceral vessels. The angiographer should always check the Teflon sleeve position with contrast medium prior to high-pressure injection of large quantities of contrast medium.

and pneumothorax, hemothorax, chylothorax, or puncture of the left ventricle may occur. Thoracic placement should be considered if the hub of the needle moves with the respiratory diaphragmatic movements of the patient. If the approach of the needle is too caudad, the advancing guidewire may enter selectively into either renal artery, into the celiac axis, or into the superior mesenteric artery. Resistance to the placement of the guidewire usually occurs under these circumstances, which warns the examiner. This resistance is not always met, however, and easy placement of the guidewire should not lull one into a feeling of security. The position of the Teflon sleeve must always be visualized fluoroscopically with contrast agent prior to a high-pressure injection of a large quantity of contrast agent.

Occasionally a very diseased atherosclerotic aorta may transmit little or no pulsation during introduction of the needle. If this situation is suspected, the examiner should proceed with caution, a gentle touch, and frequent checks for blood flow. An unsuccessful low aortic puncture (at L2 or L3) may indicate an occluded vessel, and a higher approach at T12 should then be attempted.

No more than three aortic punctures should be made at any one sitting, since severe retroperitoneal hemorrhage may occur. Five to ten percent of patients may have a moderate degree of pain following removal of the Teflon sleeve as a result of retroperitoneal hemorrhage (Fig. 3-17); the pain usually stops in approximately ½ hour and requires only analgesics for control. Because of the effects of the hemorrhage, some surgeons prefer not to operate for 6 weeks after a translumbar study.

THE AXILLARY APPROACH
Indications
The superficial position of the axillary artery facilitates puncture. However, because this approach has a higher complication rate, it should be used only when the others are not feasible or desirable.

The side entered is determined by the particular vessel or vessels under study. The left side is entered for

1. Investigation and interventional maneuvers of the descending thoracic aorta and the abdominal aorta and its branches
2. Selective splanchnic angiography; these vessels are surprisingly easy to catheterize from this approach
3. Investigation and interventional maneuvers of the pelvis or lower extremities, although catheter length may be a restriction
4. Investigation of the ascending aorta, left ventricle, and four-vessel brachiocephalic studies, if the right side is not available

Right-sided entrance is indicated for

1. Approach to the ascending aorta and the left ventricle
2. Selective coronary arteriography, particularly when femoral approaches are unsuccessful
3. Four-vessel study of the head and neck, when the femoral approach is unsuccessful or impossible
4. Studies mentioned for the left-sided approach if the left-sided entrance is impractical

Contraindications
Contraindications to the axillary approach include

1. Subclavian artery occlusive disease or aneurysms; the angiographer should check for blood

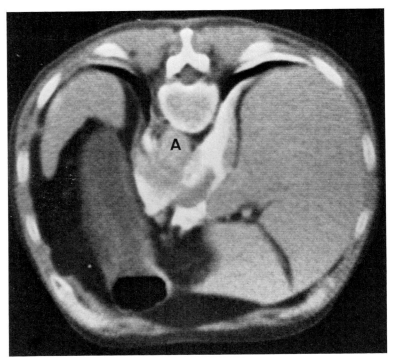

Fig. 3-17. Computed tomography scan performed following translumbar aortogram. Note the retroperitoneal hematoma at the site of the puncture. (A = aorta.)

pressure differential, pulse deficit, and supraclavicular bruits
2. Subclavian artery bypass grafts

Anatomy

The axillary artery is divided into three parts by its relationship to the overlying pectoralis minor muscle. The third portion of the artery lies lateral to the pectoralis minor, and its most distal portion extends beyond the pectoralis major, at which point it is very superficial, being covered only by fascia and skin. Branches of the brachial plexus lie in close proximity to the vessel, which adds to the hazard of the approach. Since the axillary artery is closely applied to the neck of the humerus, it can be compressed for hemostasis. Collateral circulation can develop if there is occlusion of the axillary artery; collateral branches arise from the subclavian artery, deep brachial artery, internal thoracic artery, and intercostal branches of the thoracic aorta (see Fig. 8-9). A high brachial artery approach is preferred by some and indeed may have some advantages. Continuing from the axillary artery beyond the teres major muscle, the brachial artery also lies superficially; its course is more easily palpable, and it may therefore be less difficult to puncture and compress than the axillary artery.

Moreover, the branches of the brachial plexus seem less closely applied. An added advantage is that if hematoma develops, it is not likely to be hidden within the axilla.

Technique

Palpate the radial and brachial arteries bilaterally to determine the strength of the peripheral pulses prior to the study. Listen for bruits in the supraclavicular region and compare the blood pressure in both upper extremities. Abduct the arm and position it for optimal pulsation of the high brachial artery. The point of puncture, if possible, should be just distal to the axillary fold (high brachial artery) (Fig. 3-18A). Prepare and drape the area of interest and infiltrate it with local anesthetic. A small nick in the skin is made approximately 1 to 2 cm proximal to the anticipated point of entry into the artery. Loosen the subcutaneous tissues gently with a small curved forceps to prevent hematoma accumulation. Infiltrate the vessel well, because the axillary artery often experiences spasm, and the surrounding nerves of the brachial plexus can cause considerable patient discomfort.

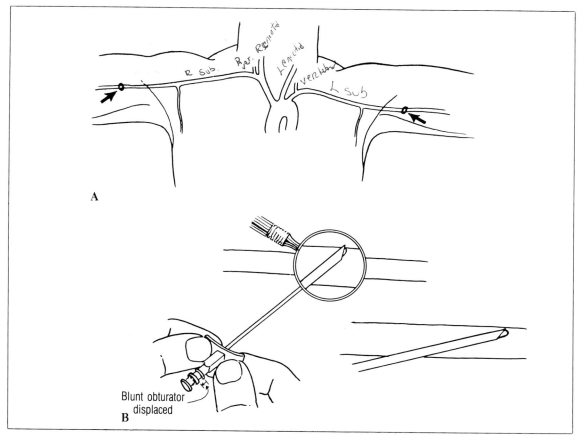

Fig. 3-18. Technique of axillary artery puncture (see text for more details).

A. Abduct the arm. The arterial puncture site is just distal to the axillary fold (*arrows*), and the puncture through the skin is 1 to 2 cm peripheral to this site.

B. The sharper needle point and less flexible shaft of the Potts needle facilitates fixation of the often mobile, rolling artery. When pulsatile flow is obtained and the sharp stylet is replaced with a blunt obturator, advance the needle using the flanges rather than the hub of the needle. The blunt obturator is left free to be pushed back if an arterial plaque or arterial intima obstructs passage.

A Potts needle should be used, since the sharper needle point and less flexible shaft of this needle facilitate fixation of this often mobile, rolling artery. Since the axillary artery is more superficial than the femoral artery, one should use a more horizontal needle approach in relation to the skin than with the latter. In addition, one should direct the needle down the long axis of the humerus rather than obliquely to it.

Following removal of the sharp stylet, withdraw the needle until pulsatile flow is obtained; then introduce the blunt obturator and gently advance the needle. To do this, one should use the flanges, so that the blunt obturator is left free to be pushed back if an arterial plaque or arterial intima obstructs passage (Fig. 3-18B). Replace the blunt obturator with a guidewire when the needle is securely in place within the artery. The guidewire often annoyingly seeks out the subscapular or lateral thoracic artery in this approach, and various maneuvers of the arm and the guidewire may be necessary to bypass them. Once the guidewire is well within the thoracic aorta, replace the needle with a 6 French or smaller catheter.

Comments and Precautions

For catheter placement in the abdominal aorta of patients younger than 50 years of age, the guidewire and catheter may be easily passed down the descending aorta using the left axillary approach. When the innominate artery takes off high on the

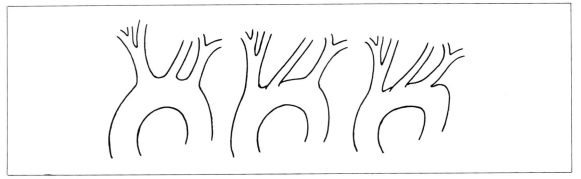

Fig. 3-19. In older patients, the left carotid and left subclavian arteries arise at ever-sharper angles from the thoracic aortic arch, making catheter manipulation more difficult.

thoracic aorta, the descending thoracic aorta may also be catheterized by the right axillary approach with ease.

DIFFICULT CATHETER MANIPULATIONS. With advancing patient age, there is an increasingly sharp angle of takeoff of the left subclavian artery from the aortic arch (Fig. 3-19). It is then difficult to pass the guidewire or catheter down the descending aorta, since the natural course is to enter the ·ascending aorta. Various maneuvers of the guidewire are often necessary. One such maneuver involves passing the guidewire down the ascending aorta, looping it over the aortic valve and back up the ascending aorta to the arch, and thence, by retracting the guidewire, advancing the loop down the descending thoracic aorta. This maneuver requires a guidewire with a long (9-in.) flexible distal portion, a curved tip with a 3- to 6-mm radius, and a gentle transition from the proximal rigid to the distal flexible portion (Fig. 3-20). Other maneuvers include the use of an acutely angled, or pigtail, catheter tip, which can be used to direct the guidewire down the descending thoracic aorta (Fig. 3-21). One must make sure that the stiff portion of the guidewire is down the descending portion of the thoracic aorta before introducing the catheter over that portion of the guidewire; failure to do this will cause the stiff catheter to withdraw the overly flexible portion of the guidewire back into the aortic arch. Sometimes several catheter changes must be made. If possible, 5 or 6 French catheters should be used because they are more likely to follow the flexible guidewires once they are properly positioned. The smaller size of the catheter ensures less trauma to the small-caliber axillary artery. The firm acute curve of an external

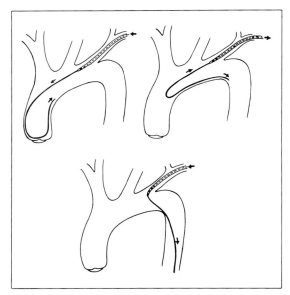

Fig. 3-20. Axillary approach for catheterizing the abdominal aorta, showing the sharp angle of the left subclavian artery with the aortic arch that is seen in older patients. The long flexible tip of the guidewire loops back over the aortic valve and up the ascending aorta to the arch. When the guidewire is retracted, it advances down the descending thoracic aorta. For successful advancement of the catheter over the guidewire, once the latter has been placed in the descending thoracic aorta, there are two requirements: a guidewire with a gradual transition from the proximal rigid to the distal flexible portion and a flexible catheter, either a Dacron catheter or a catheter of smaller caliber (6 French or smaller) made of other materials.

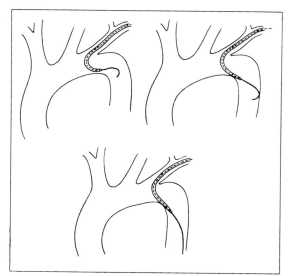

Fig. 3-21. Axillary approach for abdominal aortogram, showing an acutely angled left subclavian artery. With the guidewire in the thoracic aorta, a catheter with an acutely angled, or "pigtail," curve directs the guidewire to the descending thoracic aorta. The guidewire should have a gradual transition from the proximal rigid to the distal flexible portion. No. 6 French catheters and Dacron catheters are more likely to follow the guidewire. For similar manipulation from the right side, see Figure 8-2F.

manipulator guidewire can be used to guide a catheter down the descending aorta.

HAZARDS. The close proximity of the brachial plexus to the axillary artery makes this approach more hazardous than the femoral artery or the translumbar approach. Direct trauma to the nerves from a traumatic procedure and also compression from hematoma can cause permanent nerve damage. This vessel is often more difficult to puncture because of its small diameter, its mobility, and the fact that it is sometimes covered by the surrounding muscles. Absent pulses detected during the procedure or early symptoms of neurologic involvement should be closely watched and early surgical relief considered. Since heparin may increase hematoma formation, its use in this approach is controversial. Thrombotic occlusion is more likely to occur in smaller vessels, such as the brachial artery, particularly with interventional procedures. Careful attention to pulses, with early intervention, should minimize sequelae of these complications.

CAROTID ARTERY PUNCTURE

Indications
1. Intracranial space-occupying lesions
2. Primary intracranial vascular disease
3. Cerebral trauma

Contraindications
1. Occlusive disease of the extracranial carotid artery
2. Patients with hypertension and bleeding diathesis
3. Multiple vessel cerebral angiographic investigation is best performed by femoral artery (preferably) or by axillary artery approach catheter techniques

Technique (Fig. 3-22)
Extend the patient's head for optimal presentation of the carotid pulse and prepare the skin with povidone-iodine (Betadine). Infiltrate with local anesthetic the skin on either side of and behind the carotid artery at a point below the carotid bifurcation (approximately 2 cm below the superior margin of the thyroid cartilage). With the bevel of the Potts 18-gauge thin-walled needle pointed down, and with its shaft parallel to the long axis of the carotid artery and angled at approximately 45 degrees to the skin surface, impale both walls of the vessel. Remove the inner sharp stylet and slowly withdraw the outer cannula until blood spurts. Introduce the blunt obturator and advance the needle (using the flanges) until the needle is well placed within the artery. Remove the obturator and connect the needle hub to a transparent connecting tube that has been prefilled with 5% dextrose. Rapid washout of a test injection of 1 or 2 ml of contrast agent (checked fluoroscopically) ensures the intraluminal position of the needle. An irregular, dense stain at the puncture site means that the needle tip is extraluminal in location and requires repositioning. Frequent flushing of the needle with 5% dextrose (every 2 minutes) precludes clot formation. Follow a forceful injection of contrast agent (10 ml of Renografin-60, Conray, or nonionic contrast agent in the common carotid artery, 8 ml in the internal carotid artery) with serial films coned to the head over a period of 8 to 10 seconds. Multiple projections may be required. Compress the puncture site digitally for at least 10

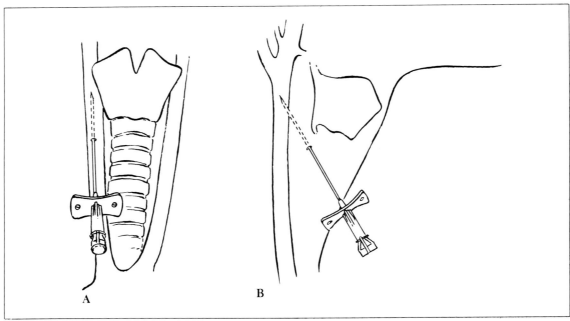

A

B

Fig. 3-22. Carotid artery puncture. (See text for details.)
A. Anteroposterior projection
B. Lateral projection

minutes after the needle has been removed to prevent hematoma formation.

After the study has been completed, the following steps should be observed:

1. Observe the patient's vital signs and watch for hematoma every 15 minutes for 1 hour, every 30 minutes for 3 hours, and then every hour until the patient is stable.
2. Order bed rest for 6 hours.
3. Apply an ice collar to the patient's neck as needed.

Comments and Precautions
1. The intracranial vessels contralateral to the side of carotid puncture may often be outlined on an anteroposterior projection by simultaneous compression of the contralateral carotid artery in the neck during injection of contrast agent. This maneuver can be dangerous and can compromise cerebral blood flow if there is significant occlusive disease on the side of the injection.
2. A puncture site that is too high may inadvertently be placed in the internal or external carotid artery. Atheromatous plaques, which are more likely to occur at or just above the carotid bifurcation, may thus be dislodged.
3. The patient should be forewarned and, if nec-

essary, restrained to avoid inadvertent needle displacement.
4. Hematomas in the neck can cause tracheal deviation and respiratory embarrassment, particularly if the punctures are bilateral. Be wary of patients with hypertension or bleeding diathesis and those who cannot be restrained. If a hematoma develops, compress the puncture site longer and try to disperse the hematoma into the mediastinum, where it has less effect on the trachea.
5. Failure to opacify intracranial vessels following an injection may be a result of vessel occlusion, increased intracranial pressure, or subintimal placement of the carotid needle. Fluoroscopic or film evaluation of the neck vessels soon points out subintimal placement. If increased intracranial pressure is the cause, the point of arterial obstruction is seen where the internal carotid artery penetrates the dura at the carotid siphon. Under these circumstances, delayed films often show late intracranial vascular filling.
6. Avoid embolization of thrombi formed at the tip of the needle, and avoid air bubbles caused by faulty technique.

BRACHIAL ARTERY PUNCTURE

Indications

Indications for the use of brachial puncture include

1. Arteriography in primary vascular diseases of the upper extremities
2. Evaluation of the arterial and venous components of renal dialysis shunts
3. Retrograde brachial angiography for evaluation of cerebral atherosclerosis and of other intracranial diseases in which direct carotid puncture or femoral cerebral catheterization is not feasible

The left brachial approach is used to study the left vertebral artery, the basilar artery, and the posterior fossa; the right brachial approach is used to study the right vertebral artery, the basilar artery, the posterior fossa, and the right anterior circulation.

Anatomy

The brachial artery in the lower third of the upper arm lies on the anteromedial aspect of the humerus. It is superficial, being covered anteriorly only by fascia and skin. The median nerve lies just medial to the artery at this level, having crossed it somewhat higher in the arm. The radial nerve lies posterior to the artery and the ulnar nerve lies in a somewhat more remote posteromedial location. Two venae comitantes lie alongside the brachial artery, and the basilic vein lies medial to it, separated by the deep fascia. The brachial artery is best palpated in the lower mid-third of the arm, just above the antecubital fossa, and this is the site designated for puncture.

Technique (Fig. 3-23)

The patient's arm is extended and supinated. Following preparation, draping, and administration of 10 to 15 ml of local anesthetic, a small entrance hole is made in the skin with a No. 11 blade. The arterial puncture is made with a 16-gauge, 2½-in., thin-walled Cournand needle or Potts needle (with a metal shaft and sharp inner stylet but without an overlying Teflon sleeve). While palpating the course of the brachial artery with the three fingers of the left hand, thrust the needle downward parallel to the artery to the point of maximum impulse,

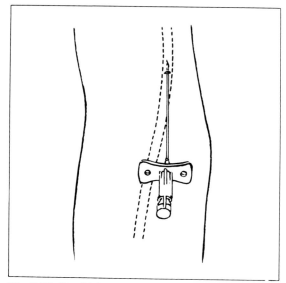

Fig. 3-23. Brachial artery puncture. (See text for details.)

as palpated by the middle finger. Pierce both anterior and posterior walls, remove the inner sharp stylet, and slowly withdraw the cannula until blood spurts from the cannula hub. Introduce the dull-tipped obturator and, using the flanges and with the needle parallel to the artery, slowly advance it to the hilt. Carefully watch the hub of the dull-tipped obturator during this maneuver (as in Fig. 3-18B) for any posterior dislocation of the hub from the metal cannula, which could mean abutment against an obstruction. Attach a prefilled transparent connecting tube and flush it every 1 or 2 minutes. The needle and flushing tube should be firmly secured to the patient's arm in order to prevent dislodging during the injection. Confirm proper placement of the needle fluoroscopically, by means of a test injection with 2 or 3 ml of contrast material.

During the high-pressure injection of contrast medium, a sphygmomanometer inflated to 50 mm above the systolic pressure at a position high in the forearm (distal to the puncture site) helps to force more contrast agent into the brachiocephalic vessels and it also helps to alleviate the pain arising from contrast medium flowing into vessels of the hand. Thirty to forty milliliters of low-concentration contrast medium (see Appendix 3), but preferably nonionic contrast agent, is injected in 2 seconds in order to visualize the left vertebral system.

Forty-five milliliters at a rate of 15 ml per second is necessary on the right side, since two circulations (the right vertebral and right carotid) are to be filled here. The patient is in a supine or right posterior oblique position during filming.

Comments and Precautions
1. Brachial puncture is a safe technique for studying intracranial structures, since the needle site and site of injection are remote from the intracranial structures. Central and neurologic sequelae from this study are rare.
2. The contrast medium in the basilar artery is usually diluted by unopacified blood from the opposite vertebral artery, causing suboptimal filling of the vertebral basilar system. This effect can be partially overcome by simultaneous compression during the injection of the opposite vertebral artery low in the neck, near its point of origin.
3. Occasionally the median or radial nerve may be damaged by the puncture. In addition, brachial arterial spasm is fairly common following puncture. Damage to the arterial wall and thrombus formation may also occur.

VENOUS PERCUTANEOUS
CATHETERIZATION
Indications
1. Study of primary venous disease
2. Catheterization of the right side of the heart, pulmonary artery, and occasionally the left side of the heart (transseptal catheterization)
3. Retrograde injection into veins of organs with suspected disease
4. IV-DSA
5. Collection of selective venous effluent for biochemical analysis
6. Percutaneous placement of inferior vena cava filters or other intravascular therapeutic maneuvers

Technique
CATHETERIZATION OF THE BASILIC OR CEPHALIC VEINS AT THE ANTECUBITAL FOSSA. Introduce percutaneously a 16-gauge needle with overlying sleeve, advance the sleeve to the hilt, and introduce the guidewire to match the end-hole catheter you have chosen for percutaneous introduction. This procedure should be accomplished prior to the administration of local anes-

thetic, since the anesthetic wheal may obscure the superficial puncture site. With the guidewire in place in the vein, rapidly anesthetize the area of entry with 2 or 3 ml of 1% lidocaine. Make a small dermal incision around the wire only after the Teflon sleeve has been removed (to avoid cutting and losing the sleeve in the venous system). Alternatively, a small diameter needle (18-gauge) and a 0.032-in. (0.80-mm) guidewire may be used for the initial venipuncture. Progressively larger needle sleeves (16-gauge) and wires may replace this initial needle until a sufficiently firm guidewire (0.038-in. [0.97-mm] or 0.045-in. [1.14-mm]) is introduced for completion of the study.

A catheter having only side holes but no end hole is often used in catheterizations of the right side of the heart and the pulmonary artery. This catheter may be introduced in the following manner (Fig. 3-24): Prepare a vascular dilator having the same diameter as the proposed catheter by introducing over it a snugly fitting, paper-thin, commercially available catheter sheath. Draw the sheath to the hub of the dilator. Percutaneously introduce into the vein a 16- or 18-gauge needle with an overlying Teflon sleeve and replace the needle with a 12-in. long, 0.038- or 0.035-in. diameter guidewire. Advance this dilator with its overlying sheath over the guidewire well into the vein. Remove the guidewire and dilator from the sheath, using the sheath as a conduit for the catheter. After the catheter has been advanced into the vein, withdraw the sheath out of the vein to the catheter hub and clean any attached fibrin. This sheath may now be used for multiple catheter changes.

Surgical exposure of the vein may be necessary (Fig. 3-25); it is usually performed at the antecubital fossa. Prepare the skin and widely infiltrate the proposed area of incision with a local anesthetic. Make a superficial, transverse, 1-in. incision medially and just above the antecubital fossa. The basilic vein lies in this area; if it is not available, the brachial veins lie in close contact with the somewhat lateral and more deeply placed brachial artery. The basilic vein is separated from these deeper vascular structures by the deep fascia. Use a curved mosquito forceps to separate the tissues gently in a direction parallel to that of the vessel. When the thin-walled, bluish-colored, nonpulsatile vessel is uncovered, free its walls from surrounding tissues by inserting the closed forceps

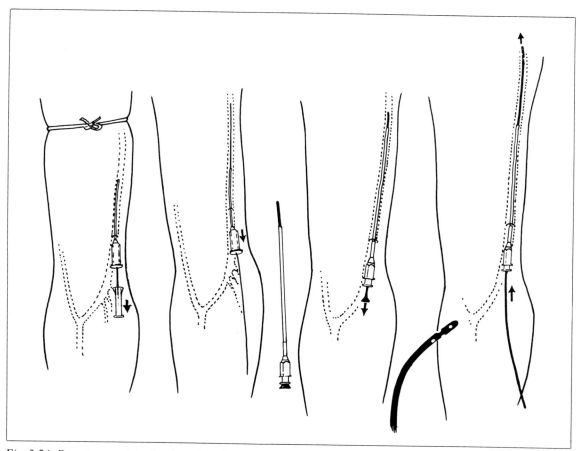

Fig. 3-24. Percutaneous introduction of a catheter with no end holes into the venous system. An ultra-thin-walled sheath covers a vascular dilator, which is introduced in the usual percutaneous fashion over a guidewire. The dilator and guidewire are removed, leaving the sheath as a conduit for the chosen catheter.

deep to the vein and spreading the jaws of the forceps. Place two ligatures around the vein, tying the distal ligature and loosely knotting the proximal one. Keep the flushed, fluid-filled catheter ready nearby for insertion. Compress and gently retract the vein upward with toothless thumb forceps and make a measured transverse incision on its anterior surface, making sure to penetrate through to the intima (see Fig. 3-25B). Insert a small, plastic, right-angled "vein elevator" centrally into the incised vein with one hand; this implement widens the venous opening to permit catheter insertion with the other hand (Fig. 3-25C). The nerves are shiny and white, and the arteries are thicker walled and pulsatile; it should present no problem to differentiate them from the

vein. During the catheterization procedure, tie the central ligature snugly over the catheter to prevent suction of air into the vein and undue bleeding at the catheterization site. Following catheter removal, tie off the proximal suture and close the skin wound with interrupted sutures.

CATHETERIZATION OF THE FEMORAL VEIN. The femoral vein lies just medial to the femoral artery at the inguinal area. Following skin preparation and adequate infiltration of the area with a local anesthetic, make a cutaneous nick with a No. 11 blade. Palpate the femoral artery with the fingers of one hand and with the other introduce a 3- or 4-inch needle (either 16- or 18-gauge with sharp obturator and overlying Teflon sleeve) just medial to the vessel. Remove the inner stylet and apply suction with an attached syringe while slowly withdrawing the needle. An easy flow of dark venous blood is obtained when the vein is entered. With suction still applied, advance the overlying Teflon sleeve. If easy flow is still maintained, the Teflon

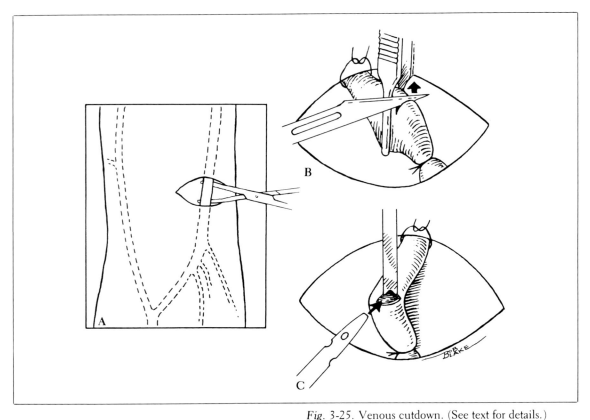

Fig. 3-25. Venous cutdown. (See text for details.)

sleeve is well within the vein and the metal needle can be replaced with guidewire and catheter in the usual percutaneous fashion. A closed-end catheter can be inserted in the same manner as described for the antecubital vein.

CATHETERIZATION OF THE INTERNAL JUGULAR VEIN (Fig. 3-26). At the base of the neck, the internal jugular vein lies anteriorly on the lateral aspect of the common carotid artery and just beneath the triangular interval between the medial (sternal) and lateral (clavicular) attachments of the sternocleidomastoid muscle. It can be made more prominent by a slight Trendelenburg position and Valsalva maneuver. Prepare the skin, palpate the carotid pulse, and infiltrate with local anesthetic an area just lateral to this approximately 5 cm directly superior to the clavicle down to the level of this triangular interval. Use a 2½-inch or longer 20- or 21-gauge needle, alternately aspirating and injecting the anesthetic. By this means, one can identify the depth and location of the internal jugular vein. Make a superficial nick in the skin. Using the same needle and suction syringe assembly described in the femoral vein approach, advance

the needle in the same direction as the identified vein. This is usually angled slightly posteriorly (approximately 30 degrees) and caudad toward a point just deep to the junction of the middle and medial thirds of the clavicle. During the maneuver one may retract the carotid artery medially and line up the point of entry in the general direction of the ipsilateral iliac crest. The right jugular vein approach is preferred, for there is a more or less straight line to the right atrium. On the left side, the course is more circuitous and in addition one may unwittingly puncture the thoracic duct as it enters into the junction of the left internal jugular and subclavian vein. During the puncture, an easy return of blood signals successful cannulation. The Teflon sleeve is then advanced, the inner metal cannula is removed, and the guidewire is introduced. This procedure opens the direct passage to the right side of the heart, and fluoroscopic monitoring is required for subsequent percutaneous catheter replacement. Care should be taken not to enter the carotid artery or to introduce a pneumothorax. Catheter exchanges should be per-

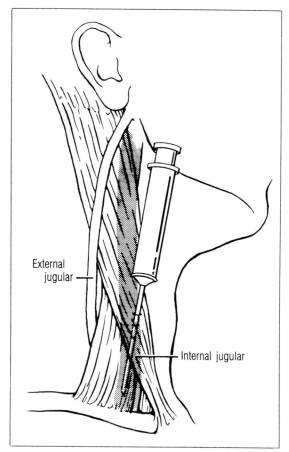

Fig. 3-26. Puncture of the internal jugular vein. (See text for details.)

formed with extreme care in this location to avoid aspiration of air into the venous system. Be sure that the patient holds his breath, preferably in inspiration, during crucial phases of catheter exchange. If air is sucked into the venous system, causing symptomatic obstruction to the inflow of the right cardiac chambers, immediately place the patient in the left lateral decubitus position and suction out the air through the indwelling catheter.

The internal jugular vein at the base of the skull may be angiographically demonstrated by direct puncture of the vein low in its cervical portion, but this time with the needle directed cephalad. Approach the vein at the same level, keeping the needle pointed lateral to the carotid pulse. An overlying Teflon sleeve is advanced once the vein has been entered; it may be exchanged for a 6 French end-hole catheter with side holes. A pref-

erable approach is selectively catheterizing the jugular vein from a femoral venipuncture site.

CATHETERIZATION OF THE EXTERNAL JUGULAR VEIN. Catheterization of the external jugular vein often requires surgical exposure for successful cannulation with a catheter of adequate size. This vein lies superficially in the neck, being covered by skin, subcutaneous fascia, and platysma muscle. It runs perpendicularly down the neck in the direction of a line drawn from the angle of the mandible to the middle of the clavicle (Fig. 3-26). This vein has two valves in the low neck, one of which lies at its entrance to the subclavian vein. The angle of the junction of the external jugular vein with the subclavian vein is often 90 degrees or less; catheter manipulation is therefore required for successful placement within the chambers of the right side of the heart.

CATHETERIZATION OF THE SUBCLAVIAN VEIN. The subclavian vein extends from the lateral border of the first rib to the sternal end of the clavicle, lying anterior and just inferior to the subclavian artery, being separated from it by the anterior scalene muscle. In its medial two-thirds, it lies just behind the clavicle, where it is immobilized by small attachments to both the clavicle and the rib. The patient should be supine with the head 15 degrees in Trendelenburg. A somewhat lateral infraclavicular approach is best used for cannulating this vein. Prepare and infiltrate the skin with anesthetic at a point two fingerbreadths lateral to the midclavicular line and one fingerbreadth below the clavicle. Advance the 6-in. Teflon-covered needle assembly (with attached syringe for suction) medially and slightly cephalad behind the clavicle toward the posterior superior aspect of its sternal end. Placing the index finger into the supersternal notch locates the deep side of the superior aspect of the clavicle and acts as a reference point. The needle should be directed slightly behind this fingertip. When blood is successfully withdrawn, advance the Teflon sleeve and replace the metal cannula with a guidewire and subsequently with the catheter. On removal of the catheter, secure hemostasis by firm infraclavicular pressure at the site where the catheter enters the vein.

CATHETERIZATION OF THE AXILLARY VEIN. The axillary vein lies slightly posterior to the axillary artery and partly overlaps its medial side. Many nerves overlie these two vessels, including the medial cord of the brachial plexus, the median ulnar nerve, and the pectoral nerve. With the patient's arm outstretched and abducted, infiltrate the area with local anesthetic. With the fingers of one hand palpating the most distal portion of the axillary artery, and with the same needle assembly used for femoral vein puncture (with attached syringe for suction), advance the needle just posterior to the artery in a central direction. Replace the metal cannula with guidewire and catheter when the vein has been successfully entered.

Selective Catheterization

GENERAL PRINCIPLES

Selective catheterization is usually, but not always, performed after a midstream aortic injection. It is used to avoid confusion resulting from overlying vessels and to obtain optimal opacification of the target organ vessel. The best filling of vessels occurs when the contrast bolus is given close to the area of interest. Selective catheterization of vessels requires that the catheter curves be preshaped according to the anatomy of the vessel to be studied. The curve is applied to the distal tip of the catheter, which allows placement within the lumen of the target vessel. Vessels may also be selectively catheterized by imposing a desired angle on a catheter tip with an internal wire that is externally controlled by a wire deflector. For selective placement, the wall of the aorta is gently probed with the catheter tip at the anticipated level of the takeoff vessel. If the catheter shape is correct, its tip will engage the orifice of the primary branch. Its position should be checked fluoroscopically with a small test injection of 2 or 3 ml of contrast agent. Once placed, the catheter must be capable of accepting a bolus of contrast agent that is sufficient to opacify the vascular bed.

As a general rule, small-diameter catheters (5 or 6 French or smaller) are preferred for selective placement deep within the arterial branches. Spasm of vessels and wedge injection are less likely to occur and better flow is maintained under these circumstances. The smaller catheters are sometimes more difficult to manipulate, however, for they often have less torque control. Smaller catheters do have the advantage that they follow a selectively placed guidewire more easily than do the larger catheters. Larger catheters have been used in the past for the large volume midstream injections

performed prior to the selective procedures. This introduces the problem of substituting the larger catheter for the smaller selective catheter, with a potential for subsequent bleeding at the site of catheter introduction. Currently manufactured thin-walled, high–tensile-strength catheters with multiple side holes at their tips now permit high-volume midstream injections through catheters with small outer diameters. If a still smaller selective catheter must be used, the initial midstream catheter may be replaced with a thin-walled sheath of equal diameter, through which the smaller catheter may be introduced. Special valves in the hub of the sheath help to prevent leaking (hemostasis valves) and side arm connectors allow positive pressure infusions through the sheaths to prevent clot formation.

CHOICE OF CATHETER TIP

Factors that influence the choice of a preformed catheter tip for a given study include

1. The angle of the vessel takeoff from the aorta. Generally within the abdominal aorta, the angle of the primary curve of the catheter tip should be similar to that of the vessel takeoff (Fig. 3-27). The primary curve of the catheter (the curve closest to the tip) (Fig. 3-28) should be not much longer (no more than 10 percent) than the diameter of the aorta. A gentle secondary curve in the catheter will help to force the primary curve of the tip deeper into the selected vessel once its origin has been engaged. If the distal tip is long, the desired angle

Fig. 3-27. Catheter shapes.
A. "Cobra head" curve for obtuse angle.
B. "Shepherd's hook" curve for acute-angle take-off vessel. Note side holes near distal tips to prevent catheter whip when a large vascular bed requires a large, rapidly administered dose of contrast agent.

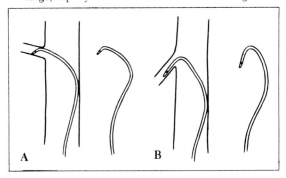

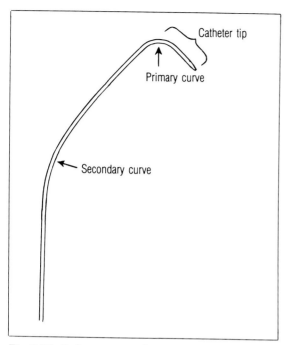

Fig. 3-28. Catheter terminology. The primary curve is that closest to the tip. From the primary curve to the tip should be approximately 10 percent longer than the diameter of the aorta. The secondary curve helps to force the primary curve and the catheter tip deeper into the selected vessel once its origin has been engaged.

Fig. 3-29. The primary curve of the catheter is longer than the diameter of the aorta. The catheter is therefore straightened and its original curve reimposed by introducing the tip into the orifice of a branch of the aorta.

of the catheter tip cannot be maintained because it is straightened by the smaller diameter of the aorta. This difficulty may sometimes be overcome by advancing the tip into a vessel orifice to reimpose the original curve (Fig. 3-29). If the angle of the takeoff vessel from the aorta is 60 degrees or greater, certain catheter shapes are easily advanced not only into the primary branch but also into the secondary or tertiary branches. For instance, the cobra head catheter shape [14] (see Fig. 3-27) has a primary curve that is short (1 cm or less) and obtuse (greater than 90 degrees). A gentle, sweeping secondary curve helps to introduce the catheter beyond the primary curve into the selected vessel once its origin has been engaged (see Fig. 13-6). A 4.5, 5, 6, or 6.5 French catheter with maximum torque control (braided polyurethane or polyethylene) is helpful for this manipulation.

2. The site of the puncture (approach). The catheter tip shaped for a given selective artery catheter placement that is approached from the axillary artery varies from that approached from a femoral artery. An acute-angled vessel takeoff from the femoral approach will be an obtuse-angled takeoff from the axillary route (see Figs. 13-1, 13-2).

3. The site of vessel takeoff. An artery arising from the aortic arch requires a catheter shape that accommodates itself to the curve of the arch (see Fig. 14-5). This need is obviously different from the requirements for selective abdominal visceral catheter placement.

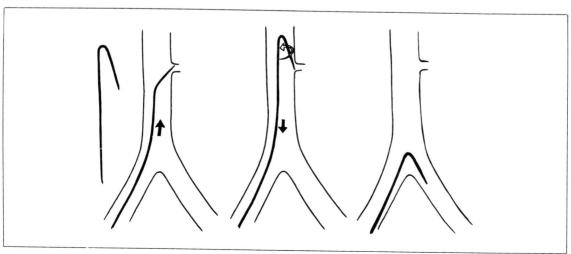

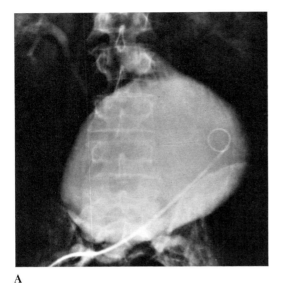

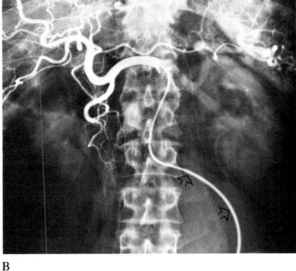

A   B

Fig. 3-30. Patient with a large abdominal aortic aneurysm requiring selective catheterization of the celiac axis. Catheterization could only be performed after placement of a sheath across the region of the aneurysm (B, arrows).

4. The size of the vascular bed being fed by the selected artery. The larger the vascular bed, the larger the bolus of contrast and the more rapid the delivery required. Higher doses and rates cause greater catheter recoil, which in turn displace the catheter tip from a selected vessel. Side holes aid mixing and help to prevent recoil, and thus permit a more rapid rate and a larger bolus injection. The holes should be placed within 2 mm of the distal tip. The angiographer should watch for clot formation within the side holes, which could lead to embolization on subsequent injection. Clot formation is less likely to occur if the patient is heparinized during the study. The procedure should be completed rapidly. Forceful flushing is essential.

5. The configuration of the iliac arteries and aorta. An ectatic aorta will require a wider primary and secondary curve. Marked tortuosity of the iliac vessels requires catheters with good torque control, guidewires with rigid shafts over which catheters will follow, or occasionally overlying sheaths through which the catheters can pass more easily (Fig. 3-30).

SUPERSELECTIVE CATHETERIZATION

If more superselective placement of the catheter tip is desired (to a second- or third-order branch), a different principle of catheter curve formation is required from that of placing the catheter tip in a

primary branch of the aorta. If the secondary branch artery is one that follows the general direction of the parent vessel, it can be entered by slowly advancing the catheter tip and using rapid, very small, back and forth "seesaw" motions of the catheter. If this maneuver is unsuccessful, a flexible guidewire may be carefully advanced well out into the vessel; the guidewire acts as a leader over which the catheter may be advanced. Care must be exercised in deeply advancing a catheter over a guidewire with a tightly curved tip which has been positioned in a peripheral vessel. On withdrawing the wire, the tip of its curve may become trapped between the end of the catheter and the arterial wall, stripping the endothelium and causing permanent damage (Figs. 3-31, 3-32). One solution is selecting a guidewire with a more gentle distal curve. Superselective maneuvers are generally more successful when small caliber catheters (5 or 6 French) are used (see Fig. 13-8).

If superselective catheterization is required of the vessel arising at an acute angle from the aorta, multiple curves to fit the anatomy may have to be used. The primary curve of the catheter will not be able to enter the vessel as it arises from the aorta unless it is altered to a single curve by means of an externally controlled catheter tip deflector (see Fig.

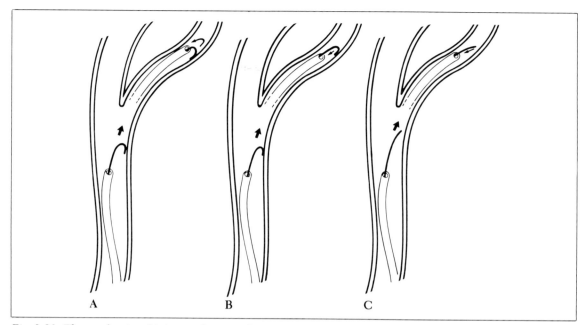

Fig. *3-31.* The mechanics of injury to the arterial intima by a J-shaped guidewire. (See text.)
A. As the guidewire tip is withdrawn, it scrapes the intima.
B and C. Scraping is prevented by using a guidewire with a smaller diameter J tip (B) or a straight tip (C).

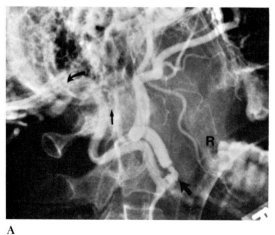

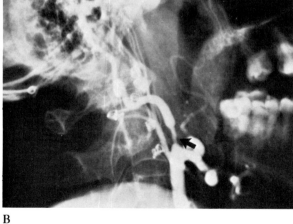

A   B

Fig. 3-32.
A. Arterial injury to internal maxillary artery (*large arrow*) during embolization of vessels (*small curved arrow*) feeding a large arteriovenous malfunction (AVM).
B. Persistent narrowing of internal maxillary artery (*arrow*) 6 months later.

13-4) [14]. Once the catheter tip is placed in the origin of the primary vessel, the catheter is "paid out" over the fixed curve of the wire tip into the vessel. When the deflector wire is removed, the preformed shape seeks out the more distant vessels.

TYPES OF EXTERNAL CATHETER
MANIPULATORS

The external catheter manipulator described in Figure 13-4 is perhaps the simplest to use.[2] Other types of external catheter manipulators are commercially available (see Fig. 2-6). The Muller USCI Guide System[3] uses a very soft-tipped, movable Dacron catheter, with or without side holes. This manipulator (rotoflector) is an entirely closed system that can impose an angle of varying degrees anywhere along the distal 6 in. of the catheter tip. It can rotate the catheter longitudinally and pay out the distal tip of the catheter deep into a selected vessel. Contrast medium can be injected during manipulation.

The MediTech[4] catheter deflecting system requires specially built catheters with four ultrathin movable steel wires attached to the distal tip and lying within the catheter wall. The proximal ends of these steel wires (at the hub of the catheter) are attached to four sides of an easily manipulated, rigid but movable plate. A change in direction of the plate imposes a curve on the catheter tip; the greater the change, the greater the degree of deflection.

COAXIAL CATHETER SYSTEM

A coaxial catheter system is simply the passage of one catheter through the lumen of a larger catheter. By this means, no. 2 to 4 French catheters may be passed deep into third- and fourth-order branches. They are used primarily for therapeutic purposes (e.g., intraarterial chemotherapy or embolization with rapidly polymerizing substances). No. 3 French and larger catheters have been adapted for placement of tiny microcoils with attached Dacron strands. No. 2 French catheters are generally too small for manipulative purposes, are usually formed of soft, pliable catheter material, and may be injected deep into a vascular system

through an outer larger caliber catheter. As a rule, a standard 8 or thin-walled 7 French catheter will accommodate a 4 French coaxial catheter, whereas a standard 6 French or thin-walled 5 French catheter will accommodate a 3 French coaxial catheter. The tip of the outer catheter should be untapered to allow easy passage of the inner catheter. The entire system should therefore be introduced into the vascular system through an overlying sheath to avoid trauma at the site of puncture. A special flushing adapter at the hub of the outer catheter and also at the hub of the introducing sheath prevents fibrin from collecting between the surfaces of the coaxial catheters. The inner core of special open-ended guidewires may be removed, providing a coaxial system with a small inner lumen for injectables. Small, 0.015 to 0.018-in., platinum tipped steerable guidewires may be introduced through these open-ended guidewires. This combination can be very useful for bypassing severely stenotic lesions and selecting very small branches (Fig. 3-33).

A coaxial system of catheters may be used as a guiding system for eventual peripheral placement of a large-bore catheter. The inner guidewire is advanced out to the vessel of choice, closely followed by the inner catheter, the major function of which is to act as a leader for the overlying, larger caliber catheter. A special flushing chamber at the hub of the outer catheter prevents fibrin collection between the surfaces of the coaxial catheters (see Fig. 13-8).

SHAPING THE CATHETER

Preformed catheter shapes for specific studies have been acquired from the experiences of many different angiographers. Various shapes can perform the same task. The angiographer should be prepared to shape catheters to fit his needs at all times. Boiling water or steam (preferably under pressure) or sterile glycerine heated to well over 100°C should be kept at hand, together with sterile catheters, for formulation during any arteriographic procedure. As a general rule, polyethylene catheter material is easy to form, requiring only seconds to acquire a shape,

---

[2] Manufactured by Cook, Inc.
[3] Manufactured by United States Catheter and Instrument Corp., Box 787, Glens Falls, NY 12801.
[4] Manufactured by MediTech Division, Cooper Scientific Corp., 372 Main St., Watertown, MA 02172.

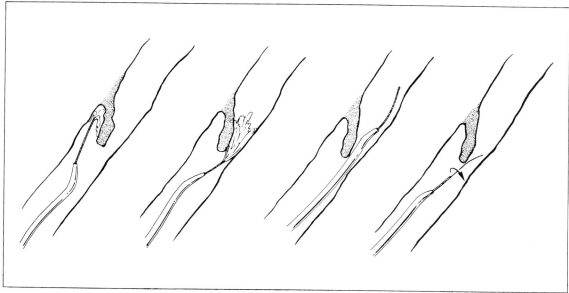

Fig. 3-33. Bypassing a severely stenotic plaque using a coaxial open-ended injectable guidewire system. Contrast injected through the guide outlines the position of the plaque, which can be bypassed. Alternatively, a small steerable guidewire can be introduced through the injectable guidewire for easier manipulation.

whereas polyurethane requires several minutes of immersion in boiling water or hot glycerine. Teflon catheters cannot be shaped with these standard techniques.

CAUSES OF FAILURE

Advancing and manipulating a catheter into selected positions is more difficult through elongated, angled vessels with intervening areas of stenosis, dilatation, and tortuosity. This is due in part to the friction or shear forces induced by the greater contact between the vessel wall and that of the catheter under these circumstances [9]. Loss of torque control of the catheter wall and improper catheter shapes are additional factors contributing to failure. These problems may sometimes be overcome by replacing the catheter with one that has a snugly fitting overlying thin-walled sheath, which tends to absorb some of these forces and allows successful catheter placement (see Fig. 3-30). A hemostatic valve (with flushing side port) on the hub of the sheath helps prevent backbleeding and fibrin accumulation.

DO'S AND DON'TS OF SELECTIVE CATHETERIZATION

The "do's and don'ts" of selective catheterization are as follows:

Do

1. Choose the catheter material, size, and shape carefully.
2. Use side holes only when a large vascular bed is to be opacified or when a forceful injection is anticipated.
3. Check the catheter closely for clots. Systemic heparinization (see Prevention of Thrombus Formation) and catheters that have been previously treated with nonthrombogenic material will lessen this difficulty.
4. Following placement or advancement of the catheter over a guidewire, forcefully withdraw and discard the contents of the catheter before flushing with a clean syringe. This procedure precludes inadvertent flushing of small clots into the arteries. Before injecting anything, always withdraw any small collection of air that may be hidden in the catheter hub.
5. Always use test injections of contrast medium to prevent subintimal injection or injection into a catheter that is wedged into an artery.

6. When catheterizing vital arteries such as the carotid or coronary arteries, a closed system may be used. In such a system, the catheter is attached to a manifold made of three 3-way stopcocks welded together. Two of these stopcocks are connected by tubes to bottles, one containing heparinized, sterile, 5% dextrose and the other containing contrast medium. The third stopcock is connected to a pressure monitoring gauge. A syringe at the hub of the manifold may withdraw either 5% dextrose for flushing or contrast medium for vessel opacification. Pressures at the tip of the catheter may be constantly monitored at times when injections are not being made. Dampened pressures forewarn of a wedged catheter, a catheter tip within a stenotic vessel, or a clot at the catheter tip.

7. Change larger for smaller catheters. If a 6 or 7 French catheter was used for a prior aortogram, smaller catheters for selective work may be replaced without leaking at the sites of arterial entry by use of a thin catheter sheath. Simply introduce a guidewire into the 7 French catheter and replace it with a 6 French catheter having an overlying, snugly fitting 7 French sheath near its hub. One such sheath has a diaphragm at its base together with a small flushing attachment to prevent fibrin accumulation.

Don't

1. Introduce air emboli or clots and do not dislodge plaques into vital organs. Do not dissect the vessel wall. Gentle manipulations are always necessary.

2. Wedge the catheter too deeply into an artery or into a stenosed vessel. Slow washout of contrast medium with a test injection and parenchymal stain forewarn of possible complications. Flow through and around the catheter tip must be present at all times.

Complications of Catheterization

Complications of catheterization may be caused by the contrast agent, by improper techniques, or by a variety of other causes [3, 8].

REACTIONS TO CONTRAST AGENTS

Complications caused by contrast agents may be either chemotoxic or allergic (see Chap. 2, Reactions to Contrast Media) [10]. Chemotoxic reactions may be seen in specific organs (e.g., heart, brain, kidney) following injection or overinjection of contrast agents. The combination of angiography with poor hydration and either impending or frank renal failure will compound the renal problem. If the study cannot be delayed, a well hydrated patient and use of restraint in the total dose of contrast medium (no more than 5 ml per kilogram) will minimize the likelihood of renal complications. A judicious combination of IA-DSA and nonionic contrast agents may provide answers at considerably lower risk.

If the patient has had a bona fide allergic reaction to contrast media in the past, he has 17 times as great a chance of a recurrence of such a reaction as the general population. Precautions must be taken with such patients [5, 11, 13, 18]; they include

1. Reevaluate the indications for the study.
2. Change the type of contrast agent from that used on the previous examination, preferably to nonionic agents, if available.
3. Have a tracheostomy tray, emergency drug tray, airways, oxygen, and suction equipment immediately available.
4. Pretreat the patient with antihistamines and corticosteroids. Give prednisone 20 to 50 mg PO every 6 hours for 24 hours. When the patient is called to the radiology department, give Benadryl, 50 mg, and cimetidine, 300 mg IV. The efficacy of this method has yet to be proven in a prospective study, but it has been used safely in a small series [13].
5. Institute an intravenous line at the start of the study in case a severe reaction necessitates urgent administration of atropine or adrenalin. Give intravenous adrenalin cautiously. Mix 1 mg in 10 ml of sterile saline. Pause after administering 3 to 4 ml of this mixture to determine its effect on the allergic manifestations and also on the systemic circulation. These patients must be differentiated from those with hypotension and bradycardia due to vasovagal attacks, who respond to intravenous injections of 0.5 to 1 mg of atropine.

6. Alert the anesthesiology department to be on stand-by.

COMPLICATIONS CAUSED DURING ARTERIAL PUNCTURE OR CATHETER MANIPULATION

Hematoma Formation

The most frequent complication is hematoma formation at the puncture site, which is usually caused by inadequate compression following catheter withdrawal. It may also be caused by multiple traumatic punctures, a catheter with an inordinately large diameter, prolonged or excessive catheter manipulation, or perforation of a retroperitoneal artery. Although they are unsightly and painful, hematomas are usually self-limiting. If progressing in size, and difficult to control, surgical consultation and correction is advised. If neurologic deficit occurs as a result of compression of adjacent nerves by the hematoma (as in the axilla), immediate surgical evacuation must be undertaken. Pelvic retroperitoneal hematomas may

Fig. 3-34. Retroperitoneal hematoma within the pelvis, causing bladder displacement. This condition occurred following a too-high percutaneous femoral puncture on the right side in a patient with poor clotting factors.

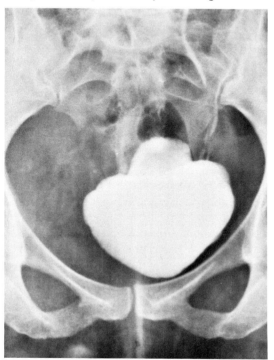

be detected fluoroscopically by bladder displacement (Fig. 3-34).

Absent Pulse

The pulse at the site of catheterization may disappear either during or after completion of a study. This complication may be caused by arterial spasm or by thrombus. Thrombus almost always forms on the surface of intravascularly placed catheters and is usually reabsorbed by the body's natural defenses. Despite meticulous technique, this condition may progress to occlude the punctured artery (Fig. 3-35). It is particularly likely to occur in diseased vessels or those having incurred intimal injury, in patients with hypercoagulable states, and in children or young people, whose vessels appear to be more spastic. Embarrassment of the extremity circulation may result. The patient should be closely watched with frequent doppler examinations of the peripheral pulses. Premature surgical intervention must be avoided, yet one cannot wait too long if the occlusion is caused by thrombus. If the patient complains of pain, exhibits pallor or mottled discoloration, and has a cold extremity that is unresponsive to treatment, prompt interven-

Fig. 3-35. Iatrogenic occlusion of the axillary artery following axillary artery catheterization. Pull-out arteriogram shows complete occlusion at puncture site (*arrow*). Surgical intervention was necessary. (From I. Johnsrude and R. Lester, Abdominal Visceral Arteriography as a Guide to the Surgeon. In *Monographs in the Surgical Sciences*, Vol. 3, No. 2. Baltimore: Williams & Wilkins, 1967. Reproduced with permission of the Williams & Wilkins Co.)

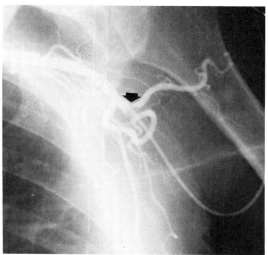

tion is necessary. If the limb is cool and painless or has mild paresthesias, one can afford to watch the patient for periods up to 12 hours or more.

If an absent extremity pulse is detected prior to withdrawal of the catheter, place the catheter tip near the puncture site and inject heparin to prevent clot progression. As much as 3000 or 4000 IU may be given intraarterially, and an additional 15,000 IU intravenously. If arterial thrombus develops, it may also be treated with a thrombolytic enzyme such as streptokinase or urokinase. These agents work best on acute thrombus and may be very effective in this setting. Particular attention must be given, however, to potential extravasation and hematoma formation at the puncture site. One method of accomplishing this is to infuse streptokinase through the catheter in place and allow blood flow to carry it to the clot. However, lysis will be more effective if the infusion catheter is buried in the clot, and this often requires a new vascular entry. For details of treatment, see Chapter 7. To relieve any spasm that may be present, inject up to 20 ml of 1% lidocaine periarterially and 100 to 300 μg of nitroglycerine intraarterially at the site of occlusion. As described earlier, a milking action of the artery just above the puncture site and release of a short spurt of blood immediately following pull-out of the catheter may extrude a small clot (see Fig. 3-10). Early consultation with a vascular surgeon is essential if problems arise.

Other Complications

Arterial or venous dissection is most likely to occur if the catheter tip does not lie freely in the vessel (Fig. 3-36) or if the jet from the catheter tip is directed at right angles to the vessel wall. Superior vena cava or right atrium injections (used in IV-DSA) may be better performed with a pigtail catheter tip configuration. Embolization of a blood clot (Figs. 3-37, 3-38), air, dislodged particles of atheromatous plaque or cholesterol, or foreign bodies may also occur. Faulty aseptic technique may result in infection. Other potential complications include false aneurysm formation at the puncture site, arteriovenous fistula formation at the puncture site, and retroperitoneal hematoma.

Midstream descending thoracic and abdominal aortic injections during a low flow state (congestive heart failure, Valsalva maneuver or other causes

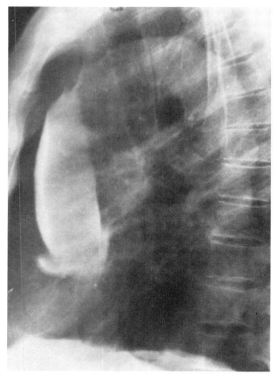

Fig. 3-36. Iatrogenic dissection of the thoracic aorta. This film was obtained 1 hour after an aortic root injection. The catheter tip was placed within the aortic lumen, but no final check was made prior to high-pressure injection. Massive subintimal injection of contrast material occurred, accompanied clinically by severe pain and mild cardiac ischemic changes. The patient survived the procedure. (From I. Johnsrude and R. Lester, Abdominal Visceral Arteriography as a Guide to the Surgeon. In *Monographs in the Surgical Sciences*, Vol. 3, No. 2. Baltimore: Williams & Wilkins, 1967. Reproduced with permission of the Williams & Wilkins Co.)

for low cardiac output) may cause stagnation of the contrast column with flooding of spinal branches arising from intercostal and lumbar arteries. Neurologic sequelae and the "medullary shock" syndrome may ensue. Here, uncontrolled, frightening, and very painful spastic contractions of the lower extremities occur immediately following the injection and persist for minutes to hours. To avoid permanent neurologic damage, no further injection of contrast medium must be given. Direct intravenous injection of Valium 5 to 10 mg (with careful monitoring of respiration and vital signs) gives almost immediate relief [4].

Following translumbar aortography, perinephric abscess, pneumothorax, hemothorax (Fig. 3-

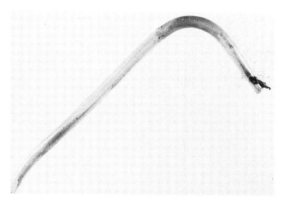

Fig. 3-37. Clot lying within side hole of catheter. The catheter can be easily flushed through the nonobstructed end hole. Subsequent high-pressure injection can cause embolization; this can be prevented with heparinization of the patient, heparin-treated catheters, frequent flushing of the catheter, and a rapid, efficient catheterization procedure.

Fig. 3-38. Iatrogenic embolization to the right renal artery.
A. An aortogram was performed subsequent to a selective renal arteriogram. There is a filling defect and nonopacification of the lower pole of the right kidney (*arrow*). The patient did not complain of pain and did not suffer from hematuria.
B. Complete resolution of embolus following 4 days of active heparin therapy. (Courtesy of Dr. William McConnell, Greenville, NC).

39), chylothorax, and periaortic hematomas may occur. There are occasionally reports of neurologic sequelae of paresis due to cord damage, but such an occurrence is usually a result of inadvertent administration of large doses of contrast agent directly into the arteries supplying the spine (the intercostal and lumbar arteries) (Fig. 3-40). Congestive heart failure, myocardial infarction, cardiac arrhythmias, and cardiac arrest have been known to occur.

Complications may also be caused by equipment failures. A faulty guidewire tip may break off and lodge within an artery. Improper electrical grounding may result in ventricular fibrillation.

Complications are more frequent in patients with severe arterial disease, congestive heart failure, polycythemia (thrombosis), renal, myocardial, or cerebral ischemia, and in those with blood dyscrasias. Patients being treated with heparin who have a clotting time above 20 minutes or a partial thromboplastin time above 45 seconds can be corrected with protamine sulfate. This is administered in a ratio of 1 mg of protamine per 100 IU of heparin. Rather than relying on protamine, however, we prefer to begin arteriography 4 hours after stopping heparin.

An abnormal prothrombin time (15 or 16 seconds compared with a control of 11 or 12 seconds) may also be reversed. Vitamin K may take several

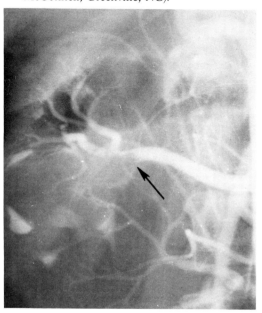

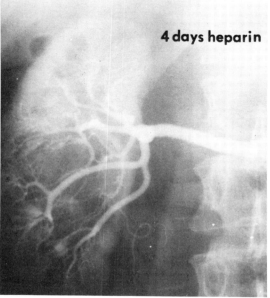

A   B

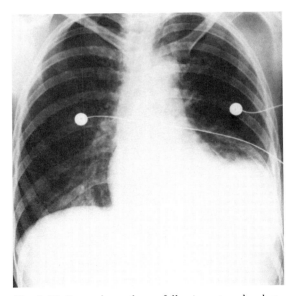

Fig. 3-39. Severe hemothorax following a translumbar aortogram. Needle placement was at T12 in a patient with a low-lying diaphragm. The patient moved from the catheterization table within 3 minutes of termination of procedure. One should allow at least 10 minutes for fibrin accumulation at the aortic puncture site prior to patient movement and should check patient anatomy carefully prior to the study.

days to be effective, and if urgent arteriography is needed, fresh frozen blood plasma should be administered.

Summary of Safe Guidelines

1. Be aware of the physical and mental state of the patient, his laboratory findings, and his state of hydration. Remember that the patient is naked and frightened and that his life is in your hands. Treat him gently and respectfully, and always be aware of his dignity.
2. The longer a patient is on the table, the more chance he has of becoming tired or of having complications, and the greater is the chance of not completing the study. Start timing the study when the patient first gets on the table.
3. Preliminary scout films ensure good radiographic technique. Use basic concepts of radiology. Know the surface anatomy. Cone down to the field of interest. Use a voltage range of 60 to 80 kV. One cannot guess proper radiographic factors outside the range of 5 kV difference on the preliminary film. Add 3 kV for coning from a large to a small field. Add 3 kV when changing to an oblique position

Fig. 3-40. Large dose of contrast medium inadvertently injected into the lumbar arteries during axillary approach aortograms. This caused pain but no neurologic damage.
A. Anteroposterior projection shows densely opacified lumbar arteries (*arrows*).
B. Lateral projection shows catheter tip in lumbar artery and densely outlined lumbar branch.

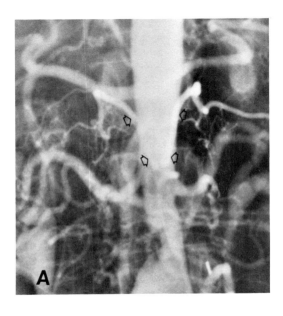

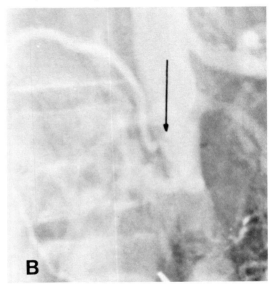

from the anteroposterior position (30 to 40 degrees). Within the abdomen add 2 to 3 kV for increased body density when previous large doses of contrast agent have been injected.

4. Check the equipment prior to the study. The needle assembly must be intact. Choose the guidewire diameter and length carefully to ensure proper fit with the catheter. The guidewire length should be at least several inches longer than the sum of the catheter length and the total flexible wire tip. The catheter tip must be tapered and not frayed. The correct catheter size, length, and shape must be selected.

5. Choose the puncture site carefully. Too high a puncture (external iliac arteries, midportion of axillary artery) may cause difficulty in securing hemostasis following catheter removal. Infiltrate the arterial puncture site thoroughly and *slowly* with procaine hydrochloride or lidocaine to prevent pain and arterial spasm.

6. Never force a needle, guidewire, or catheter up a vessel. Gentle manipulation and easy needle passage are particularly important.

7. Never pass a catheter up an arteriosclerotic vessel unless it is introduced over a guidewire. Never introduce a guidewire through a needle into an artery unless there is a good flow.

8. Remove the guidewire from the catheter as soon as possible to prevent fibrin accumulation. Intravascular heparin administered at the start of the study (45 IU per kilogram) in patients without contraindications will help in this regard.

9. Efficiency decreases blood loss during the study. Avoid excessive spillage of blood or fluid on the patient's drapes, because this reduces sterility and, more important, provides a dangerous electrical pathway to ground. Use 5% dextrose solution instead of saline solution for flushing, because it is a much poorer electrical conductor. Good lighting is important.

10. Watch closely for possible clots or air emboli. Always keep the handle of the syringe (with its possible small collections of air) pointing upward, away from the distal end of the syringe. Never inject the whole bolus that is in a syringe (allow any collections of air to be trapped in the syringe).

11. When selective catheters with side holes must be used, work rapidly to prevent clot formation within one of these side holes, because, on a forceful injection, the clot may embolize to critical areas.

12. Use test doses of contrast agent efficiently and keep them to a minimum.

13. Beware of overhydration of young children with too much flushing or fluid.

14. Never administer a high-power injection without a small preliminary hand injection (fluoroscopically checked) of contrast agent. This prevents infarction from a wedged catheter or a dissection from a subintimal location. The catheter should lie free in the lumen. There should be rapid washout of contrast medium from a selectively injected artery.

15. Beware of the inherent dangers in the high-pressure injector. Used injudiciously, it is a lethal machine.

16. Consistently good studies will be obtained if the catheter is correctly positioned and if a *safely* large bolus of contrast medium is introduced in a short period of time. Exceptions are in angiography of the extremities, in which a fairly prolonged injection is preferred. The best studies are obtained with the catheter tip closest to the site of interest.

17. Choose the type and volume of contrast agents carefully. Be aware of the new nonionic agents and the decreased requirements of IA-DSA and consider their use in high-risk or painful studies. Renal failure, congestive heart failure, and prolonged dehydration predispose to loss of renal function. If reduced renal function is suspected, a 24-hour radiograph of the abdomen may show a prolonged renal nephrogram. This finding is a signal for prompt clinical confirmation and medical intervention. Delay proposed surgery until this condition is corrected.

18. Beware of the dangers of radiation both to yourself and to the patient. Use safety features and proper coning.

19. Postangiographic care is as important as the care you render in the angiographic room.

20. Do not hesitate to consult other physicians in case of trouble. Never hide your mistakes.

References

1. Alfidi, R. Informed Consent. In T. Meaney, A. Lalli, and R. Alfidi (eds.), *Complications and Legal*

Implications of Radiologic Special Procedures. St. Louis: Mosby, 1973.

2. Eldh, P., and Jacobsson, B. Heparinized vascular catheters: A clinical trial. *Radiology* 111:289, 1974.

3. Formanek, G. Arterial thrombus formation during clinical percutaneous catheterization. *Circulation* 41:833, 1970.

4. Gordon, D., and Levin, D. Treatment of angiographically produced cord seizures by intraarterial diazepam. *Cathet. Cardiovasc. Diagn.* 2:97, 1976.

5. Greenberger, P., et al. Administration of radiographic contrast media in high risk patients. *Invest. Radiol.* 15(6 suppl.):S40, 1980.

6. Grollman, J., and Marcus, R. Antegrade translumbar aortography. *Radiology* 153:249, 1984.

7. Jacobsson, B., and Schlossman, D. Thromboembolism of the leg following percutaneous catheterization of femoral artery for angiography: Predisposing factors. *Acta Radiol. [Diag.]* 8:109, 1969.

8. Kelly, J. F., et al. Radiographic contrast media studies in high-risk patients. *J. Allergy Clin. Immunol.* 62:181, 1978.

9. Kinney, T., Fan, M., and Chin, A. Shear force in angioplasty: Its relation to catheter design and function. *A.J.R.* 144:115, 1985.

10. Lalli, A. Reactions to Contrast Media. In T. Meaney, A. Lalli, and R. Alfidi (eds.), *Complica-tions and Legal Implications of Radiologic Special Procedures.* St. Louis: Mosby, 1973.

11. Lasser, E. C., et al. Steroids: Theoretical and experimental basis for utilization in prevention of contrast media reactions. *Radiology* 125:1, 1977.

12. Maxwell, S., Kwan, O., and Millan, V. Translumbar carotid anteriography. *Radiology* 148:851, 1983.

13. Myers, G. E., and Bloom, F. L. Cimetidine (Tagamet) combined with steroids and H1 antihistamines for the prevention of serious radiographic contrast material reactions. *Cathet. Cardiovasc. Diagn.* 7:65, 1982.

14. Rosch, J. Superselective arteriography in the diagnosis of abdominal pathology: Technical considerations. *Radiology* 92:1008, 1969.

15. Seldinger, S. Catheter replacement of the needle in percutaneous arteriography: A new technique. *Acta Radiol.* 139:368, 1953.

16. Thomas, M., and Fletcher, E. Large volume translumbar aortography in aortic occlusion. *A.J.R.* 109:541, 1970.

17. Wallace, S., et al. Systemic heparinization for angiography. *A.J.R.* 116:204, 1972.

18. Zweiman, B., Mishkin, M. M., and Hildreth, E. A. An approach to the performance of contrast studies in contrast material-reactive persons. *Ann. Intern. Med.* 83:159, 1975.

Technical Considerations

Basic Concepts of Injection Rates and Doses

Doses of contrast media and their rates of injection vary considerably with the procedure being performed. Rates as high as 30 ml per second are required in thoracic aortic midstream injections, while rates of 1 to 2 ml per second may be appropriate in many small subselective arterial injections.

In the adult, a dose as high as 50 to 60 ml of contrast material per injection may be used in midstream aortic studies. A dose of 100 ml or more can be delivered at the aortic bifurcation to outline lower extremity vessels. However, no more than 2 to 3 ml can be given in certain small organ beds (e.g., the intercostal or lumbar arteries). There are intermediary situations, which will be discussed in appropriate subsequent chapters. In the child, dosages usually do not exceed 1.0 to 1.5 ml per kilogram of body weight per injection. In large midstream injections in children, the dose should be administered within 1 to 1½ seconds. Repeat injections may be given when required, but one should keep in mind that toxic effects are directly related to total dosage and elapsed time between injections. With children one should try to wait 20 minutes between injections.

The rate and the amount of contrast agent must be tailored to the size of the vascular bed and the lesion under investigation. For example, a hypervascular lesion or one with increased flow, such as an arteriovenous malformation, may require 2 to 3 times the volume of contrast agent and 2 to 3 times as rapid a rate of injection as an ischemic process involving the same area. The total dose of contrast medium should not exceed 5 ml per kilogram of body weight, and it should be lower in patients with renal failure. Somewhat larger total doses of more dilute contrast medium (30 to 42%) may be allowed. Detailed guidelines for various procedures will be presented in subsequent chapters.

The rate and dose of contrast medium injected using *digital subtraction angiography* (DSA) varies from that used during conventional arteriography. In general, during intraarterial DSA (IA-DSA) the contrast enhancing capabilities of the technique allow smaller doses of less concentrated contrast medium to be used. Often, small hand injections, with the catheter at the orifice of the target vessel will suffice. Also, less time need be spent on technical maneuvers than is required to achieve the stable catheter position necessary for the higher volume, higher rate injections. These features result in greater safety and less patient discomfort during the study. During intravenous DSA (IV-DSA), however, larger doses of higher concentration contrast agent are required to accommodate the dilution that occurs during its passage through the heart and pulmonary vessels before entering the systemic arteries. In the adult, 25 to 50 ml of a medium-density contrast agent is required per injection. The injection rate varies with the site of venous injection: 10 to 15 ml per second if injected into peripheral veins (e.g., antecubital fossa); 20 to 30 ml per second if injected into the inferior vena cava, superior vena cava, or right atrium. The total amount of contrast medium administered quickly adds up when multiple projections are required to clarify pathologic anatomy of overlapping vessels. Somewhat smaller doses may be possible if they are injected during ECG-triggered ventricular diastole.

Film Timing

Serial filming or imaging of the opacified circulation shows progressive filling of more and finer arterial radicles, followed by a contrast "blush" representing the capillary phase, and followed in turn by gradual opacification of the venous structures of the target organ. Appropriate timing of radiographic exposures is important to produce a satisfactory study and to document the following three phases:

1. The arterial phase. Standard rates during the arterial phase are 2 or 3 films per second. Rapid filming is important because some arterial changes (e.g., pathologic circulation in tumors) are fleeting events. To capture each filling of vessels, the first exposure should be near the

start of the injection, or just before the injection if a "mask" film or image is to be made for subtraction techniques (see Appendix 11). In patients with intracardiac and extracardiac shunts and those with arteriovenous malformations, rates of four or even six films per second are helpful if conventional angiography is being used. More rapid rates can be attained if photofluorography, cineradiography, or digital radiography is performed. Filming of the arteries of the extremities is performed at a much slower rate, however, since here the flow rate is slow.

2. The capillary phase. Avascular tumors and cysts in the brain, pancreas, kidney, and other organs may be seen as filling defects during the capillary phase. Tumors with a prominent capillary bed often show a tumor blush.
3. The venous phase. It is important to recognize changes in the vein, such as displacement, invasion, early filling, or varix formation.

In order to cover these three phases of the circulation, allowance must be made for the normal variations within the body, since total flow and circulation rates to a given organ vary with its functional demands as well as with the size of the vascular bed. The time required to opacify veins after an arterial injection varies in different parts of the body: in the heart and lungs, a period of 2 to 5 seconds is required; in the brain, 6 to 8 seconds; in the kidney, 10 to 12 seconds; and in the portal system, 12 to 20 seconds.

The flow of contrast medium in the arteries of the extremities is considerably slower than elsewhere in the body. This may be a result of the irritating effect of the iodine compound on the arterial wall, which leads to reflex vasospasm and in turn to increased peripheral resistance. Another cause for the slower flow may be that the heavier contrast medium layers out and moves slowly along the posterior wall of the vascular tree. If the extremity is studied on the smaller 14 × 14-in. exposure field of a rapid film changer (e.g., the Schonander AOT), sequential 6- to 8-in. movements of the tabletop over the exposure field at preset intervals will follow the vascular opacification. With the larger 14 × 36-in. or 14 × 51-in. film changers, one has the advantage of studying all phases of the circulation of the limb with less

chance of overlooking points that are proximal and distal to the area of interest. However, only a limited number of films are available with these changers (4 to 10), and the most rapid possible film rate is 1 film every 2 or 3 seconds. This rate is usually sufficient for studying obstructive disease, in which filming over a period up to 40 or 50 seconds is occasionally required, but it may be inadequate for studying rapid circulations such as are seen in arteriovenous fistulas. In arteriography of the lower extremities, the injection rate is programmed over a 4- to 5-second interval, with the first exposure at 3 to 4 seconds and subsequent exposures every 4 to 5 seconds.

In children and young adults, the flow rate is generally more rapid, and the film rate should be appropriately adjusted (e.g., three or even four films per second during the arterial phase of an abdominal aortogram).

For IV-DSA, the timing of exposures must be programmed to allow for the pulmonary circulation time, in addition to the transit time of the contrast agent from the left atrium to the target vessels. It must also provide exposures for masks prior to the arrival of the contrast media to the area of interest. Generally one can allow a delay of at least 3 to 4 seconds without any exposures to accommodate this pulmonary circulation time. At this point, mask exposures are obtained at one exposure per second for 2 to 4 seconds if a rapid injection is made into the right atrium. Exposures of one per second for 6 to 8 seconds may be necessary if the injection occurs in an antecubital vein. As soon as the contrast column becomes visually evident on the screen, more rapid arterial exposures, preprogrammed to accommodate the arterial, capillary, and finally the slower venous phase of the target organ circulation, may be instituted. These capabilities will depend on the sophistication of the equipment used, and the matrix size of the programmed image. For example, a 1024 × 1024 matrix allows fewer images, but much higher resolution than a 256 × 256 matrix.

For IA-DSA the same principles are used as for film timing of conventional angiography. At least one or two exposures must be programmed prior to the injection of contrast agent to allow for the masks used for subtraction. If the software allows flexibility in the program, a mask from the end of the contrast run may also be used.

Ancillary Methods to Enhance Studies

VALSALVA MANEUVER

Straining hard against a closed glottis for 10 to 15 seconds increases intrathoracic pressure and slows the return of flow to the heart, thus decreasing cardiac output and systemic pressures. This maneuver slows the flow in high-rate areas, such as the abdominal aorta. In a retrograde abdominal aortogram, if contrast medium is injected at the moment of release of Valsalva maneuver, more contrast filled films are available and the contrast medium will travel further retrograde. Complications may arise from this induced slow flow, since the contrast medium layers, and with the patient in a supine position the arteries supplying the spine have a higher concentration of noxious contrast medium. One of our older patients developed transient myoclonic contractions and spasticity of the legs following this maneuver, indicating reversible neurologic damage. Valsalva maneuver should be reserved for those young patients who have a very rapid flow. It may be inadvertently invoked during IV-DSA, when the patient is asked to hold his breath for rather prolonged periods. The resultant decrease in cardiac output delays successful passage of contrast agent to the systemic circulation as a rapid, relatively dense concentrated bolus.

REACTIVE HYPEREMIA

Heat, exercise, reactive hyperemia, periarterial procaine injection, and epidural anesthesia increase the flow rate in slow flow areas (e.g., atherosclerotic narrowing of the lower extremities). Reactive hyperemia is very helpful in evaluating occlusive disease of the extremities [17]. A blood pressure cuff on the distal thigh is inflated to 50 mm Hg above the systolic level for a period of 3 to 5 minutes. Maximal vasodilatation occurs approximately 10 seconds following release of the cuff due to the response of accumulation of metabolites (including prostaglandins) in the bloodstream. The contrast medium is injected at this point and greatly increases the circulation rate in the area of interest. The accumulated metabolites appear to add an element of anesthesia (possibly related to the release of beta-endorphins [22]) making the intraarterial injection less painful than when performed without hyperemia. The effect of reactive hyperemia can be enhanced by adding work (repetitive dorsiflexion of the foot) to the reactive hyperemia. This procedure is perfectly safe in patients with chronically obstructed vessels, but it should not be used in those with acute occlusion.

Epidural anesthesia is obtained by introducing polyethylene tubing into the epidural space in the midline low back area and injecting 6 to 10 ml of 2% lidocaine. Generally excellent sensory anesthesia of the lower extremities is produced within 20 to 30 minutes of the injection, which provides not only relief from the usually painful arteriogram of the lower extremities but also vasodilatation and rapid filling of the arteries [19].

PHARMACOANGIOGRAPHY

Pharmacoangiography is the use of vasoactive drugs to enhance angiography by modifying the blood flow by either vasoconstriction or vasodilatation [14].

Vasoconstrictors

The most frequently used vasoconstrictor is epinephrine. The primitive nature of tumor vessels results in a loss of the normal response to neurohumoral stimuli. Injection of small doses of epinephrine into the lumen of a selectively catheterized artery feeding a tumor results in constriction of normal vessels, while the abnormal tumor vessels stand out in bold relief. The dose is usually 5 to 10 μg injected into the artery over a period of 10 to 20 seconds. This injection is followed within 15 to 30 seconds by a slower than usual rate of injection (2 to 5 ml per second) and much slower film timing (one film per second) (Fig. 4-1).

It is known that not only tumor vessels but also inflammatory vessels fail to constrict with epinephrine [30]. Moreover, rarely will epinephrine studies outline a lesion not seen by well collimated and adequately injected angiographic studies. For this reason, this technique is losing some popularity, particularly in the study of renal tumors. Epinephrine has a different effect on the various branches of the celiac axis; it appears to constrict differentially the branches leading to the liver and spleen more than those leading to the pancreas [2]. Its use can improve evaluation of the pancreas by directing the flow of contrast agent preferentially to this

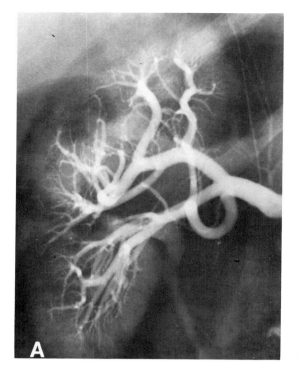

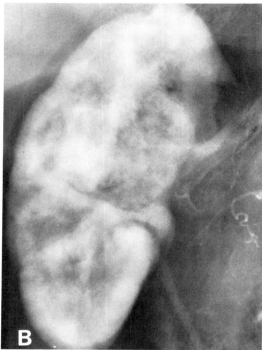

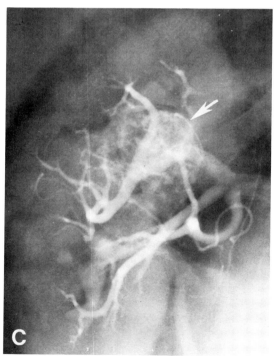

organ during a celiac axis injection. Arteries supplying the adrenal gland have a similar lack of response to adrenalin. Pathology in the adrenal gland may be better demonstrated angiographically by a prior injection of adrenalin into a renal or inferior phrenic artery (from which the adrenal arteries arise). Epinephrine does have a profound effect on the central cardiovascular system. Therefore, its dosage should be accurately measured and its use should be limited to organs below the diaphragm.

Angiotensin II, a product of the renin-angiotensin system, is a potent vasoconstrictor with a very short half-life (20 seconds). Given in very small doses, 0.5 μg, it can, like epinephrine, enhance the angiographic picture of tumor neovascularity by constricting more normal vessels [16].

Vasoconstrictive medications (epinephrine, vasopressin) are also used for treating bleeding points

Fig. 4-1. Epinephrine pharmacoangiography for evaluating right renal tumor.

A and B. Early and late phases of renal arteriogram. Although the hilar mass is clearly seen, tumor neovascularity is difficult to see.

C. After selective injection of 10 μg of adrenalin, 12 ml of Renografin-60 was injected over 4 seconds, and films were obtained at the rate of one per second. This exposure was obtained at 14 seconds and shows normal vasomotor response to vessels in areas other than the tumor with constriction and delay in circulation. Abnormal vessels indicating tumor are now seen (*arrow*).

by selective injection into the bleeding artery. This is discussed in greater detail in subsequent chapters.

Vasodilators

Vasodilators may be used when vasospasm detracts from the study (e.g., in Raynaud's disease), or when more rapid arterial flow or enhanced venous opacification is required. When placed within the superior mesenteric artery, larger doses of contrast agent can be more rapidly injected selectively into the vessel. Although there is a moderate loss in peripheral arterial detail, more intense and more rapid portal venous opacification is seen, which is particularly helpful in patients with portal hypertension. These drugs act by decreasing arterial resistance and increasing venous capacity. Portal pressures are increased by this maneuver. Vasodilators have also been used successfully in the treatment of nonocclusive mesenteric ischemia and in other vasospastic conditions [28]. Vasodilators (e.g., nitroglycerine 100 to 300 μg, tolazoline 25 mg) may be injected into a vascular bed immediately peripheral to a therapeutically dilated stenotic or occluded vessel in order to prevent or overcome vascular spasm. They may also be administered orally prophylactically (nifedipine 10 mg PO) 10 minutes prior to its anticipated need. If more rapid action is required, the capsule may be broken and its contents given sublingually. Vasodilators may also be useful in confirming or negating the hemodynamic significance of a stenotic lesion. In those patients with a questionable gradient measured across the area of narrowing, a peripheral injection of 25 mg of tolazoline may either increase the gradient, indicating a significant lesion, or leave it unchanged and therefore, insignificant. This is particularly important if angioplasty is anticipated.

Various vasodilating drugs have been used by different investigators [14]. These include

1. Isoproterenol, 2 to 4 mcg per minute for 2 minutes, given just prior to angiography.
2. Bradykinin, 5 to 10 mcg (this drug is not available in the United States).
3. Tolazoline hydrochloride (Priscoline), 25 to 50 mg, injected slowly over a period of 2 to 3 minutes immediately before injection of contrast agent. This vasodilator is commonly used in our laboratories. Tolazoline (25 mg) may also be injected intraarterially at the puncture site to treat vasospasm following catheterization. A similar dose helps reduce spasm in a more peripheral vascular bed.
4. Papaverine. The usual dosage is 30 mg intraarterially in a single dose, or an infusion of 30 to 60 mg per hour for several hours.
5. The E series of prostaglandins [21], 0.5 to 1.0 mg per kilogram. These naturally occurring, rapidly degraded, unsaturated fatty acids can be used to enhance visualization of vessels in the splanchnic viscera, kidneys, and lower extremities. Like tolazoline, they can be used to increase flow and thereby intensify a pressure gradient across an area of stenosis.
6. Dopamine.
7. Acetylcholine.
8. Nitroglycerine. This is an effective vasodilator in the coronary circulation and also in other vascular beds. It can produce prompt relief of spasm if administered directly into the affected arterial circulation in doses of 100 to 300 μg (Fig. 4-2).
9. Nifedipine, a calcium channel blocker, administered orally in 10-mg capsules. It can effectively prevent small vessel spasm if given 10 minutes prior to catheter manipulation. The capsule can be broken and the contents given sublingually if more prompt action is required.
10. Glucagon, a normal pancreatic hormone, is a helpful smooth muscle relaxant [20]. A dose of 0.2 to 1.0 mg IV decreases gastrointestinal peristalsis and eliminates the motion artifact of gas-filled loops during DSA. Its vasodilator action can be useful in pharmacoangiography of the splanchnic and renal circulation. Larger doses, however, can cause nausea and vomiting.

All vasoactive drugs must be used with caution and with full knowledge of the patient's overall cardiovascular status.

Subtraction

Conventional angiographic studies can often be enhanced by subtraction (Fig. 4-3). Overlying bony structures may be "subtracted" out of the vascular contrast-filled structures, thus permitting better visualization. In addition, smaller vessels otherwise not seen may be more clearly identified.

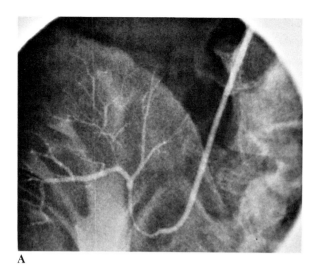

A

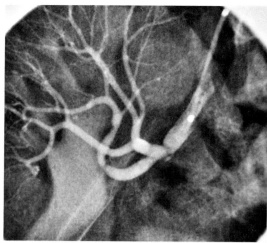

B

There are various means by which subtraction can be performed (see Appendix 11). The most sophisticated method involves computerized digital techniques, which can be used to enhance arteries opacified by injecting contrast agent intravenously (IV-DSA) or intraarterially (IA-DSA).

Although intravenous digital subtraction angiography is a useful study, its limitations indicate that its role in clinical practice should be clearly defined. Since misregistration of images due to

Fig. 4-2.
A. Diffuse spasm in transplant renal arteries due to catheter manipulation during angioplasty for renal artery stenosis.
B. Release of spasm following injection of 100 μg of nitroglycerine directly into the artery.

Fig. 4-3. Subtraction study: selective injection of right costocervical trunk.
A. Nonsubtraction film. A spinal angiomatous malformation is completely obscured by overlying bony structures.
B. The lesion is clearly identified with the bones subtracted from the picture.

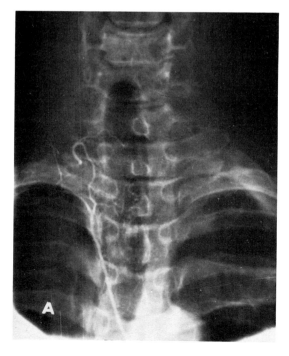

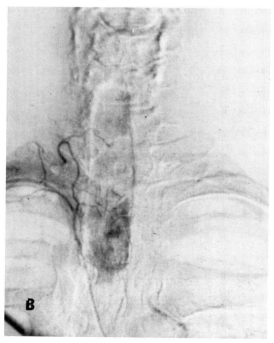

motion between the mask image and the contrast-filled image is a major drawback, it requires an alert, cooperative patient with a good cardiac output. It requires a good bolus of contrast medium (30 to 45 ml). The contrast medium may be administered through needles placed in antecubital veins or through a pigtail catheter into a large central vein (inferior vena cava or superior vena cava) or preferably into the right atrium. Optimal studies require images that are accurately positioned and collimated, with careful instruction to limit motion from various causes (e.g., breathing, swallowing). One must be careful not to incite apprehension or to induce Valsalva maneuver with its resulting lowering of cardiac output. Appropriate bolsters and/or filters must be applied to the patient or the x-ray tube in order to equalize major disparate radiographic densities over the field of exposure. Renal function and reactions to contrast agents must be considered. The study may thus be least helpful in the elderly or the very young, in whom it is most needed. Arteries cannot be selectively opacified by this technique, and superimposed vessels may prove a problem requiring injections in multiple projections. Spatial resolution is somewhat limited by DSA as compared with conventional angiography, but very adequate studies may be obtained.

Digital subtraction angiography can be useful in direct arterial studies (IA-DSA) in which decreased contrast medium requirements allow use of smaller catheters with increased safety. In patients with a previous history of severe contrast reactions, more expensive but smaller amounts of newer nonionic contrast agents or intraarterial administration of carbon dioxide [13] may be effectively used in limited areas. Although there may be less spatial resolution in IA-DSA than is seen in conventional angiography, there is increased detection of the contrast medium by its enhancing capabilities. Direct arterial digital subtraction studies can be very helpful in producing "road maps" for interventional studies. There is improved efficiency due to less required room time, and decreased cost due to reduced film handling and storage needs. Digital angiographic capabilities are therefore very useful if incorporated into a conventional angiographic suite. It is clear that the combination of DSA and newer nonionic contrast agents are opening exciting frontiers to the field of angiography and are providing information with less risk and discomfort to a broader population of patients.

Magnification

Magnification of small vessels can occur by photographic, electronic, or geometric means [3, 11]. Geometric magnification is widely used in angiography and can be achieved by decreasing the distance from the tube to the patient and increasing the distance from the patient to the film (Fig. 4-4; see also Figs. 1-2, 1-3). The magnification obtained is equal to the ratio of the target-to-film distance to the target-to-object distance. Special equipment is necessary either to lower the x-ray changer from the tabletop or to raise the tabletop from the changer.

The amount of practical magnification achieved by this geometric relationship is limited by certain factors.

1. The size of the focal spot of the x-ray tube. Unless the effective focal spot is small, the penumbra is exaggerated, which impairs image resolution. A 0.3-mm effective focal spot allows magnification of approximately $2\times$. An effective focal spot of 0.1 mm allows linear magnification up to $4\times$, but this requires a grid biased tube. The practical limit of resolution is approximately twice the anode size; thus, 0.6-mm vessels can be clearly resolved with a 0.3-mm effective focal spot tube. Although smaller vessels can be seen, they are distorted by penumbra. Small focal spots have a limited tube capacity; therefore, lower radiographic factors are available for exposures. Lower permissible amperage requires longer exposures. High voltage (well outside the optimum range of x-ray absorption for iodine) detracts from film contrast. Both of these factors are detrimental in a pulsatile, rapidly flowing, contrast filled vascular system, since fewer films and a slower rate of exposures are allowed per angiographic run. This situation can be helped by bringing the tube as close as possible to the patient, thus making lower demands for radiation. The tubes with smaller focal spots (0.1 mm or less) portray only a small area of anatomy on the film due to the sharp angle of the anode that is required for the small effective focal spot.

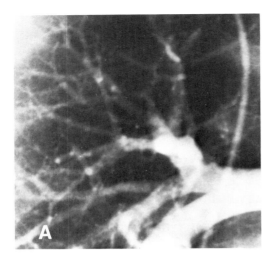
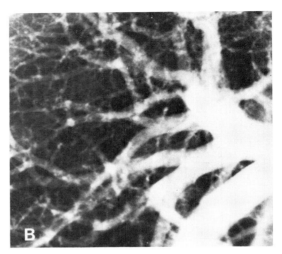

Fig. 4-4. Pulmonary arteriogram.
A. Nonmagnification study.
B. Linear magnification film following injection of equal amounts of contrast agent at approximately the same phase of circulation. There is a marked improvement in detail. A 0.3-mm focal spot tube was used.

2. The dose of radiation to the patient's skin is increased as a result of the shorter tube-object distance that is required in order to stay within the tube capacity.
3. Inherent motion in the serial film changer is magnified and must be corrected.
4. The air gap between the patient and the film helps to reduce scatter, and sometimes no grid is necessary. If the object is less than 15 in. away from the film, a low-ratio grid (5:1) is required to clean up scatter. Special carbon fiber material has replaced the aluminum alloy used for backing the film screens. This, together with rare earth screen and film combinations, decreases radiation requirements considerably, widening the scope of magnification angiography. Faster films and screens, however, mean increased mottle. In addition, the energy demands are nonlinear, with approximately 1½ to 2 times increase in radiographic density over that obtained with conventional high-speed screens in the 60 kV range, but a fivefold increase in density at 120 kV. It is generally considered that, despite certain limitations, rare earth screen-film combinations offer significant advantages in imaging [25].

General Considerations in Film Interpretation

Interpretation of the appearance of the vessels on the films in the normal flow pattern is usually not difficult, since there is a gradually increasing opacification of progressively more and finer vessels. This increase is followed by a gradual and progressive decrease in opacity due to dilution with unopacified blood. A generalized blush of capillary flow then occurs, followed by progressively increasing density of venous effluent. Occasionally the full impact of the retrograde high-pressure injection of contrast agent into an artery may occur during diastole, in which case the contrast agent may pass retrograde through connecting arterial channels.

Each phase of vascular filling—the larger arteries, the arterioles, the capillaries, and finally the veins—should be carefully evaluated for dynamic or morphologic abnormalities with the needle or catheters still in place. A second injection with a different projection or with different timing might help to resolve a questionable point.

There are many variations to the anatomic configuration of vessels supplying specific parts of the body. There is a functional or territorial anatomy of vessels rather than a traditional textbook appearance. The patient may be born with these variations, or they may be due to a vascular demand by a high-flow lesion or a surgical ligation, or may be due to a previous incomplete endovascular therapeutic attempt. The traditional vascular supply of a given territory by one broad vascular trunk may therefore be hypoplastic and the supply instead derived from another source. Instead of memorizing the usual points of origin of a given vessel, it seems more reasonable to study all possible feeding arteries to the territory under investigation. It is only by keeping these functional vascular anatomic concepts in mind that one can selectively catheterize the appropriate vessels both for completeness of a diagnostic procedure and for endovascular therapeutic endeavors.

DYNAMIC ABNORMALITIES

Hemodynamic abnormalities present primarily as changes in rate and direction of flow. Angiographic manifestations of delayed flow include a slower than normal arterial appearance time; continued opacification of a vessel or vessels after clearing of surrounding ones (stagnation); and layering of the hyperbaric contrast material in the vessel due to diminished flow.

Extravascular causes for delay in blood flow are systemic hypotension, decreased cardiac output, and increased regional parenchymal resistance (e.g., increased intracranial pressure can cause absent filling of intracranial vessels).

Intravascular factors include obstruction (either partial or complete) at the arterial, capillary, or venous level. It is important to recognize that there can be delayed flow in normal-appearing vessels; there can also be fairly considerable arterial narrowing without significant impediment to flow. These situations can occur because we are not dealing with a simple system of tubes and the flow of fluid through tubes; rather we are dealing with a pulsatile stream, distensible vascular walls, and an ever-changing vascular resistance that is dependent on both central and peripheral vasomotor controlling mechanisms. Many variables are thus introduced, and a lesion that may be significantly narrowed in one patient may not be significantly so in another.

Angiographically speaking, we claim that a narrowing is significant if there is at least 70 percent stenosis; 80 to 85 percent stenosis causes a 50 percent reduction in the flow through a vessel (in the aortoiliac region). When computing the percent stenosis of a segmental narrowing, consider the area involved (πr^2) rather than the diameter alone. Thus an 8-cm diameter vessel narrowed concentrically to a 4-cm diameter has its diameter reduced

by 50 percent but its cross-sectional area reduced by 75 percent (see Appendix 15). Other significant findings include stagnation or slowing of flow, an obvious infarction or ischemia, or poststenotic dilatation (considered to be due to turbulence). The most significant angiographic finding, however, is the presence of collateral flow. In this situation, the smaller adjacent arteries become larger when blood is diverted into them once the major vessel occlusion has changed the pressure relationships.

Abnormally rapid flow is manifested by early dilution of the contrast material and rapid venous filling. This finding may be seen in patients with an increased cardiac output or with arteriovenous communication. The latter condition includes congenital arteriovenous malformations, traumatic or inflammatory arteriovenous fistulas, and arteriovenous communications seen in tumors (Fig. 4-5).

Retrograde filling of arterial vessels can occur under special circumstances. This condition is manifested by gradual and progressive increase in the density of the artery via the collateral vessels, while the surrounding circulatory bed has advanced to the capillary or venous phase. It may be caused by obstruction near the origin of the patent artery or by an anomalous origin of this vessel from a low-pressure system.

In the bilateral organs the circulation of one side should be compared with that of the other. In a solitary organ, the circulation of one portion may be compared with that of another to determine normalcy. One should beware of artifacts caused by preferential streaming of contrast medium resulting from the position of the catheter tip or the side holes.

MORPHOLOGIC ABNORMALITIES

Morphologic abnormalities of the arterial circulation are best appreciated if seen in at least two projections (Fig. 4-6). There may be absence of or an anomalous number and origin of vessels. Arteries may be displaced as a result of extrinsic masses. They may have smaller than normal caliber, as is seen in hypoplasia, in spasm, and with decreased tissue requirements. Arteries may have a larger than normal caliber due to greater tissue demand, as is seen in tumors or in arteriovenous communications, or when they are supplying collateral flow. Irregularities in the arterial wall include atherosclerosis, coarctation, extrinsic

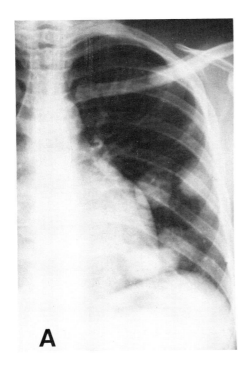

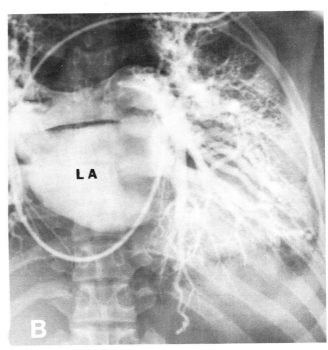

Fig. 4-5. Abnormally rapid flow in multiple pulmonary metastatic nodules.
A. Metastatic choriocarcinoma to the lung.
B. Pulmonary arteriogram shows hypertrophied peripheral vessels and premature pulmonary venous filling, indicating shunts through the tumors. (LA = left atrium.)

bands, and unusual narrowings like those seen in fibromuscular dysplasia. Arterial dilatation is found in aneurysms, arteriovenous communications, and certain tumors. An abrupt termination of a vessel may be caused by thrombus or embolus.

Tumors involve vessels in various ways. Benign cystic lesions are typically avascular or hypovascular. They are usually well marginated and manifest themselves by a smooth displacement of the adjacent vessels.

Benign vascular lesions, typified by heman-

Fig. 4-6. Two projections at right angles to each other give more accurate information than a single projection.
A. Normal opacified vessel.
B. Vascular narrowing seen en face. The only abnormality is a decrease in opacity.
C. Vascular narrowing seen in profile.

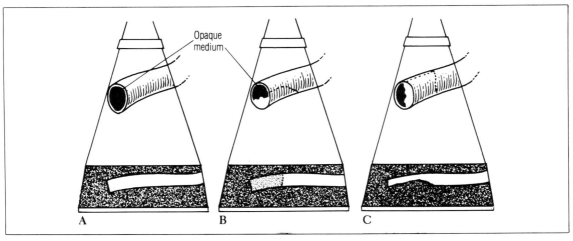

giomas, may have normal feeding vessels. They usually show moderately dense and homogeneously opacified, regularly walled, closely packed vessels. The capillary stain of these benign tumors often persists well into the venous phase, but the venous filling time is normal because there are no abnormal arteriovenous communications. Benign vascular tumors may also have enlarged feeding vessels.

Malignant hypervascular tumors show large feeding vessels and major vessel displacement. The walls of the arteries are usually irregular, and the vessels often travel in a bizarre direction. Frequently, there is pooling of contrast medium in poorly marginated and irregularly shaped vascular lakes. In contrast to the benign lesions, there are usually numerous arteriovenous communications, which cause filling of larger than normal draining veins.

Hypovascular malignant tumors may also show larger than normal feeding vessels and arterial dis-

Fig. 4-7. Artifacts: arterial spasm at the catheter tip and "stationary arterial waves." Selective arteriogram in a patient with glomerulonephritis.
A. The main renal artery is narrowed (*large arrow*), and there is a wavelike pattern of a segmental branch to the lower pole (*small arrow*).
B. Subsequent injection after the catheter position has been changed shows that neither artifact is now present.

placement. The walls of both the large and the small arteries are irregular. This irregularity is caused not by neovascularity but by extrinsic compression and periarterial invasion (encasement) by the tumor. The draining veins, with their more delicate vascular walls, often show invasion, displacement, and obstruction before these effects are seen on the corresponding arteries.

Multiple examples of these abnormalities are given in subsequent chapters of this book.

ARTIFACTS

During angiography, artifacts in vessel contour and flow may be produced. They are not indicative of disease and must be identified as being caused by the procedure itself.

There may be a transient localized narrowing in the wall of the artery at the site of the catheter tip [7]. It occurs only transiently at the time of high-pressure injection, and it is caused by the high circumferential negative pressure resulting from the positive forward pressure of the jet. Collapse of vessel walls with subsequent extravasation of contrast material and blood has been demonstrated experimentally.

Arterial spasm may be seen as a localized response to catheter placement and manipulation (Fig. 4-7, see Fig. 4-2). It may also present as a narrowing near the catheter tip, but it is usually

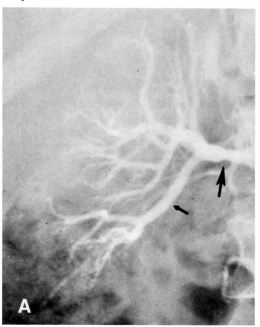

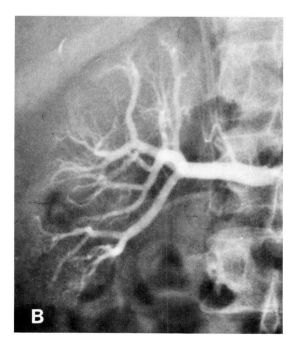

more persistent and is relieved only by removal of the catheter. This condition can also be reversed by intraarterial injection of nitroglycerine (100 μg).

A transient arterial outpouching at the site of the catheter tip may be seen during high-pressure injection. It is caused by the positive pressure of the jet being angled toward a distensible arterial wall. When a high-pressure injection is made during diastole, the bolus of contrast material may pass in retrograde fashion through anatomically normal connecting arterial channels.

Laminar flow is common where opacified and unopacified blood blend. It is caused by uneven mixing of the two substances (Fig. 4-8). "Stationary arterial waves" are seen as a fine, even, rippling, wavelike pattern (Fig. 4-9). When first observed, these waves were explained on the basis of arterial spasm. However, this seems to be less tenable than the explanation advanced by Theander

Fig. 4-8. Laminar flow: selective carotid arteriogram with the patient lying supine. The contrast medium layers on the dependent portion of the carotid artery (*arrow*).

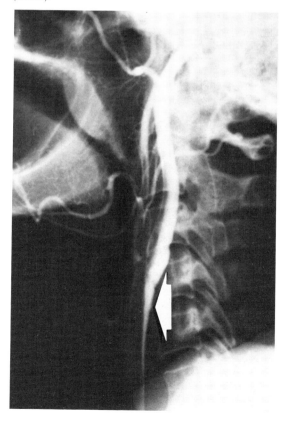

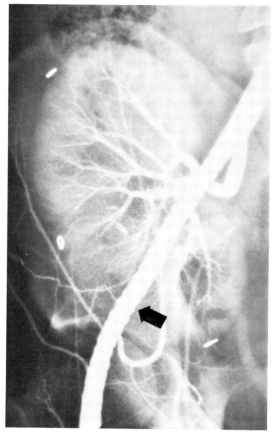

Fig. 4-9. "Stationary arterial waves" (*arrow*). This effect is purely an artifact of flow and is more often seen when there is an increase in resistance to the peripheral flow.

[27], who noted that the waves were usually seen proximal to a peripherally obstructed vessel and believes that this is a resonance phenomenon of the amplified pulse wave transmitted to the elastic arterial wall. This theory is also disputed, and it is evident that the true nature of the arterial wave is yet to be uncovered [1].

DIGITAL ARTIFACTS

A number of artifacts can occur during digital angiography. Most of these are related to misregistration due to motion incurred between the exposure of the mask image, and those exposures made after the arrival of the contrast agent in the systemic vessels. Inappropriate breathing, motion in the neck induced by swallowing, motion due to patient discomfort or inability to cooperate, bowel peristalsis, and the motion of vessels with heavily calcified walls are the usual causes of these artifacts. Vessels may not opacify at the expected time or with the expected density, due to errors in volume or rate of contrast injected, or due to a low cardiac output (e.g., heart failure, aortic or mitral valve disease, cor pulmonale, a vasovagal attack, a simple Valsalva maneuver). Uneven densitometric exposures over the field of interest can cause vascular defects, which must not be confused as morphologic abnormalities.

Ancillary Uses of Catheter Techniques

Techniques employing the percutaneous introduction of needles and catheters have been broadened to encompass a wide variety of diagnostic and therapeutic endeavors. These have not been limited to the vascular bed but include direct organ punctures and manipulations. The intravascular therapeutic maneuvers are covered in subsequent chapters. The use of extravascular techniques is beyond the scope of this book.

In the venous system, one can collect selective venous samples for assay. The most widely used assay is renal vein renin, which is elevated in patients with renovascular hypertension [12, 26]. It is also used for study in patients with functioning tumors of the adrenal glands [4, 8, 9] and parathyroid glands [5, 6, 23, 31] and the gonads. Medullary cell carcinoma of the thyroid gland and its metastatic deposits secrete higher than normal levels of thyrocalcitonin. Selective venous samplings for assay gives an accurate measure of the extent of the patient's disease [10]. Innovations in selective catheterization of the pancreatic veins through a transhepatic approach [15, 18, 24, 29] allow radioimmunologic determination of insulin in islet cell tumors as well as specific hormone assays for the rarer pancreatic islet cell tumors.

With computed tomography, ultrasonography, and radiographic biplane or C-arm photofluorographic facilities, percutaneous needle biopsies can be performed in virtually every part of the body. Added safety is ensured by using a variety of different needles, most with a small outside diameter (22 French). Puncture and subsequent drainage of intraabdominal, intrathoracic, and pelvic abscesses, cysts, and hematomas are common. One can perform transhepatic diagnostic and therapeutic maneuvers, such as simple parenchymal biopsy, biliary drainage and stenting, removal of stones, and dilating biliary strictures. Percutaneous transrenal removal of renal calculi, drainage of obstructed urinary tracts, and dilatation and stenting of strictured ureters has also become common practice.

References

1. Bergquist, E., et al. Stationary waves of segmental vasoconstriction. *Acta Radiol. [Diagn.] (Stockh.)* 11:497, 1971.
2. Boijsen, E. Pancreatic Angiography. In H. Abrams (ed.), *Abrams Angiography: Vascular and Interventional Radiology* (3rd ed.). Boston: Little, Brown, 1983.
3. Bookstein, J., and Voegeli, E. Critical analysis of magnification radiography. *Radiology* 98:23, 1971.
4. Cho, K. J. Current role of angiography in the evaluation of adrenal disease causing hypertension. *Urol. Radiol.* 3:249, 1982.
5. Doppman, J. L. The treatment of hyperparathyroidism by transcatheter techniques. *Cardiovasc. Intervent. Radiol.* 3:268, 1980.
6. Doppman, J. L., and Hammond, W. The anatomic basis of parathyroid venous sampling. *Radiology* 95:603, 1970.
7. Doumanian, H., and Amplatz, K. Vascular jet collapse in selective angiocardiography. *A.J.R.* 100:344, 1967.
8. Dunnick, N. R., et al. Preoperative diagnosis and localization of aldesteronomas by measurement of corticosteroids in adrenal venous blood. *Radiology* 133:331, 1979.
9. Dunnick, N. R., et al. Localization of functional adrenal tumors by computed tomography and venous sampling. *Radiology* 142:429, 1982.
10. Goltzman, D., et al. Calcitonin as a tumor marker. *N. Engl. J. Med.* 290:1035, 1974.
11. Greenspan, R. Magnification Angiography. In H. Abrams (ed.), *Abrams Angiography: Vascular and Interventional Radiology* (3rd ed.). Boston: Little, Brown, 1983.
12. Harrington, D., et al. Determination of optimum methods for renal venous renin sampling in suspected renovascular hypertension. *Invest. Radiol.* 10:452, 1975.
13. Hawkins, I. F., Jr. Carbon dioxide digital subtraction arteriography. *A.J.R.* 139:19, 1982.
14. Hollenberg, N. D., Garnic, J. D., and Harrington, D. P. Pharmacoangiography. In H. Abrams (ed.), *Abrams' Angiography: Vascular and Interventional Radiology* (3rd ed.). Boston: Little, Brown, 1983.
15. Ingemansson, S., et al. Portal and pancreatic vein catheterization with radioimmunologic determination of insulin. *Surg. Gynecol. Obstet.* 141:705, 1975.

16. Jekell, K., Sandqvist S., and Castenfoos, J. Angiotensin effect in the human kidney. *Acta. Radiol. [Diagn.] (Stockh.)* 19:329, 1978.
17. Kahn, P. Reactive hyperemia in lower extremity angiography: An evaluation. *Radiology* 90:975, 1968.
18. Krudy, A. G., et al. Localization of islet cell tumors by dynamic CT: Comparison with plain CT, arteriography, sonography, and venous sampling. *A.J.R.* 143:585, 1984.
19. Miller, P., et al. Epidural anesthesia in aortofemoral arteriography. *Ann. Surg.* 192:227, 1980.
20. Miller, R., et al. Gastrointestinal response to minute doses of glucagon. *Radiology* 143:317, 1982.
21. Moncada, S., et al. E Series of Prostaglandin and Derivatives. In A. G. Gilman, et al. (eds.), *The Pharmacological Basis of Therapeutics* (7th ed.). New York: Macmillan, 1985.
22. Mooring, F. J., Hughes, G. S., and Johnsrude, I. S. Role of beta-endorphins in analgesia associated with reactive hyperemia. *Invest. Radiol.* 1985.
23. Obley D. L., Parathyroid adenomas studied by digital subtraction angiography. *Radiology* 153:449, 1984.
24. Roche, A., Raisonnier, A., and Gillon-Savouret, M. C. Pancreatic venous sampling and arteriography in localizing insulinomas and gastrinomas: Procedure and results in 55 cases. *Radiology* 145:621, 1982.
25. Rossi, R., Hendu, W., and Ahrens, C. An evaluation of rare earth screen/film combinations. *Radiology* 121:465, 1976.
26. Schambelan, M., et al. Role of renin and aldosterone in hypertension due to a renin secreting tumor. *Am. J. Med.* 55:86, 1973.
27. Theander, G. Arteriography demonstration of stationary arterial waves. *Acta Radiol.* 53:417, 1960.
28. Tindall, J., Whalen, R., and Burton, E. Medical uses of intra-arterial injections of reserpine: Treatment of Raynaud's syndrome and of some vascular insufficiencies of the lower extremities. *Arch. Dermatol.* 110:233, 1974.
29. Viamonte, M., Jr., et al. Selective catheterization of the portal vein and its tributaries. *Radiology* 119:457, 1975.
30. Viamonte, M., Jr., Roen, S., and Lepage, J., Nonspecificity of abnormal vascularity in the angiographic diagnosis of malignant neoplasms. *Radiology* 106:59, 1973.
31. Wells, S., et al. The preoperative localization of hyperfunctioning parathyroid tissue utilizing parathyroid hormone radioimmunoassay of plasma from selectively catheterized thyroid veins. *N.C. Med. J.* 35:678, 1974.

II

Interventional Catheterization

There are a number of comprehensive textbooks and articles on the subject of both intra- and extravascular interventional procedures. In this book we consider only those interventional procedures that are related to the vascular system. The three chapters of Part II describe the general principles involved in these techniques. The procedures performed in specific vascular beds will be discussed in the appropriate chapter of Part III.

Therapeutic Embolization

Intravascular embolization developed from surgical techniques by which arteriovenous malformations involving peripheral vessels were more successfully obliterated by embolizing with small particles than by surgical ligation [6]. Embolizing vessels by intravascular catheters is a natural expansion of diagnostic angiography and has been developed to treat a number of acute and chronic vascular abnormalities. First used to control acute gastrointestinal bleeding or life-threatening hemorrhage from other sources, other applications soon developed. These include: temporary or definitive treatment of aneurysms, arteriovenous fistulas, and arteriovenous malformations; temporary alleviation of vascular complications of trauma; palliation or treatment of complications of tumors; preoperative occlusion of hypervascular tumors; decrease of functioning tumor hormone production; and intravascular treatment of certain large central arteriovenous shunts (e.g., closure of a patent ductus arteriosus).

General Principles of Embolization

There are two major equipment components to an embolization procedure, the embolic material and the system used for delivering the emboli [2, 3, 4, 11, 12, 25, 31, 38].

The best *embolic agent* is nontoxic, easy to deliver, safe to inject, radiopaque for easy localization, and produces a complete permanent occlusion of vessels. There is no single embolic agent that can be used for all purposes.

The *delivery system* varies to accommodate the differing size and consistency of embolic material required for a given vascular bed. It also depends on the location of the target lesion and the ease with which it can be approached. The catheter must be large enough to allow the embolic material to pass easily, and the catheter shape should allow its tip to be firmly lodged into the orifice of the target vessel.

Various methods for catheterizing vessels are described in the preceding chapter and in later chapters; with few variations, these same techniques are used for therapeutic catheterization.

Meticulous catheterization technique is necessary during embolization procedures. Single-wall punctures are preferable, since bleeding around the puncture site is not well tolerated in the long-term catheterization sometimes required for therapy. Heparin cannot be administered if the patient has an ongoing or potential source of bleeding. Because catheters delivering embolic material may become obstructed and require exchanging, they are best introduced into the femoral artery through a thin-walled sheath (Fig. 5-1). These catheters are available with a hemostasis valve to prevent back-bleeding, and a side arm that is continuously or intermittently flushed to prevent clot from forming around the catheter.

Technique should include use of state-of-the-art fluoroscopy to monitor proper positioning of the catheter tip, the transport of the emboli, and the earliest hemodynamic changes that occur subsequent to occluding the vessels.

Embolic Materials

The number of different types of embolic materials available is constantly growing. In general, those currently in common use can be divided into 3 broad categories: (1) Particulate absorbable materials causing temporary occlusion of the vessels (autogenous clot, Gelfoam, Oxycel, Avitene), (2) Particulate nonabsorbable materials causing permanent occlusion (Ivalon [polyvinyl alcohol], coils with attached Dacron strands, detachable balloons, autogenous muscle, barium-impregnated Silastic beads, Silastic-coated metal beads, and others), and (3) Liquid embolic materials, which usually pass through into the arteriolar or capillary bed, causing permanent vascular occlusion (absolute alcohol, tissue adhesives). The embolic material chosen depends on the following factors [3, 25]:

1. Whether long- or short-term occlusion is desired. Gastrointestinal bleeding and tumors that are embolized preoperatively require only short-term occlusion, whereas arteriovenous malformations (AVMs) or certain other tumors require permanent occlusion. Autogenous

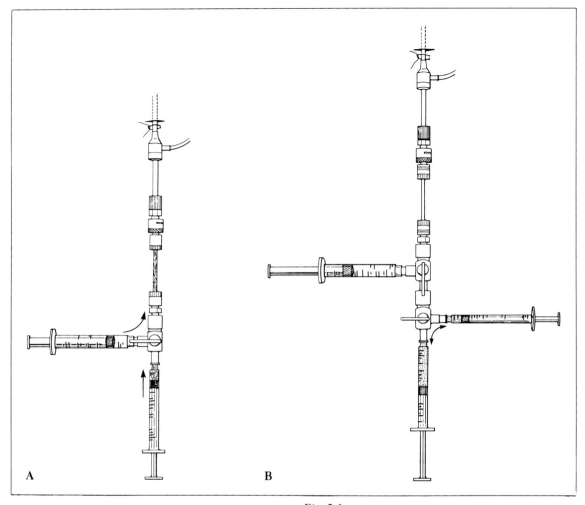

A   B

Fig. 5-1.

stabilized clots occlude vessels for short periods of time before lysis intervenes. Gelfoam occludes for longer periods, whereas Ivalon, coils, detachable balloons, and tissue adhesives provide more permanent occlusion.

2. The pathologic nature of the circulation being embolized, its collateral supply, and the effects of acute occlusion of tissues beyond the site of embolization. Total occlusion of the vascular bed of a tumor requires microparticles or a liquid polymer. A focal occlusion of a single vessel or an arteriovenous fistula may require a detachable balloon or coil.

3. The patient's ability to form clot. Deficiency of clotting factors requires an exogenous embolic agent.

A. Catheter sheath sutured in place at the femoral artery puncture site. Side arm connected to constant positive pressure flush. Hemostasis valve prevents leaking around the catheter. A small-gauge, short connecting tube is attached directly to the catheter hub; a three-way stopcock controls injection of particulate emboli followed by flush with dilute contrast agent. Low-dose heparin is administered unless contraindicated. A similar arrangement is used for injecting a liquid polymer except when connected to an inner coaxial catheter.

B. An additional three-way stopcock and syringe provides means for agitating Ivalon particles, keeping them in suspension during injection.

4. The toxicity of the embolic material. Certain tissue adhesives [46, 47] rapidly and permanently occlude blood vessels. When forcefully injected into a closed system, they may penetrate deeply into the microcirculation, induce a perivascular inflammatory response, and cause subsequent tissue infarction. These adhesives are more prone to form a perivascular inflammatory response than are inert materials such as Ivalon or silicone rubber.

5. The location and vascular anatomy of the lesion or target organ. The requirements for occluding small branches of a peripheral lesion are sometimes different from those of a proximal major vessel.

6. Plans for future treatment may affect the choice of materials and location of embolization. If serial occlusions are required, the primary feeding vessel must be left intact.

PARTICULATE ABSORBABLE MATERIALS

Most particulate absorbable materials can be introduced directly through a standard 5 to 7 French catheter with tapered preformed tip. Materials of a known larger diameter may require the tip of the catheter to be untapered.

Stabilized Autogenous Clot

Stabilized autogenous clot [5] is rapidly absorbed. The clot is more resistant to lysis if stabilized by adding 300 NIH units (5 drops) of thrombin. The thrombin clots the fibrinogen directly. Epsilon aminocaproic acid (Amicar)[1] inhibits fibrinolysis. One milliliter (250 mg) of this material may be added to 10 ml of the patient's blood. The stabilized clot is easily delivered through the catheter into the target vessel when injected with a syringe.

Gelfoam

Gelfoam gelatin sponge[2] (Fig. 5-2) is easily available, nonirritating, and nonantigenic and occludes vessels by forming a matrix for developing clot [1, 33]. It provides a more stable occlusion of vessels than does blood clot, usually being resorbed and

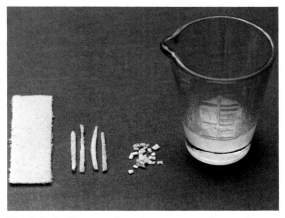

Fig. 5-2. Gelfoam in sheet form; sectioned; mixed with contrast medium to form a slurry.

the vessel recanalized within 6 weeks [33, 47]. Gelfoam may be obtained in small sheets or in powdered form. Strips of the Gelfoam sheets 2 × 5 mm or 2 × 10 mm may be cut and immersed in saline solution or contrast medium for 15 to 30 minutes to form a gelatinous sludge that is easily injected through small standard diameter (5, 6, or 7 French) catheters [1]. Antibiotics may be added to counter infection, and tantalum powder to make the material radiopaque.

A short, translucent, small diameter connecting tube between the syringe and catheter hub provides some control of the quantity of sludge injected (see Fig. 1B). Small amounts are introduced followed by a slow controlled injection of 30 to 40% contrast medium. By this means the emboli may be seen traveling to their destination, and the earliest sign of reflux detected.

Larger particles of Gelfoam ("torpedoes") may be placed directly into a tuberculin syringe and injected slowly, forcing the embolus through the catheter to its tip. There is some resistance to the injection up to this point. When this resistance is suddenly decreased, the embolus has extruded into the vessel and the force of the injection should be eased to avoid reflux.

Gelfoam powder is rarely needed. It may pass into peripheral arterioles and cause tissue infarction.

Figure 5-3 shows bleeding sites and arteriovenous fistula in the mesenteric and celiac circulation occluded with Gelfoam.

---

[1]Manufactured by Lederle Laboratories, Pearl River, NY 10965.
[2]Manufactured by Upjohn Co., Kalamazoo, MI 49001.

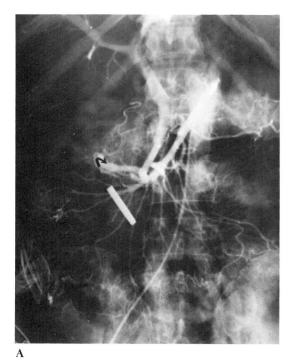

A

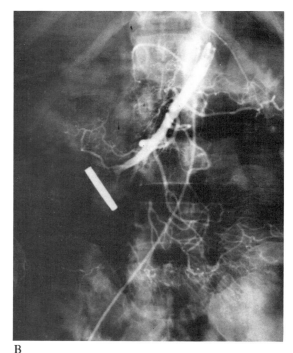

B

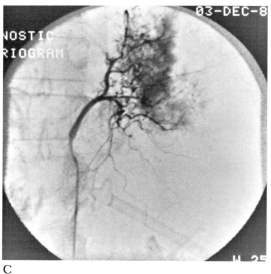

C

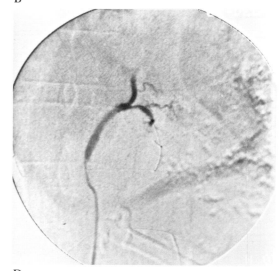

D

Fig. 5-3. A and B. Embolizing an exsanguinating gastrointestinal bleed.

A. Extravasation of contrast medium due to bleeding and arteriovenous fistula in a postoperative patient operated on for bowel malignancy (a nonsurgical candidate).

B. The fistula is occluded and the bleeding stopped following Gelfoam embolization. The patient survived without bowel ischemia (likely due to collaterals through intestinal arcades).

C and D. Bleeding from a nonresectable large gastric tumor.

C. Left gastric arteriogram demonstrates hypervascular tumor.

D. More permanent occlusion obtained with multiple Ivalon microparticles. Intraarterial digital subtraction angiograms expedite the procedure.

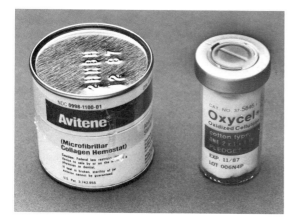

Fig. 5-4. Oxidized cellulose (Oxycel) and microfibrillar collagen (Avitene).

Oxycel

Oxycel (oxidized cellulose)[3] (Fig. 5-4) also occludes vessels by forming a matrix for the development of clot, much like Gelfoam.

Avitene

Avitene[4] [15] is microfibrillar bovine collagen. It is also prepared by soaking in saline or dilute contrast agent. The thin slurry can be easily injected through small catheters. It occludes vessels at the arteriolar level primarily by platelet aggregation and subsequent clot formation.

PARTICULATE NONABSORBABLE MATERIALS

The list of particulate nonabsorbable materials is continually expanding and currently includes Ivalon (polyvinyl alcohol),[5] spring coils of varying helix size with attached Dacron threads, stainless steel coils with barbs, metallic "spiders" [8] with or without attached Ivalon, tufts of silk, and plastic brushes, autogenous fat and muscle, barium-impregnated Silastic beads, Silastic-coated metallic beads of varying diameter, and a variety of detachable balloons. Only the more commonly used embolic agents will be described here. Others are included in Appendix 16 or are described in cited references.

---

[3]Manufactured by Parke-Davis, Div. Warner-Lambert Inc., 201 Tabor Rd., Morris Plains, NJ 07950.
[4]Manufactured by Alcon Laboratories, Inc., P.O. Box 1959, 6201 South Freeway, Fort Worth, TX 76134.
[5]Manufactured by Unipoint Laboratories, High Point, NC 27260. Also by Ingenor Medical Systems, 70 rue Orfila, 75020 Paris, France.

Ivalon

Ivalon [31, 36, 43, 46, 51] is an inert plastic foam that occludes the vessel and becomes ingrown by granulation tissue to become an integral part of the body. It comes in sheet form or small particles of varying grain size. When the sheet is soaked in saline solution, compressed in a vise and allowed to dry, it is reduced 15-fold in size; it returns to its original size in 3 minutes when replaced in a solution. Because of this feature, relatively small Ivalon pellets may pass through standard diameter catheters to produce vascular occlusion when they make contact with blood. Smaller Ivalon particles in nonuniform grain diameters are commercially available and are most popular in our laboratory. They are available in the following ranges of grain size (1 mm = 1000 μm):

190 to 250 μm
250 to 400 μm
400 to 590 μm
590 to 1000 μm

A 5 French thin-walled catheter easily accepts particulate emboli of up to 590 μm. A 4 French catheter accepts particulate matter of up to approximately 400 μm, and a 3 French particulate emboli up to 250 μm. Therefore, most of these, up to 590 μm, can be delivered through standard size tapered 5 to 7 French vascular diagnostic catheters. Larger emboli require larger diameter nontapered catheters introduced percutaneously through a sheath.

The Ivalon traps air and the particles have a high surface tension, which makes them difficult to inject. They are easier to deliver if stabilized by suspending the mixture in saline or low molecular weight dextran, mixing in a blender at high speed (10 minutes) and then slow speed (an additional 10 minutes), and then sterilizing. The mixture is added to equal parts of 60% contrast agent prior to injection.

The delivery system for Ivalon particles is similar to that for Gelfoam. The particles are agitated by rapid transfer from one 3-ml syringe to another through a three-way stopcock (see Fig. 5-1A), which further improves the suspension. A short connecting tube allows the particles to be seen as they pass to the catheter. The flow of particles to the lesion is monitored fluoroscopically while the system is flushed with controlled injections of 30% contrast medium.

Combined Ivalon and Gelfoam Emboli

Small Ivalon particles mixed with a slurry of Gelfoam [28] provides the combined ease of delivering the Gelfoam with the permanent occlusion of the Ivalon. Ivalon and Gelfoam should be mixed in equal parts. The mixture slides easily through the catheter, but its delivery should be tested prior to use in the patient.

Steel Coils

Commercially available steel coils [9, 10, 22] with attached Dacron streamers are made from 5-cm lengths of stainless steel guidewires from which the central core has been removed. The Dacron streamers provide the matrix for clot formation and permanent occlusion. They come prepared in color-coded cartridges[6] (Fig. 5-5).

When the catheter tip engages the target vessel, the cartridge is introduced into the hub of the catheter and the coil is advanced into the catheter shaft using the stiff end of a 0.038-in. straight tipped guidewire. After removing the empty cartridge, the flexible end of the straight tipped guidewire is substituted for its stiff end, to advance the coil around curves to eventually extrude into the target vessel (Figs. 5-6, 5-7). If the coil is not in the precise desired location once it is released, it can be pushed further into the vessel with the guidewire or the catheter tip.

There are varying diameters of the helix of the coils (3 mm, 5 mm, 8 mm), which may be advanced only through standard tapered catheters that accept a 0.038-in. guidewire (6.5 French or thin-walled 5.5 French). A 5-mm helix diameter is chosen to occlude a vessel of comparable diameter. If the vessel diameter is much smaller than that of the helix, the coil elongates and may back out into an undesirable location (Figs. 5-8, 5-9); if the vessel diameter is larger than that of the helix, the coil does not snugly fit the vessel wall and either migrates to a more peripheral location or refluxes out into the general circulation (see Fig. 5-8). Minicoils constructed with a 2.5-mm helix pass through an inner 3 French coaxial catheter, with a 0.018-in. guidewire used for delivery.

[6]Manufactured by Cook Inc., P.O. Box 489, Bloomington, IN 47401.

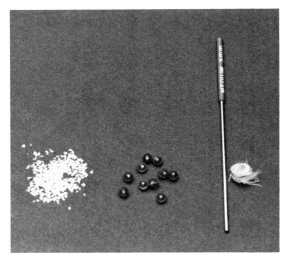

Fig. 5-5. Particulate nonabsorbable material. Left, Ivalon (polyvinyl alcohol sponge), prepackaged emboli of varying sizes. Center, Silastic-coated metal beads. Right, steel coils, within the introducer and uncoiled; these come in four separate sizes.

An improved delivery system may place the coils more distally beyond the end of the catheter. The proximal end of the coil is attached to the distal end of the specially modified guidewire [34]. The tethered proximal and distal tips of a 0.025-in. guidewire are clipped, thereby allowing the inner core to move freely within the outer coiled spring layer. A 10-cm length of the inner safety wire is exposed by clipping off an equal length of its outer coiled spring layer. The Gianturco coil is gently pushed retrograde through the cartridge (using a straight guidewire), thereby exposing 1 millimeter proximally. A 5-cm length of the wire core is next advanced through the straightened Gianturco coil and is anchored down its length. The Gianturco coil may be more firmly attached to the introducing guidewire core by uncoiling each presenting spring layer and meshing the two together. The assembly is sterilized and made ready for use. If the desired location for embolization is more remote than where the catheter tip can be advanced, the 0.025-in. wire/Gianturco coil assembly is advanced through the catheter beyond its tip to the target area. The Gianturco coil is released by withdrawing the inner guidewire core against the leading edge of its outer layer.

Problems arising during delivery of these coils may be avoided by choosing the correct catheter,

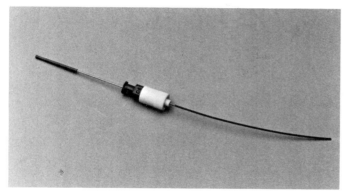

A

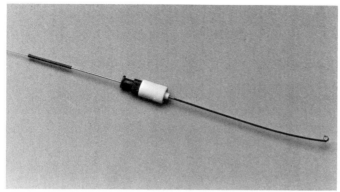

B

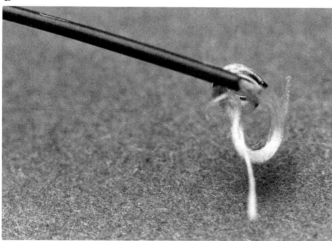

C

Fig 5-6. Steel coil introduced through a 3 French
catheter. Choose correct inside diameter of catheter
recommended for introducing the coil. (See text.)
A. Capsule holding the coil is introduced into the hub
   of the catheter.
B. Coil is pushed through with a 0.018-in. guidewire
   and extruded from the distal catheter tip.
C. Close up view.

guidewire, and coil, and by properly positioning
the catheter tip.

1. A coil may become unraveled, jammed, and
   difficult to displace from the catheter. This
   happens when the coil is advanced through a
   catheter larger (7 or 8 French) than the recommended diameter (thin-walled 5 or standard

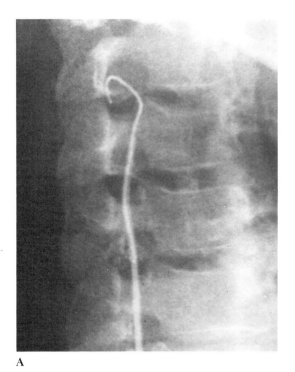

A

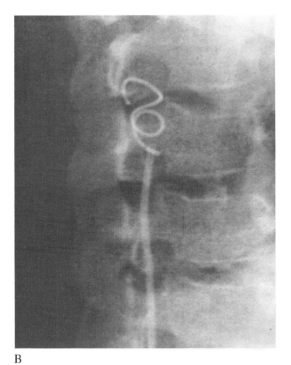

B

Fig. 5-7. Coils curl as they eject from the distal tip of the catheter introduced high in the vertebral artery.

6.5 French). It also occurs if a 2.5-mm coil is advanced in a catheter larger than 3 French. If the jammed coil remains entirely within the catheter, the catheter should be withdrawn through the overlying sheath.
2. If the coil is caught in the catheter tip and is only partially ejected, it may be dislodged into the target artery by injecting normal saline at high pressures.

Fig. 5-8. The diameter of the helix of the coil must closely match the diameter of the artery. If too small, the coil may embolize peripherally. If too large, the wire coil elongates.

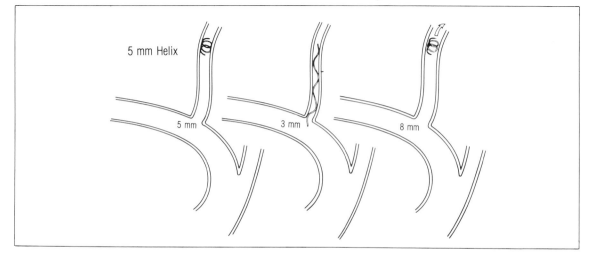

final closure of the orifice of the vessel being with the coil. A limiting factor in using coils is that they cannot be flow-guided down to a remote target area. They must be delivered at the catheter tip or advanced further by being attached to the inner core of a modified 0.025-in. guidewire.

Silastic-coated Metal Beads

Silastic-coated metal beads and barium-impregnated Silastic beads[7,8] [35] are inert nonantigenic particles that are produced in many sizes (0.5 to 3.0 mm). A special apparatus [7] (NYU introducer sheath) is used for the safe introduction of the larger particles into the vascular system (Fig. 5-10) [27].

BALLOON CATHETERS

Balloon catheters have balloons that are (1) permanently attached, (2) permanently attached with a calibrated leak, or (3) detachable. Those with permanently attached balloons are occlusive balloon catheters. Those with the calibrated leak are used for delivering liquid agents into the microcirculation. Detachable balloons are left behind in the vessel and used as an embolic agent.

Occlusive Balloon Catheters

These may have either a single lumen (used solely for inflating the balloon) or two lumina (one for inflating the balloon and the other for injecting contrast medium or other injectables).

The single-lumen occlusive balloon (Fogarty) *catheter* is introduced coaxially and advanced through the selectively placed outer catheter. A 2 French (0.66-mm) Fogarty balloon may be inflated up to a 4-mm diameter using 0.05 ml contrast agent. It can pass through a standard 6.5 or thin-walled 5 French catheter, which accepts a 0.038-in. guidewire. A 3 French (1-mm) Fogarty catheter can pass through a 7 French untapered catheter with an inside diameter of 0.05 in. (1.37 mm).

An occlusive balloon catheter with two lumina requires a catheter sheath at the puncture site for introduction. It allows both diagnostic contrast studies and temporary therapeutic occlusion of a

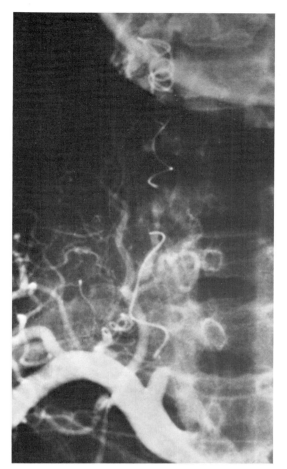

Fig. 5-9. Multiple coils and Ivalon microparticles are introduced into a right vertebral arteriovenous malformation (AVM) (see Fig. 14-34). Coils high in the AVM are in good position. The proximal coil is elongated due to stenosis of the vessel and to mismatched diameters of the coil and the vessel lumen.

3. The Dacron strands may become bunched into the catheter tip, causing withdrawal of the coil from its intended position when the catheter is removed. The coil must be retrieved (see Chap. 7). If the catheter tip is not properly fixated into the vessel orifice prior to releasing the coil, the coil may reflux into the general circulation. In this instance also the coil must be retrieved.

Despite potential problems, complications are rare, and coils are an excellent way to permanently occlude vessels in very precise focal areas. They may be used as the only means of occluding a vessel. Coils may also be combined with smaller embolic agents delivered more peripherally, the

---

[7]Manufactured by Brunswick Manufacturing Co., Quincy, MA 02171.
[8]Manufactured by Heyer Schulte, P.O. Box 946, Goleta, CA 93017. Also by Ingenor Medical Systems.

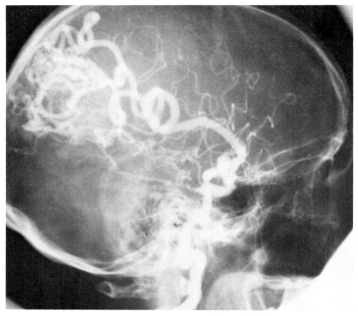

A

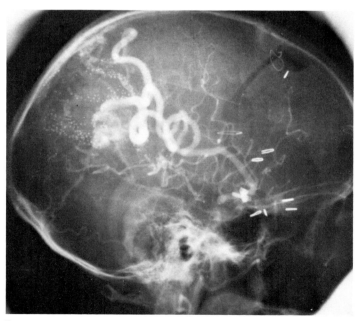

B

Fig. 5-10. A large intracranial arteriovenous malformation (AVM) supplied by branches of the middle cerebral artery. There is a berry aneurysm in the supraclinoid portion of the internal carotid artery.

A. Preembolization. The large internal carotid artery permitted selective placement of a 10 French catheter from a percutaneous femoral approach; this allowed the use of 2.5-mm Silastic-coated metallic beads.

B. Embolization of the AVM with 294 metallic beads. (Embolization followed surgical correction of the berry aneurysm.)

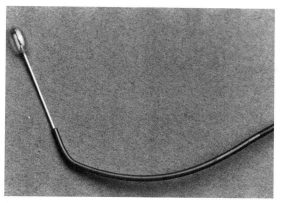

A

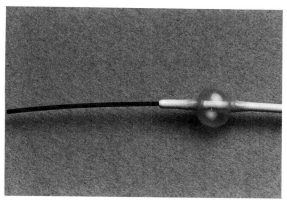

B

Fig. 5-11.
A. A 2 French Fogarty balloon catheter protruding beyond the tip of the 5 French thin-walled tapered
catheter.
B. A Berenstein occlusive balloon catheter with inner
3 French catheter. Useful for injecting tissue adhesives, microcoils, and tiny particulate emboli into
more remote areas. An inner open-ended injectable guidewire useful for injecting embolic materials may be substituted for the 3 French catheter.

vessel. It may be inflated during injection of certain embolic materials to help control their flow
and final position, and to prevent reflux into nontarget areas [26]. Most double-lumen occlusive
balloon catheters have a relatively small lumen for
delivering embolic materials, but there is one[9] that
accommodates a 0.038-in. guidewire and a coaxial
3 French catheter. This catheter allows superselective placement of microcoils or other injectables
into peripheral vessels, which is helpful in occluding tumors and AVMs in critical areas, such as the
external carotid circulation (Figs. 5-11, 5-12).

Calibrated Leak Catheters
Calibrated leak catheters[10,11] are soft flow-guided
single-lumen microcatheters (2 French) with a
calibrated leak in the inflated balloon. They are
devised for selective placement of intravascular tissue adhesives [30] and are described further in Appendix 16.

---

[9]Berenstein double-lumen balloon catheter, manufactured by
MediTech Division, Cooper Scientific Corp., 372 Main St.,
Watertown, MA 02172.
[10]Kerber balloon, manufactured by Cook Inc., P.O. Box 489,
Bloomington, IN 47401.
[11]Debruns jet controlled catheter system, manufactured by Ingenor Medical Systems, 70 rue Orfila, 75020 Paris, France.

Detachable Balloon Catheters
Detachable balloon catheters are useful when the
target vessel is in a distal location. The balloon
catheter may be injected beyond the introducing
catheter or flow-guided to the region. The vessel is
occluded by inflating the balloon. If its position is
not satisfactory, the balloon may be deflated and
repositioned. Once accurately positioned, the balloon is inflated (with isosmolar or nonionic contrast agent) and released for permanent placement.
An example of this application is closure of a
carotid cavernous fistula, where imprecise placement and dislodgement would result in significant
neurologic damage.

There are a number of detachable balloons, and
their delivery systems have been described [13, 14,
38, 42, 45]. Two of these are more widely used,
and they are available and approved for commercial release [13, 45]. The delivery systems for detachable balloons are more complicated than other
methods. Further details are described in Appendix 16.

LIQUID OR SEMILIQUID EMBOLIC MATERIALS
Liquid and semiliquid embolic materials (Fig.
5-13) include tissue adhesive (isobutyl 2-cyanoac-
rylate [bucrylate][12]), ethanol, sclerosing agents,
contrast agents, and silicone rubber.

Bucrylate
Bucrylate, or isobutyl 2-cyanoacrylate, is a controlled substance and requires an Investigational

---

[12]Manufactured by Ethicon, Route 22, Sommerville, NJ
08876.

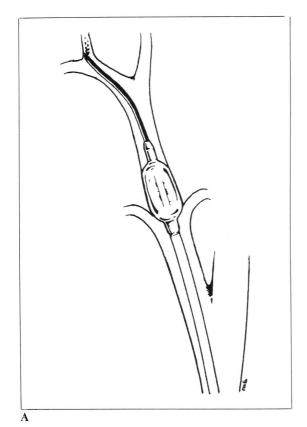

A

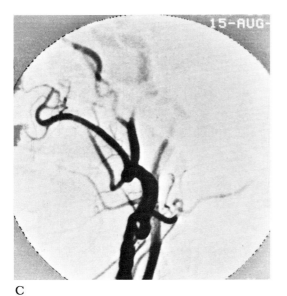

C

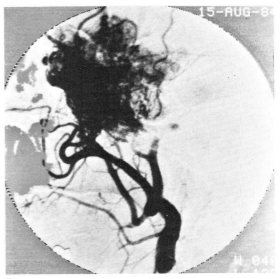

B

Fig. 5-12.
A. Line drawing showing a Berenstein occlusive balloon catheter in external carotid artery, with coaxial
   3 French catheter protruding.
B and C. Multiple external carotid branches feeding an
   arteriovenous malformation occluded with bucrylate. IA-DSA monitoring.

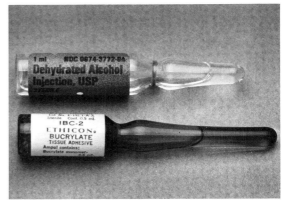

Fig. 5-13. Liquid embolic materials: 95% ethanol (*top*)
and isobutyl 2-cyanoacrylate (bucrylate) (*bottom*).

New Drug (IND) number. It is a rapidly acting
monomer tissue adhesive that forms a polymer on
contact with blood, tissue, or any ionized material
[19, 24, 27]. Within 1 second, a rapid and permanent occlusion of blood vessels results with varying
degrees of perivascular inflammatory response. A
recent report by the manufacturer describes a possible carcinogenic potential when used experimentally in rats. This limits its availability and suggests

that it should be used only in very limited circumstances.

The tissue adhesive may be made radiopaque without influencing its polymerization time by adding small amounts of nonionized sterilized tantalum[13] (1 g per milliliter of bucrylate). Tantalum is available in a 5-μm size and is charcoal gray in color. If skin or subcutaneous structures in light-skinned patients are being embolized, the tantalum powder should be exchanged for white tantalum oxide. The bucrylate may also be opacified by adding equal volumes of Pantopaque. This increases the polymerization time of the adhesive to 3 seconds, which provides greater penetration into the vascular system and allows time for withdrawing the catheter after its delivery. These radiopaque materials should be mixed with the bucrylate immediately prior to injection.

In order to avoid premature hardening, the tissue adhesive must be completely separated from ionic materials until it enters the bloodstream, where there is almost instant occlusion. If certain precautions are not observed, the bucrylate hardens within the catheter and can adhere its tip to the vessel wall.

It is best to use a 3 French coaxial catheter passed through a 5 French thin-walled or standard 6.5 French tapered catheter, in turn inserted through a sheath at the puncture site. However, the inflated balloon of an outer 6 French Berenstein occlusive balloon catheter helps to regulate the flow and final position of the adhesive injected through the more distally located 3 French inner coaxial catheter. Only very small measured amounts of bucrylate are injected from a tuberculin syringe attached by a three-way stopcock to the 3 French catheter. A 5-ml syringe filled with 5% dextrose (ion-free) is attached to the same stopcock and is used to flush the catheter system both prior to and after introducing the bucrylate. A small measured dose of bucrylate (0.2 to 0.4 ml) is injected and is immediately flushed from the catheter to the artery with a controlled injection of small amounts of 5% dextrose. The 3 French inner catheter is immediately withdrawn.

PRECAUTIONS. If the adhesive is flushed in too slowly, the catheter tip may stick to the vessel wall. Slowly withdrawing the 3 French catheter during the second flush of 5% dextrose helps to prevent this. Know the precise volume of the 3 French catheter, for this determines the volume and rate of each injection. Liberally cover the tip of the catheter with a coating of sterile silicone ointment, which prevents adhesion of the catheter tip. Avoid large rapid injections of the adhesive. It may not only reflux back to adhere to the catheter tip but also may permeate down into the precapillary levels, obstructing all collateral flow and causing an occlusion so complete it causes tissue infarction. Focal precise areas of occlusion may be achieved. Important variables in controlling the injection are (1) the polymerization time, which is lengthened, permitting greater penetration, by adding Pantopaque to the adhesive; (2) the rate and volume of injection—0.2 to 0.4 ml is recommended but varies, gauged by a prior controlled contrast injection; and (3) an inflated balloon limits peripheral flow.

An angiogram is performed by injecting contrast medium through the outer catheter after removing the 3 French catheter. If further embolization is required, insert another 3 French catheter.

Bucrylate is used to occlude vascular tumors and AVMs in the brain (through a calibrated leak balloon); to control bleeding (upper gastrointestinal tract, esophageal varices, trauma); to occlude the splenic artery in patients with hypersplenism or esophageal varices; to occlude arteriovenous fistulas, AVMs, and aneurysms; to preoperatively devascularize vascular tumors; to perform medical nephrectomies. Bucrylate can be injected transcutaneously directly into certain cutaneous vascular lesions.

Complications of tissue adhesives include: infarction of tissue with necrosis or abscess formation; embolization of nontarget areas; and adhesion of the catheter within the vessel wall.

Alcohol

The denaturing proteins of 95% ethanol [20, 21, 41, 50] cause vasculitis, which damages vascular walls and occludes vessels down to the small artery and capillary level.

Advantages of ethanol are that it is cheap, easily available (obtained in ampules from the hospital pharmacy), nonviscous, and therefore easily delivered. It causes little or no damage when diluted. Therefore, reflux into the general circulation is not as great a danger, as with other agents.

---

[13] Manufactured by Keana Metal, 55-T, Concord Road, Warminster, PA 18974. Also by Ingenor Medical Systems.

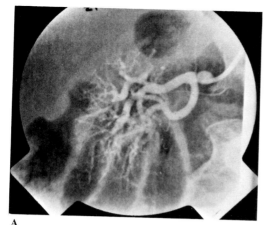

A

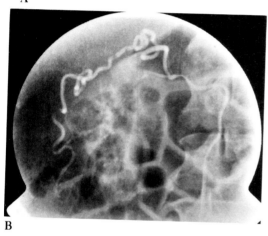

B

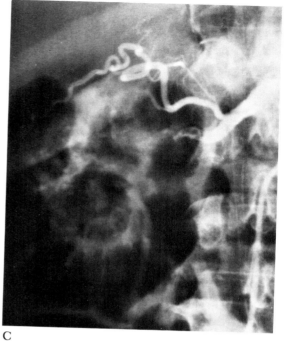

C

Fig. 5-14.
A. Double-lumen occlusive balloon catheter inflated in renal artery while embolizing renal vascular bed with absolute alcohol.
B. Capsular feeding artery embolized using open-ended guidewire.
C. Renal artery and peripheral capsular branch occluded. Patient was a nonsurgical candidate with a renal tumor and uncontrollable hypoglycemia and accompanying renal failure.

Disadvantages relate to its penetration into the microcirculation, causing tissue infarction, sloughing when too near the skin surface, or neural damage if it is injected near major nerves. This limits the sites where ethanol may be used. Its injection is always associated with considerable discomfort, which lasts during and some time after its injection. Narcotics, sedation, or sometimes general anesthesia are required.

Absolute alcohol is used to ablate an organ, a tumor (e.g., unresectable renal tumor), certain AVMs, and esophageal varices, by direct injection into the involved vessels.

The amount injected depends on the size of the vascular bed requiring occlusion. In large vascular tumors, a bolus of 10 to 15 ml is injected at a steady rate over a period of 3 to 5 seconds. Use of small volumes of ethanol, with repeat injections if necessary, avoids injury to neighboring organs due to reflux.

A coaxial system, together with an occluding balloon, limits the area injected and prevents reflux into the aorta (Fig. 5-14). The balloon should remain inflated to allow total occlusion of the vascular bed.

Sclerosing Agents

Sclerosing agents are 50% glucose; sodium decadrol. Esophageal varices are occluded when these agents are delivered mixed with Gelfoam.

Contrast Agents [16, 18]

Parenchymal necrosis results when certain small organs with end organ vessels (parathyroid adenomas) are overinjected with large doses of contrast agents of high concentration. This is due to direct chemotoxicity and hyperosmolarity of the contrast agent. Similar parenchymal staining and necrosis is induced in certain organs with a limited and fragile venous bed (e.g., adrenals) by retrograde overinjection of contrast agent. To ensure maximal cell contact with the vascular endothelium, the catheter tip should be wedged into the vessel during and for some time after the injection. The volume of contrast agent should be 2 to 3 times that for a diagnostic study.

Contrast agents may be heated to boiling and injected directly into the venous system. This induces intimal damage and an inflammatory response with subsequent thrombotic occlusion [12]. It has been used successfully in sclerotherapy of varicoceles.

Silicone Rubber

Silicone rubber [3, 17, 32] is a high-viscosity, biocompatible liquid that, when injected and polymerized, forms a nonadhesive cast of the vascular bed into which it is injected, causing permanent occlusion. It is most helpful in the treatment of AVMs. Silicone rubber[14,15] for this application is an investigational material, requiring an IND number, is difficult to obtain, and requires experimental laboratory animal experience prior to use in a patient. Further details are described in Appendix 16.

Other Substances

Other liquid experimental materials are described in Appendix 16 (Polyurethane Bayer) [37]; Ethibloc occlusion gel[15] [49].

ELECTROCOAGULATION

Transcatheter electrocoagulation has been successfully used to occlude vessels both experimentally and clinically [7, 23, 39, 44] (Fig. 5-15). DC current is safer than AC current because AC current acutely disrupts the vessel's wall. DC current may cause thrombosis by altering the polarity of the negatively charged endothelial cells, thereby attracting rather than repelling similarly charged platelets. Low amperage (less than 50 mA) is required to produce the clot safely. Unfortunately, this requires the current to be applied for prolonged periods (up to 20 or 30 minutes in vessels of 4- or 5-mm diameter). The tip of the electrode (a routine steel angiographic flexible tip guidewire) often remains at the site of electrocoagulation due to erosion by electrolysis. Cardiac arrhythmias are

not induced if the current flow pathways are directed away from the heart. The clot that forms remains firmly adherent to the vessel wall at the precise level of the electrode.

More durable flexible electrodes of smaller diameter and a better power source are required to shorten coagulation time and make this approach more practical.

General Comments

The most commonly used, easily available, and easy to use embolic agent is Gelfoam. Gelfoam is used if prolonged occlusion is not required (e.g., bleeding, preoperative occlusion of vascular tumors). Ivalon is preferred over Gelfoam if permanent occlusion is sought, as in certain vascular abnormalities or occlusion of vessels feeding tumors. The communicating vessels between arteries and veins must be small enough to trap the emboli. Since Ivalon is not pliable, the size of the emboli must be smaller than the inside diameter of the delivery catheter. Combining Gelfoam with Ivalon provides permanent occlusion and a greater ease in delivery. Autogenous clot is rarely used, and then only if there is severe hemorrhage demonstrated beyond the point where the catheter tip can be easily positioned. Clots pass easily through the catheter, often being trapped in the bleeding vessel and stopping the bleeding. Their rapid lysis prevents severe damage caused by emboli into other vessels.

Coils are used to occlude relatively large vessels, much as with surgical ligation. Arteriovenous fistulas and bleeding sites are permanently occluded with coils. Threatened normal peripheral vessels, fed by collaterals, may be protected with an occluding coil, which helps to divert subsequent emboli to a pathologic area.

Nondetachable balloons are used to temporarily occlude vessels, guide the flow of emboli, and prevent their reflux.

Detachable balloons are flow-guided and are reserved for those lesions more peripheral or remote in location. They may be deflated and repositioned if improperly placed before being permanently detached. Their use requires experience and careful technique.

Liquid embolizing materials can be introduced through small coaxial catheters positioned in small vessels in remote areas. They are used in areas

---

[14]Ingenol A + B silicone modified reactive monomers polymerize at body temperatures in 15 minutes.
[15]Manufactured by Ingenor Medical Systems.

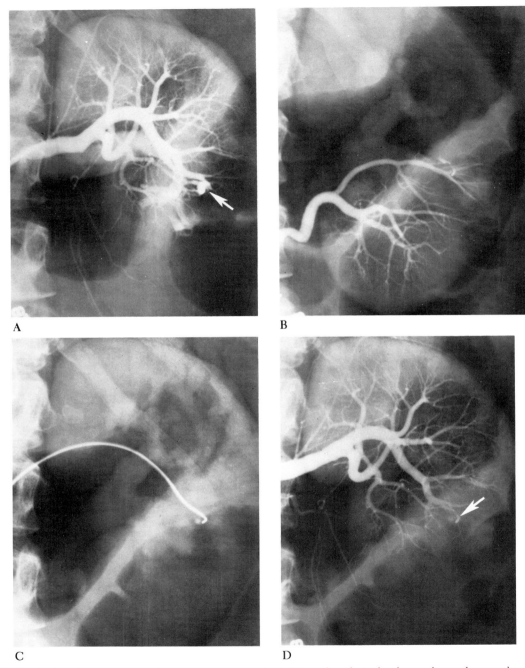

A

B

C

D

Fig. 5-15. Occlusion of postbiopsy renal arteriovenous fistula by means of selective intravascular electrocoagulation. There was severe hematuria for 2 weeks after the biopsy in this 21-year-old woman with a nephrotic syndrome.

A. Selective renal arteriogram demonstrating the precise area of the fistula (*arrow*).

B. The lower pole is supplied by another renal artery.

C. A 5 French catheter has been advanced out to the fistula, and a 0.035-in. guidewire (the electrode) protrudes 2 mm beyond its tip.

D. Renal arteriogram following occlusion of the fistula by electrocoagulation. Remnant tip of the guidewire electrode used during the procedure is seen at the site of the occluded fistula (*arrow*). The patient's bleeding promptly stopped.

Table 5-1. Particulate embolic agents and delivery systems

Lesions treated	Particulate embolic agents	Catheter delivery systems

Temporary occlusion: e.g., acute bleeding, bleeding tumor, preoperative vascular tumor, selected vascular beds (with a capillary barricade) in trauma	Gelfoam particles 1–2 mm (preferred)
	
	Gelfoam powder (40–60 μm) (mixed with contrast agent to form slurry)
		Tapered thin-walled 5 to 7 French
		
		Occlusive balloon 5 to 7 French
		Coaxial
		    Nontapered 7/4 French
		    Thin wall 5/3 French
		    Standard 6.5/3, 2.7, or 2.2 French*
		    Modified occlusive balloon 6/3 French

Permanent occlusion: Vessels supplying vascular tumors and arteriovenous malformations. Avoid major vital vessels, e.g., vertebral or internal carotid artery, femoral artery	Ivalon
	  Microemboli
	  490–1000 μm
	  200–450 μm
	
	  100–200 μm
		
		Tapered thin-walled 5–7 French; modified 6 French occlusive balloon
		Coaxial
		    Tapered thin-walled 5 French or 6.5/3, 2.7, or 2.2 French*
		    Nontapered 7/4 French
		    Modified occlusive balloon 6/3 French

	Dry, compressed cut to desired size (expands to 10 times original size) Combination of Ivalon microemboli and Gelfoam particles (1–2 mm; 40–60 μm) mixed with contrast agent to form slurry	Nontapered 7 French Tapered thin-walled 5 to 7 French

"Ligation" type occlusion: e.g., bleeding vessel; false aneurysm; some fistulas; termination embolization procedure to prevent reflux; isolating an adjacent normal vascular bed prior to embolizing pathologic microcirculation	Steel coils
	  8-mm helix
	  5-mm helix
	  3-mm helix
	
	  2.5-mm helix (microcoil)
		Any catheter accepting a 0.038 in. guidewire, *but no larger* (e.g., 5 French thin-walled; 6.5 Headhunter; 6 French modified occlusive balloon catheter)
		In coaxial system with outer catheter accepting inner 3 French catheter

Arteriovenous fistulas and certain aneurysms: e.g., carotid cavernous fistula; pulmonary arteriovenous malformations; varicocele	Detachable balloons
	  Latex
	  Silicone
		
		Debrun's delivery system*
		White's delivery system*

*Infusion catheters, manufactured by Target Therapeutics, 2100 South Sepulveda Blvd., Los Angeles, CA 90025.

where particulate emboli may fail (e.g., large tear in a blood vessel; extensive AVM not responding to particulate emboli). Liquid polymers require an IND number and are not easily available.

See Tables 5-1 and 5-2 for summaries of particulate and fluid embolic materials, their delivery systems, and under which circumstances they may be used.

Complications of Embolization

There are complications specific to embolizing techniques [36]. The most serious of these is reflux

of emboli with occlusion of a nontarget vessel. The catheter tip must therefore be securely positioned in the vessel orifice. Reflux is a product of the rate of flow of the circulation as well as the rate of injection. The emboli enter freely at the onset of injection, but as resistance in the vascular bed increases, the speed and quantity of the injection must be decreased. Reflux occurs from overinjecting and not terminating the embolization procedure sufficiently early. This is prevented by (1) careful monitoring with good fluoroscopic guidance, (2) using a small syringe, thus allowing a more controlled injection, (3) actually seeing the

Table 5-2. Fluid embolic agents and delivery systems

Lesions treated (permanent occlusion)	Fluid embolic agents	Delivery system
AVMs, vascular tumors, false aneurysms, bleeding. Requires selective placement, e.g., left gastric; superior gluteal; extracranial and intracranial vessels	Tissue adhesives (bucrylate)[a]	1. Single-lumen flow-guided (Kerber) balloon catheter with a calibrated leak (for intracranial lesions) 2. Coaxial modified occlusive balloon catheter 6(Berenstein)/3, 2.7, or 2.2[d] French[b] or coaxial nontapered 7/4 French or coaxial 6.5/3 French[b] catheter (all three must have inner catheter tips dipped in silicone)
Renal ablation Portal varices AVMs and tumors Beware lesions near skin (skin sloughing) and near major nerves (neural damage)	Absolute ethanol	Coaxial modified occlusive balloon catheter 6(Berenstein)/3 French[b] or conventional 6.5/3 French[b] or 5 French thin-walled/3, 2.7, or 2.2[d] French[b]
Extracranial AVMs and vascular tumors, e.g., spinal; external carotid	Silicone mixture[c] (with varying viscosity and vulcanization times)	Modified 6 French occlusive balloon catheter alone or coaxial with 3 French, or coaxial conventional nontapered 7/4 French or coaxial conventional tapered 6.5/3 French

[a]Bucrylate is mixed with tantalum or Pantopaque:
(1) Add tantalum 1 g/ml (tantalum oxide if subcutaneous in light-skinned patients).
(2) Add equal parts Pantopaque for radiopacity and delaying polymerization.
[b]Can replace 3 French catheter with injectable guidewire.
[c]See Appendix 16 for details. Add tantalum for radiopacity: 1g/ml.
[d]Manufactured by Target Therapeutics, 2100 South Sepulveda Blvd., Los Angeles, CA 90025.
AVM = arteriovenous malformation.

emboli by mixing them with dilute contrast media or tantalum, and (4) both preceding and flushing the emboli with dilute contrast media. Under some circumstances, an inflated balloon catheter helps to control the flow of emboli. Reflux still occurs if the balloon is rapidly deflated in an overinjected vascular bed. This is prevented by placing a coil at the proximal portion of the embolized vessel prior to deflating the occlusive balloon.

Embolizing the head and neck requires skill and knowledge of anatomy. Lesions in the distribution of the internal carotid artery, such as carotid cavernous fistulas and aneurysms, carry the risk of cerebral infarction and hemiplegia. A lesion entirely in the distribution of an external carotid artery is still at risk for intracranial complications due to passage of microemboli through large extracranial-intracranial collaterals.

Reflux of emboli during embolization of kidneys and other organs below the diaphragm may result in ischemia of the lower extremities. Pulmonary emboli may occur if communicating channels between arteries and veins in AVMs are large.

Complications occurring in the target organ are mainly those related to tissue necrosis [40]. If large areas are occluded (tumors of the kidney or liver), pain and pyrexia almost invariably occur and may be severe enough to require narcotics for several days. Infection and abscess formation and breakdown of infarcted tissue may result, with spread into adjacent organs. Renal failure and hypertension sometimes complicate infarction of the kidney.

Vessels may rupture if there is overinflation of a balloon catheter in an artery. Less severe damage to the arterial wall may lead to aneurysm formation.

Despite these potential complications, embolization techniques may be the only means of therapy in critically ill patients with bleeding or extensive tumors. Use of this procedure sometimes gains time for more definitive surgical resection at a later date.

Embolization procedures in specific vascular beds and particular vascular abnormalities are discussed in Part III.

References

1. Bank, W. O., and Kerber, C. W. Gelfoam embolization: A simplified technique. A.J.R. 132:299, 1979.
2. Berenstein, A. Flow controlled silicone fluid embolization. A.J.R. 134:1213, 1980.
3. Berenstein, A., and Kricheff, I. Catheter and materials selection for transarterial embolization: Technical considerations. 1. Catheters. 2. Materials. Radiology 132:631, 1979.
4. Berenstein, A., and Kricheff, I. Microembolization techniques of vascular occlusion: Radiologic, pathologic and clinical correlation. A.J.N.R. 2:261, 1981.
5. Bookstein, J., et al. Transcatheter hemostasis of gastrointestinal bleeding using modified autogenous clot. Radiology 113:277, 1974.
6. Brooks, B. The treatment of traumatic arterial venous fistula. Southern Med. J. 23:100, 1930.
7. Brunell, F., Kuntslinger, F., and Quillard, J. Endovascular electrocoagulation with bipolar electrode and alternating current: A follow-up study in dogs. Radiology 148:413, 1983.
8. Castaneda-Zuniga, W. R., et al. New device for simple, fast arterial and venous occlusion. A.J.R. 136: 637, 1981.
9. Clark, R., Gallant, T., and Alexander, E. Angiographic management of traumatic AV fistulas: Clinical results. Radiology 147:9, 1983.
10. Chuang, V. P., Wallace, S., and Gianturco, S. New improved coil for tapered tip catheter for arterial occlusion. Radiology 135:507, 1980.
11. Chuang, V. P., et al. Complications of coil embolization: Prevention and management. A.J.R. 137:809, 1981.
12. Cragg, A. H., et al. Renal ablation using hot contrast medium: An experimental study. A.J.R. 148:683, 1983.
13. Debrun, G. N. Treatment of traumatic carotid, cavernous fistula using detachable balloon catheters. A.J.N.R. 4:355, 1983.
14. Debrun, G. M., et al. Endovascular occlusion of vertebral fistulae by detachable balloons with conservation of the vertebral blood flow. Radiology 130:141, 1979.
15. Diamond, N. G., et al. Microfibrillar collagen hemostat. A new transcatheter embolization agent. Radiology 133:775, 1979.
16. Doppman, J. L., Popovsky, M. A., and Girton, M. Use of iodinated contrast agents to ablate organs.

Experimental studies and histopathology. Radiology 138:333, 1981.
17. Doppman, J. L., Zapol, W., and Peirce, J. Transcatheter embolization with a silicone rubber preparation: Experimental observations. Invest. Radiol. 6:304, 1971.
18. Doppman, J. L., et al. Treatment of hyperparathyroidism by percutaneous embolization of a mediastinal adenoma. Radiology 115:37, 1975.
19. Dotter, C., Goldman, M., and Rösch, J. Instant, selective arterial occlusion with isobutyl 2-cyanoacrylate. Radiology 114:227, 1975.
20. Eklund, L., Jonsson, N., and Treugut, H. Transcatheter obliteration of the renal artery by ethanol injection: Experimental results. Cardiovasc. Intervent. Radiol. 4(1):1, 1981.
21. Ellman, B. S., et al. Ablation of renal tumors with absolute ethanol. Radiology 141:619, 1981.
22. Gianturco, C., Anderson, J., and Wallace, S. Mechanical devices for arterial occlusion. A.J.R. 124:428, 1975.
23. Gold, R., et al. Transarterial electrocoagulation therapy of pseudo-aneurysm in the head of the pancreas. A.J.R. 125:422, 1975.
24. Goldman, M., et al. Transcatheter embolization with bucrylate. Radiographics 2:340, 1982.
25. Greenfield, A. J. Transcatheter vessel occlusion: Selection of methods and materials. Cardiovasc. Intervent. Radiol. 3:222, 1980.
26. Greenfield, A. J., et al. Transcatheter embolization: Prevention of emboli reflux using balloon catheters. A.J.R. 131:651, 1978.
27. Hilal, S., and Michelson, J. Therapeutic percutaneous embolization for extra-axial vascular lesions of the head, neck, and spine. J. Neurosurg. 43:275, 1975.
28. Horton, J., et al. Polyvinyl alcohol foam—Gelfoam for therapeutic embolization: A synergistic mixture. A.J.N.R. 4:143, 1983.
29. Keller, F., Rosch, J., and Bird, C. Percutaneous embolization of bony pelvic neoplasms with tissue adhesive. Radiology 147:21, 1983.
30. Kerber, C. W. Balloon catheter with a calibrated leak: A new system for super selective angiography and occlusive catheter therapy. Radiology 120:547, 1976.
31. Kerber, C. W., Banks, W. O., and Horton, J. A. Polyvinyl alcohol foam. Prepackaged emboli for therapeutic embolization. A.J.R. 130:1193, 1978.
32. Kuntslinger, F., et al. Vascular occlusive agents. A.J.R. 136:151, 1981.
33. Leight, R., and Prentice, H. Surgical investigation of a new absorbable sponge derived from gelatin for use in hemostasis. J. Neurosurg. 2:433, 1945.
34. Lund, G., et al. Detachable steel spring coils for vessel occlusion. Radiology 155:530, 1985.
35. Lussenhop, A., and Spence, W. Clinical notes: Artificial embolization of cerebral arteries. J.A.M.A. 172:1153, 1960.
36. Miller, F. H., and Mineau, D. E. Transcatheter arterial embolization. Major complications and

their prevention. *Cardiovasc. Intervent. Radiol.* 6:141, 1983.

37. Novak, D., Wiener, S. H., and Ruekner, R. Applicability of liquid, radiopaque polyurethane for transcatheter embolization. *Cardiovasc. Intervent. Radiol.* 6(3):133, 1983.

38. Pevsner, P. Micro-balloon catheter for super selective angiography and therapeutic occlusion. *A.J.R.* 128:225, 1977.

39. Phillips, J., et al. Experimental closure of AV fistula by transcatheter electrical coagulation. *Radiology* 115:319, 1975.

40. Prochaska, J., Flye, W., and Johnsrude, I. Left gastric artery embolization for control of gastric bleeding: A complication. *Radiology* 107:521, 1973.

41. Rabe, F. E., et al. Renal tumor infarction with absolute ethanol. *A.J.R.* 139:1139, 1982.

42. Serbinenko, F. Balloon catheterization and occlusion of major cerebral vessels. *J. Neurosurg.* 1941:125, 1974.

43. Tadavarthy, S., et al. Therapeutic transcatheter arterial embolization. *Radiology* 18:13, 1974.

44. Thompson, W., et al. Transcatheter electrocoagulation: Therapeutic angiographic technique for vessel occlusion. *Invest. Radiol.* 12:146, 1977.

45. White, R. I., Jr., et al. Therapeutic embolization with detachable balloons. *Cardiovasc. Intervent. Radiol.* 3:229, 1980.

46. White, R. I., Jr., et al. Therapeutic embolization with long-term occluding agents and their effects on embolized tissues. *Radiology* 125:677, 1977.

47. White, R. I., Jr., et al. Safety of therapeutic emboli remains a problem. *J.A.M.A.* 237:204, 1977.

48. Woodside, J., Schwarz, H., and Bergreen, P. Peripheral complicating bilateral renal infarction with gelfoam. *A.J.R.* 126:1033, 1976.

49. Wright, K. C., et al. Experimental evaluation of ethibloc for non-surgical nephrotomy. *Radiology* 145:339, 1982.

50. Yune, H. Y., et al. Absolute ethanol in thrombal therapy of bleeding esophageal varices. *A.J.R.* 138:1137, 1982.

51. Zollinkoffer, C., et al. Therapeutic blockade of arteries using compressed Ivalon. *Radiology* 136:635, 1980.

Percutaneous Transluminal Angioplasty

General Comments

Percutaneous transluminal angioplasty (PTA) originated in 1964 when Dotter and Judkins [8] described recanalizing atherosclerotic vessels by means of a telescoping catheter system. Because of inherent limitations, the concept lay dormant for a number of years, but it was rejuvenated in 1974 when new methods became available [9, 10]. In the past few years, considerable experience has accumulated in the use of this procedure, which has been the basis for a number of comprehensive papers and textbooks on the subject [2, 3, 5, 9, 11, 12, 19, 22, 26].

Dotter's original technique was accomplished by advancing a guidewire followed by a small diameter catheter through an area of stenosis or occlusion, and then progressively increasing its width by telescoping larger catheters over each other. Serious disadvantages limited widespread acceptance of this technique. A major drawback of this method is the large puncture required at the site of entry. Also, the "snowplow" action of the technique is bound to break off atheromatous material and distribute it peripherally. Although somewhat dangerous in the arterial system, the concept of telescoping catheter systems has not been abandoned. It has found widespread use in dilating tracts in different organ systems (e.g., nephrostomy tracts, abscess drainage). It is more safely used in the venous system, where some veins (e.g., femoral vein, internal jugular vein) can be dilated to greater diameters for percutaneous introduction of therapeutic devices (e.g., inferior vena cava filters, removal of foreign bodies) (see Chap. 7). A modification of the technique, the Staple van Andel catheter system, is still used in arterial vessels (Fig. 6-1). These catheters have an outside diameter ranging up to 12 French. The long graduated taper to their tips gradually increases the diameter of a particularly narrowed area in small branch vessels or in arteries too narrow to initially accommodate a dilation balloon catheter.

The newer dilating catheter systems employ balloons placed strategically near the tip of the catheter [9, 10, 18]. They can be safely introduced percutaneously into the vascular system while in their deflated form, advanced over a previously positioned guidewire through the area of stenosis, and then expanded to a predetermined diameter. This offers a radial rather than a shearing force to overcome the area of narrowing.

Method of Action

There are several theories as to what is accomplished by balloon dilation of a segment of vascular stenosis. The first is that there is a redistribution of pliable plastic intraluminal and mural atheromatous material, without any significant increase in the outer diameter of the vessel, but with an elongation of the area of stenosis [9]. The second is that there is a rupture of the intima and media, with an outward displacement of atheromatous material and a consequent measurable irreversible increase in both the inner and the outer diameter of the vessel [6, 7]. Shearing of the plaque-artery interface occurs with stretching and longitudinal tearing of the arterial endothelium. This longitudinal orientation of the tears, colinear with the flow of blood, likely accounts for the rarity of complications such as vascular dissection [14]. An increase in the inside diameter of the lesion may occur through a breaking off of atheromatous debris. This dislodgement results in peripheral embolization, which is undesirable and fortunately rare.

All these theories are likely correct and are more or less invoked under different circumstances [12, 27]. A stenosis formed by soft atheromatous material can be easily displaced and redistributed throughout the length of the vessel without any grossly measurable increase in its outer dimensions. On the other hand, if there is a great deal of calcium or fibrosis in the vascular wall, an expanding balloon could rupture the intima and media, causing lateral displacement and an increase in the outside diameter of the vessel, and allowing contrast material to escape into the lining of the vessel wall. Figure 6-2 shows pre- and immediate postdi-

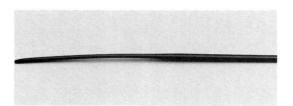

Fig. 6-1. van Andel catheter. Peripheral side holes may be added to allow injection of contrast medium during its passage through an occluded or stenotic artery.

lation angiograms on three different patients, with different angiographic manifestations demonstrating different modes of action; each had circulation successfully restored. Regardless of the method of action, soon after the procedure, neointima develops and, within several weeks, smooths out the intimal irregularities imposed by the procedure (Fig. 6-3). Restenosis can occur and is most often seen when the dilatation is incomplete [9, 27].

Poiseuille's law (see Chap. 2) states that flow in a tube increases directly with the fourth power of its radius. Thus, if we increase the diameter of a stenosed segment of a vessel by a factor of 2, the flow to that area should increase by a factor of 16. On the other hand, although the length of the stenotic lesion is also important, it is not as significant as its diameter. Dilating by a given amount a stenotic lesion that it twice as long only doubles the amount of flow in the tube. These are important concepts to keep in mind when selecting patients for transluminal angioplasty and evaluat-

ing the results following a procedure. On some occasions even though there is not a cosmetic result of restoring the lumen of a stenotic segment to its original diameter, the dilatation is sufficient to cause a significant hemodynamic improvement in the patient. Also, if there are multiple lesions, it is most beneficial to dilate the lesion that is most severely narrowed, not necessarily the longest. Dilating a less severe stenosis proximal to this tight lesion will do little to improve the flow (Fig. 6-4).

Measuring a pressure gradient across a stenosis helps to determine its hemodynamic significance [13, 24]. Although this is best accomplished by measuring the pressure proximal and distal to the stenosis simultaneously, using two separate catheters, this is sometimes not practical, for it requires two separate puncture sites and two separate strain gauges. Sequential measurements immediately before and after traversing the stenosis is often satisfactory. Sequential measurements should not be performed, however, if there is any risk of forfeiting a successful catheter placement across an area that is difficult to manipulate.

Fig. 6-2. Iliac artery stenoses in three different patients, each showing pre- and immediate postdilation appearance.
A and B. Proximal common iliac artery shows slight residual narrowing of stenotic site.
C and D. The dilated segment (postdilation photo) has a greater diameter than the adjacent vessels.
E and F. Subintimal location of contrast medium indicating intimal and medial disruption at the angioplasty site.

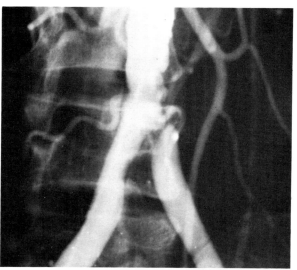

A

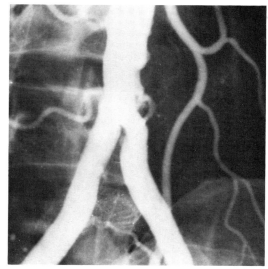

B

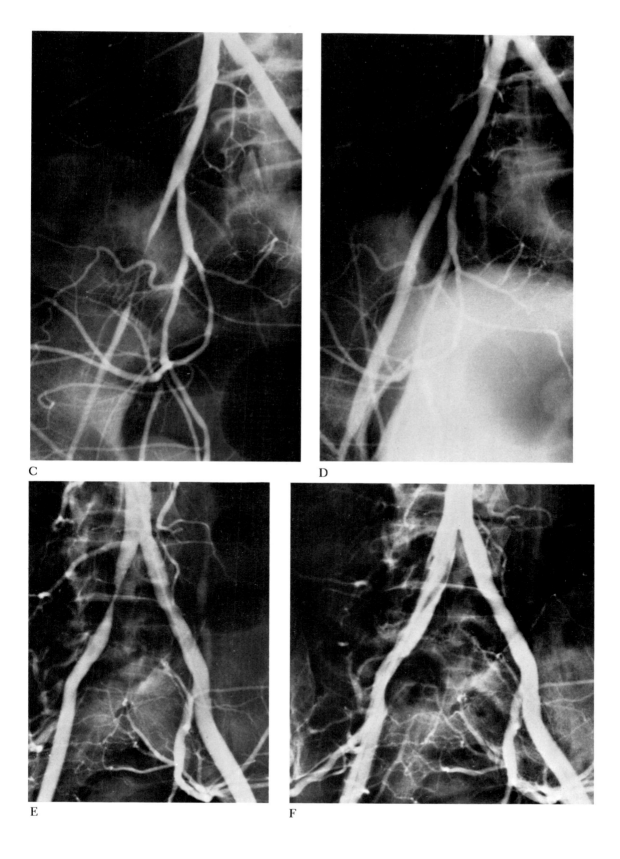

C

D

E

F

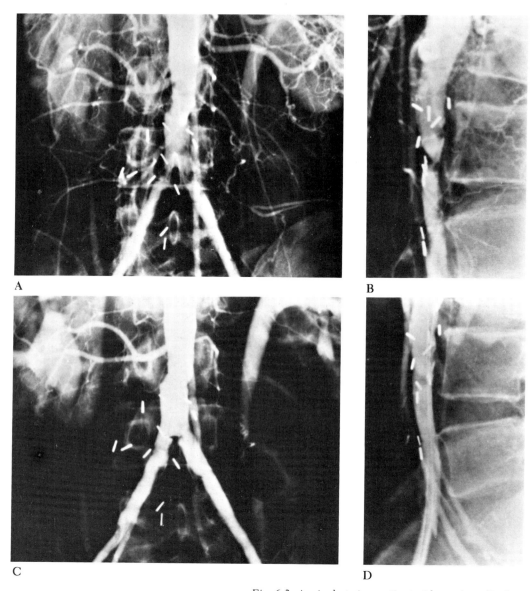

A seemingly insignificant pressure gradient measured across an area of stenosis in a vessel feeding the extremities is not necessarily a valid consideration if the patient is at rest. Generally, a peak systolic gradient of less than 10 mm Hg across an area of stenosis is not considered sufficient to warrant intervention. In patients in whom there is strong clinical suspicion but a questionable degree of stenosis seen angiographically and an insignificant pressure gradient, two additional maneuvers should be performed: (1) Angiograms should be performed in at least two or maybe even three separate projections, for a significant lesion may be

Fig. 6-3. Angioplasty in a patient with previous distal aortic endarterectomy.
A and B. Predilation anteroposterior and lateral aortograms showing tight stenosis of distal aorta.
C and D. Successful dilation.
E. Three weeks later, the roughened edges at the angioplasty site have smooth walls.

hidden if seen en face in a single projection. (2) The true significance of the lesion may be uncovered by stimulating a gradient (a) by performing reactive hyperemia (see Chap. 4) or (b) by injecting vasodilators into the vessels peripheral to the stenosis (tolazoline 25 mg; nitroglycerine 100 to 300 µg) [24].

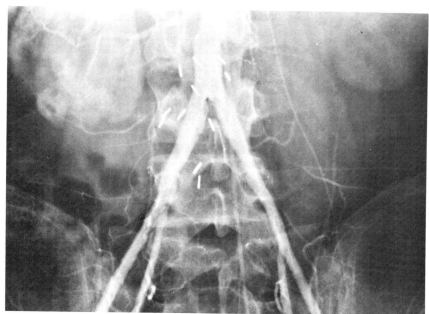

E

Laplace's law tells us that as the radius of a balloon (or blood vessel) increases, there is a progressive increase in its surface tension, as well as a decrease in its wall thickness; the balloon or vessel eventually ruptures. It is important to choose a balloon that does not expand beyond a given point and ruptures rather than further distending and endangering the vessel under treatment.

In particularly resistive focal stenotic lesions, a short balloon has a greater chance of successful dilation than a longer one. These shorter balloons, however, sometimes slip to one end or the other of the stenosis during dilation. It is more difficult to maintain their position.

One final point. When the endothelium of the artery is damaged, as it is in angioplasty, the protective layer providing antithrombogenicity is disrupted. Platelet granules are released and there is local deposition and aggregation of platelets, together with release of a number of substances, which include prostaglandins, thromboplastin, fibrinogen, coagulation factors, and serotonin. These processes, together with underlying vascular spasm, remnant stenosis, and the occlusion imposed by the balloon catheter, encourage thrombosis. Thrombosis can be prevented in part by administering antiplatelet medications (e.g., aspirin or dipyridamole) prior to angioplasty. Chances of

thrombosis can be further reduced if heparin is administered at the time of angioplasty. Heparin not only reduces thrombin activity but also decreases thrombin-induced platelet aggregation, helps induce thrombocytopenia, and has some antispasmodic action [17].

Dilating Balloon Catheters

The balloon catheter system [1][1] requires two lumina (Fig. 6-5). One of these must be large enough to accommodate standard guidewires and diagnostic columns of injected contrast medium. The lumen feeding the balloon is of much smaller caliber. The balloons are strongly bonded to the catheter shaft, and radiopaque markers define their proximal and distal limits. They vary in diameter from 2 to 3 mm (for coronary arteries, tibial and peroneal branches, and second-order visceral branches) to 12, 15, 18, and even 20 mm, and are

[1]Manufactured by American Edwards Lab, 1722 Red Hill Ave., P.O. Box 11150, Santa Ana, CA 92711; Cook Inc., P.O. Box 489, Bloomington, IN 47401; Cordis, P.O. Box 370428, Miami, FL 33137; USCI, a division of C. R. Bard, Inc., 129 Concord Road, P.O. Box 566, Billerica, MA 01898; Surgimed, Inc., P.O. Box 1403, Summerville, SC 29482; and MediTech Division, Cooper Scientific Corp., 478 Pleasant St., Watertown, MA 02172.

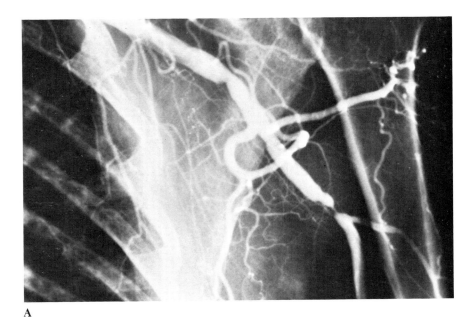

A

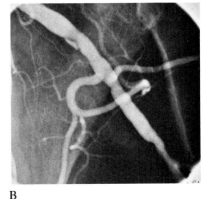

B

Fig. 6-4.
A. Mild axillary artery stenosis and severe proximal brachial artery stenosis.
B. Both were dilated, the proximal one with ease and the more distal one with resistance to inflation. Marked clinical improvement was seen despite residual stenosis.

available in varied lengths from 1 to 10 cm. The catheters carrying the balloons are sufficiently flexible to follow guidewires and easily negotiate the curves in the vascular tree. The outside diameters of the catheters measure from 1 mm (3 French) to 3 mm (9 French), and their lengths vary from 50 to 110 cm. The smallest diameter dilating balloon catheter systems require a coaxial method for successful selective placement in a coronary or visceral artery. In this coaxial system, the larger diameter outer catheter tip is placed selectively into the orifice of the target vessel and the smaller inner catheter is then passed through the area of stenosis over a leading 0.014- or 0.016-in. guidewire.

Preformed curved tips in the balloon catheters can be obtained from the manufacturer. These are constructed with the curve in the catheter shaft passing eccentrically through the balloon so that when inflated, the balloon has a straight configuration. Curves can also be safely imposed on polyethylene balloon catheters by the angiographer using a jet of hot steam if the tip of the catheter is enclosed in a firm plastic form.

The diameter of the inflated balloon must be accurately predetermined and under no circumstances should it be capable of overdistending. Early models used easily distensible latex balloons, the diameter being controlled by a "cage" composed of a focal area of stripping in the overlying Teflon catheter [18]. This was quickly replaced

with balloons made of semielastic polyvinyl with which a more fixed predetermined dimension could be accomplished. At higher pressures, however, even this material was seen to distort and overdistend with the potential for dangerous consequences to the adjacent vessel wall. Consequently, this has been replaced with less compliant materials of increasing strength (e.g., polyethylene, reinforced polyethylene, Mylar). These materials are more prone to rupture than to overdistend when

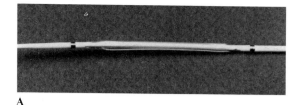

A

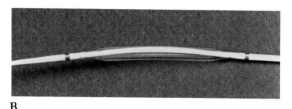

B

Fig. 6-5. Deflated (A) and inflated (B) 7 French 5-mm balloon catheter with metal markers.

too much pressure is applied. Large diameter balloons require less pressure to burst than do those with a smaller diameter. In general, balloons with a fixed inflated diameter have a high bursting pressure and produce less trauma on rupturing than do those with an expanding diameter.

Balloons will rupture if dilated well beyond the manufacturer's suggested tolerance level. Under most circumstances this causes no morbidity. The sudden release of high intraluminal balloon pressures can, however, transfer pressure to already stressed adjacent vessel walls, with the possibility of injury to the vessel wall. Arterial dissection, occlusion, and formation of false aneurysms can occur.

When the rupture in the balloon is linear and parallel to the shaft, the balloon assembly is easily removed. However, if the rupture is transversely oriented, the distal segment acts much like an inflated umbrella during withdrawal, and vascular injury may result. Fortunately, the transverse tear is a rare occurrence.

Technique of Percutaneous Transluminal Angioplasty

The basic steps of the PTA procedure are simple [1, 19]. A small diameter diagnostic catheter is advanced to a level just proximal to the narrowed vessel. Subsequently it follows a guidewire that has been gently introduced beyond the area of stenosis. The diagnostic catheter is replaced with the balloon angioplasty catheter, and the balloon is inflated as it lies directly across the lesion, thereby

dilating and correcting the stenosis. The success of the procedure is assessed, the balloon catheter withdrawn, and postdilation care is administered (Fig. 6-6).

There are special considerations not only in preparing the patient but also in the choice of approach, in performing the arterial puncture, in traversing the lesion, and in determining the hemodynamic significance of the lesion. The following are general comments on the technique of PTA. Technical points and problems specific to a given area are discussed in Part III.

BEFORE THE PROCEDURE

Inform the patient of what to expect, possible complications, and various alternatives. Surgical colleagues should be a part of the team making the decisions and should be on stand-by in case surgical intervention is required. The patient should fast for 6 hours in case emergency surgery is required. If possible, institute antiplatelet therapy 1 to 2 days prior to the procedure (aspirin 300 mg qd and dipyridamole 20 mg tid); obtain bleeding studies. Administer adequate narcotics and sedation prior to the procedure.

NECESSARY MATERIALS

In addition to the routine angiographic tray and array of diagnostic catheters and guidewires (see Table 6-1), the following sterilized equipment should be available (unopened until needed).

1. Balloon angioplasty catheter: Select balloon diameter equal to or 1 mm larger than the normal vessel measured immediately adjacent to the stenotic lesion. Balloon length should be slightly longer than the stenotic lesion. Use the shortest catheter shaft required to reach the lesion. Pretest the balloon angioplasty catheter immediately prior to use. Uncover mechanical defects or kinking. Be sure the balloon inflates and deflates promptly using 30% contrast agent. A 10-ml syringe supplies sufficient pressure for inflation (smaller syringes apply dangerously high pressures). A 30-ml syringe provides adequate suction for deflation. Higher concentrations of contrast medium are not necessary, are more viscous, and may crystallize with time, causing obstruction of the small lumen feeding the balloon. Do not pretest too early. Do not use balloon catheters previously

114

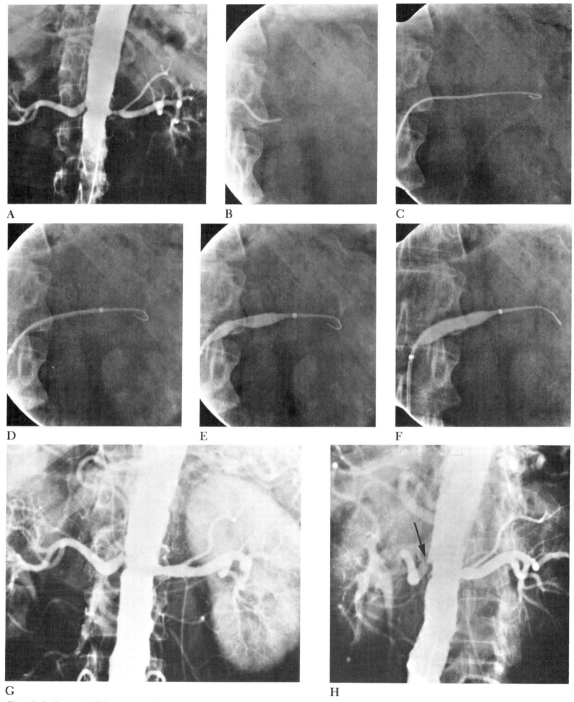

Fig. 6-6. Steps in dilating renal arteries.
A. Bilateral renal artery stenosis (right side poorly seen).
B. Mikkaelson catheter tip in left renal artery.
C. Catheter tip advanced through stenotic segment over soft-tipped guidewire; latter exchanged for stiffer heavy-duty guidewire.
D. Balloon catheter advanced over heavy-duty guidewire to straddle stenotic segment.
E. Balloon deformity due to stenotic segment.
F. Balloon inflated.
G. Successful left renal artery dilation.
H. RPO projection outlines right renal artery stenosis.
I. Both renal arteries successfully dilated.

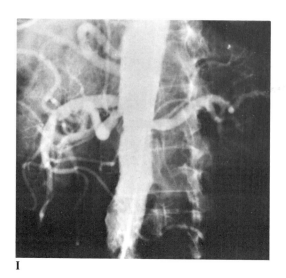

I

inflated with contrast agent. A coaxial dilating balloon system with 2- or 3-mm diameter balloons and 0.014 or 0.016-in. steerable guidewire is required for dilating small vessels [16].

2. Other catheters
   a. Staple van Andel catheters of varying lengths and diameters.
   b. Occlusive balloon catheter (in case of arterial rupture).
3. Guidewires
   a. 0.038 and 0.035-in. heavy-duty guidewires with straight tapered tip or with a 1.5-mm J-shaped tip [20].
   b. Torque-controlled guidewires of varying diameter, including 0.014 to 0.018-in. steerable guidewires.
   c. Lunderquist [15] or Amplatz exchange guidewire.
   d. Variable stiffness guidewire with Cook external manipulator.
   e. Guidewire with injectable lumen and accompanying adapter [23].

Table 6-1. Catheter inventory for percutaneous transluminal angioplasty

Balloon		Catheter		Guide-wire size (in.)	Tip curve configuration	Primary use
Diameter (cm)	Length (cm)	French size	Length (cm)			
2.5	2	4.5	90	0.018	Straight	Distal to trifurcation, coaxial distal renal or small vessel
3.5	2	4.5	90	0.018	Straight	
4.0	2, 4, 10	7	75, 100	0.038	Straight	Distal femoral, popliteal, brachial, vertebral, external carotid
5.0	2, 4, 10	5	80, 100, 110	0.028	Straight	Proximal popliteal, femoral, profunda
6.0	1, 2, 3, 4	7	60, 80, 100, 110	0.038	Straight, small and large J; Simmons	Proximal femoral, iliacs, renals, superior mesenteric, subclavian
7.0	2, 3, 4	7	60, 80, 100	0.038		Iliacs, renals, superior mesenteric, subclavians
8.0	2, 3, 4	8	75	0.038	Straight	Iliacs, renals, superior mesenteric, subclavians
9.0	3, 4	9	60, 80	0.038	Straight	Iliacs, aorta
10.0	3, 4, 10	9	65	0.038	Straight	Aorta, nephrostomy tracts, larger veins
12.0	4	9	80	0.038	Straight	Aorta
15.0	3	9	80	0.038	Straight	Aorta

Note: Tapered balloons (Motarjame, 4-, 5-, 6-, 8-mm balloon diameter) and balloon catheters with side holes (Ricketts, 5-, 6-, 7-mm balloon diameter) are available.

5. Other accessories
   a. Touhy-Borst adapter with sidearm, which has an O ring gasket that clamps around the guidewire and prevents back-bleeding. A sidearm allows injection of contrast medium and pressure measurements if the inner guidewire is of small caliber.
   b. Sheaths (with sidearms) of varying lengths and diameters (see Chap. 7).
   c. 10-ml and 30-ml plastic syringes.
6. Sterile pressure manometer (preferably able to record pressures up to 20 atm).
7. 30% contrast medium
8. Drugs:
   Heparin, 1000 IU/ml (anticoagulant and vaso-dilator)
   Xylocaine 1%, 10 mg/ml (analgesic)
   Tolazoline, 25 mg/ml (vasodilator)
   Nitroglycerine, injectable, 100 μg (vasodilator)
   Nifedipine capsules, 10 mg (vasodilator)

APPROACH

Approaches for intraarterial percutaneous translu-minal angioplasty include one or both of the common femoral arteries and either the right or the left axillary artery. The choice of approach depends on a number of factors, including the proximity of the lesion to the puncture site, the tortuosity of the vessels leading from the puncture site to the target vessel, the takeoff angle of the target vessel from the aorta, and the pulse pressure of the vessel at the anticipated puncture site (Figs. 6-7 to 6-10).

It is best to enter the common femoral artery ipsilateral to the intended target unless distance, tortuosity, or acute angulation precludes this approach.

An ipsilateral anterograde common femoral artery approach is preferable for stenoses involving the superficial femoral artery and popliteal arteries (Fig. 6-8).

A contralateral femoral approach is preferred in the iliac vessels when a lesion cannot be bypassed with the usual retrograde approach or when the stenosis is too close to the intended puncture site (Fig. 6-8). It should be used to dilate an internal iliac, a common femoral, a proximal superficial femoral, or a profunda femoris artery. It can be helpful when there is a combination of an ipsilateral iliac artery stenosis with one or more stenoses on the opposite side, or when renal transplant anastomotic sites require dilation.

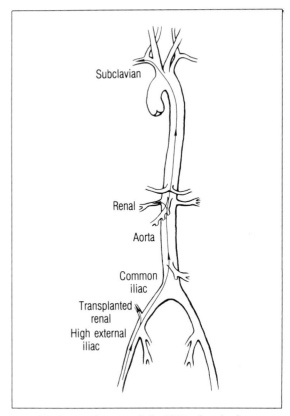

Fig. 6-7. Femoral approach for PTA of multiple areas.

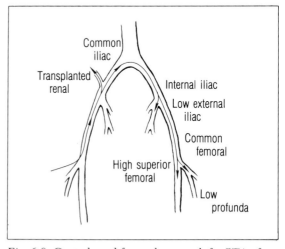

Fig. 6-8. Contralateral femoral approach for PTA of multiple areas.

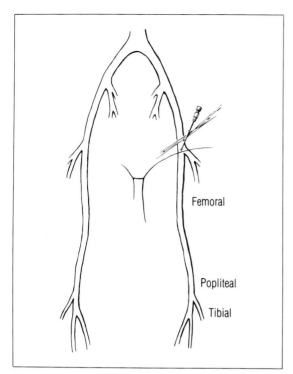

Fig. 6-9. Antegrade femoral approach for PTA of lower extremity vessels.

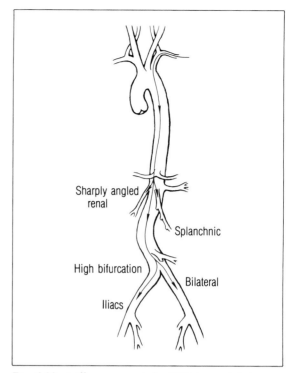

Fig. 6-10. Axillary approach for PTA in special circumstances.

Although axillary approaches are sometimes necessary, they are more hazardous. Hematomas causing brachial plexus injury occur more often with PTA than with routine angiography due to the larger bore of the balloon angioplasty catheters and the need for anticoagulation during the procedure. Axillary approaches are useful when a stenotic iliac artery cannot be crossed from below; when bilateral iliac artery dilations are anticipated; when PTA is required in a hypogastric, common femoral, or profunda femoris artery, or the arteries of some renal transplants; when a renal artery or superior mesenteric artery is acutely angled; and in some aortoiliac grafts (Fig. 6-10).

More than one puncture site may be necessary if a stenotic vessel requires two or more simultaneously inflated balloons (e.g., abdominal aorta) or when multiple sites require dilation.

Stenosis occurring in vein grafts or their anastomotic sites may be successfully dilated. If necessary, the vein graft can be entered directly at an appropriate location along its course.

Angioplasty may be performed during an operative procedure in conjunction with a surgical vascular reconstruction [19]. An example is a patient with distal popliteal artery stenosis undergoing a femoral popliteal bypass for a more proximal femoral or popliteal artery occlusion. Also, stenosis of proximal common carotid artery may be dilated, using an arteriotomy to allow back-bleeding for preventing intracranial migration of emboli.

PUNCTURE

Prior to puncture, metallic markers or familiar landmarks document the site of stenosis for easy reference during the procedure. Gently free the skin and subcutaneous tissues to allow easy passage of the catheter and its balloon. The pulse may be difficult to palpate due to occlusive disease lying proximally in the vessel. The location of the femoral artery can be found by "road mapping" using IV-DSA (see Chap. 2) or by Doppler ultrasonography. A small-caliber (5 French) catheter with a gentle distal curve is selected for initial introduction. Two side holes near the catheter tip allow injections of contrast medium around the guidewire. The catheter is advanced over a 0.035 or 0.038-in. gently J-shaped or straight flexible-

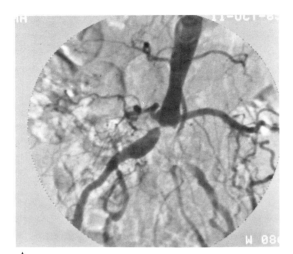

A

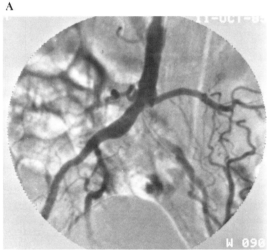

C

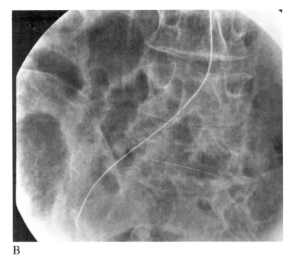

B

Fig. 6-11. Severe bilateral iliac occlusive disease in a patient who is a poor risk for surgery.
A. Occluded left common iliac artery. Subtotal occlusion of right iliac artery. Axillary approach.
B. Standard guidewires failed to cross the lesion, but a 0.016-in. steerable guidewire passed with ease.
C. Post-PTA angiogram shows widely patent right iliac system. Femoral-femoral bypass graft now possible.

tipped guidewire to a point just proximal to the stenosis. The precise position of the lesion is confirmed with injections of half-strength contrast agent.

CROSSING THE STENOSIS WITH A GUIDEWIRE

The guidewire usually crosses the area of narrowing with ease if it is concentric. If passage is not immediately successful, try a smaller gauge, but otherwise similar guidewire (0.025 or 0.021-in.). Sometimes by removing the wires altogether, the lesion can be bypassed with the catheter alone by careful fluoroscopic monitoring and small injections of contrast agent. The fluoroscopy tube should be directly over the lesion during such maneuvers to avoid distortion by parallax.

If the lesion is eccentric, the wire tip may catch under a plaque, making catheterization of the true lumen more difficult. A very flexible tipped 15-mm J-shaped guidewire will not, as a rule, be forced into a false passage, but instead will buckle away from the plaque. The buckled segment can then act as the leading point of the guidewire, which bypasses the plaque and allows the catheter to follow (see Fig. 8-10B). The captured guidewire tip may then be withdrawn slightly, released, and advanced further beyond the area of stenosis.

Problems Crossing the Stenosis with the Guidewire

If these routine measures fail, introduce the small steerable guidewire (0.014, 0.016, 0.018-in.).[2] Its small size and the clear visibility of the platinum alloy tip provide exquisite control by external manipulation. It may be used alone (Fig. 6-11) or it may be used coaxially through the injectable guidewire, which adds more body for subsequent passage of the overlying 5 French catheter.

Alternate measures include using the open-ended injectable guidewire, which may protrude

---

[2]Manufactured by USCI.

beyond the catheter tip for contrast monitored manipulations through the stenosis (see Chap. 3).

A flexible-tipped 0.038 or 0.035-in. torque-controlled guidewire is available. Rotary movements of the guidewire can be accomplished by applying an O-ring handle attachment to the external segment of wire.

Once a guidewire is across the stenosis, advance the 5 French catheter well above the lesion.

To measure pressures, replace the 0.035 or 0.038-in. guidewire with one that has a smaller diameter, inserted through a Touhy-Borst adapter with a sidearm at the catheter hub. Pressures are measured on either side of the stenosis, while advancing or withdrawing the catheter over the smaller wire, whose tip always remains well beyond the stenosis. Replace the guidewire with a heavy-duty 0.038 or 0.035-in. guidewire in preparation for the next step.

CROSSING THE STENOSIS WITH THE BALLOON CATHETER

The rigid shaft of the heavy-duty guidewire facilitates smooth passage of the balloon across the stenosis; its short tapered flexible tip does not penetrate too far into peripheral small branches, thus avoiding spasm and intimal injury [20].

Wrap the deflated balloon material around the catheter shaft, while applying suction to the lumen feeding the balloon. This minimizes trauma to the point of entry and allows the deflated balloon to be properly positioned at the site of stenosis. (Similar suction is required during the removal of the catheter at the completion of the study.) The radiopaque markers of the deflated balloon must lie on either side of the stenotic segment. The guidewire tip must remain beyond the stenosis, throughout the entire procedure, until the dilation is successfully completed. This is necessary to avoid intravascular manipulation of the guidewire through any subsequently disrupted intima.

There may be *problems associated with advancing the balloon through the stenosis:* (1) The angle of the target vessel from the aorta may be too acute to permit maneuvering (e.g., superior mesenteric artery from a femoral approach; contralateral iliac artery). (2) Sometimes there is considerable tortuosity of the vessels leading to the stenotic site, or the target vessel is some distance from the puncture site. (3) Scarring, atherosclerosis, or a graft may be present at the puncture site. (4) The narrowed segment can be rigid (as from a fibrosed plaque), very tight, or elongated.

Each problem must be solved differently. If the angle is too acute, choose another approach (e.g., axillary artery).

The catheter may be successfully advanced through the stenosis by externally compressing and fixating the guidewire (Figs. 6-12, 6-13) or by introducing a more rigid guidewire. Amplatz and long Lunderquist guidewires are available for this purpose; the marked rigidity and abrupt transformation from shaft to flexible tip of the latter must be kept in mind to avoid complications. A variable stiffness guidewire and external manipulator (Cook) may be helpful. In its flexible form, the guidewire can pass around curves and through areas of stenosis. It is stiffened by the external manipulator as the catheter is advanced, after which the rigidity is released.

If the balloon fails to pass through the stenosis due to its severity, the stenosis may be "predilated" with the gradually tapered tip of a Staple van Andel catheter. Catheters with gradually tapered balloons have been designed to help solve this problem. If these are not available, predilation with a smaller gauge balloon catheter may be required.

Scarring or a graft at the puncture may be overcome by introducing the balloon catheter through a short sheath (see Chaps. 3 and 7). If there is tortuosity, angulation, or a long vascular course, longer sheaths (now commercially available up to 80 cm in length) can help absorb the accompanying shear forces (Fig. 6-14). To accomplish this, the balloon catheter must be exchanged for a slightly larger diameter conventional catheter that lies within the sheath. The hub of the sheath should have a hemostasis valve and flushing port. The balloon angioplasty catheter replaces the conventional catheter, which advances with greater ease through the narrowed zone.

DILATING THE BALLOON CATHETER

When the balloon has bridged the stenosis, proceed rapidly so as to avoid further embarrassment of an already compromised circulation. Inject heparin 3000 IU systemically, either intravenously or directly into the artery through the Touhy-Borst adapter surrounding the guidewire within the catheter. Intraarterial vasodilators may also be injected at this time. The balloon is rapidly inflated to the maximum pressure suggested by the manu-

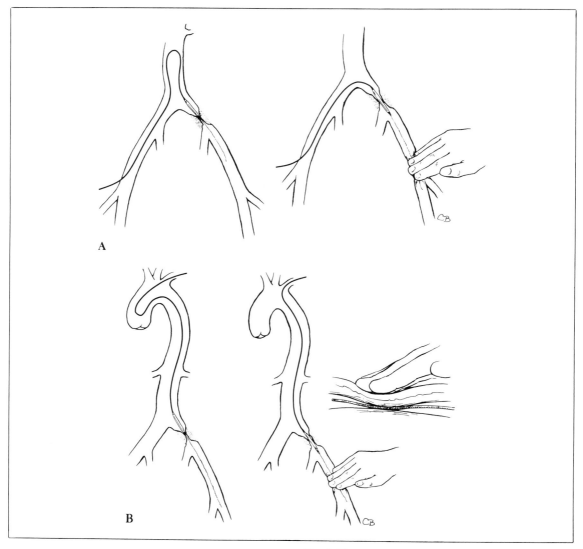

facturer by manually injecting 30% contrast material with an attached 10-ml syringe. The pressure
applied, measured through a sterilized pressure
manometer interposed between the syringe and the
balloon assembly, helps provide maximum dilating force without fear of rupturing the balloon. A
stopcock positioned between the syringe and the
pressure gauge allows uniform and easy application of pressure. As the balloon fills with contrast
agent, the deformity caused by the arterial narrowing is seen on the fluoroscopy screen to disappear
as the balloon assumes the normal tubular form of
the vessel (see Chaps. 8, 9, 10, 11, and 14). The
lesion is now successfully dilated.

Fig. 6-12.
A. Guidewire passed through stenosis, but there is resistance to passing the balloon catheter. Manually
fixate the guidewire in the groin.
B. Similar maneuver for an axillary approach.

The length of time the balloon remains inflated
and the number of dilations performed to achieve
successful dilation depend on the resistance to inflation, the residual deformity seen on the balloon
during each dilation, and to some extent on the
location of the lesion. The resistant arterial stenosis of renal transplants may require 6 or 7 dilations,
each lasting a minute or longer. A subclavian artery stenosis may require no more than a single
short period of dilation. In most vessels, three or

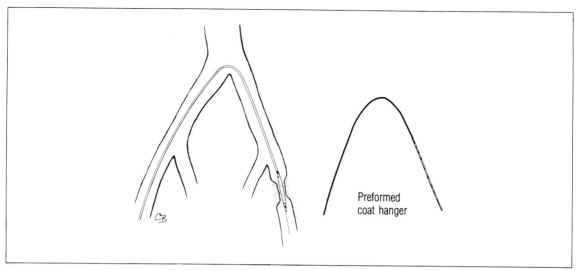

Fig. 6-13. When stenosis is traversed by guidewire, but the balloon catheter will not follow, advance a thin-walled 5 French diagnostic catheter through the stenosis, and replace the guidewire with a preformed, very rigid Lunderquist or Amplatz "coat hanger" guidewire.

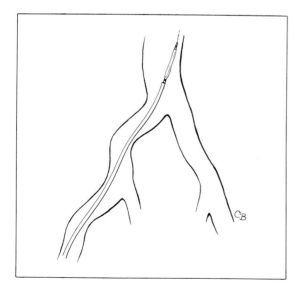

Fig. 6-14. Increased shear forces due to marked angulation and tortuosity of vessels can be absorbed by introducing the catheter through an overlying sheath. (See text.)

four dilations are performed, each lasting approximately 30 to 60 seconds.

There may be multiple or elongated narrowed segments demanding dilation of contiguous areas. The balloon must be deflated before being moved to other sites for reinflation. If there is remnant deformity during expansion of the dilating balloon, the lesion has not been completely dilated and further dilations are required. Sometimes, a slightly larger diameter balloon or one that is shorter in length may help give the desired effect.

PAIN

The patient often experiences discomfort as the vessel is being dilated. Pain that is inordinately severe or sustained after the balloon is deflated may signal impending vascular rupture. No pain whatsoever may indicate that the vessel has not been satisfactorily dilated.

FOLLOWING THE DILATATION

An angiogram and, if practical, pressure measurements document the success of the procedure, the need for further dilation, or the presence of complications. There is enough space remaining in the catheter lumen for these examinations to be performed through the balloon angioplasty catheter if the larger guidewire is replaced through the Touhy-Borst adapter with one that is smaller. All high-pressure contrast injections should be made well above the angioplasty site to avoid subintimal injury. Although the balloon angioplasty catheter is not optimal for diagnostic purposes, satisfactory studies can be obtained using IA-DSA.

If digital subtraction angiography equipment is not available, the balloon angioplasty catheter is replaced with a diagnostic catheter with multiple side holes (with a diameter 1 French size larger in order to accommodate the added diameter of the balloon material).

At all times the guidewire should remain across the dilated segment. If this is not practical, or the guidewire inadvertently slips proximal to the area of concern, careful manipulations are required to avoid intimal injury.

The postdilation angiogram might be expected to demonstrate vascular irregularities and intimal flaps, sometimes with minor degrees of residual stenosis (see Fig. 6-4). Beware of the impulse to obtain a perfect cosmetic result, for hemodynamic improvement is the desired goal. Also, as time progresses, remodeling and healing occur, and the seemingly poor immediate result often appears much improved on subsequent angiograms.

ARTERIAL SPASM

Arterial spasm due to the manipulations of the guidewire may occur in the smaller vascular beds (see Fig. 4-2). It occurs most frequently in second- or third-order branches of the renal circulation, the external carotid artery, and vessels of the lower extremity distal to the trifurcation. It can occur in larger, more proximal vessels. It can cause cir-

cumferential arterial narrowing and occasionally total occlusion of smaller branches. It is best handled prophylactically by injecting vasodilators (nitroglycerine 100 to 300 μg) [4] or tolazoline 25 mg, together with heparin 2000 IU [25] directly into the vascular bed immediately before dilating the vessel. If not given prophylactically, these same drugs should be given as soon as the spasm has been discovered on the postdilation angiogram. Administering oral or sublingual nifedipine (a calcium channel blocker) 10 mg shortly before inflating the balloon also helps to prevent arterial spasm. If vascular irregularity or occlusion persists despite antispasmodics and passage of time, there has likely been permanent intimal damage (Fig. 6-15).

REMOVING THE BALLOON CATHETER

Apply suction to the balloon during withdrawal of the balloon angioplasty catheter from the femoral artery in order to minimize trauma to the puncture site.

Sometimes prolonged manual compression is required at the puncture site following removal of the catheter due to the large bore of the catheter and the anticoagulants administered. If bleeding persists 15 to 20 minutes after withdrawing the

Fig. 6-15.
A. Fibromuscular hyperplasia of the right renal artery in a hypertensive patient.
B. Permanent intimal injury causing narrowing of renal artery branch during PTA. The narrowing persisted following intraarterial nitroglycerine.

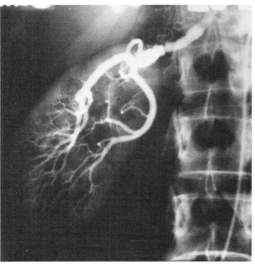

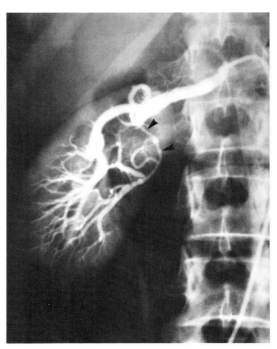

A   B

catheter, the effect of the heparin may be reversed with protamine. Protamine 10 mg is given intravenously for each 1000 IU heparin administered, assuming that 20 percent of the heparin dose dissipates every hour. Postprocedural heparin therapy is needed only in low-flow circumstances. Antiplatelet therapy (aspirin or dipyridamole) should be continued daily.

Postangiographic care includes monitoring the vital signs and checking for signs of hematoma, bleeding, and thrombosis. The patient should be allowed out of bed approximately 24 hours after the procedure.

COMPLICATIONS

Complications of angioplasty can occur at the puncture site, at the site of angioplasty, or in more remote locations. Bleeding and hematomas at the site of puncture are seen more frequently after angioplasty than after diagnostic arteriograms. Dissections, perforations, false aneurysms, arteriovenous fistulas, and thrombosis can occur both at the puncture site and at the angioplasty site. Arterial spasm, intimal damage, and peripheral embolization can occur in the distal circulation. Balloons rupture, detach, or may be slow to deflate, further embarrassing the peripheral circulation. Sepsis can occur. Patients may become hypotensive due to volume depletion following renal artery dilation, which can be corrected with intravenous fluids. Patients may also become acutely hypertensive immediately following renal arterial dilation, possibly due to a sudden release of additional renin into the circulation. Patients can go into renal failure. Those who are dehydrated may develop acute tubular necrosis and subsequent oliguria due to the contrast agents. Complications can be expected in 10 to 15 percent of patients [9, 12], but the vast majority of them are minor or self-limiting.

SUMMARY OF PROBLEMS DURING ANGIOPLASTY AND STEPS TO SOLVE THEM

The following are the most common problems that occur during angioplasty and may lead to complications or to an unsuccessful procedure, and the steps during angioplasty by which they may be overcome. Only stenotic lesions will be considered here. Occlusive lesions will be dealt with in Chapter 8.

1. *Puncturing a vessel with impalpable pulse distal to a stenosis.*
   a. Puncture blindly over the medial aspect of the femoral head.
   b. Doppler ultrasonography (use a sterilized pencil-shaped transmitter).
   c. Digital road mapping.
   d. Guidewire advanced over aortic bifurcation from contralateral puncture to act as a marker.
2. *Difficulty crossing stenosis with standard guidewires and 5 French catheter.*
   a. Use smaller gauge standard guidewire.
   b. Add "hockey stick" curve to distal tip of catheter for improved control of guidewire manipulation.
   c. Use catheter alone, without inner guidewire.
   d. Use an open-ended guidewire for manipulations and contrast agent injections.
   e. Use steerable guidewires, either alone or coaxially in an open-ended injectable guidewire. (NOTE: If focal dissection occurs, defer the procedure for 1 to 2 weeks to allow healing.)
3. *Difficulty following the guidewire across the stenosis with the balloon angioplasty catheter.*
   a. Exchange guidewire for a heavy-duty one; the Amplatz or Lunderquist exchange guidewire is the heaviest. Make all exchanges through the 5 French catheter already across the stenosis. Never forfeit a guidewire positioned beyond the lesion.
   b. Stenosis might be too tight to allow passage of the larger caliber balloon angioplasty catheter. Predilate the narrowed segment with a tapered-tip Staple van Andel catheter, a graduated-tip dilated balloon catheter, or a dilating balloon with a smaller diameter than that initially chosen.
   c. There may be scarring or a graft at the puncture site, or elongation, angulation, or tortuosity along the course of the vessel. These can be overcome by introducing an overlying sheath (1 to 2 French sizes larger than the angioplasty catheter) with an attached hemostasis valve and flushing side port.
4. *Arterial spasm of smaller peripheral vessels.*
   Avoid excess manipulation and distal advancement or wedging of the guidewire tip.

Intraarterial nitroglycerine (100 to 300 μg) or sublingual nifedipine (10 mg) may be given prophylactically immediately prior to dilation or after the spasm has been discovered.

5. *Permanent arterial damage with scarring or formation of false aneurysms by the guidewire.* Gentle manipulations and unforced positioning of flexible tipped guidewires help to limit this problem. Distal guidewire curves become trapped between the distal wall and the catheter tip (see Chap. 4). A gentle curve or a straight tip to the heavy duty guidewire limits this occurrence.

6. *Thrombosis.*

Thrombosis may occur at the angioplasty site, in more peripheral vessels, or at the puncture site. It occurs in thrombogenic patients, at angioplasty sites demanding prolonged manipulation, or in event of damage to the vessel wall. Heparin (3000 to 5000 IU) given prophylactically prior to passing the balloon across the stenosis or immediately prior to inflating the balloon may prevent it. Heparin may be given every 30 to 40 minutes if the procedure is prolonged, to a total of 8000 to 10,000 IU. The partial thromboplastin time should be measured prior to the study and, if large doses of heparin are given, should also be measured during the course of the procedure. If thrombosis occurs, and the thrombosed vessel is of small diameter or the catheter tip is close to the area, replace the balloon angioplasty catheter with one that is untapered and has a large bore (Lehman). A catheter sheath of the same diameter may be used instead. Advance it onto the clot and apply suction (see Chap. 7). If unsuccessful, treat with low-dose streptokinase intraarterially (50,000 IU as a bolus, and 5000 IU/hour), or urokinase (4000 IU/minute until clearing) (see Chap. 7). Thrombosis at the puncture site may be similarly treated. Surgical intervention is required if the circulation to the limb or organ appears to be severely compromised, or if the thrombolytic therapy does not show rapid signs of improvement.

7. *Peripheral embolization of atherosclerotic plaques.*

This problem fortunately occurs rarely (Fig. 6-16). Peripheral embolization of small plaques or blood clots may sometimes be suc-

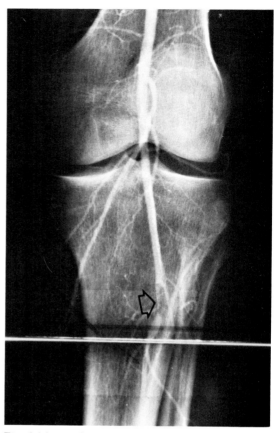

Fig. 6-16. Peripheral atherosclerotic embolus following PTA of patient in Fig. 6-3.

cessfully managed with intravenous infusion of 500 ml of low molecular weight dextran over a 6-hour period. Larger more central emboli may be removed by suctioning through a large diameter catheter or a Fogarty catheter passed through an arterial sheath (Chap. 7), but often surgical removal is necessary.

8. *Ruptured balloons.*

Balloons may rupture during dilatation if too much pressure is applied or if there is a mechanical defect. Rupture can be avoided by monitoring the inflating pressure with a pressure manometer while inflating with a 10-ml hand-held syringe. A 2- or 3-ml syringe generates much higher pressures and may be dangerous. If the balloon ruptures, gently withdraw it from the vascular system, leaving the guidewire in place over the area of stenosis. Replace the catheter with a new angioplasty catheter. Resistance to withdrawal may

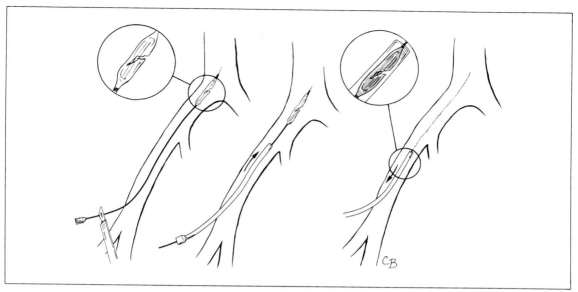

Fig. 6-17. Removing a ruptured balloon with a transverse tear. (See text.)

mean there is a transverse tear in the balloon, causing it to flare and damage the vessel walls. Under these circumstances, cut off the hub of the angioplasty catheter and advance a large-bore (10 French) catheter, or snugly fitting sheath, over the catheter shaft in an attempt to cover the ruptured balloon before it is withdrawn (Fig. 6-17). Balloon rupture transmits large forces to the surrounding arterial walls and thus carries a potential for arterial damage with resulting dissection, occlusion, or false aneurysm formation.

9. *Rupture of arterial walls with subsequent hemorrhage and shock* (Fig. 6-18).
   This situation is extremely rare, but can occur if
   a. The balloon used has a considerably larger diameter (3 mm or greater) than the caliber of the adjacent vessels [28] or the balloon is too long for a limited area.
   b. The balloon is manufactured with compliant materials (polyvinyl), which enlarge rather than rupture when increasing pressures are applied.
   c. The stenotic lesion is hard, calcified or fibrosed, and resistant to inflation.
   Institute immediate measures to counteract shock and pain. Check vital signs, force intravascular fluids, and type and crossmatch blood. Administer oxygen, have an airway handy. Deflate the balloon and reposition it in a slightly more central location and reinflate it in an attempt to temporarily secure hemostasis. Immediate surgical intervention is required to avert disaster.

10. *Difficulty deflating the balloon after angioplasty.*
   This difficulty is infrequent, but predisposes to thrombosis and can result in ischemia peripheral to the point of occlusion. Manufacturing problems, kinking of the catheter, and crystallization of contrast agent in the lumen feeding the balloon are some of the contributing causes. It can be prevented by avoiding previously used and resterilized catheters, by pretesting the balloon using only half-strength contrast agent, and by pretesting the balloon immediately prior to its insertion rather than earlier in the procedure. The catheter should be discarded if the balloon is too slow to inflate and deflate.
   If the balloon does not deflate within the vessel, try applying suction with a 50-ml syringe. If still unsuccessful, administer 3000 IU heparin intravenously and consider one of three ways to remove the balloon:
   a. If the angioplasty is being performed above the iliacs, advance a diagnostic catheter through the opposite femoral artery to the site of the inflated balloon. Introduce a

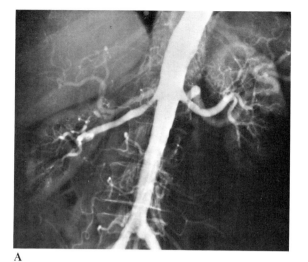

A

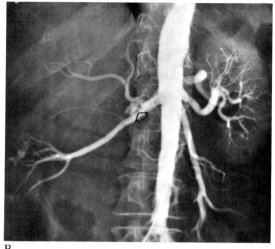

B

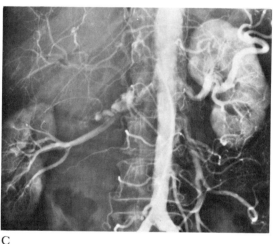

C

Fig. 6-18. This was another doctor's unfortunate experience—a ruptured renal artery following PTA. The balloon used was too long, and the guidewire was removed prior to dilation of an angulated vessel. (Printed with permission.)
A. Prior to PTA.
B and C. Post-PTA. Note extravasation of contrast (*arrow*) and lateral displacement of right kidney.

sharpened object (a metallic inner core of a guidewire) through its lumen in an effort to puncture the balloon.

  b. Puncture the balloon percutaneously through the overlying soft tissues using a thin 22-gauge biopsy needle.

  c. Remove the hub of the balloon angioplasty catheter and insert a 10 French catheter (a modified 10 French Staple van Andel

catheter with its tip removed) coaxially over the 7 French balloon catheter. Wedge the 10 French catheter at the base of the balloon, and give a sharp tug on the inner catheter. This maneuver can be dangerous, for the balloon tip may break off from the catheter shaft.

11. Avoid obstructing major collateral branches that bypass areas of severe stenosis or occlusion.

12. Do not perform angioplasty if the guidewire and diagnostic catheter pass subintimally and re-enter the major channel distally, for this may completely occlude an already compromised vessel.

13. Hematomas at the puncture site are usually self-limiting and can be followed closely. Reverse the effect of heparin by administering protamine (approximately 10 mg per 1000 IU of heparin). Dangerous retroperitoneal hematomas may form if the puncture site is above the inguinal ligament. Axillary hematomas should be followed closely with early surgical decompression in order to avoid permanent nerve damage.

References

1. Abele, J. E. Balloon catheters and transluminal dilatation. *A.J.R.* 135:901, 1980.
2. Abrams, H. *Abrams' Angiography: Vascular and Interventional Radiology* (3rd ed.). Boston: Little, Brown, 1983.

3. Athanasoulis, C. A., et al. *Interventional Radiology*. Philadelphia: Saunders, 1982.

4. Brown, B. G., et al. The mechanisms of nitroglycerine action: Stenosis vasodilatation as a major component of the drug response. *Circulation*, 64:1089, 1981.

5. Castaneda-Zuniga, W. R. (ed.). *Transluminal Angioplasty*. New York: Thieme Stratton, 1983.

6. Castaneda-Zuniga, W. R., et al. The mechanism of balloon angioplasty. *Radiology* 135:565, 1980.

7. Castaneda-Zuniga, W. R., et al. Mechanics of angioplasty: An experimental approach. *Radiographics* 1:14, 1981.

8. Dotter, C. T., and Judkins, M. P. Transluminal treatment of atherosclerotic obstruction. Description of a new technique and a preliminary report of its application. *Circulation* 30:654, 1964.

9. Dotter, C. T., et al. *Percutaneous Transluminal Angioplasty*. Berlin: Springer-Verlag, 1983.

10. Gruntzig, A., and Hopff, H. Perkutane Rekanalisation chronisher arterieller vershlusse mit einen neuen Dilatationskathete. Modifikation der Dotter-Technik. *Dtsch. Med. Wochenschr.* 99:2502, 1974.

11. Gruntzig, A., and Schoope, W. (eds.). *Percutaneous Vascular Recanalization. Technic, Application, Clinical Results*. Berlin: Springer, 1978.

12. Kadir, S., et al. *Selected Techniques in Interventional Radiology*. Philadelphia: Saunders, 1982.

13. Katzen, B. T. Percutaneous Transluminal Angioplasty (PTA) with Gruntzig balloon catheter. *Radiology* 130:823, 1979.

14. Kinney, T. B., et al. Transluminal angioplasty. A mechanical pathophysiological correlation of its physical mechanisms. *Radiology* 153:85, 1984.

15. Lunderquist, A., Lunderquist, M., and Owman, T. Guidewire for percutaneous transhepatic cholangiography. *Radiology* 132:228, 1979.

16. Meyerovitz, M. F., Levin, D. C., and Boxt, L. M. Superselective catheterization of small caliber arteries with a new high visibility steerable guidewire. *A.J.R.* 144:785, 1985.

17. Murray, P. D., Carnic, D., and Bettman, M. A. Pharmacology of angioplasty and intravascular thrombolysis. *A.J.R.* 139:795, 1982.

18. Portsmann, W., Ein neuer Korsett-Balloon-Katheter zur translumination Rekanalisation nach Dotter unter besonderer Beruksichtigung von Obliterationen an den Beckenarterien. *Radiol. Diagn. (Berl.)* 14:239, 1973.

19. Ring, E. J., and McLean, G. K. (eds.) *Interventional Radiology: Principles and Techniques*. Boston: Little, Brown, 1981.

20. Rosen, R. H., et al. New exchange guidewire for transluminal angioplasty. *Radiology* 140:242, 1981.

21. Shaver, R. W., and Soon, G. J., Angioplasty through aortofemoral graft: Use of catheter introducer shields. *A.J.R.* 138:168, 1982.

22. Sos, T. A., and Sniderman, K. W. Percutaneous transluminal angioplasty. *Semin. Roentgenol.* 16:26, 1981.

23. Sos, T., et al. A new open ended guidewire/catheter. *Radiology* 154:817, 1985.

24. Udoff, E. H., et al. Hemodynamic significance of iliac artery stenosis: Pressure measurements during angiography. *Radiology* 132:289, 1979.

25. Weiner, N. Adrenergic Nerves and Structure Innervated by Them. In A. G. Gilman, et al. (eds.), *The Pharmacological Basis of Therapeutics* (7th ed.). New York: Macmillan, 1985.

26. Wilkins, R. A., and Viamonte, M. *Interventional Radiology*. Oxford: Blackwell Scientific, 1982.

27. Wolf, G. L., LeVeen, R. F., and Ring, E. J. Potential mechanisms of angioplasty. *Cardiovasc. Intervent. Radiol.* 7:11, 1984.

28. Zollikofer, C. L., et al. The relation between arterial and balloon rupture in experimental angioplasty. *A.J.R.* 144:777, 1985.

Related Endovascular Procedures

Thrombolytic Therapy

COAGULATION PROCESS

The final step in the complex clotting mechanism that occurs in the vascular system is the production of a fibrin mesh from the fibrinogen found freely circulating in the plasma [3, 16]. This coagulation process can be interrupted, thereby preventing clots from forming, a process called *anticoagulation*. Also, once formed, the clot can be dissolved, a process called *thrombolysis* (Fig. 7-1A).

There are three major contributors to the clotting mechanism: (1) loss of integrity of the vessel wall, (2) effect of the platelets, and (3) intravascular cascades, which eventually form thrombin, which acts on the fibrinogen. The pathophysiology of thrombosis is different in the arterial system from that in the venous system.

Coagulation in the Arterial System

In the arterial system, the thrombi are predominantly white thrombi, composed primarily of closely packed aggregated platelets, with only small amounts of fibrin present. In veins, however, red thrombi form with much greater quantities of fibrin and red cell coagulum. Mixed thrombi (that is, both white and red) are found in those arterial systems in which there is stenosis. The slow turbulent flow allows aggregation of the white platelets and subsequent accumulation of red cells within the fibrin mesh, causing the red component of the clot.

In the arterial system, platelets adhere to the vessel wall and release prostaglandin endoperoxides (Fig. 7-1B), which in turn are converted by the endothelial cells to prostacyclin. This enzyme protects the endothelium of the blood vessels, where it is found in greatest concentration, for it is a vasodilator that also inhibits platelet adherence. In a second and opposing action, prostaglandin endoperoxides also convert to thromboxane A_2, which stimulates platelet aggregation and causes vasoconstriction. The thromboxane A_2 is found in greater concentration at the adventitia; the net bal-ance at the endothelial layer of the artery favors vasodilation and inhibits platelet aggregation. When atherosclerosis is present, however, the lipid peroxides inhibit the protective mechanism of prostacyclin, and the balance is tipped toward thromboxane A_2, which promotes formation of thrombosis.

Coagulation in the Veins

In veins, the coagulation process is different, and the basic theories of Virchow still hold firm. Rarely, thrombosis is induced by damage to the venous walls, as in trauma and in inflammation. Stasis and the hypercoagulable state are the most common contributors.

STASIS. Clots form in the apex of valves by platelet aggregation and then increase in size. This occurs most frequently in the calves of the legs, where there are numerous valves and a longer standing column, two factors that contribute to stasis and thrombosis.

HYPERCOAGULABLE STATE. Vessels have a fibrinolytic endothelium, which is more pronounced in veins than in arteries. Tissue plasminogen activator (tPA) is formed and stored in endothelial cells and is constantly being released into the circulation within the venous system. It has been found that tPA is not formed in the pockets of valves in the venous system, which may explain why thrombi start in this location. A dynamic equilibrium exists between tPA, which induces thrombolysis, and an inhibitor to tPA, which is also found in endothelial cells and plasma.

Anticoagulation

The coagulation process can be interrupted by a number of mechanisms. Heparin, given parenterally, is the mainstay of anticoagulation therapy. It immediately acts in several ways on the clotting mechanisms. The end result is preventing prothrombin from forming thrombin and also inactivating any thrombin that may be present. This action prevents thrombin from transforming fibrinogen to fibrin, the meshwork that forms the basis for a clot. Orally given anticoagulants (e.g.,

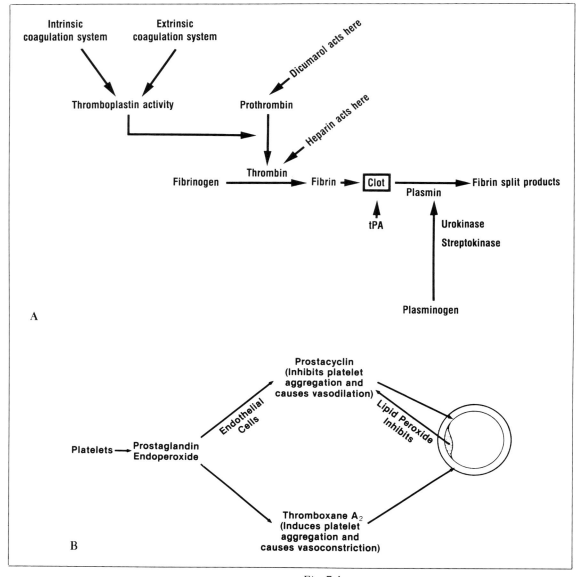

Fig. 7-1.
A. Anticoagulant and thrombolytic action. tPA = tissue plasminogen activator.
B. Prostacyclin concentrates at the endothelial layer, where it helps prevent platelet aggregation and stimulates vasodilation. The lipid peroxide of atherosclerotic plaques inhibits the protecting action of prostacyclin and allows thromboxane A_2 to induce thrombosis by aggregating platelets and constricting vessels.

warfarin) act differently and more slowly, but with similar results. Over a period of several days, they inhibit synthesis in the liver of coagulation factors that are dependent on vitamin K (factors VII, IX, and X and prothrombin). Thus, there is less prothrombin to form thrombin, and the conversion of fibrinogen into fibrin is thereby impaired. Platelet functions can be decreased by the use of antiplatelet drugs, such as aspirin.

Thrombolysis

Neither heparin nor warfarin nor antiplatelet drugs are effective in actually dissolving or reducing any existing clot. This process is left for the body to do, with its own internal system of fibrinolytic activity. This system is dependent on the circulating proenzyme, plasminogen, a substance found both circulating freely in the plasma and trapped in the clot itself. The plasminogen is converted (by a peptide bond cleavage) to form the active proteolytic enzyme, plasmin [2]. This conversion takes place both in plasma and on the surface and in the interstices of the clot. The enzyme plasmin digests both fibrinogen and fibrin and in doing so dissolves the clot. Any free plasmin formed in the circulation is inactivated by inhibitors (antiplasmin). The plasmin found in the clot, however, lyses the fibrin, unimpeded by the plasmin inhibitors. The success of this mechanism of fibrinolysis depends on the release of the plasminogen. Much of it lies trapped within the clot, where it takes time to be activated. This time period is critical for the patient, and any prolongation of it may cause the many dangerous pathophysiologic changes of ischemia.

FIBRINOLYTIC AGENTS

Streptokinase and urokinase are potent, highly purified plasminogen activators that, when in the vicinity of a clot, cause dissolution by the subsequently produced plasmin [16]. Urokinase is a naturally occurring enzymatic protein found within plasma and renal parenchymal cells and is extracted from tissue cultures of human kidneys. Streptokinase is a nonenzymatic fibrinolytic protein excreted by group C beta-hemolytic streptococci, and it acts on plasminogen found within plasma as well as within blood clots. Both streptokinase and urokinase can cause depletion in the amount of circulating plasminogen as well as of the fibrinogen. If this occurs, there will be less plasmin available for clot lysis.

New tissue plasminogen activating substances, which selectively activate the plasminogen found within clot, are under investigation [28, 30]. These are naturally occurring, circulating human proteins (serine protease) with a short half-life (5 minutes), and they do not bind avidly with the circulating plasminogen but rather with that found at the fibrin surface of the clot. Thus, selective thrombolysis occurs at the clot without the systemic thrombolytic changes that can cause bleeding at other sites. Experimental and human trials have substantiated the clot selective activity of these proteins by demonstrating clot lysis. Clot ly-

sis occurs with no change in those parameters that generally reflect a systemic fibrinolytic state (i.e., decreased plasminogen, antiplasmin, and fibrinogen levels; increased fibrinogen degradation products). Also, other tests (prothrombin time, activated partial thromboplastin time, thrombin time, and platelet counts) remain normal. Currently these tissue plasminogen activators are being purified from melanoma tissue culture supernates, are of limited supply, and are still undergoing experimental trials [30]. Recent reports of successful cloning and expression of the human gene in *Escherichia coli* suggest the possibility of large-scale production in the future [21].

THROMBOLYTIC THERAPY

Large doses of thrombolytic agents are required to lyse clots if they are administered *systemically*. There is an attendant risk of bleeding from potential bleeding sites. Intravascular fibrinolytic therapy is a means by which clots can be dissolved by injecting thrombolytic agents directly into the involved vessel or, better still, into the clot itself. The higher regional concentration afforded by injecting these agents either directly into, or close to, a clot allows clot lysis to occur with considerably smaller and, consequently, safer doses [8, 12].

Both streptokinase and urokinase are capable of lysing clots. Since urokinase is not a foreign protein and is considered nonantigenic, only mild and rare allergic reactions have been reported. Antibody mediated resistance to urokinase does not develop. The enzyme, however, is difficult to extract and very expensive. Streptokinase, on the other hand, has some reported, albeit not serious or frequent, allergic and pyrogenic reactions.

The systemic loading dose for streptokinase is 250,000 IU over the first 30 to 40 minutes, followed by 100,000 IU per hour. Selective low-dose intravascular streptokinase therapy usually calls for approximately 5000 IU per hour in peripheral extremity vessels [12], but often more within the coronary arterial circulation [22]. The systemic dose for urokinase is recommended at 4400 IU/kg/hour. Selective intravascular low-dose therapy of urokinase was initially recommended at 20,000 IU per hour; considerably higher intraarterial doses result in improved local thrombolytic results with a decreased rate of bleeding complications [17]. With this newer regimen, urokinase can be infused selectively within or as close as possible to

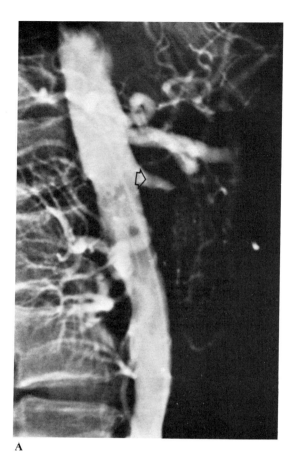

A

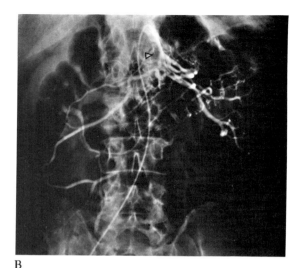

B

C

the clot with a dosage of 4000 IU per minute until antegrade blood flow is established, and then at a dosage of 1000 to 2000 IU per minute (depending on clot size and rapidity of lysis) until the clot is completely lysed.

A low-dose selective administration of fibrinolytic materials is relatively safe if the necessary precautions are taken not to administer systemic doses. It can be used to treat patients with thrombi occurring spontaneously in vessels of the extremities (see Chap. 8) and in the pulmonary arteries (see Chap. 17) [31] and it is particularly helpful in treating those with surgical grafts (see Chap. 8). It can be used in those with thrombi occurring following an arteriogram (see Chap. 8). Although intraarterial fibrinolytic therapy is most helpful in treating thromboembolic events occurring within 72 hours (Figs. 7-2, 7-3), it has been known to lyse clots of much longer duration, even to several weeks or months. Clot lysis will often uncover the underlying cause of the occlusion (severe stenosis),

Fig. 7-2. Thrombolysis of acute mesenteric thrombosis.
A. Lateral projection abdominal aortogram demonstrates occlusion of superior mesenteric artery (*arrow*).
B. Selective mesenteric arteriogram shows a large clot lying within the proximal superior mesenteric artery.
C. After 24 hours of streptokinase infusion, the superior mesenteric artery is patent.

which may then be promptly treated by either transluminal angioplasty or surgery (see Chap. 8).

Indications

Thrombolytic therapy should be considered in those patients in whom the symptoms suggest an acute occlusive process. It is helpful in those with

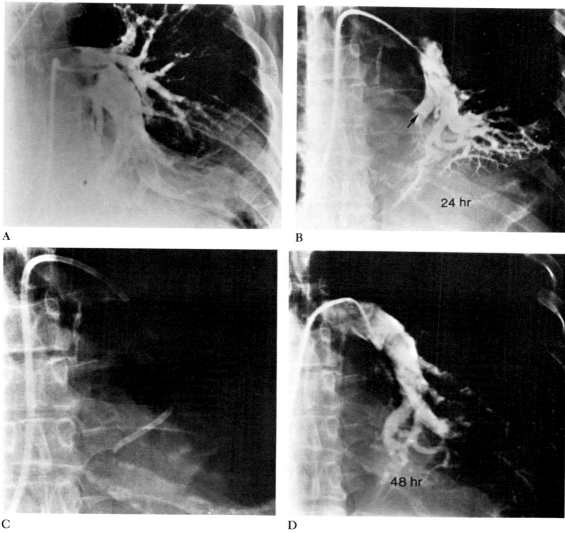

C   D

Fig. 7-3. Streptokinase therapy for large pulmonary emboli of left lower lobe. The patient experienced severe pain which prompted treatment.
A. Large filling defects of arteries to the left lower lobe.
B. Dissolution of some clots with remaining clot in posterior medial segment (*arrow*).
C. Superselective catheter placement in this clotted vessel.
D. Forty-eight hours later, all major clots have dissolved and the pain has disappeared.

accelerating claudication or rest pain. It should not be used if impending tissue death (presaged by loss of motor or sensory function) precludes a 12- to 24-hour period of treatment. Here surgery must not be delayed. Indeed, the decision to treat a patient in this manner must be considered jointly with a surgeon. Vessels with high flow (such as the renal artery, superior mesenteric artery, iliac arteries, and femoral arteries) do better than those with low flow (popliteal or tibial arteries). If the distal flow is poor, there is much less likelihood of success. Reocclusion can occur under these circumstances despite initial lysis of clot.

Factors limiting success relate, therefore, to age, size and location of the clot, and the ability to selectively position the catheter into the clot or adjacent to it. Recent clot or a small clot lying within a larger artery with good peripheral flow is more prone to success and should lyse within 10 to 12 hours. Embolic events can also be successfully treated. Sometimes, however, although the embolism may have occurred recently, the age of the embolic material may be old. Clots in infected areas (e.g., infected grafts) will usually not respond to thrombolytic therapy. The patient's endogenous supply of plasminogen is essential to lysis. Factors elevating the streptococcal antibodies preclude success with streptokinase and require the urokinase.

Contraindications to fibrinolytic therapy include a recent cerebrovascular accident (within the past 6 to 8 weeks), cerebral metastases, active bleeding from any site, recent trauma or surgery (within the past 10 days for general surgery; within the past 8 weeks for brain or spine surgery), pregnancy, blood dyscrasias, and endocarditis. Clots within the thoracic or brachiocephalic areas should not be lysed (or lysed with caution), for they may migrate to the brain. A relative contraindication would be severe hypertension.

Complications

Hemorrhagic complications have been reported in up to 23 percent of patients [1, 18]. The frequency of this complication is usually related to conditions that predispose to bleeding. These conditions include gastrointestinal bleeding, hematuria, and intracranial hemorrhage. Hematomas at the puncture site, retroperitoneal hemorrhage, and bleeding through the wall of a Dacron graft have been reported. The majority of the bleeding complications, however, are minor and are usually related to the puncture site. Thrombotic complications, with formation of new clot along the course of the catheter, and peripheral embolic events can also occur.

One can expect significant lysis to occur in up to 80 percent of patients [1, 17, 18], with a higher rate of success using urokinase. A lower success rate can be expected if the infusate is directed away from the thrombus and through adjacent collateral channels.

Treatment Techniques

PRETREATMENT. Document baseline physical and vascular factors. Obtain surgical and medical consultation. Obtain baseline complete blood count, prothrombin time, partial thromboplastin time (PTT), and fibrinogen level. If heparin is not being used concomitantly, obtain thrombin clotting times as well. Heparin always raises the

thrombin clotting time and confuses its interpretation. Obtain streptozyme levels if streptokinase is being used. These will be elevated if there has been previous exposure to streptokinase or streptococcal infection. If streptozyme levels are elevated, urokinase should be substituted.

Have cryoprecipitate or fresh frozen plasma available in case of bleeding. Type and crossmatch blood for two units of packed red cells.

CATHETER TECHNIQUE. Approach the occlusion from the most direct path available. Aspirate clot material through the catheter if at all possible. Embed a 5 French thin-walled catheter into the proximal surface of the clot or as close as possible to the clot. Try to pass the guidewire through the clot prior to infusion of the thrombolytic agent. This assures better penetration of the clot with the infusate. A coaxial system (with an attached Touhy-Borst adapter) may be used to prevent clot formation around the catheter. Under these circumstances, embed a 3 French inner catheter, or an open-ended injectable guidewire, into the clot and position the outer 5 to 6.5 French catheter tip proximal to the clot. Infuse thrombolytic agent through both of these catheters.

DOSAGE OF STREPTOKINASE. The dosage of streptokinase for an adult [1, 2, 12, 19, 23] is as follows: Add 5000 IU in 50 ml of 5% glucose solution or normal saline solution (50,000 IU/500 ml solution). If the clot is small and in a fairly large artery, infuse 5000 IU per hour. If the clot is larger or clots are present in smaller vessels, one may give a loading dose of 20,000 to 25,000 IU within the first hour. Another, more intense regimen is giving 2000 to 4000 IU per minute for approximately $\frac{1}{2}$ hour and then perform repeat arteriography to determine its effect. Following this, 5000 IU per hour may be administered. This may be increased to 10,000 or even 20,000 IU per hour if clinically success has not occurred and if the bleeding parameters permit.

Heparin may be given systemically in low doses in order to prevent clot from propagating up the catheter. A dose of 10,000 to 15,000 IU per day may be given intravenously in a continuous drip [1]. Since the infusing catheter often traverses a low-flow circulation, clot formation can be a significant problem. Some investigators avoid using heparin in order to avoid bleeding complications [12]. Decrease the heparin dosage if the PTT is much more than 100 seconds and decrease the streptokinase if fibrinogen levels are less than 100 mg.

DOSAGE OF UROKINASE. The dose of urokinase for an adult [17] is as follows: A dose of 500,000 IU urokinase is dissolved in 200 ml of physiologic saline solution and the resulting mixture is infused at 96 ml per hour (4000 IU/minute) until flow is established; then dosage is decreased to 48 or even 24 ml per hour (2000 IU or 1000 IU/minute) until complete lysis occurs.

Patient Care During Infusion

Monitor the patient in an acute care unit. Check for bleeding internally and externally. Avoid intramuscular or intraarterial injections.

STREPTOKINASE. Monitor the bleeding factors every 4 hours. Try to keep the PTT at 2 to 3 times normal if heparin is used. Thrombin clotting times are not considered interpretable if concomitant heparin is administered, for it is prolonged under these circumstances. If no heparin is administered, thrombin clotting times should be kept in the range of 1½ to 3 times normal levels. Fibrinogen levels normally approximate 400 mg. Although a low level does not necessarily correlate with hemorrhagic complications [18], this should not be allowed to decrease to much less than 100 mg. If thrombin clotting time is markedly elevated or fibrinogen levels are markedly depressed, temporarily substitute saline for the thrombolytic agent.

UROKINASE. Monitor bleeding parameters (PTT, fibrinogen, hematocrit) after the initial 2 hours of treatment and 2 hours after any change in urokinase dose. Again, fibrinogen levels should not be allowed to fall to much less than 100 mg, and this is controlled by altering the dosage of urokinase. Fibrin degradation products and euglobulin lysis times are less important parameters to follow.

Follow-up Angiograms

STREPTOKINASE. Follow-up angiograms should be performed within 1 hour if higher doses are used. Otherwise, repeat arteriograms are performed within 6 to 8 hours. If there is no change, increase the streptokinase up to 10,000 IU per hour. Check for elevated streptokinase antibodies; if they are present, change to urokinase.

UROKINASE. Angiographic documentation of the course of thrombolysis is performed following each course of 500,000 IU of urokinase. Intravenous heparin can be administered concomitantly at the rate of 1000 IU per hour, trying to maintain a PTT of 100 to 150 seconds; if PTT is much more than this, decrease the dose of heparin.

If the angiogram demonstrates improvement but persistent clot, advance the catheter further into the clot and continue the infusion of thrombolytic agent. One can continue this for up to 3 or 4 days if improvement continues. Be aware that systemic fibrinolysis occurs both with high loading doses and by accumulation from prolonged low-dose therapy.

If the clot is lysed, remove the catheter and secure hemostasis. In low-flow circulations that have been lysed, heparin must be administered at a rate of 25,000 IU per day for 4 or 5 days in order to prevent rethrombosis induced by the plasminogen depleted system. Delay the heparin treatment until thrombin time is less than 1½ times normal. Heparinization may not be necessary if there is a widely patent high-flow vascular system. If an underlying stenosis is uncovered in the patient who is a candidate for percutaneous transluminal angioplasty (PTA), dilation should be carried out immediately, for without treatment rethrombosis can occur within a very short period of time [18]. If the clot is unaffected within 24 hours, discontinue thrombolytic therapy and consider surgical means.

If the patient starts to bleed, discontinue the infusion, and administer cryoprecipitate or fresh frozen plasma and/or packed red cells.

The end point of the treatment is complete lysis of the clot, the development of intervening complications (usually related to bleeding), indications for surgical intervention, or no improvement over a 24-hour period.

Significant advances are being made in clot-selective fibrinolytic therapy by using tissue-type plasminogen activators, but these are still in an investigational stage. To date this therapy appears to be more efficient and to cause fewer complications than streptokinase or urokinase, features that make this an exciting new concept [14, 28, 30].

Aspiration of Clot by Percutaneous Catheter

Peripheral arterial clots and emboli are usually handled surgically by arteriotomy and Fogarty catheter extraction; intravascular embolectomy re-

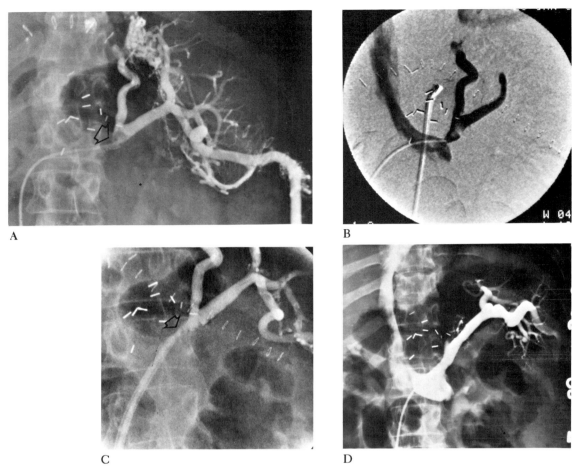

A

B

C

D

Fig. 7-4. Percutaneous aspiration of clot and subsequent PTA of stenosed Warren shunt. Ten days postoperative.
A. Almost totally occluded Warren shunt with stenosis at the anastomosis and a clot at anastomotic site (*arrow*). Catheter advanced from inferior vena cava through left renal vein into the shunt.
B. IV-DSA better demonstrates the clot and stenosis.
C. No. 10 French catheter was advanced to the stenosis and the clot was suctioned. Narrowed anastomotic site (*arrow*).
D. Shunt is widely patent after dilation with a 1-cm diameter balloon catheter.

mains firmly in the domain of the surgeon. There are select circumstances when thromboemboli can be aspirated percutaneously with catheters. Therefore, aspiration of clots should be kept in mind as a potential percutaneous therapeutic measure for management of occluded vessels, together with local thrombolytic therapy and percutaneous transluminal angioplasty.

INDICATIONS
Percutaneous aspiration of clot may be useful when the patient is at high risk for surgery or when more extensive undesirable surgical intervention might be required (Fig. 7-4) [27, 29]. It may help in the success of other endovascular procedures (thrombolytic therapy or PTA) by debulking large thrombi. It may be used when thrombolytic therapy is contraindicated (recent strokes or surgery, blood dyscrasias). It is the procedure of choice in those with thromboemboli complicating PTA or

angiography (see Fig. 8-48). It has been used by some to remove pulmonary thromboemboli. At all times, the procedure should be considered on the basis of its clinical merits and with close surgical consultation.

METHODS
Percutaneous aspiration will be more successful when clots are small and relatively acute in nature.

Long or firm clots can be broken into smaller, softer parts for easier aspiration if probed with a guidewire and if the volume is first reduced by treatment with thrombolysis.

Materials

As shown in Figure 7-5A, materials needed are as follows [29]:

1. Thin-walled, large diameter (up to 10 French) untapered catheters with special low friction walls, which are available[1] in lengths up to 80 cm. They can be trimmed to the desired length and should be long enough to reach the site of the clot. These catheters are used for aspirating the clot.
2. An overlying, snuggly fitting, thin-walled sheath of slightly shorter length, with an exchangeable hemostasis valve and a sidearm at the hub of the sheath.[2] The sheath helps confine the retrieved embolism if it is dislodged during withdrawal. The exchangeable hemostasis valve may trap fragments which may be extruded when exchanged.

Technique

The technique described is for lower extremity clot aspiration; modifications can be made for other areas.

An arteriogram (contralateral approach) outlines the location, size, and multiplicity of clots. An ipsilateral antegrade puncture is dilated to accommodate an 8 French diagnostic catheter with overlying thin-walled sheath that has been trimmed to the appropriate length. Advance the catheter with the overlying thin-walled sheath to a point just proximal to the clot. Replace the diagnostic catheter with the aspiration catheter and advance it gently into the clot while aspirating with the 50-ml syringe. When continued suction results in no further aspiration of blood, the clot has been engaged (Fig. 7-5A). Withdraw the catheter partially into the sheath, and withdraw both catheter and sheath proximally, closer to the puncture site

(Fig. 7-5B). While still applying suction to the suction catheter, remove the suction catheter from the sheath (Fig. 7-5C); apply suction to the sidearm of the hemostasis valve to remove fragments dislodged into the body of the sheath. Detach and exchange the hemostasis valve to remove trapped fragments. At this point, the sheath may be pinched closed with fingers or rubber tipped forceps (Fig. 7-5D). The hemostasis valve can be cleansed or replaced with another. Empty the syringe contents into a gauze pad to document the clots that have been removed. If suction characteristics or contrast injections through the side port of the hemostasis valve still suggest remnant clot, introduce a guidewire through the sheath and replace it with another catheter sheath system for further aspiration (Fig. 7-5E).

Percutaneous Removal of an Intravascular Foreign Body

Iatrogenic intravascular foreign bodies include a variety of intravascular devices that may be dislodged into the arterial or venous systems or into the cardiac chambers: intravenous central lines, ventriculovenous shunts, inferior vena cava filters, intravascular sheaths, intraarterial catheters, portions of coiled spring guidewires, misplaced coiled spring emboli, and cardiac pacemakers.

Sometimes these foreign bodies become extravascular in location with the passage of time, and occasionally they may finally come to rest in a small nonvital arterial branch. If inert and not infected, these may not have to be removed. In general, however, intravascular foreign bodies should be removed because of their attendant high complication rate [9]. Potential complications include sepsis, thromboembolism, cardiac arrhythmias, and even perforation of the cardiac chambers or the major vessels.

There are special precautions required during withdrawal of foreign bodies. All manipulations should be performed with retrieval catheters advanced through an introducing nontapered sheath of appropriate diameter. These vary up to 8, 9, or 10 French diameter and are of varying lengths up to 80 cm. They can be cut to the required length prior to use. A sheath is useful, for the tip may be placed close to the site of the foreign body, which can be rapidly withdrawn into its protective cus-

---

[1] Manufactured by Mallinckrodt, Diagnostic Products Division, St. Louis, MO 63134.
[2] Manufactured by USCI, a division of C. R. Bard, Inc., Box 566, Billerica, MA 01821; Cordis Corp., 125 NE 40th St., Miami, FL 33137; Angiomedics, 2905 NW Blvd., Minneapolis, MN 55441.

138

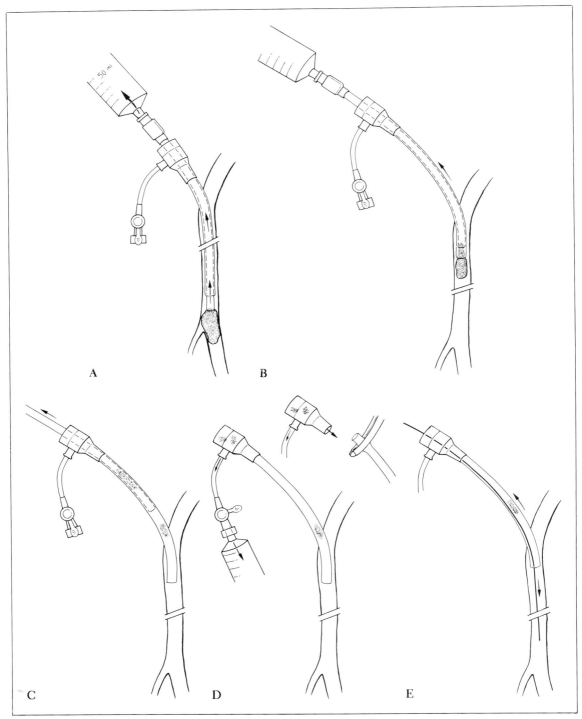

Fig. 7-5. Aspiration of clot through percutaneous catheter. (See text.)

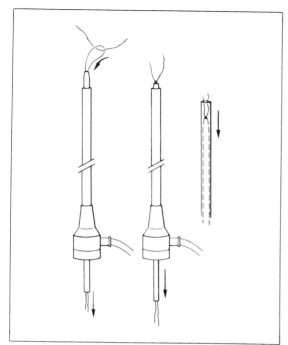

Fig. 7-6. A snare loop is introduced through a sheath with a sidearm (available in varying diameters and lengths). It is fitted with a hemostasis valve, which prevents back-bleeding during the procedure. A side port allows flushing and contrast medium injection. The hemostasis valve is easily removed and exchanged. The snare loop is available commercially (Cook Inc.) or can be manufactured in your own laboratory. A 0.025-in. guidewire can be looped on itself and advanced into a 7 French catheter. An 0.021-in. guidewire can be looped through a 6.5 French catheter. Another modification is attaching a thread or filament to the flexible tip of the guidewire and advancing both of these through the catheter lumen. The snare loop requires that the foreign body (e.g., catheter fragment, guidewire, coil) have an end be free to be snared.

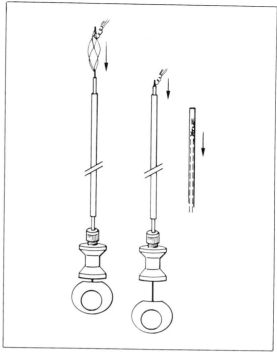

Fig. 7-7. Dormia type basket. It is advanced through the sheath, opened to engage the free end of the foreign body, and then withdrawn back into the sheath following retrieval. It is useful in trapping lost coils.

tody by the retrieval catheter. There is less fear of fragmentation, dislodgement, and peripheral embolization.

When a foreign body is being withdrawn from the arterial system, a hemostasis valve with attached side port for positive pressure flushing[3] should be placed on both the hub of the sheath and on the hub of the retrieval catheter [26]. This helps to combat loss of blood and provides constant

flushing to prevent accumulation of thrombus during a sometimes lengthy retrieval procedure.

During intracardiac manipulations, an ECG should be constantly monitored to avoid sustained arrhythmias.

A variety of retrieval devices are available [4, 6, 7, 9, 13, 20, 24, 25, 26]. These are illustrated and described in Figures 7-6, 7-7, 7-8, 7-9, and 7-10. Figure 7-11 demonstrates a catheter that had been present within the right atrium for over a year and was successfully removed using the grasping forceps shown in Figure 7-9C.

Percutaneous Management of Knotted and Coiled Intravascular Catheters

Intravascular catheter manipulations can result in severe coiling of the catheter at a number of sites along its path and occasionally in knotting at its tip. Knotting or coiling may be due to a combina-

---

[3] Manufactured by Cordis Corp., Angiomedics, and USCI.

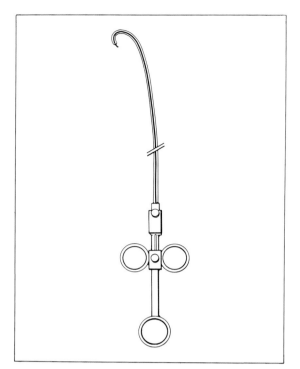

Fig. 7-8. A hook-shaped catheter (Simmons I), or an externally deflecting guidewire [24], can be used to manipulate a linear foreign body to a more favorable position or to free one end of a lost catheter or guidewire in which both ends are anchored to the vessel wall or endocardium.

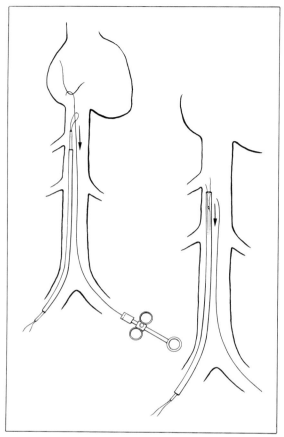

Fig. 7-9. The combination shown uses a snare introduced from one femoral vein and an external manipulator through the other. Here the lost catheter is freed by the external manipulator and is withdrawn through the loop of the snare.

tion of causes. The catheter material may be too flimsy for its required task, or it may have lost its torque control. More often, the primary curve of the catheter tip is longer than the vessel diameter, and the manipulations required to make it effective result in coiling and knotting (e.g., Simmons II curve, Chap. 14; Grollman catheter, Chap. 17). Complicated catheter configurations are most prone to occur (1) in those vessels that are elongated, ectatic, or tortuous; (2) when the site of the anticipated selective catheter tip placement is remote from the site of its introduction; and (3) when there are numerous curves to traverse for successful selective placement.

Severe coiling of the catheter is not limited only to its tip. It may occur proximally in the shaft (such as in ectatic tortuous iliac vessels or in a large aortic aneurysm) during catheterization of brachiocephalic vessels or in the subclavian vein dur-

ing catheterization of the pulmonary artery. It can even occur proximal to the point of entry into the vessel, such as in patients with thickened subcutaneous or fibrous tissues at the entry site of the groin.

Be alerted to the possibility of knotting or coiling when there is a lack of catheter response or when excessive manipulation is required. An immediate fluoroscopic examination should be made of the entire length of the catheter from its point of entry to its tip. If no deformity is present, you have three options: (1) Exchange the catheter for one of greater body and torque control and a more appropriate curve. (2) Give body to the catheter already in place by advancing a guidewire to a point just

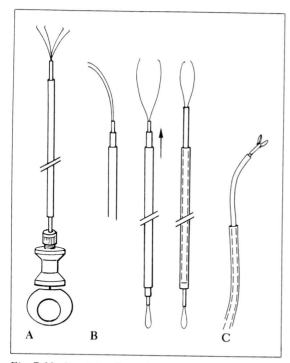

Fig. 7-10. A variety of grasping instruments.
A. The thin wires of the grasping forceps (MediTech) often do not allow a firm grasp on the object. Also, the fine steel tines can cause damage to endothelium and cardiac structures.
B. Grasping forceps made from a piano wire with shafts held immobile by a 5 French catheter. An 8 French catheter overlies this combination and acts as a protective sheath during its introduction. When in the vicinity of the foreign body, the 8 French catheter uncovers the forceps and also closes its jaws by advancing over the 5 French catheter. Once snared, the forceps and foreign body are withdrawn into a 10 French sheath. This forceps is useful when both ends of the catheter or foreign body are anchored in the vessel wall or the endocardium. It must be handled with care to prevent damage to cardiac valves and vessels walls.
C. Flexible endoscopic grasping forceps. Add a 30-degree curve to the distal end to permit directional control.

proximal to the tip during the final manipulations. (3) Remove the catheter and replace a new one through a sheath (with an attached hemostasis valve on a sidearm for flushing) of appropriate diameter and length (see Fig. 7-6).

If a *catheter deformity is present,* the most likely cause is coiling rather than knotting. Calm reflection as to the direction of the manipulation and opposing this maneuver (sometimes aided by introducing a guidewire into the catheter) is usually all that is required. Advance a heavy-duty guidewire up to and through the coiled catheter tip, thereby gently widening and eventually releasing the loop. During this maneuver, advance the coils and loops upward into the widest part of the aorta (the aortic arch) rather than withdrawing it into the more constricted proximal portions.

There are a variety of means available to unravel knots once they have formed [5, 10, 11, 15]. The simplest of these is to replace the heavy-duty guidewire with a 120-cm long 0.038-in. (0.097-cm) Lunderquist exchange wire [15]. The 8-cm long coil spring flexible portion can be advanced through the knot. As the rigid solid segment of this guidewire is gently advanced under fluoroscopic supervision, it loosens and migrates the knot to the tip of the catheter, where it is eventually untied.

Other methods for untying knots are available. A J-shaped deflector wire may be passed through the lumen of the knotted catheter to the level of the knot and locked in its first turn, and the catheter can be withdrawn or advanced over the imposed fixed curve of the deflector wire to loosen and eventually release the knot [10]. A J-shaped catheter (with or without an inner wire to give it body) can be positioned from the opposite femoral artery, advanced through the loop of the knot and fixated on a renal or other visceral vessel. The knotted catheter can then be gently pulled around this fixed point, untied, and withdrawn. A J-shaped external manipulator wire (alone, but preferably in the tip of a pigtail catheter) may be advanced through the opposite femoral artery to engage the knot loop. Simultaneous withdrawal of the hooked catheter and advancement of the knotted catheter will untie the knot [11].

There may be some catheters that cannot be uncoiled. A thin-walled 10 or 12 French sheath should be introduced through a puncture site in the opposite femoral vessel (this can be performed

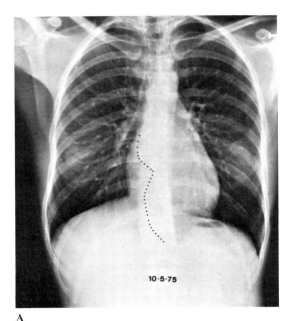

A

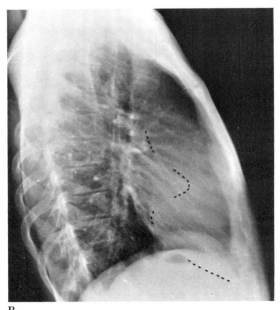

B

Fig. 7-11.
A and B. A catheter was embedded in the right atrium
    for 13 months.
C. It was withdrawn with the device described in Fig-
    ure 7-10B.

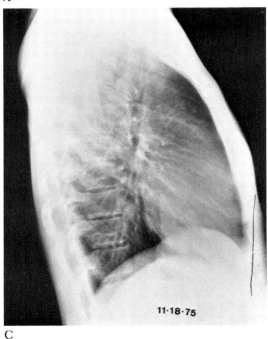

C

by gradual dilation of the puncture site using vessel
dilators of progressively increasing diameters). An
externally controlled deflector wire may then be
introduced to engage the coiled catheter, which
can be withdrawn through the sheath. Only occasionally is surgical arteriotomy or venotomy required to remove the catheter from the site of entry.

References

1. Becker, G. H., et al. Low dose fibrinolytic therapy:
   Results and new concepts. *Radiol.* 148:663, 1983.
2. Bell, W., and Meek, A. Guidelines for the use of
   thrombolytic agents. *N. Engl. J. Med.* 301:1266,
   1979.
3. Bookstein, J., Mose, K., and Houghie, C. Coagu-
   lative interventions during angiography. *Cardiovasc. Intervent. Radiol.* 5:46, 1982.
4. Castanedá-Zuniga, W., et al. Coilon removal.
   Cardiovasc. Intervent. Radiol. 5:60, 1982.
5. Cho, S. R., Tisnado, J., and Beachley, M. Percutaneous unknotting of intravascular catheters and
   retrieval of catheter fragments. *A.J.R.* 141:397,
   1983.
6. Chuang, V., et al. Complications of coil embolization: Prevention and management. *A.J.R.* 137:809,
   1981.
7. Dotter, C., Rösch, J., and Bilbao, N. Transluminal
   extraction of catheter and guide fragments from the
   heart and great vessels: 29 collected cases. *A.J.R.*
   111:467, 1971.
8. Dotter, C. T., Rösch, J., and Seaman, A. J. Selective clot lysis and low dose streptokinase. *Radiology*
   111:31, 1974.
9. Fisher, R., and Ferreyro, R. Evaluation of current
   techniques for non-surgical removable intravascular
   iatrogenic foreign bodies. *A.J.R.* 130:541, 1978.

10. Hawkins, I. F., and Tonkin, A. Deflector method for non-surgical removal of knotted catheters. *Radiology* 106:705, 1973.

11. Holder, J. C., and Cherry, J. F. The use of a tip deflecting guide in untying a knotted arterial catheter. *Radiology* 128:808, 1978.

12. Katzen, B. T., and Van Breda, A. Low dose streptokinase in the treatment of arterial occlusions. *A.J.R.* 136:1171, 1981.

13. Kim, M., and Horton, J. Intra-arterial foreign body retrieved using endoscopic biopsy forceps. *Radiology* 149:597, 1983.

14. Kominger, C., and Collen, D. Studies on specific fibrinolytic effect of human extrinsic (tissue-type) plasminogen activator in human blood and in various animal species *in vitro. Thromb. Haemost.* 46J(2):561, 1981.

15. Lo, L. O. The use of the Lunderquist exchange guidewire for non-surgical elimination of angiographic catheter knots. *Radiology* 145:835, 1982.

16. Marder, V. Pharmacology of thrombolytic agents: Implications for therapy of coronary artery thrombosis. *Circulation* 68(Suppl. I):I-1, 1983.

17. McNamara, T., and Fischer, J. The thrombolysis of peripheral arterial and graft occlusions: Improved results using high dose urokinase. *A.J.R.,* 144:769, 1985.

18. Mori, K. W., et al. Selective streptokinase and infusion. Clinical and laboratory correlates. *Radiology* 148:677, 1983.

19. Murray, P. D., Garnic, J. D., and Bettman, M. A. Pharmacology of angioplasty and intravascular thrombolysis. *A.J.R.* 139:795, 1982.

20. Padulla, G. Hook and snare technique for intravascular retrieval. *Radiology* 135:529, 1979.

21. Pennica, D., et al. Cloning and expression of human tissue-type plasminogen activator cDNA in *E. coli. Nature* 301:214, 1983.

22. Rentrop, P., et al. Selective intracoronary thrombolysis in acute myocardial infarction and unstable angina pectoris. *Circulation* 63:307, 1981.

23. Risius, B., et al. Catheter directed low dose streptokinase infusion: A preliminary experience. *Radiology* 150:349, 1984.

24. Rossi, P. Percutaneous removal of intravascular foreign bodies. In R. A. Wilkins and M. Viamonte, Jr. (eds.), *Interventional Radiology.* St. Louis: Blackwell Scientific, 1982. Pp. 359–369.

25. Rubinstein, Z., Morag, B., and Izghak, Y. Percutaneous removal of intravascular foreign bodies. *Cardiovasc. Intervent. Radiol.* 5:64, 1982.

26. Smith, P. An improved method for intra-arterial foreign body retrieval. *Radiology* 145:539, 1982.

27. Sniderman, K., Bodner, L., and Saddekni, S. Percutaneous embolectomy by transcatheter aspiration. *Radiology* 150:357, 1984.

28. Sobel, B., et al. Improvement of regional myocardial metabolism after coronary thrombolysis induced with tissue-type plasminogen activator or streptokinase. *Circulation* 69:983, 1984.

29. Starck, E., McDermott, J., and Crummy, A. Percutaneous aspiration of thromboembolectomy. *Radiology* 156:61, 1985.

30. Van de Werf, F., et al. Coronary thrombolysis with tissue-type plasminogen activator in patients with evolving myocardial infarction. *N. Engl. J. Med.* 310:609, 1984.

31. Vujic, I., et al. Massive pulmonary embolism: Treatment with full heparinization and topical low dose streptokinase. *Radiology* 148:671, 1983.

III

Arteriographic Studies

Arteriography and Therapeutic Procedures of the Extremities

Indications

Arteriography of the extremities should be performed with the mind constantly alert toward performing interventional procedures. This requires a close rapport with the attending physician and consulting surgeon, careful prior evaluation of the patient, informed consent that includes discussion of the potential for a therapeutic endeavor, and an appropriate armamentarium of both diagnostic and therapeutic intravascular equipment (see Chaps. 3 to 7).

ORGANIC DISEASES

1. Atherosclerosis (plaques, stenosis, occlusion, aneurysm, dissection, tortuosity)
2. Thrombosis
3. Embolism
4. Trauma
5. Arteritis (Buerger's, giant cell, Takayasu's, tuberculous, syphilitic)
6. Arterial dysplasia
7. Arteriovenous malformations and angiomas
8. Extrinsic diseases (tumor, thoracic outlet, popliteal artery entrapment)
9. Primary tumors of vessels, other soft tissues, and bones
10. Follow-up study of bypass grafts

FUNCTIONAL DISEASES

1. Hypertonicity
2. Raynaud's disease
3. Drug intoxication (e.g., ergot)

INTERVENTIONAL PROCEDURES

1. Percutaneous transluminal angioplasty
2. Intravascular thrombolysis
3. Therapeutic blockade
4. Intravascular removal of foreign bodies

Techniques

APPROACHES

Lower Extremities

A variety of approaches are available. The angiographer should choose the simplest and least traumatic approach before a diagnostic arteriogram and should avoid, if possible, a site requiring imminent surgery. If a therapeutic procedure is anticipated, the approach or approaches differ from those of a purely diagnostic study. Often a vessel ipsilateral to the lesion must be punctured (see Chap. 6), a choice usually based on a prior arteriogram. Approaches for a diagnostic procedure should be considered in the following order of preference:

FEMORAL APPROACH. Check both femoral pulses. If one side is weaker, avoid puncturing it, since this disparity indicates proximal occlusive disease.

For unilateral peripheral arterial disease:

1. Direct puncture of the common femoral artery on the diseased side and injection of contrast medium through the needle sleeve. This approach is used only if the disease is in the periphery and remote from the site of the puncture. One should avoid compromise of a potential site of proximal surgical arterial anastomosis.
2. Percutaneous entry of the femoral artery opposite to the diseased side and passage of the catheter across the aortic bifurcation to study vessels of the involved side (Fig. 8-1). This approach should be attempted with caution if there is significant atherosclerotic disease involving iliac vessels.

For bilateral peripheral arterial disease:

1. Unilateral femoral artery puncture with catheter tip placement at the aortic bifurcation. Either a straight-tipped catheter or a tightly

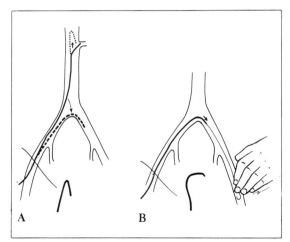

Fig. 8-1. Catheter maneuvers for studying vessels on the opposite side of the one that is punctured. No. 5 French catheters are advanced over a 0.035-in. (0.89-mm) guidewire.

A. Acutely angled catheter. Advance the catheter to the renal artery, reform the curve, and draw the catheter down to the aortic bifurcation.

B. Catheter with a "cobrahead" curve. Place the curve at the bifurcation and advance a 145-cm guidewire with a tapered core to the level of the femoral artery. Fixate the guidewire manually and advance the catheter over the wire.

coiled "pigtail" catheter may be used. Be sure that all side holes are above the aortic bifurcation (Fig. 8-2B). We prefer this approach when studying peripheral vascular occlusive disease, even when the disease would appear clinically to be unilateral.

2. Bilateral direct femoral artery puncture with simultaneous bilateral injection (Fig. 8-2A). Introduce 4- to 6-in. Teflon needle sleeves and anchor them well on the skin of the groin. Contrast medium is refluxed up to the aortic bifurcation both by the force of the injection and by the concomitant use of Valsalva maneuver. Straining against a closed glottis for 10 to 15 seconds, followed by a sudden release, reduces the cardiac output and systemic blood pressure at the moment of retrograde injection. Forty-five milliliters of 60% contrast agent injected over a period of 3 seconds through each

Fig. 8-2. Multiple approaches to aortoiliac femoral arteriography.
A. Bilateral femoral artery puncture.
B. Single catheter at aortic bifurcation.
C. High translumbar aortogram.
D. Low translumbar aortogram.
E. Left axillary approach (note catheter shape).
F. Right axillary approach.

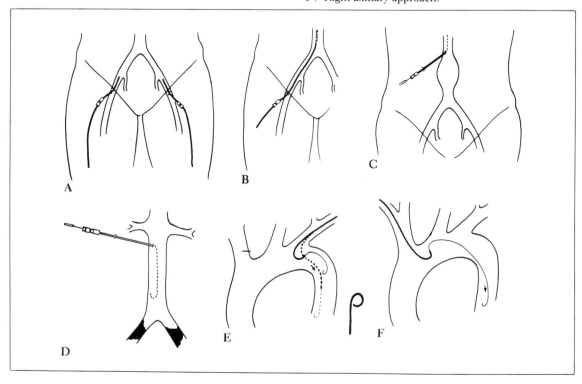

Teflon sleeve (a total of 90 to 100 ml) produces excellent opacification of the distal aorta, pelvic vessels, and, on subsequent films, the peripheral vessels of each lower extremity. A separate injector for each side is preferable to a single injector connected to a Luer-Lok Y adapter.

If a single femoral artery is available for puncture, but it is impossible to maneuver the catheter through that vessel to the aortic bifurcation, an alternate method is as follows: Apply blood pressure cuffs to both lower extremities and inject (within 2 seconds) 50 to 60 ml of contrast agent retrograde through the femoral artery sleeve following Valsalva maneuver, having just released the cuff on the opposite side to induce reactive hyperemia. Leave the cuff inflated on the side of the puncture during the injection to induce more flow to the side of interest.

Anterograde femoral artery puncture (see Chap. 3) is often required for percutaneous transluminal angioplasty or embolization procedures of lesions involving the superficial femoral artery, the popliteal artery, or trifurcation vessels.

TRANSLUMBAR APPROACH. The translumbar approach is indicated when there are severely dampened or obliterated femoral pulses on both sides, indicating occlusion or severe stenosis of the iliac arteries or the distal aorta. This approach may be used if there is a synthetic or venous bypass graft interposed at the femoral artery and if puncture is contraindicated. The angiographer should be aware of contraindications to the translumbar approach, such as blood dyscrasias, aneurysms, dissections, and high aortic grafts. Severe hypertension and also aortic insufficiency (high pulse pressure) are relative contraindications. The reader should review Chapter 3 regarding the technique of performance. Two methods are available: In the first, the aorta is punctured at the T12 level, and the Teflon sleeve is advanced upstream into the descending thoracic aorta (Fig. 8-2C). This approach should be used if one suspects high aortic occlusion, abdominal aortic aneurysm, abdominal aortic graft below L2, or renal vascular disease. When occlusive disease is suspected in the low abdominal aorta or below the bifurcation, the aorta may be punctured between L2 and L3 (a more transverse translumbar approach) and the Teflon sleeve advanced caudad (Fig. 8-2D). This

second method permits better definition of vessels with less contrast medium because it uses an anterograde injection and therefore less dilution occurs.

AXILLARY APPROACH. The axillary approach is used if the femoral approach is unavailable and the translumbar approach is contraindicated. The left side is preferred because less manipulation is required to enter the descending thoracic aorta (Fig. 8-2E). However, decreased blood pressure, dampened pulses, or supraclavicular bruits on the left may require use of the right side (Fig. 8-2F).

GRAFT PUNCTURE. The technique of graft puncture is more hazardous, because damage to pseudointima and ultimately thrombosis may occur. Moreover, infection may be introduced, which is a very serious complication. If no other approach is available, a single anterior wall puncture with very gentle manipulation using a flexible guidewire and a small diameter catheter is required [44].

Upper Extremities

1. Percutaneous femoral puncture and catheter approach (Fig. 8-3) is preferable, particularly in the absence of brachiocephalic occlusive disease.

Fig. 8-3. Femoral catheter approaches in brachial arteriography. These approaches are identical to those used in femoral cerebral catheterization (see Fig. 14-4). Engage the catheter tip into the orifice of the subclavian artery, advance the guidewire well out into the high brachial artery, and follow the catheter over the guidewire.
A. No. 5 or 6.5 French "Hincks 1" catheter shape with a 145-cm, 0.035-in. (0.89-mm) heparin-coated guidewire with a curved, flexible tip.
B. Tortuous vessels. Use a thin-walled 5 French catheter over a similar guidewire or one with a movable core.

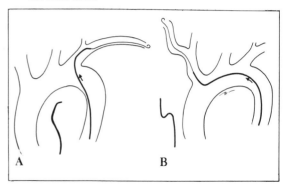

2. Direct needle puncture.
   a. Brachial, if pathology is below the elbow (see Chap. 3).
   b. Axillary (see Chap. 3).

CATHETERS

Only small catheter diameters are required in angiography of the extremities, because adequate studies can be obtained by slow delivery rates of contrast agents.

Lower Extremities

To perform an aortic bifurcation angiogram, a 50- to 65-cm 5 French straight Teflon or polyethylene end-hole catheter with multiple side holes or, preferably, a tightly coiled pigtail catheter should be used. The catheter should be introduced over a 145-cm guidewire with a flexible, curved tip and a diameter of 0.035 or 0.038 in. A 65-cm polyethylene 5 French end-hole catheter with a short hook or a "cobra-head" curve should be used for opposite internal or external iliac or femoral artery studies. This catheter is introduced over a 145-cm guidewire with a flexible, curved tip, a movable core (or a tapered core), and a diameter of 0.035 in. (0.89 mm). Straight 5 or 6 French polyethylene catheters may be advanced over the bifurcation by means of an external manipulator.

Upper Extremities

Femoral cerebral catheter shapes should be used for selective brachiocephalic studies (see Fig. 8-3); these are 100-cm 5, 6, or 6.5 French end-hole catheters without side holes. These catheters are introduced over a 145-cm guidewire with a flexible curved tip and a diameter of 0.035 or 0.038 in.

CONTRAST MEDIA, PROJECTIONS, AND RADIOGRAPHIC PROGRAMMING

Details concerning contrast agents, radiographic programs, and projections in arteriography of the extremities are given in Tables 8-1, 8-2, and 8-3. Additional comments and technical considerations are discussed in the following sections.

PELVIC OBLIQUE PROJECTIONS

Right posterior oblique (RPO) views should be used to study bifurcations of the right common iliac and left common femoral arteries (see Fig. 8-6); left posterior oblique (LPO) views open the bifurcations of the left common iliac and right common femoral arteries.

FILMS OF THE LOWER EXTREMITIES

Large Film Changers

To equalize radiographic density, the film cassettes should be placed with the thickest portion of the tapered, graduated screen toward the patient's head, the anode toward the feet, and if necessary, an appropriately wedged filter in place. Special cones or collimators are required to reduce scatter. Large film changers may provide four to ten long film cassettes, with film measurements of 14 × 36 in. or 14 × 51 in. The focal spot–film distance for 36-in. film changers is 72 in., and for the 51-in. changer, 79 in. (Fig. 8-4).

Film timing depends on the circulation time, which, in the vast majority of patients, is slow as a result of chronic or subacute occlusive disease. The technique of reactive hyperemia gives the best results. The tourniquets should be applied well above the patient's knees, 50 mm above systolic pressure for at least 3 minutes. The tourniquets are then released, and 10 seconds later the contrast medium is injected. The accumulation of metabolites in the circulation induces vasodilation and more rapid blood flow. Work-reactive hyperemia involves the same process, with the addition of exercising the legs during the pressure cuff elevation. This technique rapidly stimulates flow through developing collaterals and demonstrates vessels proximal to an obstruction as well as more peripheral reconstituted arteries. An alternative technique is the use of pneumatic cuffs or boots [17], which are now commercially available. These devices encase the leg in an inflatable boot with pressure levels that are above systolic pressure. If the boot is applied for 10 minutes and injection is made immediately on release, the vessels of the entire extremity can be opacified on a single large film. These techniques should not be applied to those patients with an acutely ischemic extremity. Similar results may be obtained by injecting vasodilators (e.g. nitroglycerine 300 µg) through the catheter immediately prior to injecting the contrast agent.

Since flow through the extremities is relatively slow, a long time period is used to inject the contrast medium (5 to 6 seconds). The initial exposure should be made approximately 1 second prior to the termination of the injection. This exposure shows the contrast medium in the proximal vessels as well as the long column of contrast medium that

Table 8-1. Technical specifications in arteriography[a] of the lower extremity (adults)

Location of arteriographic procedure	Contrast agent			Total films		Total time (sec)	Radiographic program		Projections
	Density	Volume (ml/inj)	Rate (ml/sec)	51 × 14 in.	14 × 14 in.		Films/sec	Timing	
Single leg 14 × 14-in. seriograph and moving tabletop	L	50	8	—	8	23	1 every 2 sec[b] for 4 sec at each of 4 positions 10 in. apart	Start films 1 sec after start of injection. 1½–2 sec required between each movement	Invert foot to see trifurcation Evert foot to see plantar arch
Long leg changer[c] Hyperemia[c] No hyperemia	L L	50 50	8 8	5 5		15–20 25–40	1 every 4 sec 1 every 5 or 6 sec	Start films just before end of injection	
Bilateral (hyperemia[c]) Long film changer Catheter at aortic bifurcation or low translumbar	L or M (NI)	100 80	20 16	5		20	1 every 4 sec. 1 every 5 or 6 sec without reactive hyperemia	Start films just before end of injection	
High translumbar	M	100	18	5		20			
Bilateral femoral puncture	L or M (NI)	50 40 (in each)	10 10	5		20			
Small film changer (entire extremity)		Same		—	8	23	1 every 2 sec for 4 sec at each of 4 positions 10 in. apart	Start films 1 sec after start of injection. 1½–2 sec required between each movement	
Pelvis only	L or M (NI)	40	10	—	8	9	1/sec	Start films 1 sec after start of injection	AP and both obliques (include aortic bifurcation and common femoral bifurcation)

[a] For intraarterial digital subtraction angiography, use contrast agent at half strength but same volume.
[b] See page 153.
[c] Reactive hyperemia; see page 150.
Note: M = medium density contrast agent; L = low density contrast agent; NI = nonionic (see Appendix 3).

Table 8-2. Technical specifications in arteriography[a] of the upper extremity (adults)

Location of arteriographic procedure	Contrast agent[b]			Total films 14 × 14 in.	Total time (sec)	Radiographic program		Projections
	Density	Volume (ml/inj)	Rate (ml/sec)			Films/sec	Timing	
Subclavian artery or upper arm	L	16	8	12	9	2/sec for 3 sec; 1/sec for 6 sec	Start films 0.4 sec after start of injection	Anatomic position (supine)
Forearm and hand (reactive hyperemia[c])	L or M (NI)	24	8	20	20	1/sec; delay films 2 sec	Start films 0.2 sec after start of injection	

[a]For intraarterial digital subtraction angiography, use contrast agent at half strength but same volume.
[b]Nonionic contrast agent is less painful.
[c]See page 150.
Note: M = medium density contrast agent; L = low density contrast agent; NI = nonionic (see Appendix 3).

Table 8-3. Technical specifications in arteriography of the extremities (children)

Location of arteriographic procedure	Contrast agent[a]			Total films 14 × 14 in.	Total time (sec)	Radiographic program	
	Density	Volume (ml/inj)	Rate (ml/sec)			Films/sec	Timing
Lower extremity (bilateral)	L or M (NI)	1.0–1.5 ml/kg	Total in 2 sec	18	10	2/sec[b] for 3 sec at each of 3 positions 6 in. apart	Start films 1 sec after start of injection
Upper extremity	L or M (NI)	0.5–1.0 ml/kg	Total in 2 sec	18	16		

[a]Nonionic contrast agent is less painful.
[b]See page 153.
Note: M = medium density contrast agent; L = low density contrast agent; NI = nonionic (see Appendix 3).

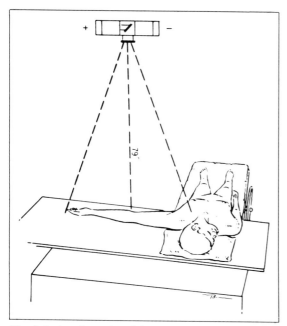

Fig. 8-4. Arteriography of the upper extremity, using a large film changer.

is extended down the extremities. If reactive hyperemia or vasodilators are used, subsequent film exposures are taken every 3 or 4 seconds and the entire study obtained within 16 to 20 seconds. Without these methods, exposures are obtained every 5 or 6 seconds with an interval to cover at least 30 to 40 seconds.

For a rapid-flow vascular problem (arteriovenous malformation, vascular tumor), film timing must be gauged according to each case but is more rapid than normal.

The 51-in. film changer requires no tabletop movement. The 36-in. film changer is not long enough to cover the entire extremity, so after the first exposure (covering the aortic bifurcation and the thighs), the tabletop and the patient must be moved 8 to 12 in. in order to cover the lower extremities. If the femoral pulses are absent, the tabletop should be moved after the second exposure to ensure viewing the point of iliac artery or femoral artery reconstitution.

Small Film Seriographs

For small film (14 × 14 in.) seriographs [1], an automatic tabletop movement programmer can be installed, which sequentially moves the patient cephalad as the column of contrast agent progresses down the extremities. The table movements are variable and can be selected for distances of 5, 6.25, 10, or 12.5 in. One can also select the length of time during which the area of interest is stationed over the film changer. A typical case would call for four or five tabletop movements, each 10 inches apart. One film taken every other second for 4 seconds at each station would sequentially outline the circulation in the pelvis, thigh, knee, and lowermost portions of the extremity. Because a period of 1½ to 2 seconds is required between each tabletop movement, the entire maneuver will occupy approximately 23 seconds.

FILMS OF UPPER EXTREMITIES

Rapid film changers (14 × 14 in.) can be placed diagonally along the axis of the upper extremity. Several injections are usually required, overlapping different segments of the extremity. For the hand and wrist, use 20 films at a rate of 1 per second. The vessels should be dilated immediately prior to injection of contrast agent by inducing reactive hyperemia, applying hot towels to the hand, a slow intraarterial injection of tolazoline (Priscoline 25 mg over a period of 30 seconds), or nitroglycerine 100 to 300 μg. For more proximal upper extremity arteriography, use approximately 12 films, 1 per second. Alternatively, the patient may lie on a stretcher perpendicular to a larger film changer, with the arm extending down its long axis (Fig. 8-4). Intraarterial digital subtraction methods are particularly helpful in the upper extremity.

DIGITAL SUBTRACTION TECHNIQUES

Digital subtraction techniques are very useful in extremity angiography [29]. This is particularly true during interventional intraarterial maneuvers, in which low-dose intraarterial dilute contrast requirements allow multiple, relatively pain-free injections and "real time" capabilities decrease procedure time. Pre- and postangioplasty and embolization procedures are thus more easily monitored, and complications such as renal failure, thrombosis, and bleeding are less likely to occur. In addition, vessels distal to a point of obstruction, which are poorly visualized due to poor collateral flow, may be more accurately assessed by intraarterial digital subtraction techniques. The limitation of digital subtraction angiography is the small field size available, which may require multiple injections in order to adequately cover the area of interest. Accurately calibrated tabletop movements decrease the number of injections required. Artifacts due to motion may occur, but motion due to pain is unlikely due to the dilute contrast agent required.

Peripheral angiography using intravenous digital subtraction angiography (IV-DSA) techniques requires a cooperative patient with a good cardiac output and good renal function. Fairly large doses of contrast medium are required using this technique, but the detail provided is often of diagnostic value. It can be helpful in special circumstances, such as severe occlusive disease, in patients who are otherwise at poor risk for angiography, and it can be used to evaluate bypass grafts and outpatients who have undergone prior angioplasty. Even the smallest amount of motion during the interval between the mask and the contrast image degrades the resultant image, and this feature must be kept in mind during patient selection.

Anatomic Considerations

LOWER EXTREMITIES

The arterial anatomy of the lower extremity is illustrated in Figures 8-5, 8-6, 8-7, and 8-8. The arterial supply to each limb commences at the common iliac artery. An important branch, the internal iliac (hypogastric) artery, supplies branches to the pelvic viscera and also provides anastomotic channels to peripheral vessels in obstruction [11].

The external iliac artery becomes the common femoral artery at the inguinal ligament. Just before this occurs, the external iliac artery gives off two small branches, the inferior epigastric and the deep circumflex iliac arteries. The latter vessel arises laterally from the distal external iliac artery, ascends laterally to the anterior superior iliac spine and then passes along the iliac crest. It enlarges as a frequent collateral in occlusive disease to anastomose with branches of the deep femoral, internal iliac, and lumbar arteries, and thus it may be inadvertently catheterized.

Approximately 2 in. beyond its origin, the common femoral artery bifurcates into the deep femoral artery (profunda femoris) and the superficial femoral artery. The latter vessel continues on to Hunter's adductor canal. In the groin, small branches of the common femoral artery (the superficial circumflex iliac and superficial external pu-

dendal arteries) may be important to the surgeon but are of little practical consequence to the angiographer. The deep femoral artery (profunda femoris) passes deep to the adductor longus muscle and gives off medial and lateral circumflex femoral branches, continuing down the extremity with several muscular perforating branches. These perforating branches, usually four in number, encircle the shaft of the femur, anastomosing with each other and the geniculate branches of the popliteal artery. The lateral femoral circumflex artery has an ascending branch and a descending branch. These branches are an important source of blood supply to the thigh muscles and, in addition, form important collaterals that link the arterial anastomosis around the pelvis, hip, and knee. Because the profunda femoris can be involved with atherosclerosis, its origin should be well outlined for the surgeon. Steep oblique views, with the patient's involved side raised, show this origin best since it is a posterior lateral branch.

The popliteal artery continues on from the femoral artery at Hunter's canal and courses down below the knee joint to its terminal branches, the anterior and posterior tibial and peroneal arteries. The proximal boundary of the popliteal artery is marked angiographically by the supreme geniculate artery. Muscular and geniculate branches form important collateral channels around the knee in obstruction. The larger of the two terminal branches of the popliteal artery is the posterior tibioperoneal trunk. This vessel has a short undivided segment, and, after giving off the peroneal artery, it descends posteromedially as the posterior tibial artery, behind the medial malleolus, terminating below the ankle in the medial and lateral plantar arteries. The peroneal artery lies closely applied to the medial aspect of the fibula; it eventually pierces the interosseous membrane to descend over the lateral malleolus and anastomoses with arteries on the dorsum of the foot. The anterior tibial artery continues laterally from its origin at the popliteal artery to course caudad, anterior to the interosseous membrane in the anterior compartment of the leg. It passes over the dorsum of the foot as the dorsalis pedis, giving off an arcuate artery to supply branches to the toes, and anastomoses with branches of the plantar arch. The trifurcation represents the segment of vessels from the popliteal artery bifurcation to the first branching of the posterior tibioperoneal trunk; it includes

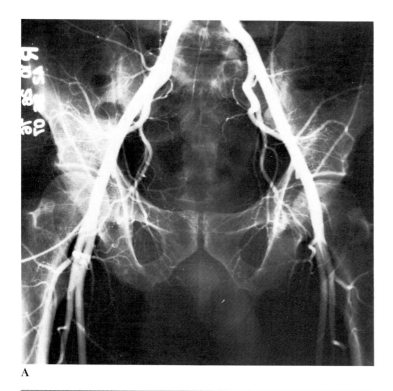

A

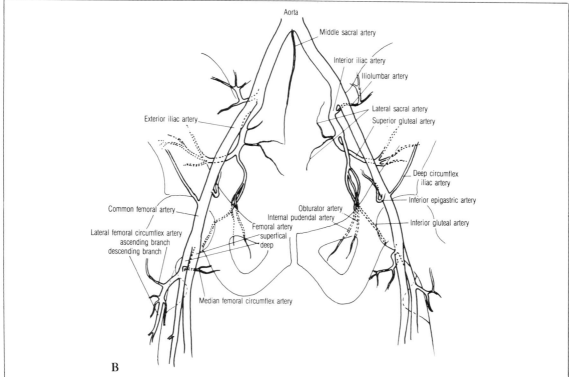

B

Fig. 8-5. A and B. Arteriographic anatomy of the pelvic and proximal femoral branches.

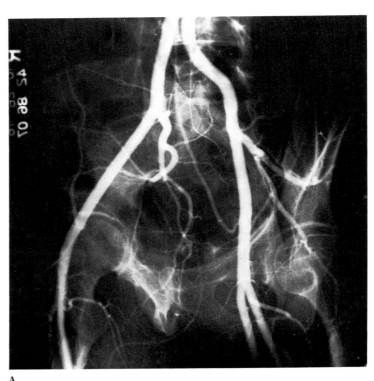

A

the proximal anterior and posterior tibial arteries
and the peroneal artery. Successful surgery for occlusive disease at or below this point is sometimes
more difficult.

UPPER EXTREMITIES

The arteries of the upper extremity are illustrated
in Figure 8-9. The axillary artery is a continuation
of the subclavian artery at the lateral border of the
first rib. It ends at the lower border of the teres
major muscle to become the brachial artery. Its
divisions and close application to the brachial
plexus have already been described (Chap. 3). Important arterial branches are the thoracoacromial,
lateral thoracic, and subscapular arteries and the
anterior and posterior circumflex humeral arteries.

The brachial artery continues to its bifurcation

Fig. 8-6. A and B. Right posterior oblique projection.
The right common iliac and left common femoral
bifurcations are better outlined in this projection. The
origin of the left deep femoral artery branch (profunda
femoris) may be hidden on the anteroposterior projection. With the patient in the supine position, elevate
the symptomatic side to uncover hidden pathology in
the profunda femoris.

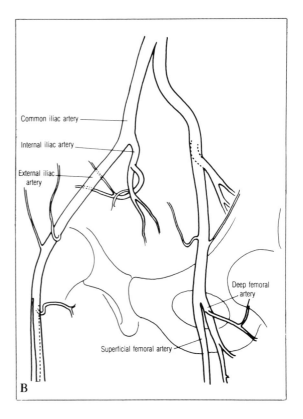

Common iliac artery

Internal iliac artery

External iliac
artery

Deep femoral
artery

Superficial femoral artery

B

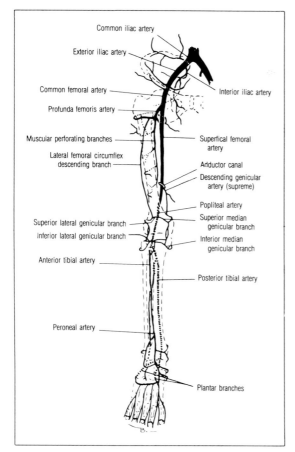

Fig. 8-7. Anatomy of arteries of the lower extremity. (See text for details.)

The interosseous artery arises from the ulnar artery near its origin, bifurcates, and sends branches down the forearm on either side of the interosseous membrane. These branches rejoin near the wrist to enter into the dorsal carpal network of vessels. Digital arteries arise from the palmar arches to supply the medial and lateral aspects of the digits. There are a number of variations in the formation of the deep and superficial palmar arches [10, 13].

Technical Considerations

The angiographer should be aware of the following additional technical considerations:

1. The injection of contrast medium into the arteries of the extremities is painful. Because the degree of pain is directly related to the osmolarity of the contrast agent, nonionic contrast agents (or, in their absence, lower osmolarity contrast agents) should be used. Very adequate studies can be achieved using conventional filming technique with 60% ionic contrast agents if larger volumes are injected over the same time interval. Thus 100 to 120 ml of 60% contrast agent (injected over 5 to 6 seconds) at the aortic bifurcation provides adequate bilateral femoral arteriography with considerably less discomfort than 60 ml of 76% contrast agent. Even lesser concentrations of contrast agent (30%) are possible if intraarterial digital subtraction angiography (IA-DSA) techniques are employed. Specially coordinated moving tabletop techniques are required here in order to counter the small film size provided by DSA. Pain is further reduced by mixing 200 mg of lidocaine (1 ml of 20% lidocaine) to the 100-ml bolus of contrast. Be sure not to inject lidocaine mixed with epinephrine. Lidocaine should not be allowed to enter arteries feeding the brain or spine. Patients in whom reactive hyperemia has been induced immediately prior to the injection of contrast agent appear to have less pain. This may be related to the concomitant release of endorphins into the circulatory system (see Chap. 4).

   Pain may be further countered by adequate medication. General anesthesia or epidural anesthesia has been used, but it is usually not necessary when lower osmolarity or nonionic contrast agent is used.

into the radial and ulnar arteries. At a variable distance along its course, it gives off the profunda brachialis and ulnar collateral arteries, which accompany the radial and ulnar nerves, respectively. The radial artery commences at the level of the radial neck, continues laterally to the wrist, and passes below the tendons of the anatomic "snuffbox" and between the first and second metacarpals to form the deep palmar arch. The ulnar artery courses peripherally on the medial aspect of the forearm and wrist to form the superficial palmar arch. Occasionally, the radial or ulnar artery may arise anomalously high; if the catheter tip is placed too peripherally during angiography, an erroneous diagnosis of an occluded vessel may be entertained. Small branches from the ulnar artery assist in forming the deep palmar arch, as do small branches of the radial artery in forming the superficial palmar arch.

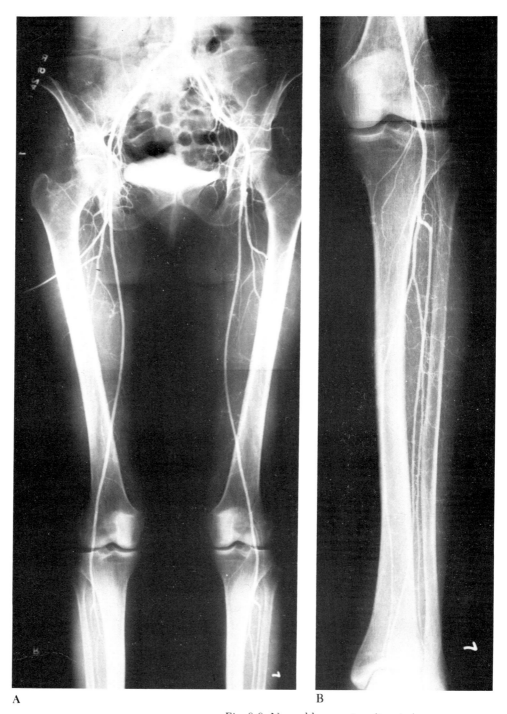

A   B

Fig. 8-8. Normal lower extremity arteriograms.

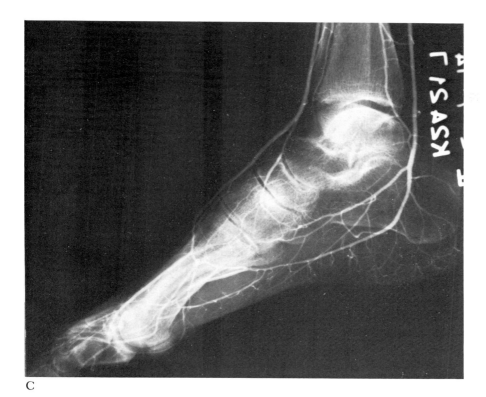

C

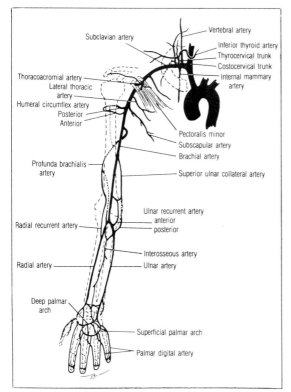

Fig. 8-9. Arterial anatomy of the upper extremity.

2. The flexible J-shaped guidewire may become coiled and impossible to pass through a particularly tortuous iliac artery (Fig. 8-10A). If a test injection excludes significant occlusion as the cause of this difficulty, advance a long (8- or 10-inch) 4 or 5 French Teflon catheter (the sleeve from the translumbar catheter needle will do well) to the point of the coiling. The wire often advances to the next sharp turn, and the sleeve follows in stepwise fashion until the guidewire is well within the descending thoracic aorta. At this point, exchange the sleeve for the catheter of choice. Atherosclerotic plaques, particularly those eccentric in nature, may be difficult to traverse. The wire tip may catch under a plaque. If the wire tip is very flexible with a gentle distal curve, it will buckle instead of being forced under the plaque; the buckled segment acts as the leading point, bypasses the plaque, and allows the catheter to follow. The captured guidewire tip is then withdrawn slightly, released, and advanced further (Fig. 8-10B). If there is still difficulty, special guidewires (injectable open-ended guidewires, steerable 0.014- to 0.018-in. platinum

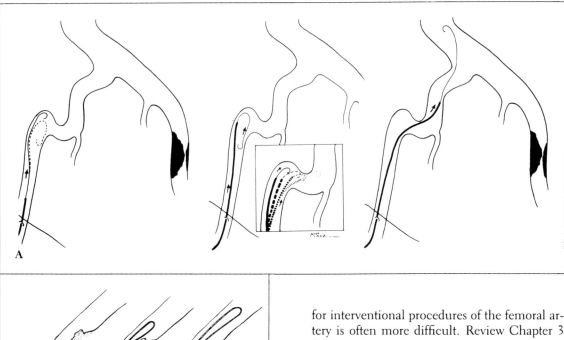

Fig. 8-10.
A. Maneuvering the guidewire in tortuous iliac vessels (see text for details). The guidewire must be flexible and should have a curved tip with a short radius (3 mm). A catheter with a narrow diameter will more easily follow the leading guidewire.
B. Bypassing an eccentric plaque with a flexible tipped guidewire. The tip is trapped in the plaque and a loop is formed, which acts as the lead point. Further advancement releases the tip.

tipped guidewires) and maneuvers may be necessary (see Chap. 6).

3. Sometimes the angiographer will see the guidewire and catheter pass with surprising ease into the abdominal aorta, only to find in subsequent arteriograms that the catheter lies deep in an atheromatous plaque (Fig. 8-11). There is usually little ill effect to the patient from this situation; however, multiple catheter exchanges and dilatation procedures should be avoided; the study should be expedited as much as possible.

4. The anterograde puncture sometimes required for interventional procedures of the femoral artery is often more difficult. Review Chapter 3 for special considerations in this approach.

5. The angiographer must be sure to see inflow to as well as outflow from diseased vessels. If the distal aorta is diseased, a separate injection involving the abdominal aorta may be required; this is particularly true if there is an aneurysm or if there is a possibility of renal artery involvement. With current surgical techniques, bypass grafts to small peripheral vessels require seeing the outflow down to the level of the foot. The sequence of filming may have to be lengthened in severe occlusive disease to 40 or 50 seconds, even with the use of reactive hyperemia. IA-DSA can be invaluable under these circumstances, for otherwise virtually indiscernible vessels can be easily visualized (Fig. 8-12) [29].

6. If the clinical disease is not explained on the basis of the anteroposterior projection angiographic findings, steep bilateral oblique or lateral views should be obtained. These views help outline en face plaques. Measurement of pressure gradients from the distal aorta to the femoral artery also helps in determining the presence of significant disease. This can be performed by simultaneous measurement of pressures proximal and distal to the lesion. A second catheter may be introduced to lie above the lesion using an approach from the opposite femoral artery, an axillary artery, or translum-

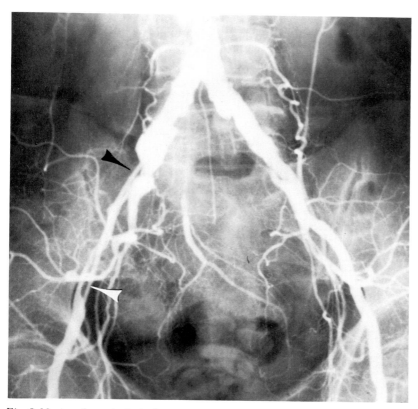

Fig. 8-11. A catheter in "subatheromatous space." Entry point of catheter (*white arrow*) into this space. Catheter reenters lumen of artery (*black arrow*).

bar aortic approach. It may be helpful to adopt the habit of documenting pressures in the femoral artery immediately after its puncture. This can be useful information in recording a gradient if a more proximal iliac or aortic stenosis is successfully crossed and the higher prestenotic arterial pressure is compared. There is another means of recording the pressure gradient across the stenosis once it has been crossed with the catheter. Simply replace the conventional guidewire with a smaller gauge guidewire, and attach a Touhy-Borst adapter with a sidearm attached to a pressure monitor. Leaving the guidewire well above the stenosis at all times, monitor the pressure as the catheter is withdrawn across the lesion.

7. The most significant collaterals to an obstructed distal aorta or proximal iliac artery may originate from subcostal or high lumbar branches, and these vessels must be opacified if

the point of reconstitution or peripheral run-off is to be seen.

8. The angiographer should pay particular attention to details of technique in performing angiography of the extremities in order to avoid complications. Use the smallest possible catheters; if the study is prolonged, heparinize the patient (45 IU/kg); use test injections to ensure proper catheter position; use adequate doses of contrast agent. Always check the peripheral pulses before withdrawing the catheter; if they are not present, check the flow in the punctured artery near the puncture site with an injection of contrast medium. Tapered occlusion of an artery around the catheter may indicate arterial spasm (see Chap. 3); filling defects or sharp cutoffs indicate thrombus formation (see Chap. 3). If either of these situations is encountered, inject nitroglycerine 100 μg or tolazoline 25 mg intraarterially. Injection of 3000 to 5000 IU of heparin directly into the artery through the catheter is also helpful. Periarterial lidocaine may be injected at the puncture site or the area surrounding the vessel if it is superfi-

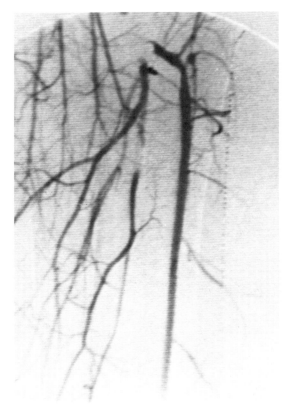

Fig. 8-12. IA-DSA showing reconstituted tibial arteries distal to an occluded popliteal artery.

cial in location. Following such treatment, removal of the catheter is often sufficient if spasm is the underlying problem. If thrombus is suspected, a vascular surgeon should be notified. If the pulse is absent, but the leg not in imminent danger of tissue damage (warm or slightly cool with minimal paresthesias), consider aspirating the clot (see Chap. 7). If clot aspiration is unsuccessful, the catheter should be withdrawn into the clot, baseline bleeding parameters obtained, and thrombolytic therapy immediately instituted. (Review Chapter 7 for precautions and contraindications.) A bolus of 20,000 to 30,000 IU of urokinase, followed by 4000 IU per minute, should be infused immediately. Follow-up angiograms should be obtained after infusion of 500,000 IU, or sooner if pulses return. If clot lysis is apparent but there is residual thrombus, the infusion dose can be decreased to 1000 to 2000 IU per minute. When the clot has been resorbed, the

catheter can be removed. Early surgical intervention is justified if the extremity is cold, mottled, or white, or if the patient complains of pain.

9. After completing the study, the angiographer should secure hemostasis. If heparin has been administered, 1 ml (10 mg) of protamine per 1000 IU of heparin, given intravenously, counteracts the anticoagulant effect if the time interval has been less than 1 hour. The effect of heparin within the body is usually depleted at a rate of 20 percent of the initial dose every hour. Postangiographic care should be given.

Noninvasive Laboratory Studies

These procedures are usually performed in a noninvasive vascular laboratory and should be considered an integral part of the preangiographic work-up of a patient with occlusive peripheral vascular disease. A brief survey of these techniques provides some insight into the hemodynamics and pathophysiology of the uncovered occlusive disease [6, 14, 54, 57].

SEGMENTAL PRESSURE MEASUREMENTS

Blood pressures are measured in the upper extremities using a conventional sphygmomanometer. A nondirectional pocket-type Doppler is exchanged for the stethoscope in order to more accurately detect the systolic pressure. If there is a slight difference measured in the upper extremities, the higher pressure reading is chosen and recorded. Similar pressure readings using appropriate size pressure cuffs (cuff diameter approximately 20% larger than limb diameter) are obtained in both thighs, calves, and ankles. Under normal circumstances, at rest the pressures in the lower extremities are equal to or slightly higher than those in the arm. They are equal at similar levels in each lower extremity and not significantly different between the thigh, calf, and ankle in the same extremity. Pressure drops of more than 20 to 30 mm Hg are abnormal. A pressure drop measured in one thigh signifies unilateral iliac disease; in both thighs, aortoiliac disease; in one calf, femoral or popliteal artery disease; in the ankle, occlusive disease below the trifurcation. An ankle systolic index (the ratio of the ankle pressure to that of the brachial artery pressure) may thus be cal-

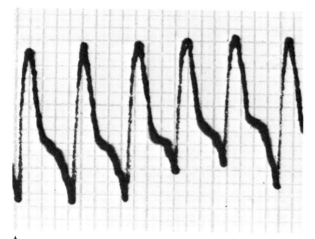

A

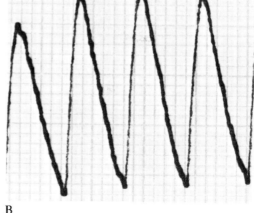

B

Fig. 8-13. Pulse volume recordings.
A. Triphasic wave form typical of a normal peripheral (thigh) artery.
B. Biphasic wave form typical of stenotic artery in a patient with iliac artery stenosis. (Courtesy Dr. Larry Lewis, Department of Surgery, East Carolina University School of Medicine, Greenville, NC.)

culated (normal is 1/1). An occlusive process of the lower extremity is represented by a lower fraction, depending on the severity of the disease.

There are several pitfalls that one must keep in mind during interpretation of these studies. Large collaterals can sometimes mask occlusive disease in the resting state, particularly in the iliac vessels. In the calf, where there are multiple vessels of similar size, the pulse measured distally may be normal while only one of the several vessels is patent; the remaining occluded vessels may go unrecognized. Often, in the presence of occlusive disease, there is no pressure gradient with the patient at rest; the increased demand for blood during exercise (as in a treadmill exercise test) or following reactive hyperemia will augment or uncover the gradient. An abnormal response occurs when the ankle pressure decreases during a standard treadmill exercise test.

PULSE VOLUME RECORDINGS [14]
As blood enters tissue during each cardiac cycle there is a small transient increase in that tissue's volume. These tiny volume changes can be detected by means of segmental plethysmography and recorded on a strip recording chart (Fig. 8-13). In the presence of a significant stenosis or occlusion, the pulse volume curves decrease in ampli-

tude and their contour changes. Since exercise or reactive hyperemia augments any abnormal findings, plethysmographic pulse volume recordings are often performed under these circumstances. This is particularly true if the patient's symptoms of claudication do not correspond with those of the noninvasive study while at rest.

A third noninvasive method of evaluation is directional Doppler analysis.

Angiographic Findings

ATHEROSCLEROSIS
Atherosclerosis [18, 31, 35, 63] tends to occur in the peripheral vascular system in regions of sharp bends in the vessels and at bifurcations; it also occurs in locations where vessels are likely to be distorted or occluded by external forces, such as beneath ligaments, at fascial planes, and around joints. Turbulence develops in these areas and energy is transformed into vibrations (clinically detected as thrills and murmurs), which lead to more stress on the arterial walls. This breaks down the protective antithrombogenic barrier on the intima's endothelial cells with subsequent deposition and aggregation of platelets. These platelets release factors that penetrate into the media to stimulate smooth muscle cells to migrate into the intima. These muscle cells proliferate, depositing a connective tissue matrix that, together with lipid collections, forms a relatively nondistensible fibromuscular plaque. The fibromuscular plaque can in turn become complicated by central necrosis,

infiltration with lipid, hemorrhage, calcification, and thrombosis. The fibrous covering may break down, causing ulceration of the plaque. Mural thrombi can form on this irregular surface, which may become organized and incorporated into the plaque, causing further stenosis or progression to complete occlusion of the vessel [63]. At areas of stress, there are numerous smaller arteries that may become collateral channels through which blood can be diverted once any major vessel occlusion changes the pressure relationships. This type of diversion occurs in the pelvis, groin, knee, ankle, shoulder, and elbow [11].

The arteriographic patterns seen in atherosclerosis depend on the following factors:

1. Stage of disease (early or late)
2. Plaques, which may be concentric, eccentric, or ulcerated
3. Degree of narrowing (localized, diffuse)
4. Occlusion (length involved)
5. Dilatation and/or elongation (localized or diffuse)
6. Presence of superimposed complications (thrombosis, embolus, dissection, rupture)
7. Viability of the surrounding vascular bed

Atherosclerosis in the Lower Extremities
In a large series of lower extremity studies performed at our hospitals, the highest frequency of vessel disease was in the femorals and then the iliacs, followed by vessels of the trifurcation, the popliteals, and then the distal aorta. The hypogastric arteries and the profunda femoris form major collateral channels in occlusive disease; fortunately, they show a lower, but still significant, frequency of involvement.

Superficial femoral artery lesions are most frequent peripherally, in the region of Hunter's canal. Thrombosis supervenes and progresses centrally to the next largest branch, the profunda femoris. The integrity of this deep femoral artery is important in sustaining collateral flow to more peripheral branches.

Diabetics have more diffuse small vessel disease, demonstrate vascular changes earlier in life, and have more frequent involvement below the trifurcation. As a result of loss of vasomotor control, the flow of contrast medium in diabetics is slightly more rapid than in nondiabetics with occlusive disease.

Patients with hyperlipemia are often younger, and lesions in these patients are sometimes limited to the distal aorta or the iliacs (Fig. 8-14).

Vessels that are peripheral to a severely occluding lesion of the abdominal aorta or the iliacs are frequently spared the ravages of increased pressure and the resultant plaques, elongation, and tortuosity associated with atherosclerosis. These vessels are often smooth and normal in appearance (Fig. 8-14A). The lumens of vessels that are peripheral to a point of occlusion may be diffusely narrowed due solely to decreased flow; they revert to normal once flow is reestablished.

Atherosclerosis of the Brachiocephalic Vessels
The reader is referred to Chapter 14 for a discussion of atherosclerosis of the brachiocephalic vessels.

Atherosclerosis in the Upper Extremities
In vessels supplying the upper extremities, atherosclerosis involves the subclavian arteries, but seldom proceeds beyond this point. If occlusion occurs proximal to the origin of the vertebral arteries, it may compromise circulation to the posterior fossa by decreasing anterograde flow up the corresponding vertebral artery. This type of occlusion can also result in a "steal" of blood from the basilar system, because blood preferentially descends retrograde from the vertebral artery due to the low pressure in the subclavian artery distal to the stenosis. Significant narrowing of the second and third portions of the subclavian artery induces ischemic symptoms in the upper extremity.

There is a marked variability in the clinical manifestations of vascular occlusion from patient to patient, depending on the presence of predominant collateral vessels. Before occlusion becomes complete, and while the stenosis is gradually progressing, the collateral circulation may not adjust rapidly enough to prevent episodes of ischemia following alterations in systemic blood pressure. This situation is particularly dangerous when the disease affects vital structures (e.g., the brain, heart, kidneys, or bowel).

EMBOLUS
An embolus (Fig. 8-15A; see also Figs. 8-52 and 8-53) may be caused by clot, plaque, myxoma, or a foreign body or by subacute bacterial endocarditis. Emboli may arise from the left atrium, aneu-

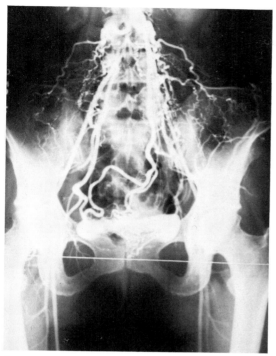

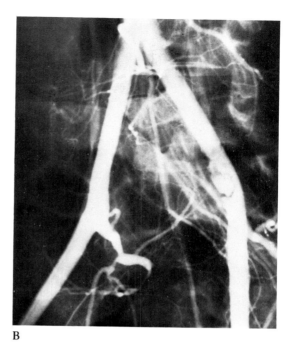

B

A

Fig. 8-14.

A. Localized occlusion of the distal aorta and the proximal common iliac arteries due to atherosclerosis in a 42-year-old woman with type II hyperlipemia. Note the large pelvic collaterals and the smooth reconstituted peripheral vessels.

B. Atherosclerotic ulcerating plaque of the left common iliac artery in a different patient.

rysms, myocardial infarcts, atheromas, cardiac tumors, or the venous system (as in paradoxical emboli). Arteriographically, emboli are frequently found at bifurcations and are seen as filling defects with straight or concave borders.

Because of the acute nature of the embolization process, there is poor collateral formation, and the peripheral vessels are often totally obstructed. After the acute episode is over, during which time restoration of circulation takes precedence, a search for the source of the embolus may be carried out. Occasionally, an immediate search for the source of the emboli may be life-saving, as is demonstrated in Figure 8-15B.

ARTERIAL TRAUMA

Causes

The causes of arterial trauma [5, 46] include the following:

1. Fracture (Fig. 8-16)
2. Dislocation
3. Penetrating wounds, e.g., gunshot and stab wounds (Fig. 8-17)
4. Blunt trauma
5. Iatrogenic causes, e.g., surgical or arteriographic
6. Temperature extremes, e.g., frostbite, burn
7. Repeated small trauma (Fig. 8-18)

Arteriographic Findings

Arteriographic studies of arterial trauma reveal the following findings:

1. Arterial spasm-tapered occlusion, delayed filling
2. Arterial intimal tears (see Fig. 8-17A) and dissection
3. Complete transection with occlusion (see Fig. 8-16C)
4. Thrombosis, sometimes with more peripheral emboli
5. Displacement (by hematoma)
6. False aneurysm (see Fig. 8-17B)
7. Arteriovenous fistula, immediate or delayed (see Fig. 8-17B)
8. Extravasation of contrast medium due to acute bleeding (Fig. 8-16C; see also Chap. 9)

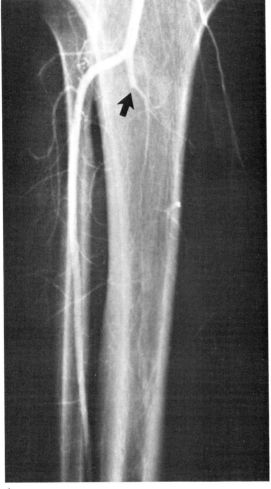

A

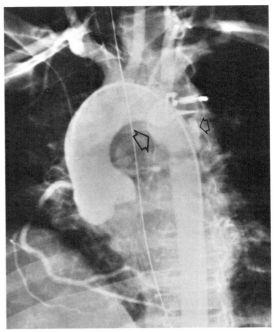

B

Fig. 8-15.
A. Embolus (*arrow*) occluding the peroneal-tibial
   trunk, immediately after an automobile accident.
B. Although clinically not suspicious, thoracic aortogram demonstrates transected aorta (*arrows*) as the
   source of the embolus.

The clinical state of the peripheral pulses distal
to the site of trauma is not always a reliable indicator of the extent of disease because the distal
pulses may be good even with fairly severe trauma
to the artery, or, conversely, the distal pulses may
be absent or diminished when only spasm and no
real arterial damage is present.

In cases of arterial trauma, the physician should
resort to arteriography freely and early. There is a
significantly higher salvage rate when surgical correction of an acutely occluded limb occurs within
6 hours of the trauma. Intervening diagnostic studies must be expeditious and accurate.

The interventional angiographer must always be
aware of potential requirements for intravascular
therapeutic interventions in traumatized vessels.
Thus vessels feeding major bleeding sites may be
temporarily or permanently occluded, and arteriovenous fistulas or false aneurysms may be embolized.

ANEURYSMS

An aneurysm is a persistent abnormal dilatation of
an artery that is usually the result of a localized
weakness and stretching of the arterial wall.

Fig. 8-16. Arteriograms on three separate patients with
fractured legs.
A. Severe fracture of left femur with displacement of
   branches of the profunda femoris due to hematoma. Major vessels are intact.
B. Cold blue leg following trampoline injury with
   fractured distal femur. Compression of the popliteal
   artery was verified at surgery with no evidence for
   intimal injury.
C. Severely fractured tibia and fibula with extravasation of contrast medium (*arrow*), indicating arterial
   disruption. Occlusion of anterior and posterior tibial arteries, and severe spasm of the peroneal artery
   proximally.

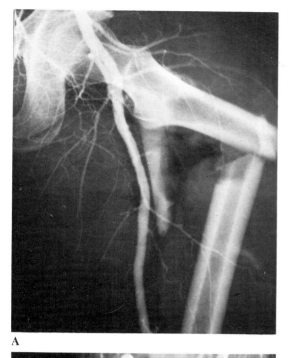

A

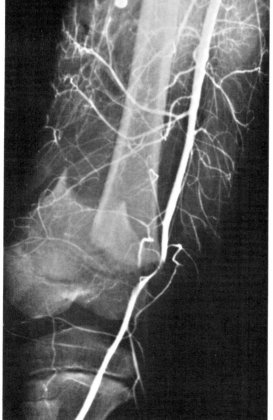

B

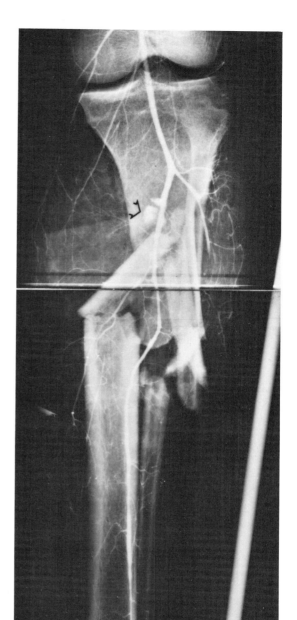

C

Types
1. Fusiform aneurysm: A rather uniform, diffuse dilatation (see Fig. 8-18B).
2. Saccular aneurysm: A localized outpouching (Fig. 8-19).
3. Dissecting aneurysm: Blood dissects between layers of the arterial wall (cystic degeneration of the media). Marfan syndrome or some abnormality of the aortic wall is seen in 90 percent of cases.
4. False aneurysm: A rent in the arterial wall communicating with a sac that is not composed of layers of arterial wall (Figs. 8-17B, 8-20B and C).

Etiology
1. Atherosclerosis (Fig. 8-19)
2. Medial degeneration
3. Congenital causes
4. Syphilis
5. Mycotic (Fig. 8-20) [68]
6. Fibrinoid degeneration (polyarteritis nodosa)
7. Developmental causes (fibromuscular hyperplasia; see Fig. 8-24B)
8. Traumatic causes
9. Behçet's disease [53] (see Fig. 8-27)

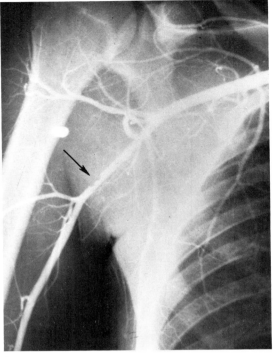

A

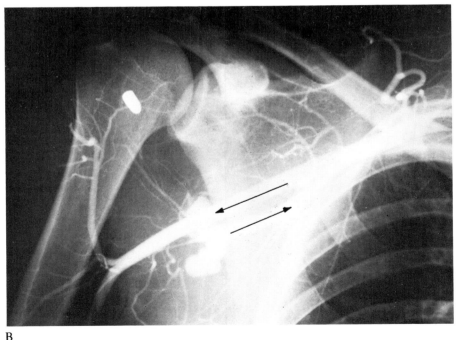

B

Fig. 8-17.
A. Gunshot wound to the right axilla with arterial laceration (*arrow*). The patient subsequently developed a false aneurysm at this site.

B. Gunshot wound to the right axilla. There is penetration of both the artery and the vein (*arrows*) with development of false aneurysms and an arteriovenous fistula.

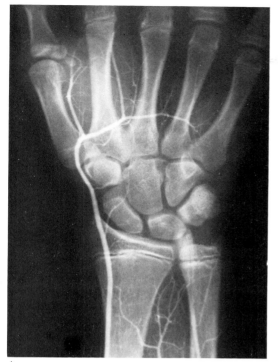

A

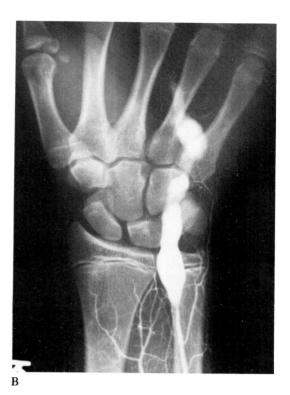

B

Fig. 8-18. Repetitive trauma to the hand (patient was a 12-year-old Little League catcher).
A. Brachial arteriogram shows preferential flow to the deep palmar arch through the radial artery. Faint filling of an ulnar artery traumatic aneurysm.
B. Repeat arteriogram following manual compression of the radial artery. The fusiform aneurysm is seen to extend over the entire wrist and into the superficial palmar arch. The interosseous artery is hypertrophied in response to impaired circulation.

Arteriographic Findings

False-negative arteriograms are possible in patients with aneurysms, because laminated clots may lie along the wall and partially fill the aneurysm. The angiographer should look carefully for telltale calcification in a clot or in the wall of an aneurysm. In such cases, ultrasonography, computed tomography, or nuclear magnetic imaging may detect the true size and configuration of the aneurysm in a safe, noninvasive technique.

ARTERIOVENOUS COMMUNICATIONS

There is a direct premature communication between artery and vein.

Etiology
1. Congenital causes [7, 45]
2. Traumatic causes (including iatrogenic [56])
3. Neoplasm
4. Infection

Angiodysplasias

Congenital arteriovenous malformations are part of the spectrum of angiodysplasias. There are three types of angiodysplasias [7, 45]:

TYPE I. Arteriovenous malformations (Figs. 8-21, 8-22)

1. Enlarged feeding arteries with increased number of small branching vessels
2. Arteriovenous shunting
3. Draining veins may be enlarged

TYPE II. Small vessel malformations (Fig. 8-23)

1. Normal size feeding arteries
2. Capillary stain
3. No significant arteriovenous shunting
4. Normal size draining veins

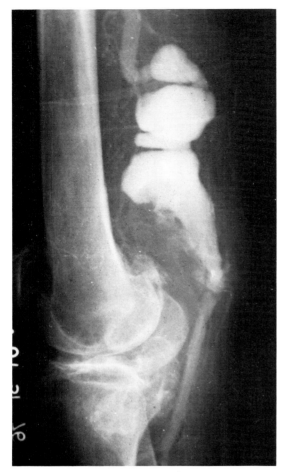

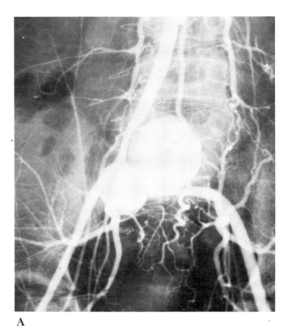

A

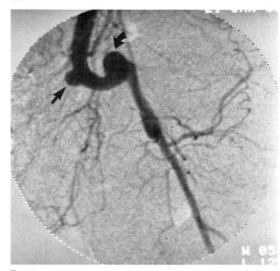

B

Fig. 8-19. Atherosclerotic aneurysm of the popliteal artery. There is a large clot lying within the inferior portion of the aneurysm. Such aneurysms are often bilateral.

TYPE III. Venous malformations (see Chap. 20)

1. Normal arteries and capillaries
2. Enlarged, tortuous veins that can best be demonstrated on venography

Larger than normal doses of contrast medium and rapid film timing (three or four exposures per second) are necessary in studying most forms of arteriovenous abnormalities. In addition, arteriography performed after the administration of tolazoline (Priscoline) may better define the capillary and venous components of type II and III lesions. Arteriovenous malformations and arteriovenous

Fig. 8-20.

A. Large, bilobate, saccular, mycotic aneurysm. There was traumatic disruption of the left iliac artery 3 months earlier complicated by infection from a perforated bowel. An anastomosis of the left common iliac artery with the intact right iliac artery was performed. The patient presented clinically with appendicitis, but aneurysms were discovered at surgery and at subsequent arteriography at the site of anastomosis.

B. IV-DSA of a false aneurysm (*curved arrow*) of the distal anastomosis of an aortofemoral graft. Occluded femoral-femoral graft remnant (*arrow*).

1. Intimal fibroplasia
2. Medial fibroplasia with aneurysms
3. Medial fibromuscular hyperplasia
4. Subadventitial fibroplasia
5. Adventitial fibroplasia

One form may be difficult to differentiate arteriographically from another, but, characteristically, medial fibroplasia with aneurysm represents the "string of beads" appearance commonly seen on angiograms. This appearance is caused by alternating areas of narrowing due to thickened segments of media partially replaced with collagen and areas of dilatation (internal elastic lamina and media partially destroyed). Tubular focal areas of stenosis are seen with intimal fibroplasia (due to circumferential localized predominant fibroplasia of the intima) and in adventitial periarterial fibroplasia (uniform thickening of adventitia by fibromuscular disease). The stenosis of fibromuscular hyperplasia responds well to percutaneous transluminal angioplasty (PTA), and this procedure should be considered if the lesion is symptomatic.

ARTERITIS

The various types of arteritis [27] are discussed in the following sections.

Thromboangiitis Obliterans
(Buerger's Disease)
Buerger's disease [30, 47] is found in young Caucasian or Asiatic males who are heavy smokers. They have a hypercoagulopathy with increased fibrinogen, decreased fibrinolytic activity, and high blood viscosity. These patients often have a migratory phlebitis. In contrast to atherosclerosis, there is a high degree of involvement of the upper extremities. No calcium is seen in the vessel walls. The lesions start distally, involving small and medium size vessels; the large central vessels are characteristically normal. The lesions migrate centrally, usually without skip areas. Arteriographically, the lesions may be totally occlusive, or they may portray a long, stringlike, narrowed appearance. Collaterals are inadequate, and occasionally they give an unusual appearance (tightly coiled and parallel to the major occluded vessel and having a "tree root" appearance, with small, inadequate, filamentous terminations) (Fig. 8-25). The pathology is that of intimal prolifera-

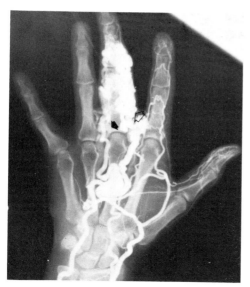

Fig. 8-21. Congenital arteriovenous malformations. This patient presented clinically with a large, warm, pulsatile third digit. There are enlarged feeding arteries (*open arrow*) and premature draining veins (*black closed arrow*) in the hand.

fistulas are particularly amenable to intravascular embolic techniques, and this subject is covered later in this chapter.

FIBROMUSCULAR DYSPLASIA
Fibromuscular dysplasia (Fig. 8-24) is more commonly seen in young females. Although the renal artery is most frequently involved, the lesion occurs in many other arteries, such as the carotids, some of the intracranial vessels, the vertebral arteries, the hepatic and other splanchnic arteries, the iliacs, and upper extremity arteries. Fibromuscular dysplasia is a developmental lesion of unknown etiology, consisting of areas of heaped-up intima and media (arterial narrowing) alternating with areas of medial destruction (localized aneurysms). The condition can be progressive. Commonly the renal arteries are involved in their middle or distal third, or in the more peripheral branches. When the internal carotid arteries are diseased, the areas involved are usually more distal in location than in atherosclerosis (see Chap. 14).

The following classification of types of fibromuscular dysplasia is based on histologic abnormalities found predominantly in intima, media, and adventitia [52, 62].

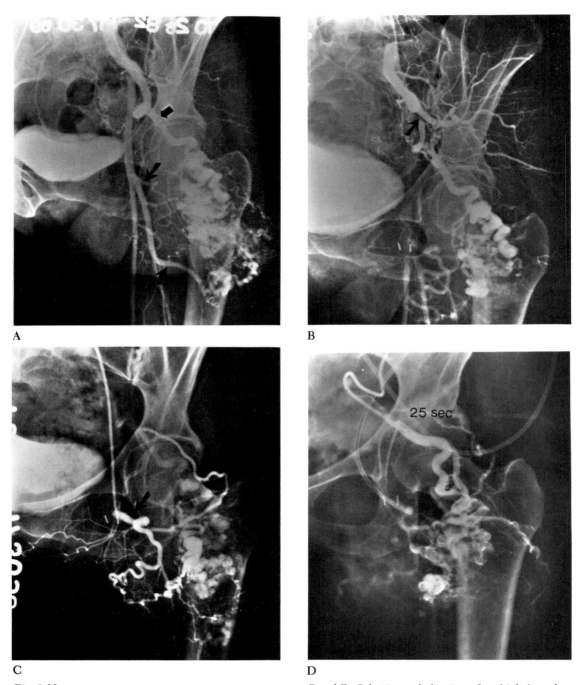

A

B

C

D

Fig. 8-22.

A. Large arteriovenous malformation (AVM) supplied by the inferior gluteal artery and multiple branches of the profunda femoris (*arrows*).

B. Surgical ligation of the inferior gluteal artery. The AVM now fills from branches of the profunda femoris artery.

C and D. Selective embolization of multiple branches with absolute alcohol and other embolic agents. The lesion was subsequently totally resected in a bloodless field.

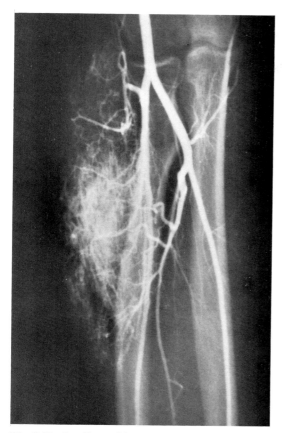

Fig. 8-23. Small vessel hemangioma. There are normal-size feeding arteries and a capillary stain with no significant arteriovenous shunting.

tion, with luminal occlusion by thrombus and granulation tissue. Regions of recanalization and, in acute lesions, microabscesses may be seen intraluminally on microscopy. Some authorities deny the existence of this disease.

Takayasu's Arteritis

Takayasu's arteritis [38] is an idiopathic inflammatory process involving arterial walls and is seen more frequently in young women. It most often involves segments of the aorta and the brachiocephalic vessels, but it can occur in the proximal portion of other major arteries of the aorta (see Chap. 18). Aneurysms are not a feature in this disease, helping to differentiate it from other forms of arteritis. The disease is usually insidious in onset, and presenting complaints are those related to vascular ischemia. The ischemic area is due to narrowing and/or occlusion caused by marked thickening of the arterial wall due primarily to intimal fibroplasia. The proximal portions of the involved vessels (e.g., coronary arteries, visceral arteries, subclavian arteries) may be amenable to transluminal dilation (see Fig. 18-34B) [20]. This should not be attempted in the acute phase of the disease.

Giant Cell Arteritis

Giant cell arteritis [32] is a self-limiting disease that is seen in elderly patients of either sex, who present clinically with malaise, fever, and headache. The temporal arteries are frequently involved (see Chap. 14), but the condition can also be seen in peripheral vessels such as the carotid, axillary, brachial, femoral, and popliteal arteries. Pathologically, the findings are inflammatory cells with disruption of elastica and intimal proliferation. Although the arteritis usually burns itself out within 6 months to 2 years, a residual arterial narrowing, sometimes with blindness and cerebral ischemia, remains. The angiographic appearance is one of multiple smooth, elongated segmental stenoses (Fig. 8-26).

Behçet's Disease

Behçet's disease [53] is a multisystem systemic disease of unknown etiology but suspected to be of autoimmune origin. It is found most often in young adults (twice as frequently in women) generally from the Mediterranean and Middle Eastern countries and the Orient. It involves the cardiovascular system in up to 30 percent of patients.

The large vessels (aorta and pulmonary artery) are the prime target, but visceral vessels and extremity vessels are also involved (Fig. 8-27). Fragmentation and splitting of medial elastic fibers, and an obliterative endarteritis of the vasovasorum are the underlying causes for aneurysm formation and vascular occlusion. Major criteria for making the diagnosis rest in the other clinical manifestations of ulcerations of the mouth, the genitals, ocular inflammatory lesions, and skin lesions. These manifestations help to differentiate the disease from Buerger's disease, fibromuscular hyperplasia, or arteritis from other causes.

Arteritis Associated with Other Conditions

Arteritis can be associated with syphilis, rheumatoid disease, rheumatic fever, Reiter's syndrome, and recurrent polychondritis.

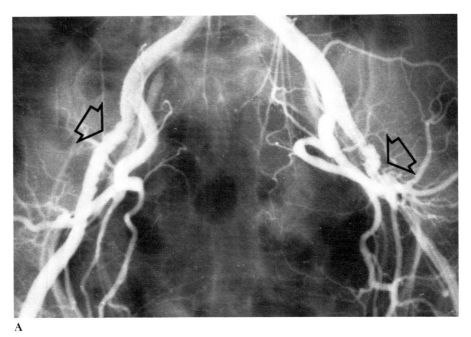

A

Fig. 8-24.
A. Medial fibroplasia with aneurysms involving the iliac vessels bilaterally (*arrows*). Similar changes were also noted in the renal arteries.
B. A young man with bilateral pulsatile masses in the palm of the hand. Note corrugated appearance to several of the branches of the superficial and deep palmar arches with an aneurysm. Similar changes were seen in the opposite hand. Aneurysms frequently accompany changes of fibromuscular hyperplasia. (Courtesy Dr. James Green, Ruston, Louisiana.)

MEDIUM AND SMALL VESSEL OCCLUSIVE DISEASE

Medium and small vessel occlusive disease of the extremities is often the end result of a varied number of diseases. Contrast studies define the site and extent of the disease, and there may be associated clues as to its cause. These findings include distinctive morphologic changes of the involved vessel, predilection of some diseases for certain sites, and distinctive changes in the remaining vascular bed. Often, however, no such clues are available. Then one must rely on the history and the clinical and laboratory findings. The following group of conditions should be kept in mind when one is faced with this problem [4, 61].

1. Chronic recurrent trauma. Typists, pianists, baseball players, carpenters, and workers using

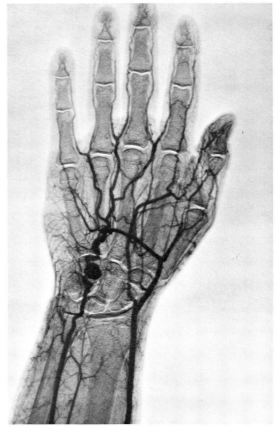

B

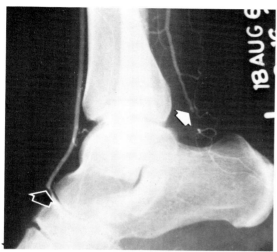

A

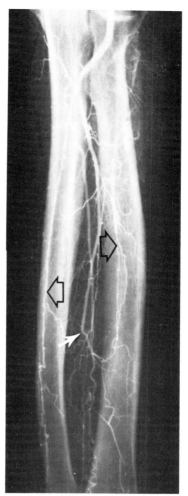

B

Fig. 8-25. Thromboangiitis obliterans (Buerger's disease).

A. A 43-year-old white man, a heavy smoker, with multiple ascending amputations of the right leg and the left hand. The peripheral pulses were absent in all four extremities. There was abrupt occlusion of the dorsalis pedis (*black arrow*) and posterior tibial arteries (*white arrow*) with inadequate collaterals.

B. Brachial arteriogram of the same patient, showing long, stringlike arterial narrowing and tightly coiled collateral vessels (*open arrows*). The interosseous branches are occluded (*white arrow*)

vibrating tools can have occlusion of the digital vessels in the upper extremities; frequent bending of the knees can lead to popliteal artery occlusion.

2. Multiple small emboli (one should search for their source).

3. Collagen diseases (Fig. 8-28). Scleroderma shows spasm and small vessel occlusion; polyarteritis nodosa displays small vessel aneurysm and occlusion.

4. Temporal arteritis.

5. Dysproteinemias (cryoglobulins; cryofibrinogens; macroglobulins as seen in leukemias, multiple myeloma, and other malignancies).

6. Polycythemia vera (Fig. 8-29).

7. Excess circulatory catecholamines.

8. Adverse reaction to warfarin (digital vessel occlusion with gangrene).

9. Pseudoxanthoma elasticum [2], a rare hereditary disease with an abnormal production of elastica resulting in widespread vessel abnor-

malities and redundant skin folds. Medium and small arteries of the extremities demonstrate narrowing and occlusion early in life, particularly in the upper extremities. This narrowing is caused by medial proliferation, disruption of elastica, and superimposed thrombosis.

CYSTIC ADVENTITIAL DISEASE OF THE POPLITEAL ARTERY

This disease [9] should be considered when ischemic symptoms of the lower extremity are seen in patients under 50 years of age. It occurs most frequently in males and is due to a focal adventitial accumulation of myxomatous material in the popliteal artery, usually just above the knee joint. This extrinsic compression of the lumen of the vessel,

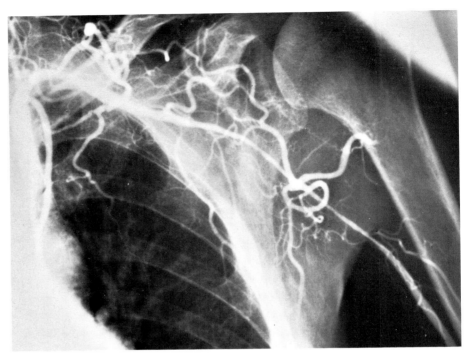

Fig. 8-26. Giant cell arteritis in a 55-year-old woman with headaches, low-grade fever, and elevated erythrocyte sedimentation rate. Blood pressure is diminished in both upper extremities. There is a long area of smooth stenosis involving the subclavian, axillary, and proximal brachial arteries.

manifested angiographically as a curvilinear or spiral narrowing, can progress to total occlusion. The cystic adventitial material may be demonstrated as an intramural sonolucent collection by ultrasonography. It should be differentiated from focal atherosclerosis, for treatment is directed toward surgical unroofing (or grafting if occluded), rather than percutaneous transluminal angioplasty. A differential diagnosis would include popliteal artery aneurysm with thrombosis, Buerger's disease, embolism, popliteal artery entrapment, and ruptured Baker's cyst.

NEUROVASCULAR COMPRESSION

Arteries and veins may be compressed extrinsically by neighboring bony, ligamentous, and muscular structures [39]. Symptoms may occur as a result of compression of the accompanying nerve rather

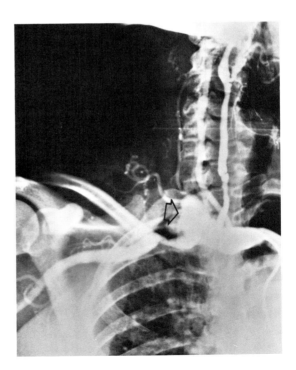

Fig. 8-27. Innominate artery injection shows areas of narrowing and aneurysm with marked irregularity of the bracheocephalic vessels in a 28-year-old Korean woman with multisystem disease. She also had occlusion of the proximal left subclavian artery, stenosis of the left common carotid artery, and occlusion of the right renal artery—likely Behçet's disease. (Courtesy Dr. G. Smyser, United Hospital, Grand Forks, ND.)

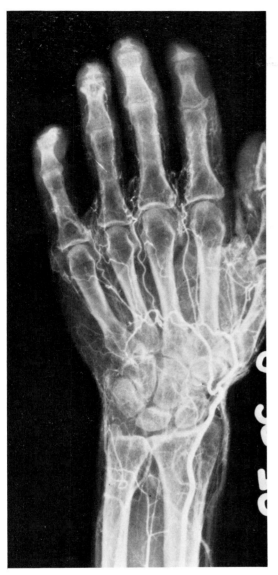

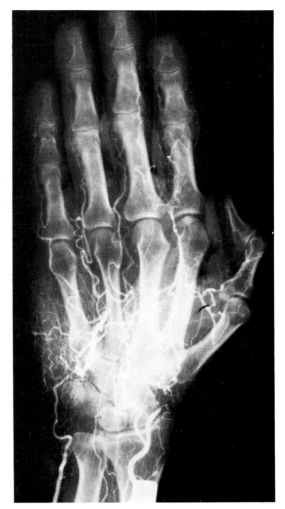

Fig. 8-29. Occlusion of radial, ulnar, and digital arteries in a patient with polycythemia rubra vera.

Fig. 8-28. Scleroderma with multiple occlusions of the digital arteries and the ulnar artery. Note sclerodactyle of second through fifth digits.

than compression of the vessel. Since arterial compression may be induced by stress maneuvers in symptomless patients, considerable clinical judgment is required to implicate an angiographically demonstrated lesion. There are several areas in the thoracic outlet where the subclavian or axillary artery may be compressed:

1. Cervical rib. In this condition there is compression of the neurovascular bundle by a cervical rib or by a fibrous band attached to a cervical rib. Cervical ribs are demonstrated on 0.5 percent of routine chest x rays, but in only approximately 5 percent of the patients does vascular compression of the vessels exist.

2. Costoclavicular syndrome (Fig. 8-30). In this condition compression occurs between the clavicle and the first rib. This is the most frequent type of neurovascular compression syndrome.

3. The scalenus tunnel syndrome. In this entity the compression occurs in the scalene triangle by the scalene muscles.

4. The hyperabduction syndrome (Fig. 8-31). In this condition the compression occurs between

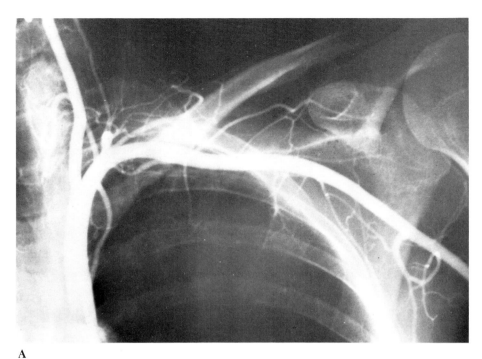

A

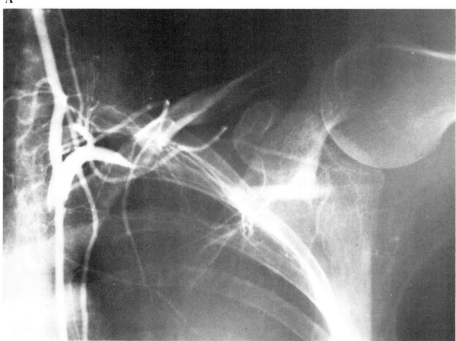

B

Fig. 8-30. Costoclavicular syndrome.

A. Patent left subclavian artery showing mild dilatation of the distal one-third, with the arm in neutral position.

B. Complete occlusion of the left subclavian artery at the point where the clavicle crosses the first rib during the stress maneuver of abduction. One should not overinject into this occluded vessel, since contrast agent is diverted into the vertebral artery. No more than 10 ml of medium-density contrast agent is required.

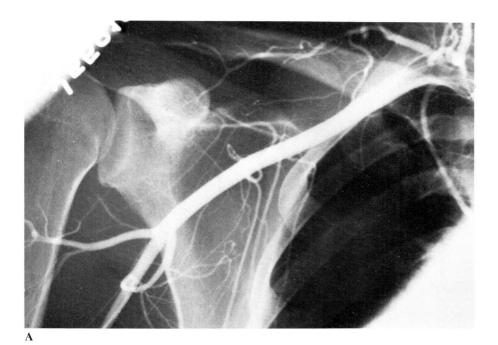

A

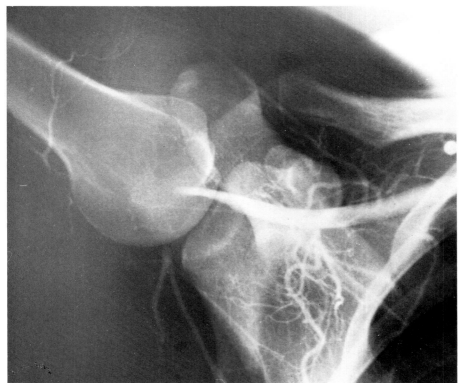

B

Fig. 8-31. Hyperabduction syndrome.
A. Normal right subclavian arteriogram in the neutral position.

B. With abduction, there is extrinsic compression of the axillary artery between the head of the humerus and the pectoralis minor.

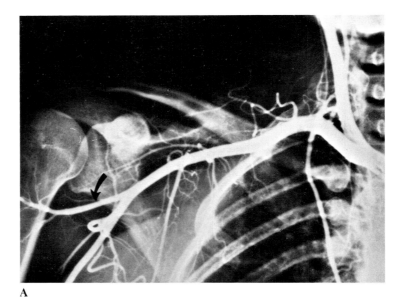

A

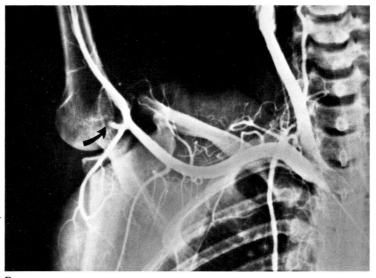

B

Fig. 8-32. Quadrangular space syndrome.
A. Normal vessels with the arm in neutral position.
B. Segmental occlusion of the posterior circumflex humeral artery with the arm abducted. (See text.)

the head of the humerus and the pectoralis minor. Since the lateral boundary of the subclavian artery is the first rib, the segment of vessel compressed is the axillary artery.

5. The quadrangular space syndrome. In this condition the posterior circumflex humeral artery and the axillary nerve pass through a space formed between the triceps heads laterally and the teres major and teres minor muscles above and below. The artery and nerve can be compressed, with resulting shoulder pain. On arteriography the posterior circumflex humeral artery fills normally in the neutral position, but it fills retrograde through collaterals because of occlusion when in the abducted position (Fig. 8-32).

Any of the above causes of compression may be seen alone or in combination. The angiographer should always try to induce the dampened pulse and to perform the angiogram with the patient's arm in the stress position. Extrinsic compression or tapered occlusion may be demonstrated angiographically with the stress position. An aneurysm due to weakening of the arterial wall, with or without clot, may be seen. Do not overinject a subclavian artery occluded in this fashion for fear of diverting too much contrast medium to the vertebral artery. This is an ideal situation for IA-DSA studies because of real-time capabilities and dilute contrast demands. Since the axillary artery may also be extrinsically compressed by overlying muscles and ligaments, this vessel should always be included in the field of exposure; this is particularly true if there is a normal subclavian arteriogram despite obliteration of pulses by the stress position.

POPLITEAL ARTERY ENTRAPMENT

The popliteal artery can be externally compressed and deviated medially from its normal position by an anomalous relationship to the gastrocnemius muscle. Normally, the medial head of the gastrocnemius muscle is inserted on the posterior aspect of the medial femoral condyle; the popliteal artery lies between the medial and lateral heads of the gastrocnemius and ventral to the popliteus muscle. Entrapment occurs when this relationship is altered. The popliteal artery may course medial to the medial head of the gastrocnemius; this muscle insertion may either be normally positioned or lie in a more lateral than normal position. The artery may pass medial to the medial head of the gastrocnemius and deep to the popliteus muscle. Occasionally the artery may be entrapped by an accessory muscular tail of the gastrocnemius. Angiographically the popliteal artery takes a more medial than normal course, may demonstrate poststenotic dilatation and aneurysm formation, occlusion, and peripheral embolization. The condition usually is observed in patients between 15 and 30 years of age and should be differentiated from diseases such as embolism, Buerger's disease, premature atherosclerosis, aneurysm, and adventitial cystic disease. Dynamic computed tomography scans of the popliteal fossa determine the precise relationship of the artery to its muscular and bony landmarks [51].

FOLLOW-UP STUDY OF BYPASS GRAFTS

Bypass grafts are composed of a variety of materials, including autogenous vein, woven Dacron,

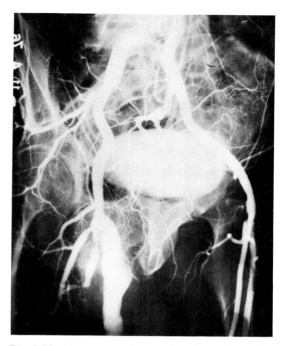

Fig. 8-33. An aneurysm has developed several months following placement of a right femoral popliteal bypass graft made of synthetic grafting material.

Gore-Tex, Teflon, and bovine carotid artery. Woven Dacron is most commonly used in the larger vessels (e.g., aorta, iliacs) and autogenous veins in smaller vessels (e.g., femoral, popliteal, aortorenal, or coronary bypass graft). Bypass grafts are subject to either acute or chronic complications [64]. These complications may occur as a result of technical difficulties at the time of surgery, but more often they are caused by inherent weakness in the grafting material and by the natural progression of the primary disease process of the host.

Grafts may occlude as a result of thrombosis, or they may stenose (see Figs. 8-54, 8-55). They may dilate and form aneurysms (Fig. 8-33). Infection or poor healing may occur at anastomotic sites, with subsequent leakage and formation of false aneurysms (Fig. 8-34), sinuses, and fistulas to surrounding structures. Aortoenteric or arterioenteric fistulas may be particularly dangerous, as are false aneurysms, *which may rupture spontaneously* (see Chap. 10). Arteriovenous fistulas may also develop. Stenosis of autogenous venous grafts can occur as a result of clamp injury at the time of surgery; it can also occur as a result of a fibroblastic intimal proliferation, which may be local or dif-

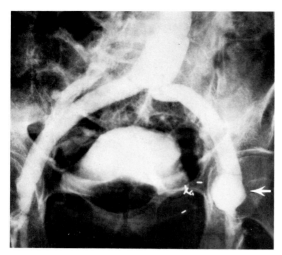

Fig. 8-34. Aortobifemoral bypass graft. A false aneurysm can be seen at the distal anastomosis on the left (*arrow*).

fuse in location. Venous grafts may also develop atherosclerotic changes.

SURGICALLY CREATED ARTERIOVENOUS FISTULAS

Surgically created arteriovenous fistulas are made to allow dialysis of patients with chronic renal failure. These fistulas may fail, and angiography can outline the cause of failure [25]. The vessels most frequently used are those of the forearm. The artery and vein may be directly connected, either end to end, side to side, arterial end to side of vein, or venous end to side of artery. A bridge may be interposed between the artery and vein; this may be composed of plastic tubing, an autogenous vein, or a piece of specially treated bovine carotid artery (a heterograft). An unwanted result of the fistula may be development of ischemia of the hand peripheral to the shunt. In addition, the surrounding veins may become varicosed. Complications may occur in the graft itself or at its anastomoses; thus stenosis or occlusion due to thrombosis may occur on the arterial or the venous side (Fig. 8-35). Aneurysms may occur in the artery, and pseudoaneurysms may develop in the graft as a result of the multiple punctures required for dialysis. Sclerosis in more remote areas of the draining veins may occur. Often the resulting stenosis leads to eventual thrombosis. Lesions such as these can sometimes be treated by intravascular techniques. Thrombosis

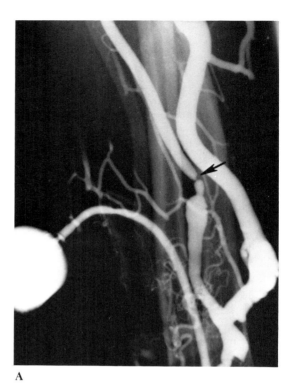

A

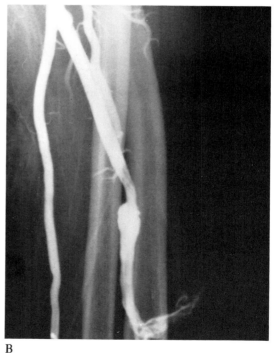

B

Fig. 8-35. Stenosis of renal dialysis fistula.
A. Fistulogram demonstrates a high grade stenosis (*arrow*).
B. After percutaneous angioplasty the gradient is alleviated.

can be lysed by low-dose thrombolytic therapy and stenotic lesions subsequently subjected to angioplasty. Infected grafts do not respond, however, and intensive medical treatment and prompt surgical intervention are required in these circumstances.

Angiography may be performed through a needle already introduced for dialysis. Another technique is the injection of 20 ml of low-density contrast agent through a 19-gauge needle directly in the graft approximately 1 cm from one or the other anastomosis. A blood pressure cuff inflated to 250 mm Hg prior to injection makes a closed system of the graft and the adjacent arteries and veins. Contrast medium can reflux both through the anastomosis and the vessels and outline them satisfactorily on seriographic films. Midway through the injection, the cuff is released, and arterial blood washes the contrast agent out so that the more remote draining veins may be visualized.

FUNCTIONAL PERIPHERAL ARTERIAL DISEASE

Functional peripheral arterial disease is a result of exaggerated vasomotor tone. There may be varying etiologies [61]. The arteriographic pattern shows delay in filling of threadlike arteries.

1. Ergotism [19, 37A]. Ergot directly stimulates smooth muscle, and it has a toxic effect on the endothelium, predisposing to thrombosis. Arteriographically there is marked delay in filling of threadlike arteries and a tapered occlusion (Fig. 8-36). Treatment of ergotism includes withdrawing the drug, heparinization, and administering a channel blocker such as nifedipine 10 mg orally 3 times a day. The channel blocker induces dilation of coronary and peripheral vessels by decreasing smooth muscle contractility. More prompt vasodilation may be required if the limb is in danger of irreversible damage and may be achieved by intravenously introducing nitroprusside. With the latter, systemic pressures must be carefully monitored to prevent profound hypotension.

2. Phlegmasia cerulea dolens [8] (Fig. 8-37). In this condition the patient develops an intensely painful, pulseless, cold, cyanotic, swollen leg. There is often an associated shocklike condition. Arteriography shows delayed flow, tapered occlusion, and threadlike vessels. Venog-

raphy shows acute massive thrombosis. The arterial occlusion may be caused by:

   a. Arterial spasm due to contiguous phlebitis.
   b. Increased periarterial tissue pressure due to edema.
   c. Release of circulatory humoral substances.

3. Raynaud's phenomenon. This condition typically consists of a transient, intermittent episode of constriction of the small vessels of the hand. There is an accompanying pallor, then cyanosis followed by rubor, with associated paresthesias. It is usually exacerbated or incited by cold or emotion. There are a number of conditions causing this problem, which have already been described. They include multiple repetitive trauma, neurovascular compression syndromes, occlusive disease (arteriosclerosis obliterans, Buerger's disease, arteritis, embolism), intoxication (ergot, heavy metals), and miscellaneous other causes. Raynaud's disease can also cause this phenomenon. It is a condition of unknown cause, is seen in young women, is bilateral, and has no associated underlying diseases or arteriographic evidence of occlusion. These patients can be temporarily helped by an intraarterial injection of 1 mg of reserpine.

PERIPHERAL TUMORS

When a peripheral tumor is suspected, imaging modalities such as ultrasonography, computed tomography, and magnetic resonance imaging give precise information regarding the size, location, and extent of the lesion [23, 40]. Angiography may also give helpful information [40, 42, 66]. Arterial and capillary neovascularity are well recognized signs of malignancy. Generally, the neovascularity of a lesion increases proportionately with the degree of malignancy. This may be in the form of coarse or fine neovascularity, a capillary blush, arteriovenous shunting and pooling of contrast material, venous prominence or displacement, and/or encasement of major branches (see Fig. 8-56). Hypovascular lesions may also be malignant, however, and areas of hypovascularity within a tumor may reflect tumor necrosis. Very malignant lesions have been known to be generally hypovascular. Also, hypervascularity is not specific for neoplasia, for it can be seen in some inflammatory processes. Benign primary bone tumors (osteoid osteoma, giant cell tumor) and hemangiomas may

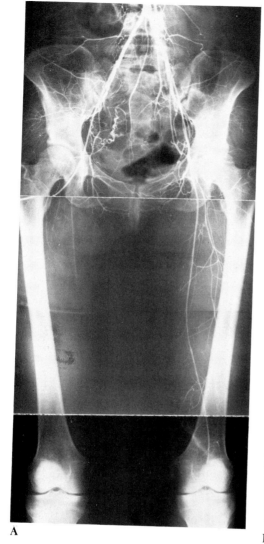

A

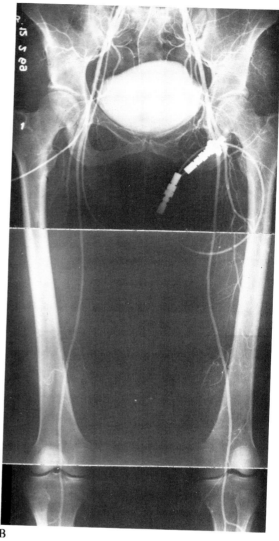

B

Fig. 8-36. Ergotism in a 41-year-old woman with a history of migraine and ergot intake. Acute ischemic changes were seen clinically in both legs.
A. Iliac femoral arteriogram showing generalized narrowing of all vessels and tapered occlusion.
B. Repeat arteriogram 1 week following withdrawal of medications. Caliber of vessels has now returned to normal.

also be hypervascular; these tumors show a homogeneous opacification due to numerous capillary vessels. This appearance contrasts with the irregular tumor vessels of malignancy. Surgical treatment of malignant lesions is now becoming more conservative [41], which in some instances includes intraarterial chemotherapy. Occasionally, some peripheral tumors are embolized [37, 67]. Because catheter placement is required for administering the drugs, an accompanying angiogram can be performed which provides a means to monitor tumor size, vascularity, and degree of necrosis both before and after chemotherapy (see Fig. 8-56).

Intravascular Therapeutic Procedures of the Extremities

PERCUTANEOUS TRANSLUMINAL ANGIOPLASTY (PTA)

Selection of Patients for PTA

There are a number of factors that determine whether or not a patient is a candidate for PTA of

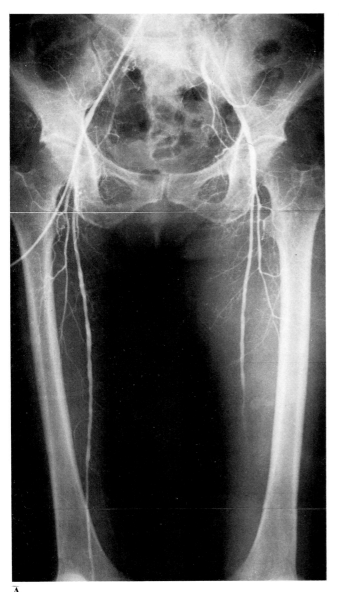
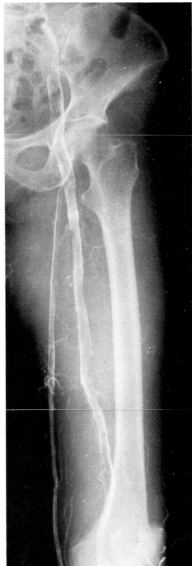

Ā   B

Fig. 8-37. Phlegmasia cerulea dolens.
A. Tapered occlusion of arteries to edematous left
   lower extremity.
B. Extensive deep and superficial vein thrombosis.

the lower extremity. These include the clinical presentation, noninvasive laboratory findings, and whether or not a patient is a candidate or a high risk for surgery. The acceptance of the procedure by the patient and attending physician, availability of a consulting vascular surgeon, and findings on angiography are important considerations. Often PTA may be considered as an adjunct to a surgical

procedure. It may be used as an alternative to surgery because of no available suitable veins for bypass procedures. It may be performed as a temporizing measure on an otherwise marginal candidate with ischemia and an anticipated short life expectancy.

The Clinical Findings
The clinical presentation indicates the general location of the occlusive process [21]. Thus, impotence and hip and thigh claudication favor distal

aortic and/or iliac lesions; calf or foot pain points to lesions in the femoral, popliteal or more distal arteries. Intermittent claudication (Fontaine stage II), pain at rest (Fontaine stage III), or nonhealing ulcers or tissue necrosis (Fontaine stage IV) indicate varying but progressive degrees of ischemia. Under circumstances in which limb salvage is of primary concern, a more aggressive approach to angioplasty may be considered, despite the unfavorable anatomy or morphology of a lesion [43].

Noninvasive Laboratory Findings [6, 57]

Noninvasive laboratory findings help to confirm the severity of the occlusive process. On occasion, they may help one choose the appropriate approach to a potential angioplasty procedure. They may also give insight into the significance of a stenotic lesion uncovered at angiography. After the procedure, they may determine the success or failure of an angioplasty procedure and provide objective evidence for long-term follow-up.

The Pathology Underlying the Occlusive Process

Although atherosclerosis is by far the most common pathologic process undergoing PTA, there are a number of other conditions producing stenosis that are also potential candidates for vascular dilation. Fibromuscular hyperplasia in the renal, carotid, and iliac arteries has been treated successfully by PTA. Angioplasty should be considered when this condition is the cause of symptoms in vessels to the extremities, particularly if the disease is localized. Other stenotic lesions that should be considered for PTA in the extremities include congenital narrowings, the inactive end-stage vascular fibrosis and stenosis due to arteritis, intimal fibroplasia found at anastomoses with arterial grafts, and stenosis produced as a reaction to radiation. Some of the lesions may prove difficult to dilate, particularly those related to anastomoses with synthetic grafts. They are all, however, potential candidates for PTA [20].

Angiographic Findings

Angiography, performed in multiple projections, allows an understanding of the pathology, and also accurately portrays the location, the degree and length and multiplicity of stenoses, the presence and length of total occlusions, and the state of the peripheral run-off. Pressures measured on either side of a lesion may demonstrate a pressure gradient, thereby providing added information as to the hemodynamic significance of the lesion. If the angiographic findings and pressure measurements do not fit with the clinical suspicion of significant stenosis, a pressure gradient may be induced by injecting tolazoline 25 mg or nitroglycerine 100 to 300 μg directly into the artery peripheral to a lesion, or by inducing reactive hyperemia (Chap. 4), and immediately rechecking the pressure measurements.

Patients may be categorized into major groups according to their angiographic findings [26, 50].

In the appropriate symptomatic candidate, PTA is the treatment of choice for the following circumstances (Fig. 8-38) [26, 36, 50].

1. A single, short-segment stenosis (less than 4 cm) in an area ranging from the distal aorta down to and including the popliteal artery. Shorter segment stenosis involving proximal tibial artery if it is not the only vessel supplying the distal leg.

Fig. 8-38. Indications for percutaneous transluminal angioplasty. (See text.)

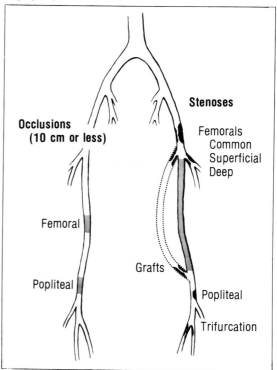

2. Stenosis of the profunda femoris in patients with occluded femoral arteries and poor distal run-off. Distal stenoses of the profunda when it is acting as a major collateral bypassing an occluded superficial femoral artery. When the stenosis of the profunda is at the origin of the vessel, and there is good peripheral run-off, surgical profundaplasty is a simple, well-tried procedure and is likely the procedure of choice [58].

3. Stenosis of the femoral artery proximal to, or the popliteal artery distal to, a femoral popliteal bypass graft. These are often uncovered following successful thrombolysis of an occluded graft (see Fig. 8-54).

4. Patients with lesions amenable to either surgery or PTA but who are poor surgical candidates or who refuse surgery.

Surgery is the treatment of choice in patients with long multiple areas of iliac occlusive disease, occlusion of the aorta or iliac vessels, long occlusions of the superficial femoral artery, and/or occlusion of the popliteal artery. Surgery is also the treatment of choice with focal proximal stenosis of the profunda with an occluded superficial femoral artery and good peripheral run-off. These lesions may be accepted for angioplasty if surgery is not possible for a variety of reasons.

Patients do well with surgery or PTA when there are short segments of occlusion of the superficial femoral artery (less than 10 cm) or proximal popliteal artery with good peripheral run-off.

Some conditions require both surgery and PTA for optimal results. One example of this would be a patient with a stenotic iliac artery on one side requiring PTA and an occluded femoral artery on the opposite side requiring a femoral-bypass graft (Fig. 8-39A). Another example would be a patient with a stenotic iliac artery on one side requiring PTA and occluded superficial femoral artery on the same side requiring femoral-popliteal artery bypass procedure subsequent to the dilation (Fig. 8-39B). A patient may demonstrate an occluded aorta or iliac vessel requiring surgical bypass, with a focal contralateral iliac artery stenosis or a distal femoral or popliteal artery stenosis which can be easily handled with an intraluminal dilatation, either prior to (Fig. 8-39D) or at the time of surgery (Fig. 8-39C).

Avoid dilating a patient with an occlusion of the superficial femoral artery or popliteal artery when the symptoms are of relatively recent origin (less than 6 weeks; preferably delay until 12 weeks or older) due to the possibility of embolizing relatively fresh clot. Avoid dilating a vessel that may endanger an essential collateral (Figs. 8-40, 8-41). Do not dilate a partially patent vessel below the knee when it is the sole provider of the circulation to that limb.

Technique of PTA in the Lower Extremities
Review Chapter 6 pertaining to preangiographic care, selection and care of angioplasty catheters, and availability of the required guidewires, adapters, sleeves, antispasmodics, and vasodilators. Review also the anterograde approach to femoral artery puncture and when it should be used. Review the manipulations sometimes required to cross the aortic bifurcation when using the contralateral femoral artery and how to overcome buckling of the catheter in an acutely angled bifurcation. Review the special considerations required for an axillary artery approach, if this is the only available route for profunda or proximal femoral angioplasty. Be aware of the precautions for both introducing and withdrawing the balloon catheter, and its accurate placement over the site of stenosis or occlusion. Familiarize yourself with the manipulations of guidewires and catheters across eccentric areas of stenosis. Be prepared to use 105-ml spot films and/or IA-DSA for adequate documentation of the procedure. Review the section on summary of problems and how to handle them during angioplasty.

SPECIAL CONSIDERATIONS IN PTA OF THE LOWER EXTREMITY. Perform the diagnostic procedure for ischemia of the leg by retrograde puncture of the contralateral artery. The aorta and peripheral arteries and pressure measurements proximal to the stenosis can be evaluated without compromising access to the affected limb.

APPROACH. An anterograde ipsilateral approach to PTA is used for lesions of the mid- or distal superficial femoral artery; surgically inaccessible sections of the distal profunda artery; the popliteal artery; or proximal tibial vessels (see Chap. 6). Exceptions to this are obese patients (in whom anterograde punctures are difficult), patients with previous surgery and grafts in the ipsilateral groin, and patients with combined lesions of the iliac artery and the femoral artery. In these the contra-

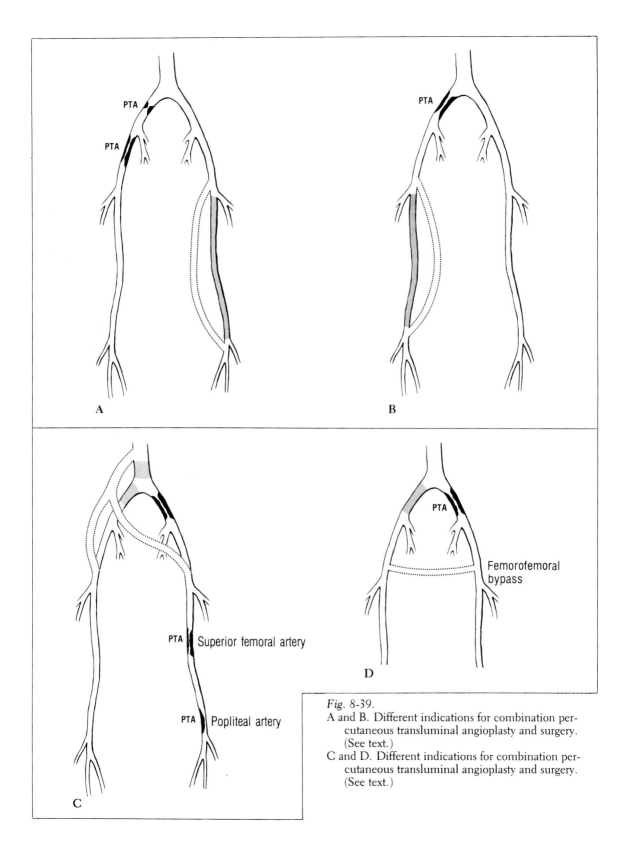

A

B

C

PTA Superior femoral artery

PTA Popliteal artery

D

Femorofemoral bypass

Fig. 8-39.
A and B. Different indications for combination per-
cutaneous transluminal angioplasty and surgery.
(See text.)
C and D. Different indications for combination per-
cutaneous transluminal angioplasty and surgery.
(See text.)

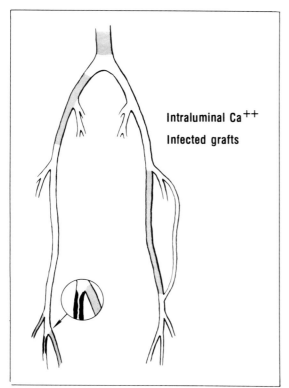

Intraluminal Ca^{++}

Infected grafts

Fig. 8-40. Avoid percutaneous transluminal angioplasty (PTA) with occlusion of the abdominal aorta, long occluded segments of the iliac arteries, and long occlusions of the superficial femoral artery. Do not dilate the only vessel feeding the leg distal to the trifurcation. Dense calcification and infected grafts usually preclude PTA.

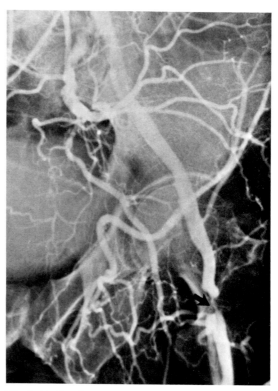

Fig. 8-41. Focal stenosis at the common femoral bifurcation with vessels patent peripherally. This lesion should be treated surgically.

lateral approach is preferred. The contralateral femoral artery (or if necessary the axillary artery) is also used for PTA of the common femoral artery, proximal superficial femoral artery, or profunda femoris artery. On some occasions, a retrograde approach may be manipulated into one that is anterograde (see Figs. 8-45, 8-46).

PRECAUTIONS. Carefully mark the surface anatomy of the occluded or stenosed segments. This helps to avoid time-consuming confusion during the procedure.

If there are multiple stenotic lesions, dilate the proximal one first. This reduces the obstructing effect of the passage of the catheter to the distal lesion (Fig. 8-47).

Arterial spasm and subsequent occlusion of peripheral vessels may occur, particularly with distal femoral, popliteal, and proximal tibial PTA [59]. All efforts to avoid this should be considered, including

1. Antiplatelet therapy (aspirin 300 mg qd and dipyridamole 50 mg tid) for 2 or 3 days prior to the procedure.
2. An adequate amount of 1% xylocaine surrounding the femoral puncture site not only provides anesthesia but achieves sympathetic blockade.
3. Antispasmodics. Nifedipine 10 mg PO several minutes prior to catheter manipulation or dilation. An immediate effect can be had by breaking the capsule into the mouth. Tolazoline 25 mg or nitroglycerine 100 to 300 μg should be injected intraarterially immediately after the diagnostic catheter has bypassed the lesion and prior to dilation.
4. Heparin 5000 IU should be administered through the diagnostic catheter tip as it approaches the stenotic lesion, realizing the 10 minutes required for the effect of anticoagulant actions and heparin's added antispasmodic actions.

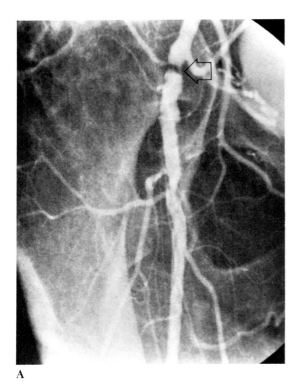

A

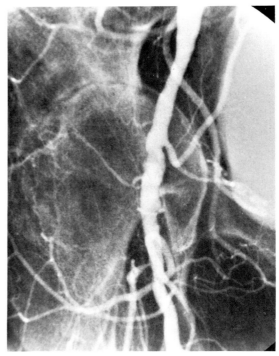

B

Fig. 8-42.
A. Focal stenosis of right common femoral artery with occluded superficial femoral artery.
B. Successful PTA from contralateral femoral approach.

5. Gentle manipulation of the guidewire and catheter through the lesions.

If the occlusive process is in the superficial femoral or popliteal artery, avoid advancing the guidewire or catheter beyond the trifurcation, for this induces vasospasm and invites thrombosis.

Figures 8-42 through 8-48 show both short- and long-segment stenotic lesions successfully dilated.

PASSING THROUGH AN OCCLUDED SEGMENT. The artery is negotiated with a 5 French catheter with a tapered slightly curved distal tip and two proximal side holes. A Touhy-Borst Y adapter at the catheter hub accepts the tapered 0.032 or 0.035-in. straight-tipped (alternatively, an 0.035-in. movable core, 3-mm J-tipped) guidewire which protrudes just beyond the catheter tip. The guidewire and the catheter are passed together down the artery to and beyond the diseased area. Repeated test injections of 30% contrast agent can be made through the sidearm of the Y adapter during catheter-guidewire manipulations. They outline the course of the vessel lumen and side and peripheral branches. The guidewire follows the path of least resistance across the lesion. At the point of occlu-

sion, gentle forward probing during test injections of contrast agent usually discloses the soft central part of the atheroma. Occasionally, the guidewire meets strong resistance due to (1) a heavily calcified chronically occluded segment, (2) passage of the guidewire and catheter tip into a smaller side branch, or (3) perforation of the vessel wall (Fig. 8-50). The latter is less apt to occur if the advancing catheter guidewire assembly has a blunt leading edge, as occurs with a J-shaped guidewire (Fig. 8-49). Injection of contrast agent through the adapter sidearm determines the cause. Fluoroscopic monitoring and multiple projections may be necessary.

If the guidewire and catheter appear to remain in the vessel lumen and resistance to its passage persists, the guidewire may have to be exchanged for a heavy-duty guide with a gentle 15-mm J curve. Sometimes exchanging the guidewire for one with a 2- or 3-mm J curve (or one with a movable core) with its tip projecting just beyond

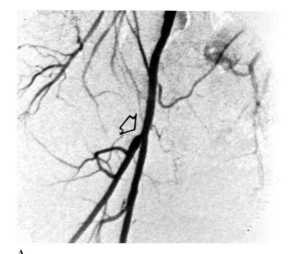

A

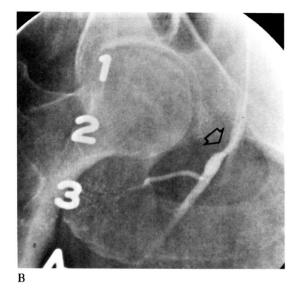

B

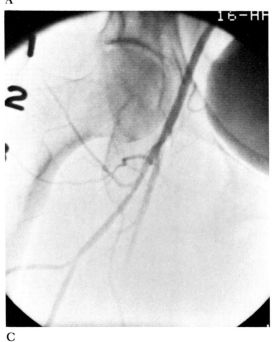

C

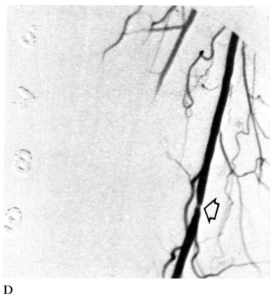

D

Fig. 8-43. Multiple stenoses involving proximal
femoral branches. Contralateral femoral approach.
A and B. Stenosis of profunda femoris.
C. Its successful dilatation.
D and E. Successful PTA of proximal superficial
    femoral artery.

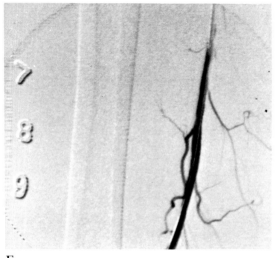

E

192

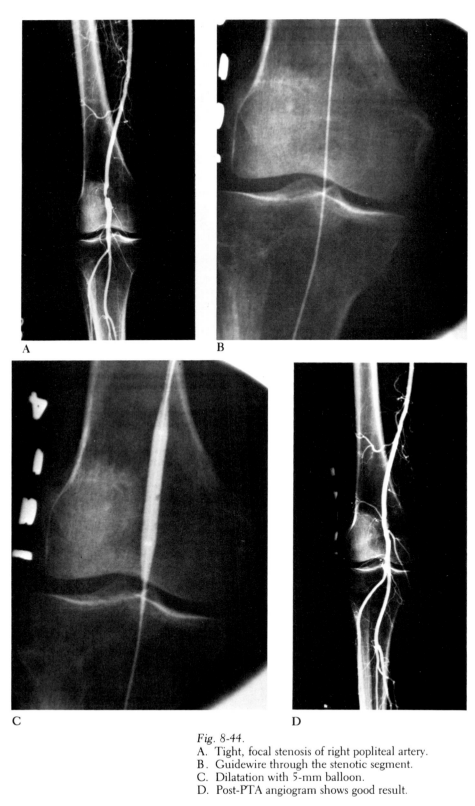

Fig. 8-44.
A. Tight, focal stenosis of right popliteal artery.
B. Guidewire through the stenotic segment.
C. Dilatation with 5-mm balloon.
D. Post-PTA angiogram shows good result.

the catheter will be helpful. Occasionally, a modified Lunderquist exchange guidewire must be used. Steady forward advancement of this catheter-guidewire combination through the occluded segment, with careful fluoroscopic monitoring of contrast injections, is required to avoid vascular damage.

If the catheter-guidewire tip has advanced into a side branch, it must be withdrawn and redirected into the central lumen.

If the guidewire has perforated the artery, the catheter-guidewire assembly often annoyingly searches out the same path and on subsequent manipulations cannot bypass it. The procedure may have to be abandoned at this point. Usually there is little or no damage, and no perivascular hematoma ensues, for the vessel was totally occluded in the first place. A surgical option must then be employed.

After traversing the lesion, and before introducing the dilating balloon catheter, a series of Teflon dilating catheters up to a diameter of 7 French gradually dilates the vessel lumen. Alternate methods include using the gradually tapered tip of

the 7 French Staple van Andel catheter (with side holes near its tip) or a specially constructed tapered-tip dilating balloon catheter with two distal side holes [3].

Once the guidewire has crossed the stenotic lesion, it should never be withdrawn until the entire procedure has been completed (Fig. 8-51). The initial heavy-duty guidewire may have to be exchanged for one with a smaller diameter in order to provide an adequate lumen in the catheter for injectables and for pressure monitoring. It should only be replaced once the catheter has traversed the lesion and lies well beyond its distal limits.

Some investigators inject heparin during the passage of the catheter through the occluded or stenotic segment rather than proximal to it. At this point, nitroglycerine (100 to 300 μg) is administered through the catheter tip and the appropriate diameter angioplasty balloon catheter is chosen.

The diagnostic or preliminary dilating Teflon catheter is replaced with a balloon catheter of choice. No. 7 French balloon catheters of 4 to 6 ml diameter and 2 to 10 cm length are available for distal extremity angioplasty. Six-millimeter diame-

Fig. 8-45. Turning a retrograde to an antegrade approach.

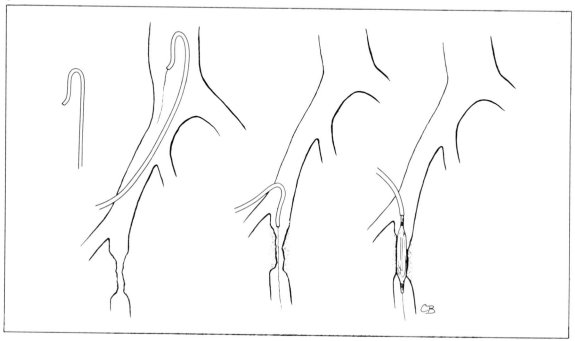

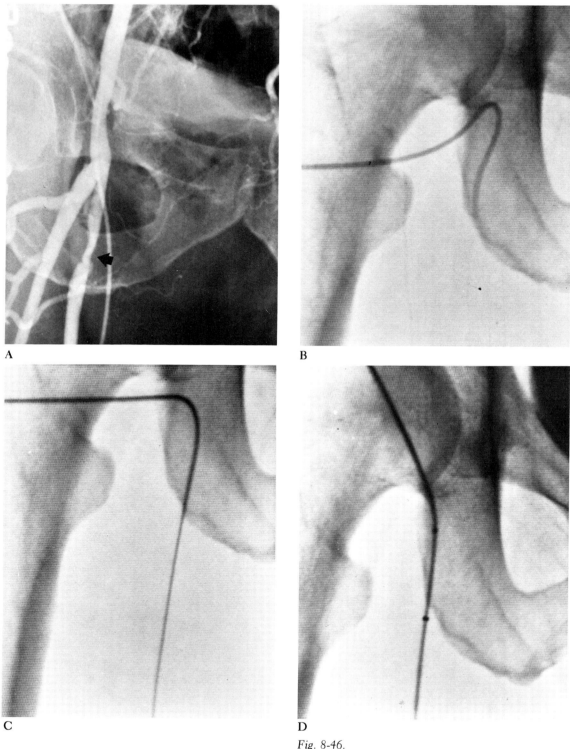

Fig. 8-46.
A. Stenosis of right proximal superficial artery. Retro-
grade approach to arteriogram.
B, C, D, E, and F. Steps in successful PTA.

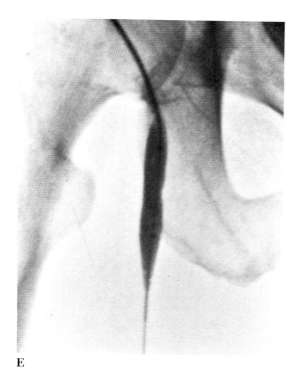

E

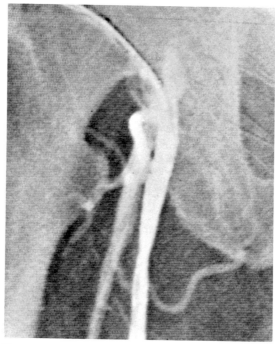

F

ter balloons of varying length are employed for proximal superficial femoral artery lesions; 5-mm diameter balloons are employed for distal superficial femoral and proximal popliteal artery lesions; 4-mm diameter balloons are used for more distal popliteal lesions.

Dilating balloon catheters with side holes proximal to the balloon are available. These catheters permit contrast agent injection to document the relation of the balloon to the stenosis and the effectiveness of the subsequent dilation without having to withdraw the deflated balloon catheter.

Buckling of the guidewire at the puncture site during introduction of the balloon catheters can be avoided either by introducing them over a modified Lunderquist guidewire or through a sheath placed in the groin.

With some distal lesions, 6 or 7 French Staple van Andel catheters provide sufficient diameter for successful dilation.

PTA OF VESSELS DISTAL TO THE TRIFURCATION. Distal small-lumen vessels may be dilated using the 2- to 3.6-mm diameter balloon catheters made primarily for coronary artery and distal visceral artery branch angioplasty. In the latter procedures

they are used coaxially, being advanced to their destination over a 0.014- or 0.016-in. steerable guidewire and through an overlying guiding catheter. In the lower extremity, however, they can simply be dropped anterograde down the femoral artery through a 5 French sheath, over a steerable 0.014- to 0.016-in. guidewire previously manipulated across the stenotic segment.

FOLLOWING ANGIOPLASTY. An angiogram should be performed following the angioplasty. This can be done with the deflated balloon catheter in position if it has side holes proximal to the balloon. If it does not, replace the guidewire with one of smaller caliber and withdraw the balloon catheter proximal to the dilated segment, leaving the guidewire in position across the stenosis. Intraluminal pressures may be measured during this maneuver.

Make a preliminary IA-DSA evaluation using 30% contrast agent. If there is persistent stenosis, repeat angioplasty must be performed. If the result is satisfactory, the guidewire is removed, the catheter is withdrawn far proximal to the dilated lesion, and a conventional angiogram is performed using 60% contrast agent. Avoid a high-pressure contrast injection through a catheter without side holes di-

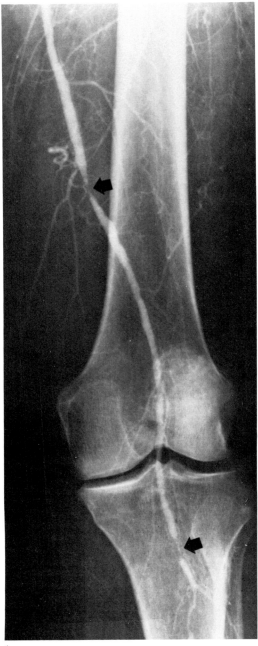

A

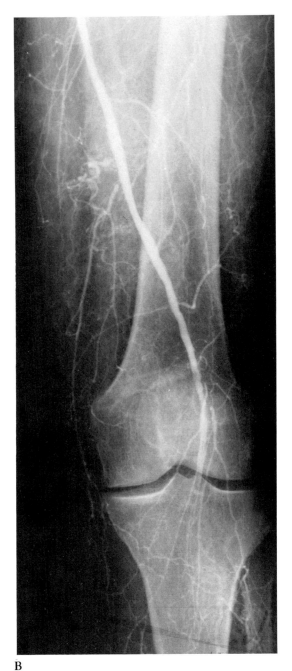

B

Fig. 8-47.

A. Multiple stenoses of popliteal artery. Always dilate the proximal lesion first.

B. Here the distal lesion was dilated first, then the proximal lesion. Note thrombotic occlusion of the popliteal artery.

C and D. Vessel now patent following suctioning of thrombus.

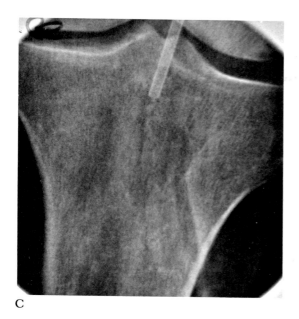

C

rectly into a vascular area recently traumatized by a balloon dilation to avoid damage to the arterial walls.

The angiogram provides precise information regarding the angioplasty procedure and determines whether complications have occurred. If angioplasty is successful, there is an increase in the caliber of the stenotic lesion, improved peripheral flow, and absent or decreased pressure gradients across the lesion.

HEPARIN. If the PTA involved an area of occlusion or multiple diffuse long areas of stenosis, heparin should be given in the form of an intravenous drip (15,000 IU qd) [33]. Otherwise, heparin may be discontinued after the procedure. Antiplatelet therapy should be continued post-PTA.

Clinical improvement is reflected by an improvement in the patient's symptoms of ischemia and is documented by an increase in the Doppler ankle-arm systolic pressure index and pulse volume recordings.

Results

The result of angioplasty in the lower extremity [16, 28, 36, 59, 60, 69, 70] depends on the stage of the disease. In experienced hands, patients with intermittent claudication (Fontaine stage II) due to superficial femoral artery stenosis may enjoy an initial success rate of 90 percent and a 3-year patency rate of 80 percent. Almost as good results

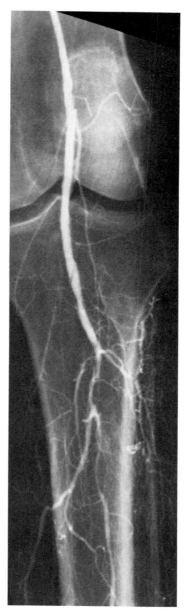

D

may be expected in those with superficial femoral artery occlusions less than 10 cm in length. This success rate drops to 60 percent or less initial patency when longer occlusions are dilated, with two-thirds or less of these stenoses remaining open at 3 years. There is less success in patients with rest pain and gangrenous changes (Fontaine stages III and IV).

In patients with lesions in the *popliteal artery*, an initial success rate of 80 to 90 percent for steno-

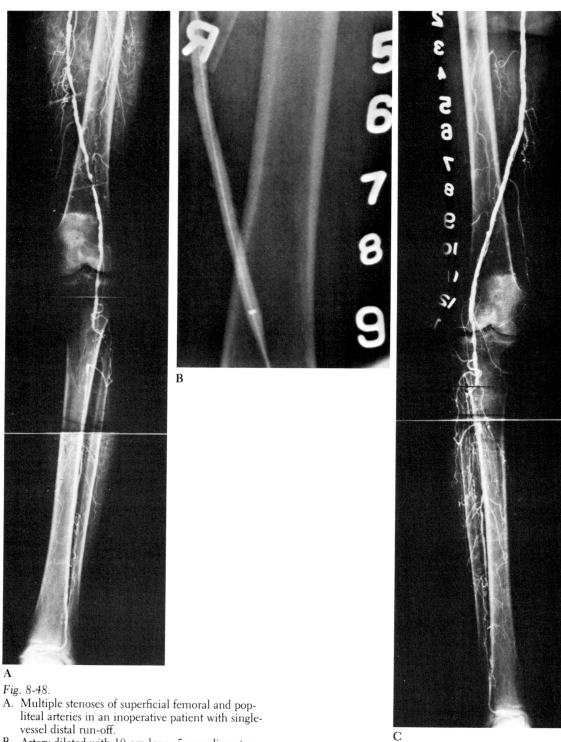

A

Fig. 8-48.

A. Multiple stenoses of superficial femoral and popliteal arteries in an inoperative patient with single-
   vessel distal run-off.

B. Artery dilated with 10-cm long, 5-mm diameter
   balloon.

C. Improved flow to the lower leg following PTA.

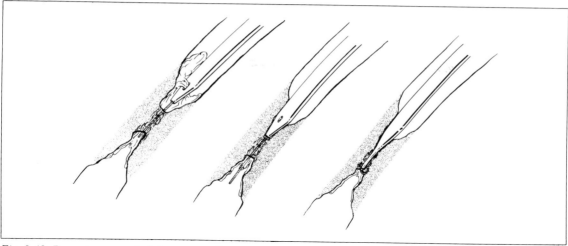

Fig. 8-49. Bypassing an occluded segment. (See text.)

sis, and 70 to 75 percent for short occlusions can be achieved. Two-year follow-ups show patency of 70 to 75% for stenoses and 60 to 70 percent for occlusions.

Vessels below the trifurcation are approached cautiously, in the hope of improving limb salvage. Amputation was avoided in one series in approximately 70 percent [43].

Complications

Complications during PTA of the extremities occur in 3 to 5 percent of patients and are as de-

Fig. 8-50. Problems bypassing an occluded segment.
A. Heavy calcification.
B. Catheter-guidewire combination enters a tributary.
C. Artery is perforated.

scribed in Chapter 6. They include thrombosis at the angioplasty site, distal embolization, perforation of the vessel, occasionally rupture of the artery, and significant hematomas at the puncture site.

PTA of the Upper Extremities

Atherosclerosis is frequently found in the subclavian arteries, both proximal and distal to the origin of the vertebral artery. Significant occlusive disease of the axillary or brachial artery from this disease, however, is rare. When present, and symptomatic, focal lesions may be treated by PTA using the same principles applied elsewhere, as may arterial lesions of other etiology. A femoral artery approach is most often used.

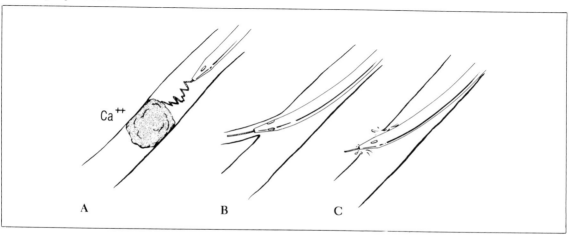

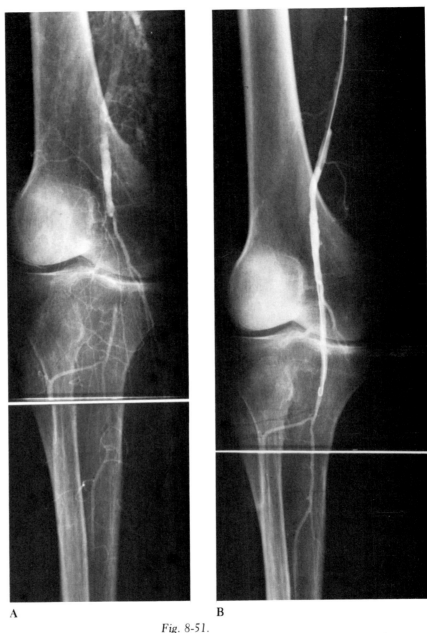

A   B

Fig. 8-51.
A and B. PTA-occluded popliteal artery. Guidewire remains distal to the occluded segment but proximal to the trifurcation during the post-PTA contrast medium injection in B.

PTA IN OCCLUSIVE COMPLICATIONS OF SURGICAL ARTERIOVENOUS DIALYSIS ACCESS FISTULAS [22, 34]. Stenoses on the venous side and immediately adjacent to the anastomoses are usually due to intimal hyperplasia and perivascular fibrosis. They are often resistant to dilation, and sometimes require balloon diameters 2 or more times greater than that of the adjacent normal vein. Dilations that are prolonged (up to 1 minute), multiple (up to 8 or 10), and use reinforced high-pressure balloons (up to 10 atm pressure) may successfully dilate these lesions in some patients. Only stenoses shorter than 4 cm should be attempted (see Fig. 8-35). Lesions more remote from the anastomotic site are more easily dilated. Stenoses underlying a thrombosed fistula may be uncovered by prior intravascular thrombolytic therapy.

TECHNIQUE. A 5 French catheter is introduced percutaneously, preferably into the vein just distal to the narrowed segment. It may be introduced directly into the graft, upstream from the area of stenosis. The lesion is first crossed with a probing 15-mm J-shaped guidewire, followed by the 5 French catheter and subsequently the balloon catheter. The balloon is dilated immediately after administering 5000 IU of heparin. In order to relieve accompanying pain, xylocaine 1% should be introduced into the tissues surrounding the areas of dilatation. Up to 70 percent of these grafts may be initially dilated, although long-term patency rates are not high (33 percent at 3 years).

THROMBOLYTIC THERAPY IN THE EXTREMITIES

Thrombolytic therapy is covered in Chapter 7. It is useful to treat patients with spontaneously occurring thromboemboli of the extremities (Figs. 8-52 and 8-53) by thrombolysis. It is particularly helpful in those with thrombosed surgical grafts, where it may uncover an underlying stenosis that can be corrected by transluminal angioplasty or surgery (Fig. 8-54). Infected grafts do not respond well and must be treated surgically (Fig. 8-55). It can be curative in those with thrombi subsequent to an angiographic or intravascular therapeutic maneuver. Although best results are obtained with clots of less than 72 hours' duration (up to 90 percent success rates in postprocedural cases), chronic occlusions of 3 months' to several years' duration may show response [55]. Thrombolytic therapy may be used in those with accelerating claudication and rest pain, but should be avoided if impending tissue death supervenes; here emergency surgery is necessary.

Acute embolism to the upper extremities may be successfully lysed [65]. If streptokinase is used, a high loading dose of 100,000 IU or more is introduced into the brachial artery, proximal to the point of occlusion, over a period of 30 minutes, followed by a low dose of 5000 IU per hour for a number of hours. Figure 8-54 demonstrates suc-

cessful thrombolysis of the arteries of the right upper extremity with intraarterial urokinase. There was partial lysis after the first 4 hours of treatment (500,000 IU), which prompted continued treatment over the next 48 hours (see Chap. 7 for details).

THERAPEUTIC INTRAVASCULAR EMBOLIZATION

Therapeutic embolization of the extremities should be performed only if there is close consultation with an attending vascular surgeon. Indications include angiodysplasias, complications of trauma (bleeding, arteriovenous fistulas, false aneurysms, avulsed vessels), and occasionally peripheral tumors.

Angiodysplasias

Factors determining the therapeutic approach to angiodysplasias include [48]:

1. The nature and size of the lesion:
   a. Arteriovenous malformations (AVMs) fed by large tortuous arteries and rapidly draining veins are often symptomatic, disfiguring, or complicated by ulceration, hemorrhage, or an increased cardiac output.
   b. Small-vessel malformations of the capillary venous level.
   c. Venous malformations.
2. The location of the lesion (proximal or peripheral) and whether it is local or diffuse in nature.

Avoid intervention in those with small asymptomatic uncomplicated lesions.

Large, symptomatic, or complicated AVMs located in the proximal portion of the limb usually require a combination of embolization followed shortly thereafter by surgical excision (see Fig. 8-22). Surgery alone, with ligation of major feeding vessels and partial excision, is not curative. Embolization alone can be equally unrewarding. With time, residual vascular abnormalities grow at the small-vessel level despite an apparent total ablation of the lesion.

Larger AVMs in the periphery of the extremities are usually symptomatic, develop complications, and are difficult to manage. Again, surgical ligation or excision alone is rarely curative. These lesions are best treated palliatively by repetitive in-

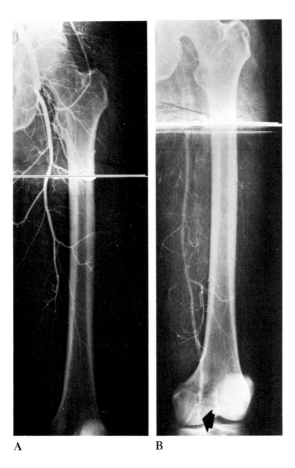

A   B

travascular embolizations performed sequentially in small steps to avoid ischemic complications and necrosis. The emboli are lodged as peripherally as possible to conserve more proximal vessels for future embolization.

Capillary venous malformations that break down and bleed may be treated by either intraarterial or direct injection of sclerosing materials (absolute alcohol, if not in the vicinity of major nerves, or isobutyl cyanoacrylate).

TECHNIQUE. Prior to intervention, the limb must be thoroughly evaluated with arteriography and sometimes with venography or lymphography and computed tomography scanning. The embolic material should be nonresorbable and should penetrate deeply into the malformation to ensure its complete ablation. These include:

Fig. 8-52. Thrombolytic therapy of acute embolic occlusion.
A. Superficial artery.
B. Popliteal artery. Delayed flow through a peripherally patent superficial femoral and proximal popliteal artery.
C and D. Infusion of urokinase through coaxial system. Thin-walled 5 French catheter in left common femoral artery and injectable guidewire in popliteal artery (*arrows*).
E. After 48 hours of treatment, pulses returned and two-vessel patency distal to the trifurcation was seen. No underlying stenosis was uncovered.

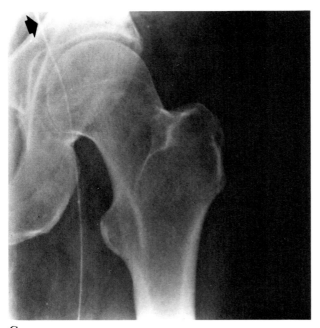

C

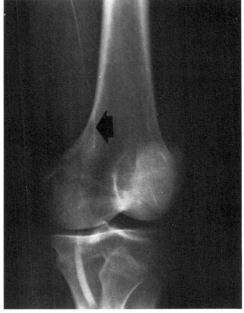

D

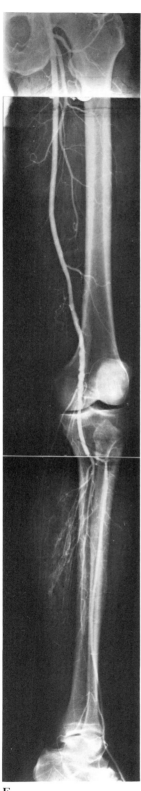

E

1. Liquid or semiliquid material (absolute alcohol, isobutyl cyanoacrylate, or silicone rubber [if available]).
2. Small Ivalon particles, either alone or mixed in a Gelfoam slurry.
3. Liquid materials may be combined with particulate emboli.
4. Coils can be introduced to act as a ligature, in order to protect a neighboring vascular bed as emboli are diverted to the AVM. They can be injected at the end of the procedure to prevent reflux of emboli into nontarget areas.

The delivery system depends on the size and location of the target vessels and the embolic material chosen to do the job. Small peripheral lesions, and use of liquid emboli require coaxial catheter systems; the open-ended injectable guidewire is particularly helpful under these circumstances. The Berenstein 7 French catheter with 5 French distal 10 cm has excellent torque control and accepts a 3 French coaxial catheter, through which liquids and microcoils can be inserted. Occlusive balloon catheters may help divert the flow of emboli to proper channels and prevent their reflux from others.

All these systems should be introduced through an appropriate size sheath, sutured firmly at the puncture site. Intraarterial heparin (low dose) during the study (when not contraindicated) and measures to prevent arterial spasm should be undertaken.

THE APPROACH. The approach depends on the site of the lesion. An ipsilateral anterograde femoral approach is used for peripheral lesions of the lower extremities; a retrograde contralateral approach for proximal femoral, profunda, or combination iliac and proximal femoral lesions; a femoral approach for lesions of the proximal upper extremity; an anterograde brachial or selective radial or ulnar approach for more peripheral lesions. Review Chapter 5 for details of technique.

Embolization in Trauma
Embolization can control bleeding from lacerated or avulsed arteries by occluding vessels either temporarily or permanently [5, 15]. Patients may be stabilized for subsequent surgery. False aneurysms and arteriovenous fistulas may be permanently occluded.

PRECAUTIONS. Rapid, firm decisions and easily

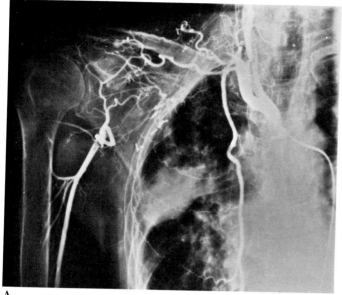

A

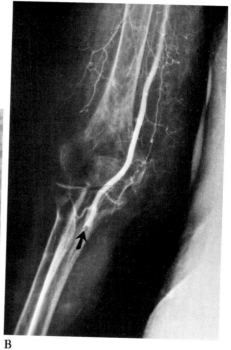

B

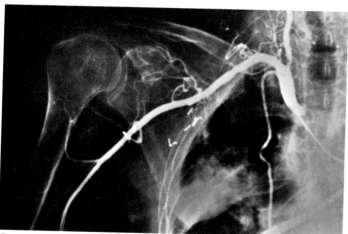

C

Fig. 8-53.

A and B. Acute embolism of right subclavian artery
and right brachial artery.

C. After 12 hours of intraarterial urokinase infusion,
right subclavian artery was patent.

D. After 36 hours of urokinase infusion, branches to
the forearm were opening. Pulses and color returned to the hand.

available and deliverable occlusive devices are
needed in acutely bleeding patients with critical
needs. The fear of ischemia to healthy areas precludes permanently occluding major vessels such
as the superficial femoral, popliteal, tibial, or brachial arteries (temporary occlusion with nondetachable occlusive balloons may be life-saving).

Less critical branches such as the hypogastric,
profunda femoris, geniculate, or subscapular
branches may be safely occluded. Similarly, arteriovenous fistulas and false aneurysms involving
vessels other than the main channels supplying the
extremities may be permanently embolized.

EMBOLIC MATERIALS

1. Gelfoam—easy to obtain and to deliver.
2. Ivalon particles or Gelfoam-Ivalon mixtures—
   provide permanent occlusion.
3. Isobutyl cyanoacrylate (tissue adhesive)—
   provides permanent occlusion but requires a
   more complicated delivery system under emergency circumstances.

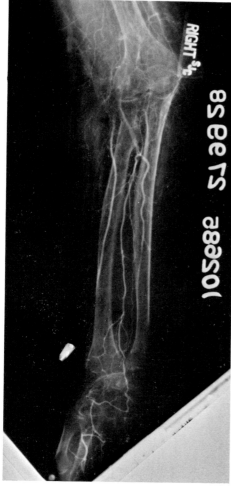

D

4. Coils—for larger, lacerated arteries. They may also act as ligatures, to divert flow of smaller emboli away from otherwise critical, uninvolved areas.
5. Detachable balloons (or coils)—for occluding fistulas or large false aneurysms.
6. Occlusive balloon catheters—for temporary life-saving occlusion of major vessels.

Musculoskeletal Tumors

Musculoskeletal tumors can be embolized. The resulting vessel obliteration and tumor infarction provide a relatively bloodless field for local surgical excision of the tumor and, in some instances, slow the progression of and even shrink the size of the lesion over a period of time, making an originally unresectable lesion easier to remove. Emboliza-

tion has been used as the primary method of treatment when surgical resection would result in unacceptable loss of limb or severe disfigurement. Embolization of bone tumors can decrease the pain related to the stretching of periosteum by the tumor mass. Both benign primary (giant cell tumor and aneurysmal bone cyst) and malignant primary and secondary bone tumors have been embolized [24, 37, 67] using a variety of liquid and particulate embolic materials.

Complications from Embolization of Extremity Lesions

Necrosis of healthy tissues adjoining the lesions and peripheral embolization to nontarget areas can be avoided by selective placement of the catheter. Do not embolize if there is risk of damaging neighboring healthy areas. Peripheral nerve damage can occur if embolizing materials such as alcohol penetrate through to the vaso nervosum of major nerves (this apparently does not occur when isobutyl cyanoacrylate is used, because the rapid polymerization of this liquid occurs before it reaches the precapillary areas of the nerves [49]).

Self-limiting pain usually is present for 1 or 2 days following the embolization. It can be controlled with narcotics.

INTRAVASCULAR CHEMOTHERAPY

Malignant neoplasms can be subjected to higher concentrations of chemotherapeutic agents without increasing toxicity by administering them selectively to the feeding vessels through an indwelling arterial catheter. The catheter may be left in place for several hours to several days. Special care must be instituted to prevent thrombosis surrounding the catheter. Systemic heparinization and antiplatelet therapy should be used. The chemotherapeutic agents used include cisplatinum, methotrexate, Adriamycin, actinomycin D, among others [12, 67] (Fig. 8-56).

INTRAVASCULAR VASODILATORS

Patients with vascular diseases with a significant vasospastic component, such as seen in patients with Raynaud's syndrome or Raynaud's disease, may obtain temporary relief from the intraarterial injection of reserpine into the involved vascular bed. One milligram of the medication is given, shortly after the diagnostic arteriogram and before removal of the catheter.

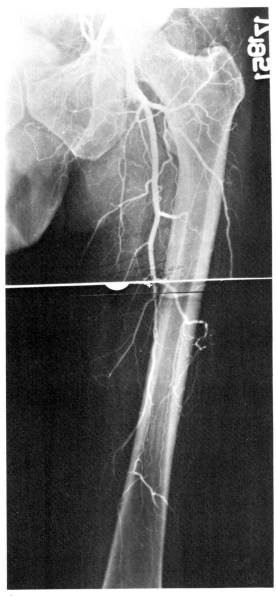

A

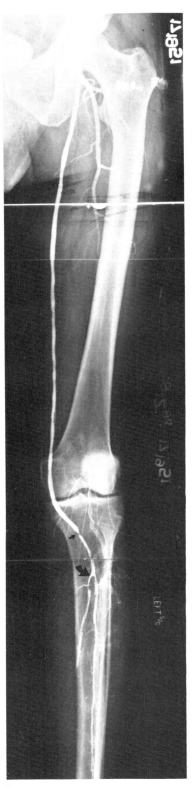

B

Fig. 8-54.

A. Acute thrombosis of femoral popliteal bypass graft.

B. After 22 hours of intraarterial streptokinase, proximal vessels were widely patent except for severe stenosis of distal anastomosis (*arrow*). There is still clot below the trifurcation (*broad arrow*).

C. At 36 hours, most of the distal clots have disappeared.

D. After PTA of distal anastomosis.

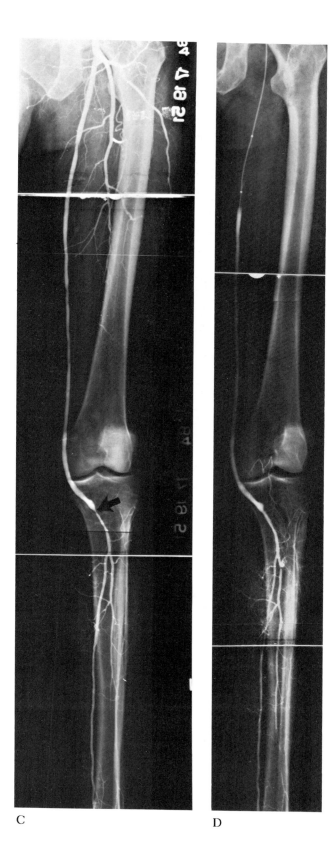

C

D

208

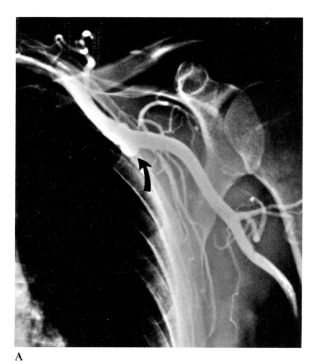

A

Fig. 8-55.
A. Occluded left axillobifemoral graft.
B and C. Limbs of the graft are patent after intraarterial streptokinase. Graft was infected and reocclusion occurred.

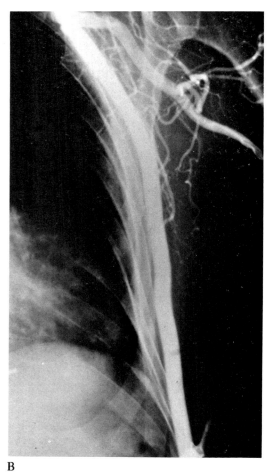

B

C

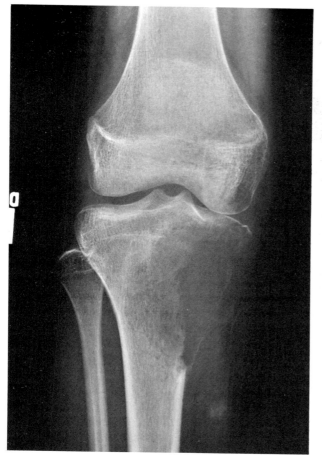

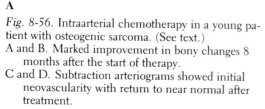

A

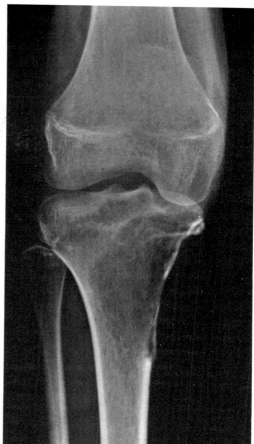

B

Fig. 8-56. Intraarterial chemotherapy in a young patient with osteogenic sarcoma. (See text.)

A and B. Marked improvement in bony changes 8
    months after the start of therapy.

C and D. Subtraction arteriograms showed initial
    neovascularity with return to near normal after
    treatment.

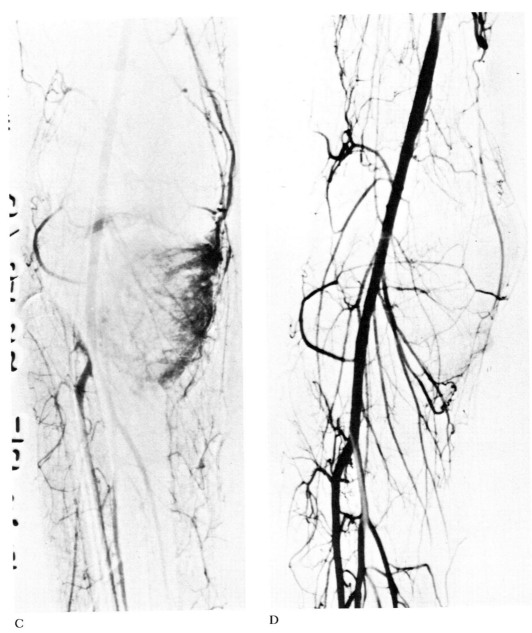

C

D

Fig. 8-56 (continued)

References

1. Agee, O. Arteriography of the pelvis and lower extremities with moving table top technique. *Am. J. Roentgenol.* 106:400, 1969.
2. Bardsley, J., et al. Pseudoxanthoma elasticum: Angiographic manifestations in abdominal vessels. *Radiology* 93:559, 1969.
3. Barth, K. H. A modified catheter for transluminal angioplasty of the femoral popliteal artery. *Radiology* 149:598, 1983.
4. Benedict, K., Change, W., and McCready, F. The hypothenar hammer syndrome. *Radiology* 111:57, 1974.
5. Ben-Menachem, Y. *Angiography and trauma.* Philadelphia: Saunders, 1981.
6. Bernstein, E. F. (ed.). *Noninvasive Diagnostic Techniques in Vascular Disease.* St. Louis: Mosby, 1978.
7. Bliznack, J., and Staple, T. Radiology of angiodysplasias of the limb. *Radiology* 110:35, 1974.
8. Brockman, S., and Vasko, J. Phlegmasia cerulea dolens: Collective review. *Surg. Gynecol. Obstet.* 121:1347, 1965.
9. Bunker, S. R., Lauten, G. J., and Hutton, J. E., Jr. Cystic adventitial disease of the popliteal artery. *A.J.R.* 136:1209, 1981.
10. Calenoff, L. Angiography of the hand: Guidelines for interpretation. *Radiology* 102:331, 1972.
11. Chait, A. Collateral arterial circulation in the pelvis. *Am. J. Roentgenol.* 2:392, 1968.
12. Chuang, V. P., et al. Multimodal approach to osteosarcoma. Emphasis on intraarterial cisdiamine chloroplatinum II and limb preservation. Presented at the Society of Cardiovascular Interventional Radiology, 1985.
13. Coleman, S. S., and Anson, B. J. Arterial patterns in the hand based upon a study of 650 specimens. *Surg. Gynecol. Obstet.* 113:409, 1961.
14. Darling, R. C., et al. Quantitative pulsed volume recorder: A clinical tool. *Surgery* 72:873, 1972.
15. Dedrick, C. G., and Athanasoulis, C. A. Localization and control of osteoarticular hemorrhage. In R. A. Wilkins and M. Viamonte, Jr. (eds.), *Interventional Radiology.* Oxford: Blackwell Scientific, 1982.
16. Dotter, C. T., et al. (eds.). Percutaneous transluminal angioplasty. Technique, early and late results. Berlin: Springer-Verlag, 1983.
17. D'Souza, V., et al. Peripheral angiography: Enhancement by longleg pneumatic boots. *Radiology,* 120:209, 1976.
18. Eastcott, H. G. *Arterial Surgery* (2nd ed.). Philadelphia: Lippincott, 1973. Chapter 3.
19. Fagerberg, S., Jorulf, H., and Sandberg, C. Ergotism: Arterial spastic disease and recovery, studied angiographically. *Acta Med. Scand.* 182(FASC6): 769, 1967.
20. Fallon, J. T. Pathology of arterial lesions amenable to percutaneous transluminal angioplasty. *A.J.R.* 135:913, 1980.
21. Fontaine, R., et al. Long-term results of restorative arterial surgery in obstructive disease of the arteries. *J. Cardiovascular. Surg.* (Torino) 5:463, 1964.
22. Glanzs, G. D., et al. Dialysis access fistulas: Treatment of stenoses by transluminal angioplasty. *Radiology* 152:637, 1984.
23. Golding, S. J., and Husband, J. E. The role of computed tomography and the management of soft tissue tumors. *J. Radiol.* 55:740, 1982.
24. Goldman, M., et al. Transcatheter embolization with bucrylate (in 100 patients). *Radiographics,* 2(3):340, 1982.
25. Gothlin, J., and Linstedt, E. Angiographic features of Ciminobrescia fistulas. *Am. J. Roentgenol.* 125:582, 1975.
26. Greenfield, A. J. Femoral, popliteal and tibial arteries: Percutaneous transluminal angioplasty. *A.J.R.* 135:927, 1980.
27. Grollman, J., Lecky, J., and Rosch, J. Miscellaneous diseases of arteries; or, all arterial lesions aren't fatty. *Semin. Roentgenol.* 5:306, 1970.
28. Gruntzig, A., and Zeitler, E. Cooperative study of results of PTA in 12 different clinics. In E. Zeitler, A. Gruntzig, and W. Schoop (eds.), *Percutaneous Vascular Reconstruction.* Berlin: Springer-Verlag, 1978. Pp. 118–119.
29. Guthaner, D. F., et al. Evaluation of peripheral vascular disease using digital subtraction angiography. *Radiology* 147:393, 1983.
30. Hagen, B., and Lohse, S. Clinical and radiologic aspects of Buerger's disease. *Cardiovasc. Intervent. Radiol.* 7:283, 1984.
31. Haimovichi, H. Patterns of arteriosclerotic lesions of the lower extremities. *Arch. Surg.* 95:918, 1967.
32. Hauser, W., et al. Temporal arteritis in Rochester, Minn., 1951–1957. *Mayo Clin. Proc.* 46:597, 1971.
33. Horvath, L. Percutaneous transluminal angioplasty: Importance of anticoagulant and fibrinolytic drugs. *A.J.R.* 135:951, 1980.
34. Hunter, D., et al. Failing arterial venous dialysis fistulas: Evaluation and treatment. *Radiology* 152:631, 1984.
35. Juergens, J., and Bernatz, P. Arteriosclerosis Obliterans. In E. V. Allen, N. W. Barker, and E. A. Hines (eds.), *Peripheral Vascular Disease* (4th ed.). Philadelphia: Saunders, 1972.
36. Katzen, B. T. Percutaneous transluminal angioplasty for arterial disease of the lower extremities. *A.J.R.* 142:20, 1984.
37. Keller, F., Rosch, J., and Bird, C. Percutaneous embolization of bony pelvic neoplasms with soft tissue adhesive. *Radiology* 147:21, 1983.
37A. Kemerer, V. et al. Successful treatment of ergotism with nifedipine. *A.J.R.* 143:333, 1984.
38. Lande, A., and Berkmen, Y. Aortitis: Pathologic, clinical and arteriographic review. *Radiol. Clin. North Am.* 142:219, 1976.
39. Lang, E. Arteriography of the thoracic outlet syndrome. In H. Abrams (ed.), *Abrams' Angiography: Vascular and Interventional Radiology* (3rd ed.). Boston: Little, Brown, 1983. P. 1001.

40. Levine, E., et al. Comparison of computed tomography and other imaging modalities in the evaluation of musculoskeletal tumors. *Radiology* 131:431, 1979.

41. Lindberg, R. D., et al. Conservative surgery and postoperative radiotherapy in 300 adults with soft tissue sarcomas. *Cancer* 47:2391, 1981.

42. Lois, J. F., et al. Angiography in soft tissue sarcomas. *Cardiovasc. Intervent. Radiol.* 7:309, 1984.

43. Lu, C. T., et al. Percutaneous transluminal angioplasty for limb salvage. *Radiology* 142:337, 1982.

44. Main, R., and Costin, B. Catheter angiography through aortofemoral grafts: Prevention of catheter separation during withdrawal. *Am. J. Roentgenol.* 128:328, 1977.

45. Malan, E., and Puglionisi, A. Congenital angiodysplasias of the extremities. *J. Cardiovasc. Surg.* 5:87, 1964.

46. McDonald, E., Goodman, P., and Winestock, D. Clinical indications for arteriography and trauma to the extremity: A review of 114 cases. *Radiology* 116:45, 1975.

47. McKusick, V., et al. Buerger's disease: A distinct clinical and pathologic entity. *J.A.M.A.* 181:93, 1962.

48. Merland, J. J., Riche, M. C., and Melki, J. P. Selective arteriography and embolization in vascular malformations of the limbs. In R. A. Wilkins and M. Viamonte, Jr. (eds.), *Interventional Radiology*. Oxford: Blackwell Scientific, 1982.

49. Miller, F. J., and Mineaud, E. Transcatheter arterial embolization. Complications and their preventions. *Cardiovasc. Intervent. Radiol.* 6:141, 149, 1983.

50. Motarjeme, A., et al. Percutaneous transluminal angioplasty and case selection. *Radiology* 135:573, 1980.

51. Müller, N., et al. Popliteal artery entrapment demonstrated by CT. *Radiology* 151:157, 1984.

52. Palubinskas, A., and Ripley, H. Fibromuscular hyperplasia in extrarenal arteries. *Radiology* 82:451, 1964.

53. Park, J., Han, M. C., and Bettman, M. A. Arterial manifestations of Behcet's disease. *A.J.R.* 143:821, 1984.

54. Raines, J. K., et al. Vascular lab criteria for management of peripheral vascular disease of the extremities. *Surgery* 79:21, 1976.

55. Risius, G., et al. Catheter directed low dose streptokinase infusion: A preliminary experience. *Radiology* 150:349, 1984.

56. Rossi, P., et al. Iatrogenic arteriovenous fistulas. *Radiology* 111:47, 1974.

57. Rutherford, R. B., Lowenstein, D. H., and Klein, M. F. Combining segmental systolic pressures and plethysmography to diagnose arterial occlusive disease of the legs. *Am. J. Surg.* 138:211, 1979.

58. Schwarten, D. E. Percutaneous transluminal angioplasty of the iliac arteries: Intravenous digital subtraction angiography for follow-up. *Radiology* 15:363, 1984.

59. Sniderman, K. W., and Sos, T. A. The popliteal artery and its branches. In W. Castaneda-Zuniga (ed.), *Transluminal Angioplasty*. New York: Thieme-Stratton, 1983. Pp. 118–127.

60. Sos, T. A., Sniderman, K. W. Percutaneous transluminal angioplasty. *Semin. Roentgenol.* 130:617, 1979.

61. Spitell, J. Raynaud's phenomenon and allied vasospastic conditions. In E. V. Allen, N. W. Barker, and E. A. Hines (eds.), *Peripheral Vascular Disease* (4th ed.). Philadelphia: Saunders, 1972. P. 387.

62. Stanley, J., et al. Arterial fibrodysplasia: Histologic character and etiologic concepts. *Arch. Surg.* 110:561, 1975.

63. Stemerman, M. B. Atherosclerosis: The etiologic role of the blood elements and cellular changes. *Cardiovasc. Med.* 3:17, 1978.

64. Thompson, W., et al. Late complications of abdominal aortic reconstructive surgery: Roentgen evaluation. *Ann. Surg.* 185:326, 1977.

65. Tisnado, J., et al. Low dose fibrinolytic therapy in hand ischemia. *Radiology* 150:375, 1984.

66. Voegeli, E., and Uehlinger, E. Arteriography in bone tumors. *Skeletal Radiol.* 1:14, 1976.

67. Wallace, S., and Chuang, V. P. Transcatheter management of musculoskeletal neoplasms. In R. A. Wilkins and M. Viamonte, Jr. (eds.), *Interventional Radiology*. Oxford: Blackwell Scientific, 1982. Pp. 225–238.

68. Weintraub, R., and Abrams, H. Mycotic aneurysms. *Am. J. Roentgenol.* 102:354, 1968.

69. Zeitler, E., Richter, E., Seyferth, W. Primary results. Leg arteries. In C. Dotter et al. (eds.), *Percutaneous Transluminal Angioplasty. Technique, Early and Late Results*. Berlin: Springer-Verlag, 1983.

70. Zeitler, E., et al. Results of percutaneous transluminal angioplasty. *Radiology* 146:57, 1983.

9

Arteriography
and Intervention
of the Pelvis

Indications

1. Primary vascular diseases of the pelvic vessels (e.g., occlusions, stenosis, aneurysms, trauma, congenital and acquired arteriovenous malformations [see Chapter 8], vasculogenic impotence)
2. Tumors
   a. Gynecologic tumors: benign and malignant tumors of the uterus and adnexa (particularly choriocarcinoma). Angiography is infrequently required because clinical evaluation and imaging methods are usually accurate.
   b. Occasionally, lower urinary tract tumors (urologic and urographic procedures largely take precedence here)
   c. Primary bone and soft tissue tumors
3. Interventional angiography
   a. Angioplasty of stenotic iliac vessels: thrombolysis of occluded pelvic vessels
   b. Selective hypogastric artery catheter placement for embolic occlusion of bleeding vessels, arteriovenous malformations, and tumors
   c. Selective catheter placement for chemotherapy of malignant lesions

Techniques

APPROACHES

1. Percutaneous femoral artery (Fig. 9-1). For selective hypogastric artery catheterization, the femoral artery ipsilateral to the lesion may be used (Fig. 9-1A, B). The same approach is available for contralateral iliac artery (common, internal, external) catheterization by feeding the catheter over the bifurcation of the aorta (Fig. 9-1C, D, E, F).
2. Percutaneous left axillary artery. This approach should be used if the femoral artery is unavailable as a result of occlusive disease. A gentle curve on the distal catheter tip allows selective common, internal, and external iliac artery placement.
3. Translumbar. This approach should be used only when there are bilaterally dampened femoral pulses, when selective aortic branch catheterization is not anticipated, and when there are no contraindications to its use. Contraindications include blood dyscrasias, severe hypertension, aortic insufficiency, aneurysms, dissections, and interposed grafts in the proposed site of the puncture. The reader should review Chapter 3 regarding technique of performance.

CATHETERS

1. A 5 French 65-cm straight or pigtail catheter with side holes should be used for midstream aortic bifurcation injections (Fig. 9-1G). The catheter should be introduced over an 0.035-inch (0.89 mm) or 0.038-inch (0.97 mm) 145-cm guidewire with a flexible, curved tip.
2. A 4 or 5 French 50- to 65-cm polyethylene catheter with a small shepherd's crook, Simmons curve, or an exaggerated cobra curve should be used for selective catheterization of the ipsilateral hypogastric artery (Fig. 9-1).

   A catheter with a cobra-head curve, one with a 45-degree-angle primary curve that is 2 cm proximal to the tip, or one with a Simmons curve may be fed over the aortic bifurcation to engage the opposite iliac vessels (Fig. 9-1D, E, F). This catheter should be fed over an 0.035- or 0.038-inch (0.89 or 0.97 mm) 145-cm guidewire with a flexible, curved tip. The guidewire may be advanced down the opposite iliac artery by opening the pigtail catheter curve across the bifurcation. Once the stiff portion of the guidewire is across the bifurcation, it prevents the catheter from flipping back over the bifurcation (Fig. 9-1C). In difficult cases the guidewire can be fixed by compression of the contralateral femoral artery (Fig. 9-1F). Stiffer-core Coons guidewires, Lunderquist or heavy-duty Amplatz guidewires with a pre-

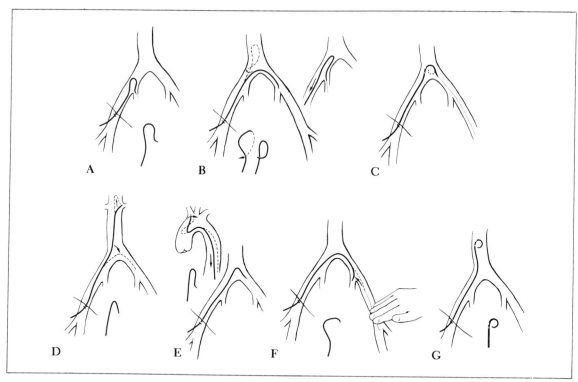

Fig. 9-1. Approaches for pelvic arteriography.

A. Selective internal iliac catheterization ipsilateral to the side of puncture.

B. Selective internal iliac catheterization ipsilateral to the site of puncture using exaggerated cobra-curve manipulation.

C. Pigtail catheter helps to direct the guidewire down the opposite iliac artery.

D. Acutely angled catheter. A curve is formed in a branch of the aorta (e.g., the renal artery) and the catheter withdrawn caudad to hang over the bifurcation.

E. Simmons catheter advanced to the aortic arch where the curve is formed. The catheter is withdrawn to hang over the bifurcation.

F. Selective catheterization of the internal iliac artery contralateral to the side of puncture. A cobra-head catheter is positioned over the aortic bifurcation and the guidewire advanced to the opposite common femoral artery and manually fixed. The catheter is threaded over the guidewire, the guidewire is then removed, and the catheter retracted to the orifice of the internal iliac.

G. Pigtail catheter at aortic bifurcation. All side holes must be above the bifurcation.

formed curve to match the angle of the aortic bifurcation (see Fig. 9-5), and variable stiffness wires with an external manipulator (Cook) can be used to prevent buckling of a catheter as it crosses the bifurcation.

CONTRAST AGENTS, PROJECTIONS, AND RADIOGRAPHIC PROGRAMMING

Details concerning contrast agents, projections, and radiographic programs in arteriography of the pelvis are given in Table 9-1.

DIGITAL SUBTRACTION ANGIOGRAPHY

1. Intravenous digital subtraction angiography (IV-DSA) is useful for outlining pelvic vessels, particularly when dampened or absent pulses require planning for more conventional angiographic procedures, surgery, or for percutaneous transluminal angioplastic intervention. In addition to primary angiographic screening for suspected or known peripheral vascular disease, IV-DSA can be used to evaluate the results of therapeutic maneuvers.

The advantages of IV-DSA include (1) a less invasive procedure than intraarterial angiogra-

Table 9-1. Technical specifications in conventional arteriography of the pelvis. [a]

Arteriographic procedure	Contrast agent			Total films	Total time (sec)	Radiographic program		Projections
	Density	Volume (ml/inj)	Rate (ml/sec)			Films/sec	Timing	
Adult								
Aortic bifurcation	L	40–50	12	14	15	2/sec for 4 sec; 1/sec for 2 sec; 1 every 2 sec for 8 sec	Start 1 sec after start of injection	AP and both obliques RPO: right iliac bifurcation LPO: left iliac bifurcation
Selective catheterization								
Common iliac artery	L	24	8	12	12	2/sec for 3 sec; 1/sec for 3 sec; 1 every 2 sec for 6 sec	Start 0.5 sec after start of injection	
Hypogastric artery	L(NI)	30	4–5	20	30	1/sec for 10 sec; 1 every 2 sec for 20 sec	Start at the start of injection	RPO: left internal iliac; LPO: right internal iliac
Child [b]								
Aortic bifurcation Infant	L	1 ml/kg to maximum of adult dose	Total within 1–1½ sec	14	8	3/sec for 2 sec; 2/sec for 2 sec; 1/sec for 4 sec	Start 0.5 sec after start of injection	

[a] For IA-DSA studies, use half concentration of contrast agent but the same volume and injection rates.
[b] Amount of contrast agent varies with body weight in children.
Note: M = medium density contrast agent; L = low density contrast agent; NI = nonionic contrast agent (this is less painful) (see Appendix 3).

phy, (2) improved patient tolerance, (3) outpatient capabilities, and (4) less cost. There are certain limitations. Patients must be able to cooperate and have adequate cardiac output and good renal function. Smaller field size imposed by the size of the image intensifier requires multiple injections of high-concentration contrast agent. Usually four injections (40–50 ml of 370–400 mg iodine/ml injected into the vena cava or right atrium at a rate of 20 to 25 ml/second) are necessary to show the distal abdominal aorta, pelvic vessels, and reconstitution of obstructed pelvic and proximal femoral vessels. Even more injections are required if peripheral extremity vessels must be seen. The largest field image intensifier mode and a movable tabletop, with accurate computerized, pre-programmed masking capabilities, helps to decrease the number of injections required. Intravenous glucagon (1 mg) immediately prior to the injection and extrinsic abdominal and pelvic compression during the injection, or performing the study with the patient prone decreases motion artifacts.

2. Easy performance, less contrast requirements, and real time display of contrast filled vessels make intraarterial digital subtraction angiography (IA-DSA) invaluable during diagnostic and intraarterial interventional studies in the pelvis. Lesions can be seen in multiple projections prior to the intervention and can be adequately evaluated to determine results following embolization or angioplasty. Reconstructed vessels peripheral to a point of obstruction may be difficult to see on conventional angiograms but are frequently outlined with IA-DSA using smaller doses of contrast agent.

"Road mapping" may be performed during interventional procedures using digital subtraction techniques. An arterial injection is made in the region of the lesion and displayed on the fluoroscopic screen. With the patient remaining immobile, the interventional catheter (therapeutic blockade, balloon angioplasty) is shown in an image that is reversed to that of the angiogram stored and seen on the screen. Thus, the position of the catheter and its relationship to the area of interest and surrounding branches can be accurately judged. By seeing the diameter of the vessel, expanding balloon diameters may be accurately assessed, precluding overexpansion and misplacement.

Anatomic Considerations

The anatomy of the pelvic arteries is shown in Figure 9-2 (see also Figs. 8-5 and 8-6). The common iliac artery bifurcates at a variable distance from the aortic bifurcation into the internal iliac artery (hypogastric artery) and the external iliac artery. The course of the latter vessel is a continuation of the common iliac artery. As the external iliac artery emerges from the pelvis, it becomes the common femoral artery.

The internal iliac artery on each side passes posteromedially into the true pelvis where it divides into two major divisions, the posterior division which supplies muscles of the buttocks, lower extremities, body wall and the posterior trunk of the body, and the anterior division which supplies the pelvic viscera and the perineum. There are a number of variations in the distribution of these vessels.

In the posterior division, the first muscular branch to arise is the iliolumbar branch, which forms important anastomoses with the lumbar branches of the aorta and the iliac circumflex branches of the common femoral artery. The superior gluteal artery has a large branch that is easy to recognize because it passes posterolaterally, perpendicular to the axis of the common and external iliac arteries. The superior gluteal artery passes through the greater sciatic notch and eventually anastomoses with the lateral femoral circumflex branch of the deep femoral artery. Other muscular branches from the posterior division are the superior and inferior lateral sacral branches. They anastomose with those on the opposite side of the pelvis and with the middle sacral artery. The latter arises from the aortic bifurcation and travels down the long axis of the sacrum. These branches form important collaterals in obstructive disease of the internal iliac or common iliac arteries. Although the inferior gluteal branch is usually a branch of the anterior division of the internal iliac artery, it can sometimes arise from the superior gluteal artery or directly from the internal iliac artery.

The anterior division of the internal iliac artery gives off the umbilical artery (in turn, the superior vesical branch), the uterine artery in the female, and the middle rectal artery (which anastomoses with the superior rectal branch of the inferior mes-

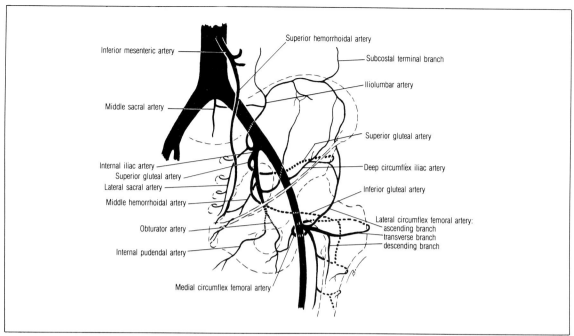

Fig. 9-2. Anatomy of the pelvic arteries and predominant anastomotic channels (see also Figs. 8-5 and 8-6).

enteric artery). The anterior division also gives off muscular branches. The inferior gluteal artery exits from the greater sciatic foramen, passes posteriorly and laterally, close to the posterior medial margin of the femoral head. The obturator artery frequently has anomalous points of origin and supplies the obturator internus as its branches pass through the obturator foramen. Both of the gluteal arteries and the obturator artery anastomose with the femoral circumflex branches of the profunda femoris artery.

The internal pudendal artery is the vessel supplying erectile tissue both in the female and in the male. There are pelvic, gluteal, ischiorectal, and perineal segments to this vessel. After giving off muscular, inferior rectal, urethral, and bulbar branches, the internal pudendal artery terminates (in the male) in the dorsal artery to the penis (which runs along the upper border of the penis to the glans) and the cavernosal or deep artery. An accessory internal pudendal artery may arise separately from the internal iliac artery. The entire course of the internal pudendal artery, in addition to the more proximal iliac vessels, must be studied and evaluated for vasculogenic impotence.

COLLATERALS

When the distal aorta and the iliac arteries are involved in occlusive disease, anastomotic vessels supplying the extremities take on added significance [2]. Segmental stenosis of some of the major branches feeding these collaterals may be improved either surgically or by transluminal angioplasty in order to enhance peripheral circulation. It is, therefore, important to define these branches angiographically, which sometimes requires multiple views. These branches include:

1. The internal iliac artery (hypogastric artery). This artery helps to bypass occlusions of
   a. the distal aorta and/or common iliac artery by lumbar, iliolumbar, lateral sacral, hemorrhoidal, and vesical arterial anastomoses
   b. the external iliac and femoral arteries, by anastomoses of the muscular branches with the deep circumflex iliac branch of the common femoral artery and the medial and lateral femoral circumflex branches of the deep femoral artery
2. The deep femoral artery (profunda femoris). This artery supplies the medial and lateral femoral circumflex branches, which form crucial anastomoses with branches of the hypogastric artery and the popliteal artery.

3. The inferior mesenteric artery. This artery, through its superior hemorrhoidal–middle hemorrhoidal anastomoses, bypasses aortic occlusion and common and internal iliac artery occlusion.

The angiographic findings in many primary vascular diseases involving the arteries of the pelvis are described in Chapter 8.

Vasculogenic Impotence

ARTERIAL CAUSES FOR IMPOTENCE

Arterial insufficiency to the penis is the most frequent cause of organic impotence [6, 13]. Doppler pressure measurements may provide the initial clue to the vascular occlusive disease. Vascular studies are required for anatomic definition.

TECHNIQUE OF ARTERIOGRAPHY

A urethral catheter keeps the bladder empty of overlying contrast agent. A midstream pelvic arteriogram is followed by selective internal iliac arteriograms. Posterior oblique projections during midstream injections open up the ipsilateral common iliac bifurcation (see Fig. 8-6). For selective studies, the side injected is obliqued anteriorly (Fig. 9-3). A water bag placed over the penis equalizes radiographic densities. Immediately prior to injection of contrast medium, inject 25 mg of tolazoline (Priscoline) or 100 to 200 μg of nitroglycerine to dilate the vessels. Because ionic contrast agent injections are painful, nonionic agents are preferable. They are injected at a rate of 4 to 5 ml/second for 8 to 10 seconds. In their absence, 30 to 40 ml of low-density (60%) ionic contrast agent (to which 2 mg of lidocaine per milliliter of contrast is added [0.4 ml of 20% lidocaine]). Twenty films are obtained at 1 per second (starting 4 seconds after an initial contrast-free film is obtained for a subsequent subtraction study) for 10 seconds, followed by one every other second for the remainder.

Although vasculogenic causes of impotence can be due to trauma (see Fig. 9-3), embolism, thrombosis, "steal" or diversion of blood from the internal pudendal artery (due to an arteriovenus malformation [AVM] or an AV fistula or some collateral supplying an adjacent ischemic area), the most frequent problem is occlusive disease due to atherosclerosis. Varying degrees of occlusion in the distal aorta or proximal common iliac vessels (Leriche's

syndrome) (see Chap. 8 and Fig. 9-4) or in proximal or distal branches of the internal pudendal artery (Fig. 9-5) can occur. Diabetics are more prone to this peripheral form of disease (Fig. 9-6).

Correction of proximal lesions (aorta, common or internal iliac arteries, or lesions providing a steal phenomenon) may help restore potency. Distal atherosclerosis is not, however, amenable to endarterectomy. Surgical revascularization techniques have been tried with some success.

VENOUS CAUSES FOR IMPOTENCE

There is another cause for impotence which is unrelated to the arterial inflow to the penis [20]. Under normal circumstances, with the penis flaccid, drainage from the erectile tissue of the corpora cavernosa is by veins draining along the length of the shaft of the penis to the dorsal vein of the penis. A greater number of veins, however, pass out through the root of the penis to empty directly into the prostatic plexus. During normal erection, the expanding walls of the corpora cavernosa mechanically obliterate the perforating venous branches draining the corpora cavernosa along its shaft, maintaining tumescence by trapping the blood within the nonexpansile fibrous tunica. The only venous drainage during a normal erection is by those veins at the root of the penis entering into the prostatic plexus.

In some patients, tumescence is not maintained due to inadequate closure of the veins along the shaft, a condition which can be corrected by surgical venous ligation. The condition can be detected by performing a corpora cavernosagram (Fig. 9-7). A single, 21-gauge butterfly needle is introduced into the distal half of either corpora cavernosa (the corpora communicate peripherally), which is then distended by rapidly injecting 50 to 100 ml or more of normal sterile saline. Penile turgidity can sometimes be better maintained by prior direct corporal injection of nitroglycerine 300 μg or 60 mg papaverine. Another combination of drugs providing a firm erection is 30 mg papaverine and 0.5 mg phentolamine (Regitine). These agents directly act on the draining veins and occlude them. When the penis is rigid, 25 to 50 ml of 60% Conray or preferably a nonionic contrast agent (300 mg iodine) is injected into the needle and a number of serial spot films are rapidly obtained at 2- to 3-second intervals.

Under normal circumstances the entire length

of the corpora cavernosa opacifies and drains through the prostatic plexus at the root of the penis. The glans also commonly opacifies, but there should be no drainage along the dorsal or ventral aspect of the penile shaft (Fig. 9-7A). If venous drainage is seen along the shaft, the veins are incompetent, preventing maintenance of tumescence, and require surgical correction (Fig. 9-7B).

Usually the erection subsides spontaneously after the injection, particularly if there is abnormal drainage. If not, a solution of 20 ml of normal saline containing 20 to 50 μg of epinephrine is flushed and then withdrawn through the needle in the corpora cavernosa inducing flaccidity.

Interventional Procedures

PERCUTANEOUS TRANSLUMINAL ANGIOPLASTY OF PELVIC VESSELS

Patients with significant iliac occlusive disease have hip and buttock claudication, a decreased or disappearing femoral or peripheral pulse following exercise, abnormal Doppler studies, and abnormal pulse volume recordings. In general, focal concentric short segments of iliac artery stenosis are the most optimal candidates for dilatation (Figs. 9-4, 9-5, 9-8, and 9-9). Longer lesions, multiple stenosis, and even occlusions of the common and external arteries may be successfully dilated [1, 3, 8] (see Chap. 10).

Special Considerations

1. Ipsilateral approach. A severely stenotic common or external iliac artery lesion may cause the femoral pulse to be almost impalpable or absent, making puncture difficult. It may be outlined by prior angiography (IV-DSA or arteriography from a different approach). "Road mapping" here may be helpful. An aspirating arterial puncture needle can be accurately guided by a strong ultrasound signal. If the vessel cannot be entered, an alternate approach may be required.

Measure intraarterial pressures distal to the lesion once the needle or overlying sheath is in position in the vessel prior to traversing the stenosis.

An internal iliac artery stenosis is usually approached from an axillary artery puncture site, and occasionally from the opposite femoral artery.

2. Crossing a stenotic lesion. Standard techniques include a floppy-tip guidewire, a more rigid guidewire, or catheter alone without a preceding guidewire. Sometimes these require IA-DSA or "road mapping" in multiple projections for successful crossings. If unsuccessful, torque controlled guidewires, guidewires with an injectable lumen, or small gauge (0.014–0.018 inch) steerable platinum tipped guidewires can be used (see Fig. 6-11). A coaxial system of steerable guidewire passed through the lumen of an injectable lumen guidewire gives flexibility and excellent torque control yet body to the guiding system for subsequent passage of the catheter. Sometimes changing to an anterograde approach (axillary artery or over the bifurcation from the contralateral femoral artery) succeeds if passage from the retrograde direction is impossible (see Figs. 6-11, 9-5, and 9-10). With the catheter above the lesion, measure pressures and compare to pressures in the poststenotic area to determine the gradient. A gradient of 10 to 15 mm at rest is significant. If there is no gradient present, but there is strong clinical suspicion, a gradient may be induced when a significant lesion is present by using either reactive hyperemia (inflating blood pressure cuffs for 3 minutes to a level 20 mm or more than the systemic systolic pressure and then releasing the cuffs) or by injecting a vasodilator such as Priscoline (25 mg) directly into the artery distal to the stenosis.

3. Review Chapters 6 and 8 on how to overcome difficulties in passing both the initial 5 French diagnostic catheter and the subsequently replaced balloon catheter through an area of tight stenosis. Have available a variety of stiffer body guidewires (Lunderquist, Bookstein modification of a Lunderquist, Amplatz, Rosen, Coons, and variable stiffness guidewires). A low profile, tapered balloon catheter is also helpful. Predilatation with a Staple van Andel dilating catheter or a smaller caliber balloon catheter may be necessary.

4. Chronically or acutely thrombosed iliac vessels and grafts may be opened by intraarterial low-dose thrombolytic therapy (see Chap. 7). We prefer intraarterial urokinase, 4000 IU/minute, until a channel is opened, followed by lower

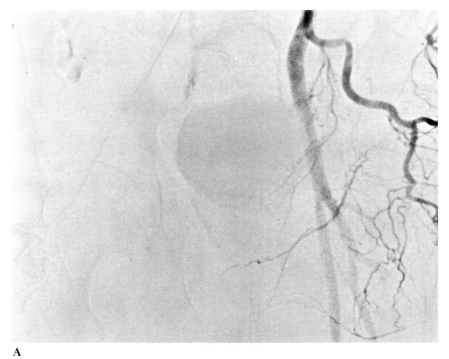

A

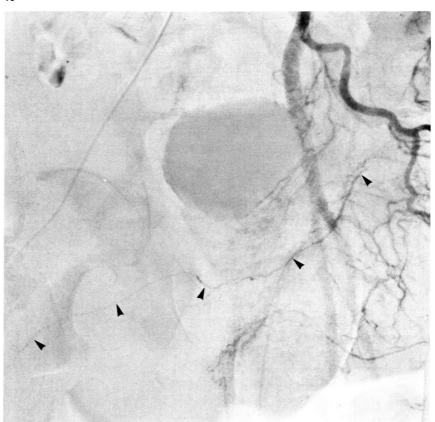

B

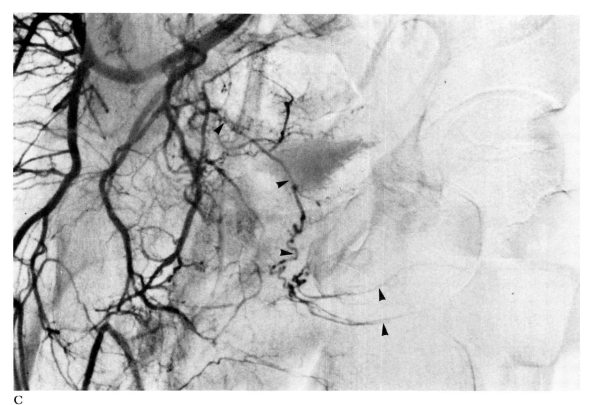

C

Fig. 9-3.
A and B. Traumatic occlusion of major vessels of the
  anterior division of the left internal iliac artery in a
  young man with impotence (*arrows*).
C. Right internal iliac arteriogram in same patient.
  Arrows point to the distal internal pudendal artery,
  the dorsal artery to the penis, and the cavernosal
  artery (see text).

doses of 1000 to 2000 IU/minute until there is
complete lysis [12]. There should be simultaneous administration of 500 to 1000 IU of heparin per hour. Angiograms and bleeding parameters are checked after each aliquot of 500,000
IU urokinase. If an underlying stenosis is uncovered, this should then be dilated.

Iliac occlusions are not routinely crossed and
dilated for fear of peripheral embolization and
retroperitoneal bleeding. An occluded iliac artery may, however, be traversed with a catheter, whether occluded acutely or chronically
[3]. It may be attempted if the patient is a poor
operative candidate and requires limb salvage.
The occluding mass of thrombus in large arteries is composed of inelastic, gum-like acellular fibrosed material with a rather slow process

of organization. This can sometimes be traversed and dilated with relative ease. As a rule,
there is at least one underlying, firm, stenotic
atheromatous plaque which initiates the
thrombotic process. Once traversed, the occluded segment can be dilated. To cross the
lesions, a small hockey-stick-shaped catheter is
passed retrograde directly into the thrombosed
vessel, guided by intrathrombic injections of
contrast. The catheter guidewire combination
must be in the center of the vessel. This can be
monitored with multidirectional fluoroscopy.
Once the clotted area is bypassed, it is dilated
with a balloon of a diameter chosen by measuring neighboring or ipsilateral iliac vessels. Long
segments of occlusion and stenosis are less
prone to remain open than shorter lesions following dilatation.

5. During dilatations, the balloon should be inflated for several periods, each lasting at least 1
   minute. Multiple dilatations are usually necessary. Administer heparin (3000–5000 units)
   into the vessel prior to the dilatation. Dilate the

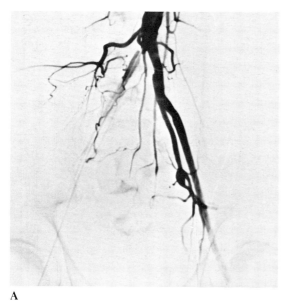

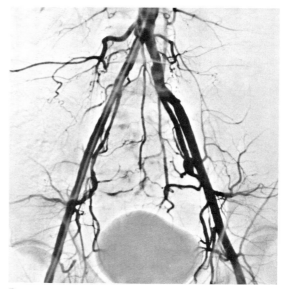

A

B

Fig. 9-4.

A. Subtotal occlusion of right common iliac artery due to focal stenosis. The patient was impotent (possibly due to a hypogastric artery steal).

B. Postdilatation. There was symptomatic improvement.

Fig. 9-5.

A. Focal stenosis of left common iliac bifurcation. (Stenosis of left internal iliac and occlusion of right internal iliac.)

B. Lunderquist guidewire across the bifurcation.

C and D. Balloon dilatation of left common iliac stenosis.

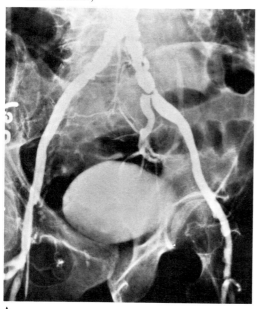

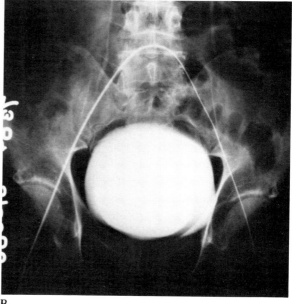

A

B

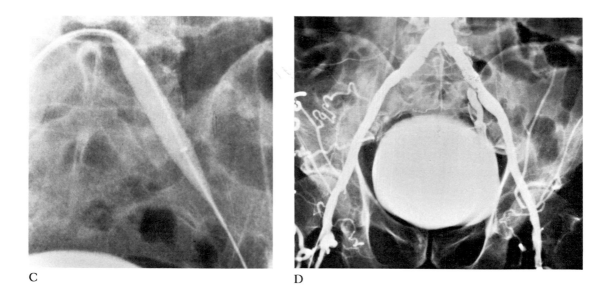

C   D

Fig. 9-6. Small vessel distal occlusion (*arrows*) of the dorsal artery to the penis in a diabetic patient.

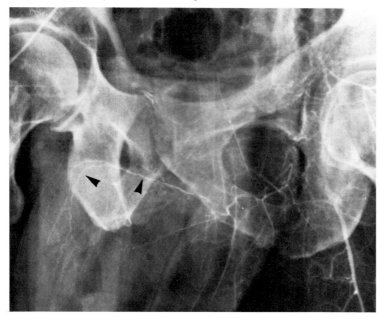

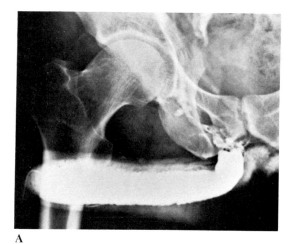

A

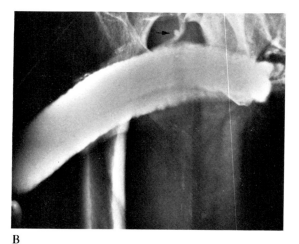

B

Fig. 9-7. Corpora cavernosagrams on patients suspected of venous leak.
A. Normal study showing drainage through root of penis into the prostatic venous plexus.
B. Venous leak with an abnormally draining vein on the dorsal side of the penile shaft (*arrow*).

entire length of the lesion, usually from its most proximal aspect first down to its distal area of narrowing. Do not withdraw the guidewire proximal to the dilated area until after the post-dilatation arteriogram and pressure measurements document success. If IA-DSA is available, exchange the guidewire for one with a small gauge (with the catheter tip well beyond the lesion), attach a Touhy-Borst adapter, and inject the contrast agent. If conventional angiography alone is available, exchange the balloon catheter for an 8 French Teflon straight catheter with multiple side holes; this provides a diagnostic bolus of contrast agent despite the inner guidewire. Do not inject directly into the newly dilated lesion because the disrupted intima may be undermined. If there is residual stenosis or gradient present, the vessel should be redilated.

6. After the study, administer aspirin 300 mg daily and 50 mg of pyridamole 3 times daily for several weeks. If the dilated iliac vessel was originally thrombosed and successfully dilated, 12,000 to 15,000 IU of heparin should be given systemically daily for 2 days.

7. There should be an immediate high success rate from dilating iliac artery stenosis (93%). Three-year cure rates range from 64 to 86 percent [5, 15]. The results for iliac artery occlusion are less easy to document due to the few procedures reported but are surprisingly high (94%) in a limited series [4].

Fig. 9-8. Indications for percutaneous transluminal angioplasty in the pelvis.

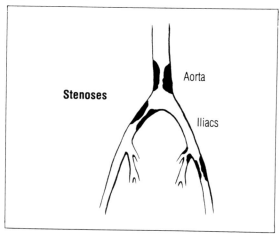

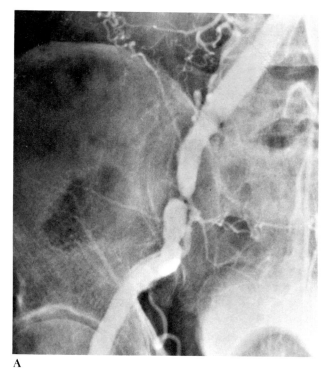
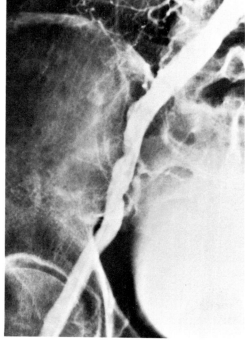

A
B

Fig. 9-9. Dilatation of right external iliac artery stenosis.

THERAPEUTIC EMBOLIZATION

Transcatheter embolization can be used to stop postoperative bleeding, bleeding in patients with pelvic trauma (Fig. 9-11), postpartum hemorrhage, or bleeding from pelvic tumors [10, 16, 17]. Embolization has been used for bony tumors of the pelvis. It reduces blood loss during surgery, bone pain in nonresectable cases, and occasionally is the definitive therapy in patients with aneurysmal bone cysts [9, 18, 19]. Pelvic arteriovenous malformations can be treated by embolization alone. Combining embolization with surgery, however, seems to give the best results [14] (see Fig. 8-22). There are case reports of successful treatment of priapism by embolization.

Special Technical Considerations
in Embolization

Review Chapter 5 for details of embolization techniques. Prior to embolization procedures within the pelvis, there should be complete angiographic evaluation of both internal iliac arteries as well as extra pelvic potential collateral vessels. This is because the superior rectal branch of the inferior mesenteric artery, middle sacral artery and lumbar arteries from the aorta, and medial and lateral femoral circumflex branches of the profunda femoris artery freely anastomose with branches of the internal iliac arteries; they may require embolization if they supply an AVM or the vascular supply to a pelvic neoplasm.

Selective catheterization of the hypogastric artery can be accomplished by techniques illustrated in Fig. 9-1. Five French catheters, placed through a sheath in the femoral artery, are usually necessary for embolization with particulate material (e.g., Gelfoam, Ivalon). More peripheral branches may be catheterized using either 3 French or injectable-lumen guidewires coaxially through a 5 French thin-wall catheter. Both coaxial systems can be positioned accurately with the help of the small caliber (0.014 to 0.018 inch) steerable guidewire. The small internal diameter of the open-ended injectable wire limits its use to liquid in-

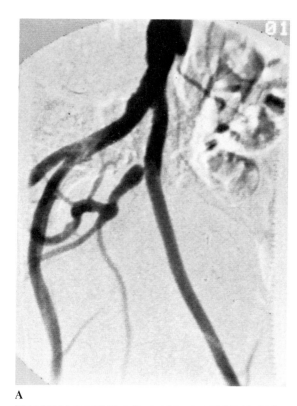

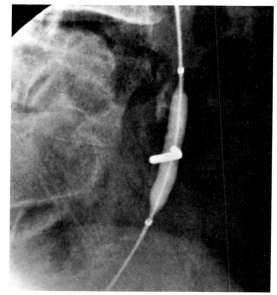

B

Fig. 9-10.
A. Left internal iliac artery stenosis (oblique view of IA-DSA).
B. Metallic marker identifies location of stenosis. Balloon dilatation.
C. Balloon catheter withdrawn into common iliac artery. Successful dilatation.

A

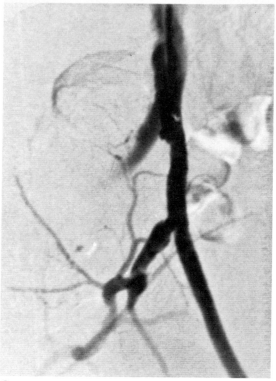

C

jectables (absolute alcohol, bucrylate mixed with Pantopaque). The smallest Ivalon particles, Gelfoam powder emulsions, and microcoil spring occluders can be introduced through 3 French catheters.

When a suitable catheter position cannot be achieved, protection of noninvolved distal vessels with spring coil occluders prior to injection of smaller particulate or liquid injectables helps avoid embolization of nontarget areas. Avoid being too aggressive in embolizing the hypogastric arteries for ischemic neuropathies may result. This is prone to occur when using liquid embolic agents such as ethanol and can be a serious complication if the sciatic nerve is involved [7].

Certain pelvic neoplasms can benefit from intraarterial chemotherapy [11] (Figs. 9-12 and 9-13).

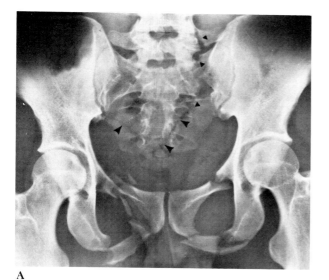

A

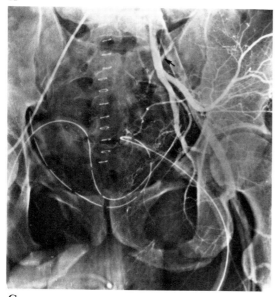

C

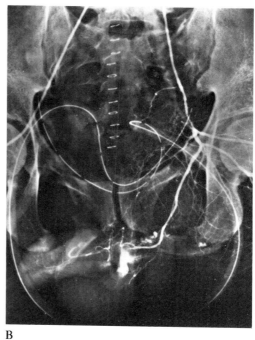

B

Fig. 9-11. Severe pelvic bleeding following automobile accident.
A. Multiple pelvic fractures (*arrows*).
B. Extravasation from internal pudendal artery.
C. Postembolization. Bleeding stopped from internal pudendal artery. More proximal bleeding (*arrow*) embolized with stabilized autogenous clot.

Fig. 9-12. Choriocarcinoma of the uterus. Bilateral selective internal iliac catheterization was performed for chemotherapeutic purposes. Note the prominent uterine arteries (*arrows*) and the hypervascular blush within the uterus.

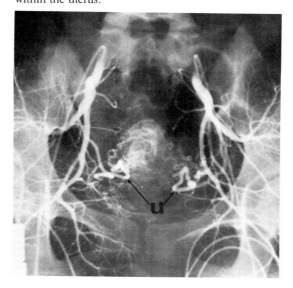

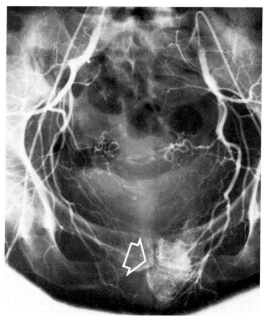

Fig. 9-13. Malignant tumor of the vagina (*open arrow*). Selective catheter placement in the internal iliac arteries was performed for chemotherapeutic purposes. Compare the normal-sized uterine arteries with those seen in Figure 9-12.

References

1. Auster, M., et al. Iliac artery occlusion: Management with intrathrombus streptokinase infusion and angioplasty. *Radiology* 153:385, 1984.
2. Chait, A., Moltz, A., and Nelson, J. The collateral arterial circulation in the pelvis: An angiographic study. *Am. J. Roentgenol.* 102:392, 1968.
3. Colapinto, R. Percutaneous recanalization of complete iliac artery occlusions. In W. Castaneda-Zuniga (ed.), *Transluminal Angioplasty*. Stuttgart: Thieme, 1983. Pp. 93–102.
4. Colapinto, R. Long-term results of iliac and femoral popliteal angioplasty. In C. Dotter, et al. (eds.), *Percutaneous Transluminal Angioplasty. Technique, Early and Late Results*. Berlin: Springer, 1983. Pp. 202–206.
5. Gailer, H., Gruntzig, A., and Zeitler, E. Late results after percutaneous transluminal angioplasty of iliac and femoral popliteal obstructive lesions.

A cooperative study. In C. Dotter, et al. (eds.) *Percutaneous Transluminal Angioplasty. Technique, Early and Late Results*. Berlin: Springer, 1983. Pp. 215–218.
6. Gray, R., et al. Investigation of impotence by internal pudendal angiography: Experience with 73 cases. *Radiology* 144:773, 1982.
7. Hare, W., and Holland, C. Paresis following internal iliac artery embolization. *Radiology* 146:47, 1983.
8. Katzen, B. Transluminal angioplasty of the iliac arteries. In W. Castaneda-Zuniga (ed.), *Transluminal Angioplasty*. Stuttgart: Thieme, 1983. Pp. 93–102.
9. Keller, F., Rosch, J., and Bird, C. Percutaneous embolization of bony pelvic neoplasms with tissue adhesive. *Radiology* 147:22, 1983.
10. Lang, E. K. Transcatheter embolization of pelvic vessels for control of intractable hemorrhage. *Radiology* 140:331, 1981.
11. Maroulis, G., et al. Arteriography and infusional chemotherapy in localized trophoblastic disease. *Obstet. Gynecol.* 45:397, 1975.
12. McNamara, T., and Fischer, J. Thrombolysis of peripheral arterial and graft occlusions. Improved results using high dose urokinase. *A.J.R.* 144:769, 1985.
13. Miller, K., et al. Radiology of male impotence. *Radiographics* 2:131, 1982.
14. Palmaz, J. C., et al. Particulate intra-arterial embolization in pelvic arteriovenous malformations. *A.J.R.* 137:117, 1981.
15. Reiger, H., et al. Late results of percutaneous catheter treatment in iliac stenosis. A retrospective study. In C. Dotter, et al. (eds.), *Percutaneous Transluminal Angioplasty. Technique, Early and Late Results*. Berlin: Springer, 1983. Pp. 194–198.
16. Ring, E., et al. Angiography in pelvic trauma. *Surg. Gynecol. Obstet.* 129:375, 1974.
17. Sclafani, S., and Becker, J. Traumatic presacral hemorrhage: Angiographic diagnosis and therapy. *A.J.R.* 138:123, 1982.
18. Wallace, S., et al. Arterial occlusions of pelvic bone tumors. *Cancer* 43:322, 1979.
19. Wallace, S., and Chuang, V. Transcatheter Management of Musculoskeletal Neoplasms. In R. A. Wilkins and M. Viamonte, Jr. (eds.), *Interventional Radiology*. Oxford: Blackwell, 1982. Pp. 225–240.
20. Wespes, E., and Shulman, C. C. Venous leakage: Surgical treatment of a curable cause of impotence. *J. Urol.* 133:796, 1985.

10

Arteriography and Interventional Procedures of the Abdominal Aorta

Indications

1. Primary vascular diseases of the aorta
   a. Atherosclerosis (aneurysms, stenosis, thrombosis, arteriovenous [AV] fistulas, tortuosity)
   b. Aortic dissection
   c. Thromboembolism
   d. Trauma (aneurysms, occlusion, arteriovenous fistulas)
   e. Coarctation (congenital, arteritis, neurofibromatosis)
   f. Complications of grafts
2. Evaluation of major branch stenosis
3. Retroperitoneal soft tissue and bony tumors
4. Prelude to the study of visceral pathology (individual visceral entities are discussed in subsequent sections)
5. Interventional procedures: percutaneous transluminal angioplasty (PTA) of distal abdominal aorta; thrombolysis of occluded grafts and an occluded aorta; therapeutic blockade of abdominal aortic aneurysms, AV fistulas, bleeding sites from aortic branches; selective intraarterial chemotherapy

A number of diseases of the aorta may be best studied by noninvasive imaging methods. Ultrasound, computed tomography (CT), and magnetic resonance imaging (MRI) can be used to study aortic aneurysms, grafts, or their complications (hematoma, infection, aortoenteric fistula, false aneurysm, occlusion).

On some occasions, intravenous digital subtraction angiography (IV-DSA) provides adequate pathologic anatomic detail in those with an occluded or stenotic aorta or disease of some of its major branches. This obviates a more invasive and sometimes technically difficult and risky intraarterial approach. Intraarterial DSA studies are necessary in circumstances requiring more precise anatomic detail, more selective studies, and more information about peripheral run-off which may sometimes not be adequately found by IV-DSA. It is helpful in monitoring a number of intravascular therapeutic endeavors.

Technique

APPROACHES

The reader should review the approaches described in Chapter 3. The following approaches are used in arteriography of the abdominal aorta:

1. Femoral. Either side may be used if the femoral and peripheral pulses are equal bilaterally. If a difference is detected, the side with the stronger pulse should be used.
2. Translumbar. This approach should be used only when there are dampened or obliterated femoral pulses bilaterally, when selective aortic branch catheterization is not anticipated, if IV-DSA is unsatisfactory or unavailable, and when there are no contraindications to its use. Contraindications include blood dyscrasias, severe hypertension or aortic insufficiency, aneurysms, dissections, and interposed grafts in the proposed site of puncture. The reader should review Chapter 3 regarding the technique.
3. Axillary. This approach is used if the femoral approach is unavailable and a translumbar approach is contraindicated. The left side is preferred because less manipulation is required to enter the descending thoracic aorta (see Chap. 3).

CATHETERS

In the femoral approach, several different types of catheters may be used (Fig. 10-1):

1. A 65-cm 5 or 6.5 French straight Teflon or polyethylene catheter with a long, tapered tip and multiple side holes.

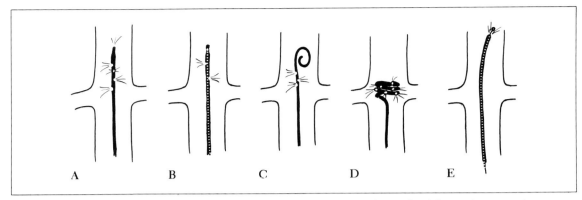

Fig. 10-1. Catheters for abdominal aortography.
A. End-hole catheter with multiple side holes.
B. Catheter with an end hold and multiple side holes. An indwelling filamentous wire with a bulbous tip occludes the end hole and forces contrast medium through the side holes.
C. Catheter with a "pigtail" curve.
D. A ring-shaped catheter, which directs most of the contrast medium to the renal arteries.
E. Cope catheter system. The single curved catheter is straightened by an inner wire for aortography. The inner wire is replaced by one with a curve for subsequent selective studies.

2. A 65-cm 5 or 6.5 French polyethylene, "pigtail tip" catheter with multiple side holes. This type of catheter prevents unwanted retrograde flow of contrast agent into the descending thoracic aorta and allows more contrast agent to enter the abdominal visceral vessels. Its disadvantages include difficulty in keeping the distal tip free of clot except by forceful flushing, and occasional difficulty in exchanging the catheter. If the catheter tip is not properly coiled during the injection, it may enter a lumbar or intercostal artery, and could result in a forceful injection of contrast agent into the artery feeding the spinal cord. Paraplegia has been reported as a complication in such cases [4].

3. A 65-cm 5 or 6.5 French polyethylene catheter with a ring-shaped tip with multiple side holes which directs contrast medium into the adjacent renal arteries. These first three types of catheters may be advanced over a 145-cm stainless-steel guidewire with a curved, flexible tip and a diameter of 0.035 inch (0.89 mm) or 0.038 inch (0.97 mm). Difficulty may be encountered in exchanging the ring catheter because the guidewire may pass out through a side hole or may not advance through to the tip. This difficulty can be overcome by straightening the coils of the catheter by withdrawing it to the iliac artery prior to inserting the guidewire.

4. A 3 or 4.5 French catheter suffices if the aorta distal to the renal arteries or the abdominal aorta of children is being studied. This catheter may be advanced over a guidewire with diameters ranging from 0.028 inch (0.71 mm) to 0.035 inch (0.89 mm) with a flexible, curved, or straight tip.

With an axillary approach, an 80-cm 5 or 6 French Teflon or polyethylene end-hole catheter with multiple side holes easily follows the guidewire into the descending thoracic aorta to the abdominal aorta. Catheters with larger diameters are more likely to cause complications of spasm and thrombosis of the axillary artery and are less able to follow the guidewire. Shorter catheters reach only to the level of the T10 or T11 vertebra. Longer catheters (100 cm) require a longer guidewire (180 cm) than the standard (145 cm) in order to retain their position low in the abdominal aorta while advancing the catheter into the axillary artery. Adequate injection rates (17–20 ml/second) are possible through these longer, narrower catheters. If the guidewire descends into the descending thoracic aorta easily, a straight-tipped catheter may be selected; if the guidewire does not descend with ease, a pigtail-shaped catheter tip allows manipulation of the guidewire into the descending aorta (see Fig. 8-2). One must be wary of high-pressure injections through pigtail catheters advanced into the abdominal aorta because of possible recoil into lumbar arteries and subsequent spinal cord damage. For this reason, a straight catheter of similar diameter may be preferable.

CONTRAST AGENTS, PROJECTIONS, AND RADIOGRAPHIC PROGRAMMING

Details concerning contrast agents, radiographic programs, and projections are given in Table 10-1. Lateral projections help to outline the origin of splanchnic vessels, the anteroposterior diameter of abdominal aneurysms, the presence of en face plaques, and to determine suspected pathology of aortic grafts. Oblique projections, on the other hand, better define the origin of renal arteries (Fig. 10-2). If lateral exposures are required, the anteroposterior AOT changer should be filled with 12 films loaded in every other slot, and the lateral changer should be filled with six films in alternate slots. Film timing of four exposures per second for 3 seconds, two per second for 2 seconds, and one per second for 8 seconds gives anteroposterior exposures as shown in the first program in Table 10-1. This program allows biplane exposures without film fog due to scattered radiation. If the patient's size precludes alternate film loading, one should load biplane changers simultaneously and cone severely to reduce fog from scattered radiation. Separate injections for each plane may also be made.

DIGITAL SUBTRACTION ANGIOGRAPHY

Digital subtraction angiography is helpful in evaluating the abdominal aorta. The major limitations are the relatively small size of the image amplifier field in some units and some loss of spatial resolution.

Intravenous Digital Subtraction Angiography

This avoids more risky axillary or translumbar techniques in patients with occlusion of the aorta or iliac vessels. Four separate contrast injections (35–40 ml each at 20–25 ml/second) through a catheter placed in the right atrium may provide all the information a surgeon requires (Fig. 10-3). The study sites are centered consecutively over the aorta, with renal arteries at the top of the field, the pelvis, and, subsequently, over each femoral area [27]. Not only the point of occlusion, but the area of vascular reconstitution may be seen, for all potential collaterals (including those from above the

diaphragm) are filled with this technique. Motion artifacts from gas are minimized by intravenous glucagon (1 mg) and abdominal compression. A prone position is particularly helpful, for gas in the gastric antrum is displaced into the fundus and that in the small bowel or colon is displaced laterally away from the origin of the aortic vessels. Adequate renal function and cardiac output are required for this technique. Overlapping vessels are a disadvantage, and small vessel detail is often not provided.

Intraarterial Digital Subtraction Angiography

Intraarterial digital subtraction angiography (IA-DSA) expeditiously provides entirely adequate studies of the aorta and its major branches [12]. The required field is chosen fluoroscopically and almost instantaneous subtraction studies may be obtained. Much smaller doses of less concentrated contrast agents are needed than in standard angiography or IV-DSA. Smaller catheters are required than by other techniques. Overlapping vessels, poor cardiac output, and motion artifacts are not as critical as with IV-DSA. Patients with poor renal function may be studied more safely, and those with a past history of contrast reactions can be examined using carbon dioxide as the contrast agent (see Chap. 2). Intraarterial DSA can evaluate patency of vascular grafts and anastomoses and abdominal aortic aneurysms prior to operative repair. There is a considerable saving of time and contrast material in interventional procedures such as embolization or angioplasty using IA-DSA.

Anatomic Considerations

The abdominal aorta commences at the diaphragm at the T12 level and ends by bifurcating into the common iliac arteries, usually at the L4 vertebral body. It lies directly on the anterior aspect of the vertebral column and slightly to the left. The inferior vena cava lies just to its right. From superior to inferior, the pancreas, the left renal vein, the third part of the duodenum, and the coils of the small intestine lie anteriorly. The diameter of the abdominal aorta decreases rather abruptly after the renal arteries, since one-quarter of the cardiac output goes to the kidneys.

Table 10-1. Technical specifications in conventional arteriography of the abdominal aorta.[a]

Arteriographic procedure	Contrast agent			Total films	Total time (sec)	Radiographic program		
	Density	Volume (ml/inj)	Rate (ml/sec)			Films/sec	Timing	Projection
Adult								
Femoral approach above renal artery	M	40–50	25	12	12	2/sec for 3 sec; 1/sec for 3 sec; 1 every other sec for 6 sec	Start 0.4 sec after start of injection	Biplane
Alternate program[b]	M	40–50	25	12	11	3/sec for 2 sec; 1/sec for 3 sec; 1 every other sec for 6 sec[b]		
Femoral approach below renal artery	M	40	10	12	12	2/sec for 3 sec; 1/sec for 3 sec; 1 every other sec for 6 sec		
Axillary approach	M	50	20	12	12	Same as for femoral approach		
Translumbar approach								
High	M	60	20	12	12	Same as first program for femoral approach	Start 1 sec after start of injection	
Low	M	40	15	12	12	Same as femoral approach, below renals		
Child[c]								
Infants	L	1.0–1.5 ml/kilo	Total within 1–1.5 sec	12	8	3/sec for 2 sec; 2/sec for 2 sec; 1 every other sec for 4 sec	Start 0.4 sec after start of injection	
Others	M							

[a] For IA-DSA studies use one-half concentration of contrast agent but the same volume and injection rates.
[b] Use this program if flow is rapid, as in young people, or if the origin of major branches is of prime importance.
[c] Amount of contrast agent varies with body weight in children.
Note: M = medium density contrast agent. Nonionic contrast agents are less painful. L = low density contrast agent (see Appendix 3).

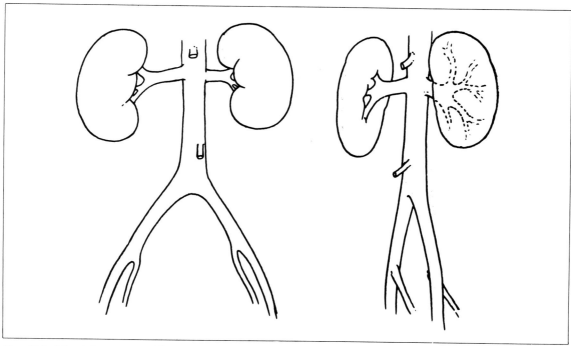

Fig. 10-2. The right posterior oblique projection outlines the origin of the renal arteries on both sides in profile.

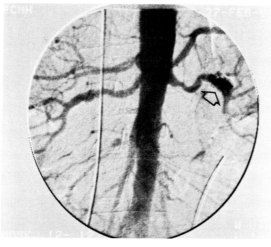

Fig. 10-3. IV-DSA abdominal aorta. An artifact due to gas obscures the left renal artery branch (*arrow*).

BRANCHES OF THE AORTA

The branches of the abdominal aorta may be divided into three groups (Fig. 10-4).

1. Three anteriorly arising, unpaired splanchnic branches
   a. The celiac axis, which arises at approximately the level of T12 and slightly to the left of the midline, gives branches to the liver, spleen, stomach, pancreas, duodenum, and gallbladder.
   b. The superior mesenteric artery, which arises just below or up to 2 cm distal to the celiac axis, feeds the small bowel and right and middle colon.
   c. The inferior mesenteric artery, which arises approximately at the L3 vertebral body anterolaterally to the left, gives branches to the descending and sigmoid colon and the rectum.
2. Three lateral paired visceral branches
   a. The renal arteries arise laterally at the L1 to L2 vertebral body with the right slightly more anterior and the left slightly posterior. A right posterior oblique (RPO) projection brings both these vessel origins into profile (see Fig. 10-2).

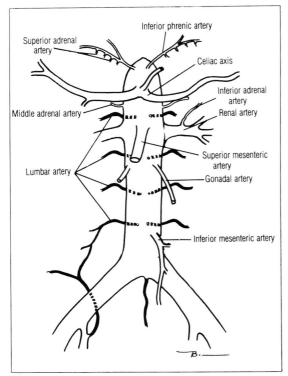

Fig. 10-4. Branches of the abdominal aorta (see text for details.)

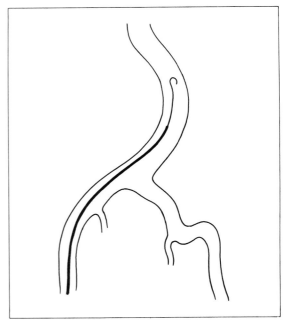

Fig. 10-5. Elongation and tortuosity of the aorta to the left. The right femoral approach is usually more successful and easier than the left.

b. The middle adrenal arteries, which are small inconstant vessels, arise just above the renal arteries.

c. The gonadal arteries arise anterolaterally just below the renal arteries.

3. Five paired muscular branches

a. The inferior phrenic arteries arise just above the celiac axis anteromedially or alternatively from the superior margin of the celiac axis near its origin from the aorta. The superior adrenal branches are important vessels that supply the superior pole of the adrenal glands.

b. Four lumbar branches arise posterolaterally, loop upward, and then downward as they pass inferolaterally along the retroperitoneal muscles. One or more of these branches can supply important radicular branches to the spine.

Because the patient is usually supine during aortography, and because the specific gravity of contrast agent is greater than that of blood, the contrast agent layers out on the most dependent (posterior) portion of the aortic lumen. Those vessels arising from the posterior and lateral portions of the aorta are often more densely opacified than the splanchnic vessels, which arise from the anterior wall. In addition, the lumbar arteries remain opacified for longer periods. These arteries can be traced back to their origin by studying the later films in the angiographic series and can, thus, be differentiated from other small branches such as the adrenal, accessory renal, or gonadal vessels. When the contrast agent leaves the major vessels 5 or 6 seconds after the injection, the parenchymal phase of the opacified organs can be seen, followed in several seconds by the venous phase. Often the latter phase is only faintly seen.

With advancing age of the patient, the aorta may elongate and arch anteriorly and to the left. This tends to straighten the right iliac vessels but makes the left iliac vessels more tortuous; therefore, it is often more difficult to advance the catheter from the left femoral approach (Fig. 10-5).

There are variations in the origin of vessels from the abdominal aorta which are discussed in subsequent sections.

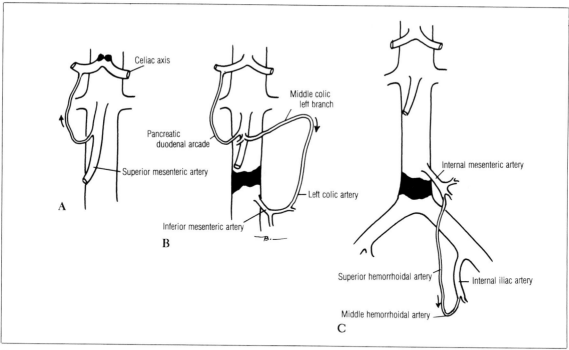

Fig. 10-6. Collateral flow through the visceral vessels (see text for details).
A. The pancreaticoduodenal arcade. There is stenosis of the celiac axis.
B. Anastomosis between the left branch of the middle colic artery of the superior mesenteric artery and the left colic branch of the inferior mesenteric artery. There is occlusion of the aorta.
C. Anastomosis between the superior hemorrhoidal branch of the inferior mesenteric artery and the middle hemorrhoidal branch of the internal iliac artery. There is occlusion of the distal aorta.

COLLATERAL FLOW

Collateral vessels supplying an area distal to aortic occlusion may be either visceral or parietal.

1. Visceral branches. Branches from the celiac axis, the superior mesenteric artery, and the inferior mesenteric artery may all take part in collateral flow (Fig. 10-6).
   a. The pancreaticoduodenal arcade (and sometimes fetal circulation remnants such as the arc of Buhler) forms important collaterals between the celiac axis and the superior mesenteric artery when there is stenosis or occlusion of the origin of these vessels or of the aorta in between (Fig. 10-6A; see Chap. 13).
   b. The middle colic branch of the superior mesenteric artery and the left colic branch of the inferior mesenteric artery form anastomoses when there is stenosis or occlusion of the origin of these vessels or of the aorta in between (Figs. 10-6B, 10-7, 10-8).
   c. The superior hemorrhoidal branch of the inferior mesenteric artery and the middle hemorrhoidal branch of the internal iliac artery form anastomoses when there is stenosis or occlusion of the origin of the inferior mesenteric artery, the internal iliac artery, or the aorta and the common iliac artery in between (Figs. 10-6C, 10-9).
2. Parietal branches (Fig. 10-10). The intercostal, subcostal, lumbar, and middle sacral branches of the aorta form anastomoses with branches of the internal iliac and deep femoral arteries. The superior epigastric branches of the internal mammary arteries sometimes anastomose with the inferior epigastric branches of the external iliac arteries. These anastomoses, which run along the anterior abdominal wall, may be missed if the contrast agent is injected below their origins.

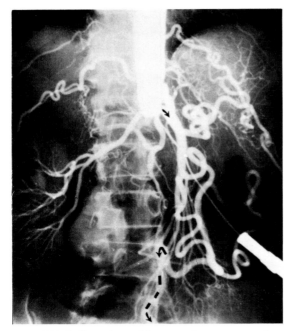

Fig. 10-7. Collateral vessel between the superior and inferior mesenteric arteries in a patient with occlusions of the aorta, inferior mesenteric origin, and iliac arteries. This large channel provides major supply to the lower extremities. There are also large subcostal collateral branches.

Angiographic Findings

ATHEROSCLEROSIS

Although atherosclerosis is seen primarily in patients over age 50, it can be symptomatic in patients in younger age groups, particularly those with hyperlipidemia and diabetes mellitus. There is a clinical syndrome of distal aortic occlusive disease in younger women (particularly smokers in whom the aortic and iliac vessels are generally smaller than the usual caliber) [11]. The most common manifestations of atherosclerosis in the abdominal aorta are varying degrees of occlusion, tortuosity, and the formation of aneurysms.

OCCLUSION

Atheromatous plaques form, and stenosis and occlusion of both the aorta and its major visceral

Fig. 10-8.
A. Lateral aortogram showing occlusions of the celiac axis and the superior mesenteric artery (*arrowheads*).
B. An anastomotic branch from the inferior mesenteric artery supplies all of the small bowel (*arrows*). Many smaller collaterals (adrenal, retroperitoneal, and inferior phrenic arteries) help to supply the celiac axis.

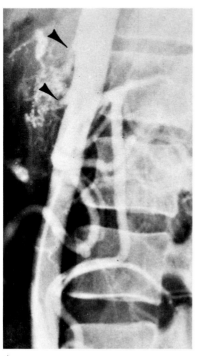

A

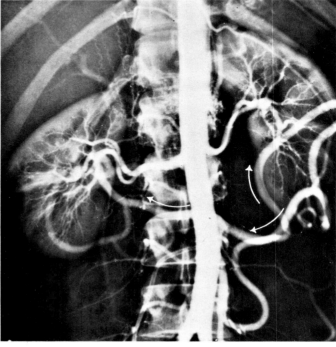

B

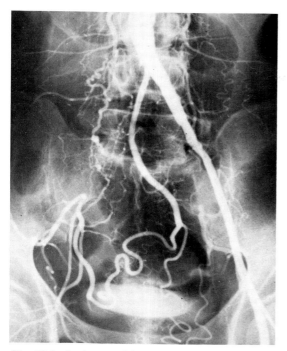

Fig. 10-9. Occlusion of the right common and external iliac artery and the left internal iliac artery. The prominent superior hemorrhoidal artery anastomoses with hemorrhoidal branches of the internal iliac arteries bilaterally. There is retrograde flow with eventual filling of both internal iliacs.

Fig. 10-10. Collateral flow through parietal branches with occlusion of the aorta or the iliacs.

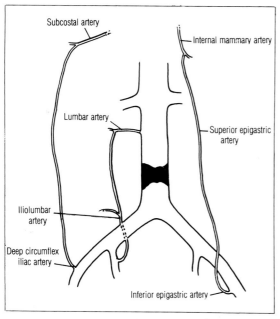

branches may occur. Disease occurring below the level of the renal arteries is most common and often extends down into the iliac arteries and beyond. Patchy, irregular vascular calcification on preliminary films often forewarns of significant atherosclerosis. Arteriography shows either diffuse or localized, eccentric or concentric luminal narrowing, sometimes with irregular filling defects, short constrictions (see Figs. 10-33, 10-34), or segmental occlusions. There may be small saccular outpouchings indicating ulcerating plaques. With significant occlusion, collaterals develop; their demonstration attests to the chronicity of the problem. It has been estimated that the flow of blood through aortoiliac vessels remains unchanged until 70 percent of the luminal diameter is decreased, and a narrowing of more than 80 percent of the diameter is required to decrease the flow by 50 percent.

It is important to demonstrate angiographically for the surgeon not only the site and nature of the disease but also, if there is occlusion, the point of reconstitution of the peripheral vessels. The point of reconstitution is not seen if the collateral vessels are not opacified, and it is, therefore, important to be aware of the major collateral pathways. Often two projections are required to uncover an en face plaque because the only abnormality on one plane may be a localized thinning of contrast density. Knowledge of the anatomic relationship of the disease to essential visceral vessels (e.g., renal, splanchnic) is necessary for planning reconstructive surgery. Complications of atherosclerosis such as mural thrombi, thrombotic or embolic occlusions, and intramural dissection may be uncovered by angiography.

ANEURYSMS

The formation of aneurysms [3, 13] is a dangerous manifestation of atherosclerosis and occurs more frequently below the renal arteries. Aneurysms may be localized and saccular in appearance, but they are sometimes fusiform and may diffusely involve the entire abdominal aorta with extension into the iliac arteries (Fig. 10-11).

Complications of Aneurysm
Abdominal aortic aneurysms may leak or rupture. This may represent a surgical emergency. Large aneurysms (greater than 5 cm in outer diameter) are more prone to do so, but this can occur in

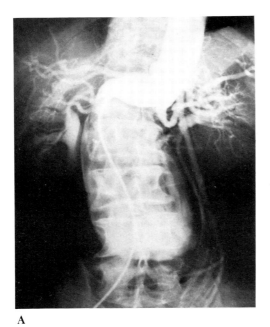

A

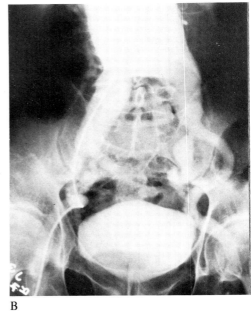

B

Fig. 10-11. An abdominal aortic aneurysm that arises below the renal arteries (A) and extends to the common iliac arteries (B).

smaller aneurysms. Aneurysms larger than 7 cm diameter should be operated upon promptly. Aneurysms usually rupture into the retroperitoneal space but can also extend into the psoas muscle (see Figs. 10-12 and 10-16). They can rupture directly into the inferior vena cava (IVC), creating AV fistulas (Fig. 10-13), or into the duodenum as an aortoenteric fistula [8]. Although primary aortoenteric fistulas are most often seen only when there is an underlying abdominal aortic aneurysm (0.1 to 0.8% of abdominal aortic aneurysms), they can be associated with other lesions [23]. These include previous irradiation to the area, perforating duodenal ulcer or diverticulitis, and pancreatic malignancy or pseudocysts. They can occur anywhere from the esophagus to the colon but most frequently (80%) in the third portion of the duodenum.

Imaging methods help in the diagnosis of those patients suspected of aortoduodenal fistulae by uncovering the presence of periaortic fluid collections. Endoscopy, followed by angiography, is usually required for diagnosis in the acutely bleeding patient. If a bleeding site is not uncovered by selective splanchnic angiography, a biplane abdominal aortogram should be performed to exclude this remote but real possibility as a bleeding site. Prone positioning of the patient may help to demonstrate the lesion.

Fig. 10-12. Ruptured aortic aneurysm. There is an accumulation of contrast medium outside the lumen of the aortic aneurysm, and delayed washout from this area was seen on subsequent films. The right kidney is markedly displaced by an unopacified retroperitoneal hematoma.

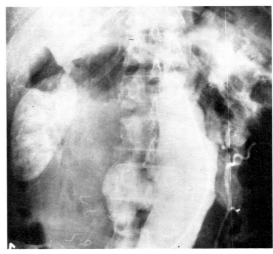

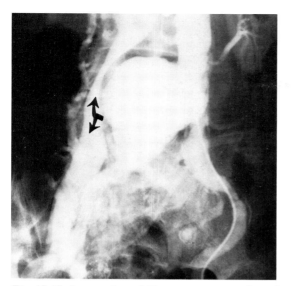

Fig. 10-13. Low aortic and iliac aneurysm complicated by a fistula to the inferior vena cava. The catheter is in the left iliac artery. Systemic aortic pressure forces the contrast medium retrograde down the right iliac vein before it ascends to the inferior vena cava (*arrows*).

An unusual complication of abdominal aortic aneurysms is the perianeurysmal collection of a rind of fibrous or chronic inflammatory tissue, a process similar to retroperitoneal fibrosis [14] (Fig. 10-14).

Imaging Techniques

Imaging techniques are preferable to angiography as the initial examination of patients suspected of abdominal aneurysms.

ULTRASOUND. Ultrasound is easily available and inexpensive and can be used to detect or confirm (in more than one plane) the diagnosis of aortic aneurysms (Fig. 10-15). It can also determine its size, extent, its true outer border, and sometimes its relationship to the renal arteries. It can often define the presence or absence of clot within the aneurysm walls. In pulsatile abdominal masses, ultrasound can discriminate between aneurysms and periaortic masses, such as pancreatic malignancy or enlarged periaortic lymph nodes.

COMPUTED TOMOGRAPHY. Computed tomography can be used to supplement information by ultrasound. It is most helpful in evaluating complications of aortic aneurysms such as suspected leakage or rupture (Fig. 10-16). It is the preferred imaging device when there is clinical suspicion of infection of the aortic aneurysms or associated graft (see Fig. 10-25), perianeurysmal inflammation, and contiguous retroperitoneal disease processes such as tumors, hematomas, or abscesses. It is often more reliable than ultrasound in defining the upper and lower border of the aneurysm.

MAGNETIC RESONANCE IMAGING. If early results are confirmed by larger series, MRI will be the imaging procedure of choice in evaluating abdom-

Fig. 10-14. "Inflammatory" abdominal aortic aneurysm. A and B. Enhanced study of the abdominal aorta and iliac vessels demonstrates contrast filled lumens, unopacified blood clot along the wall, and thickened densely staining walls of the vessels likely due to an inflammatory process.

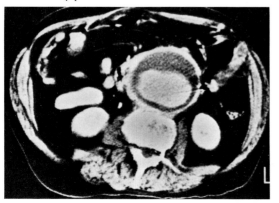

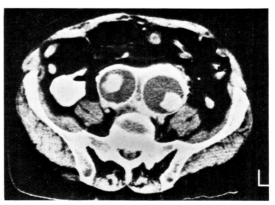

A

B

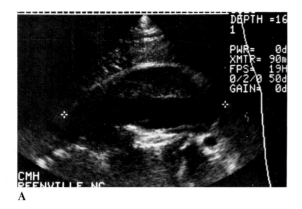

A

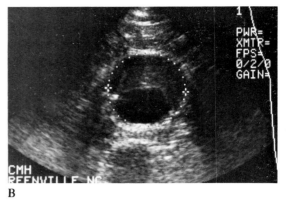

B

Fig. 10-15. Ultrasound imaging of abdominal aortic aneurysms demonstrating clot within the wall.
A. Longitudinal sagittal section.
B. Transverse section.

inal aortic aneurysms when the procedure becomes more available and less expensive. The virtual absence of intraluminal signal from blood flowing at normal velocity contrasts sharply with signals obtained from the vessel wall. This provides a natural image of large intraabdominal vessels without the need for ionizing radiation, contrast agents, or invasive techniques [1, 2, 17, 18, 21]. It provides an accurate measure of the diameter and length of the aneurysm and the thickness and constituents of the aortic wall (Fig. 10-17). It also shows the relationship of the aneurysm to major aortic branches and its effect on contiguous periaortic structures. Other vascular lesions such as intramural and intraluminal clots, atherosclerotic plaques, dissections, and even walls thickened by inflammatory changes as in arteritis have been described by MRI [1].

Angiography in Abdominal Aortic Aneurysms

This should be limited to those occasions when surgery is contemplated and

1. There is suspected involvement of the renal arteries (hypertensive patient, impaired renal function, high location of aneurysm)
2. There is associated claudication of the lower extremities, or diminished or absent femoral pulses. Because grafts may have to be extended down to the femoral arteries to bypass areas of iliac occlusion, the iliac, common, and femoral arteries should be demonstrated angiographically
3. There is suspected suprarenal extension of the aneurysm or presence of associated thoracic aneurysm
4. There is suspected mesenteric ischemia
5. There is suspicion of certain complications of aneurysms such as dissection, thrombosis, or an arteriovenous fistula

Fig. 10-16. Ruptured abdominal aortic aneurysm. Enhanced CT scan showing contrast extravasating into the left retroperitoneum from the abdominal aortic aneurysm.

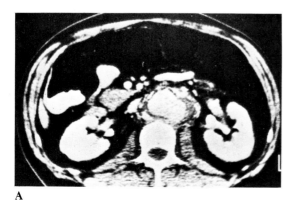

A

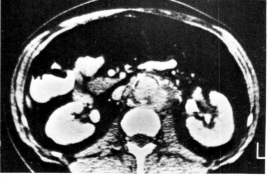

B

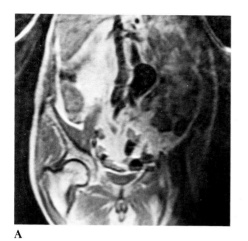

A

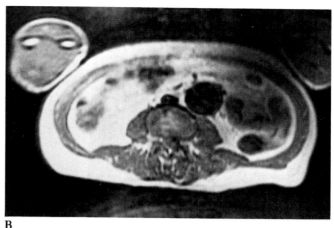

B

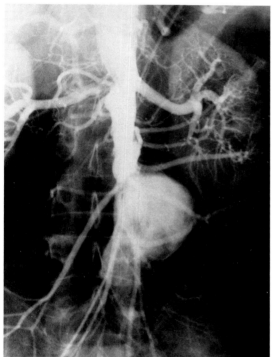

C

Fig. 10-17.
A and B. Abdominal aortic aneurysm outlined by MRI
   sagittal and transverse projections.
C. Arteriogram of the same patient outlines the aneurysm and renal artery stenosis on the right.

The angiographer should beware of pulsatile abdominal masses in which no aneurysm is identified angiographically. A clot may lie within the
wall of the aneurysm, obscuring its true identity
(Fig. 10-18). Tumors lying contiguous to the aorta
may be clinically confused with an aneurysm, par-

ticularly in the presence of carcinoma of the pancreas. In the absence of angiographic signs of such
tumors, the imaging modalities should be employed.

The study may be approached from the femoral
route if the iliac vessels are not occluded. A catheter may be safely advanced through the lumen of
the aneurysm if it is introduced over a floppy
guidewire. Sometimes an injection of contrast medium into the aneurysm is necessary to see the
major branches.

AORTIC DISSECTIONS
Aortic dissections usually have their origin in the
thoracic aorta (see Chap. 18). They can be clinically silent; therefore, their demonstration may be
a complete surprise (Fig. 10-19). Clues to the extent of aortic dissection are provided by imaging
techniques and may suffice if surgical intervention
is not being considered. Magnetic resonance not
only demonstrates the intimal flap as a linear structure but also the presence of flow and the relative
velocity in each of the lumens. It can determine
the origin of major aortic branches from either of
the lumens [1]. Compromise of vessels to vital
structures and insufficiency of the aortic valve is
best studied by angiography in the emergent preoperative patient.

AORTIC GRAFTS
Prosthetic abdominal aortic grafts are surgically introduced to treat abdominal aortic aneurysms or
occlusions (Fig. 10-20). Late complications of

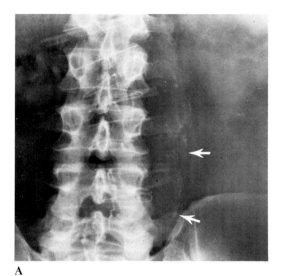

A

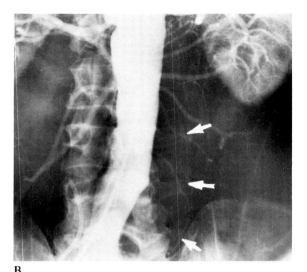

B

Fig. 10-18. False negative arteriogram in the evaluation of an abdominal aortic aneurysm.
A. The KUB shows calcium (*arrows*) outlining aneurysm.
B. This calcium is lateral to the opacified aortic column. At least 3 cm of clot is present in the left
lateral wall of the aneurysm (*arrows*); this can be
easily identified by ultrasound.

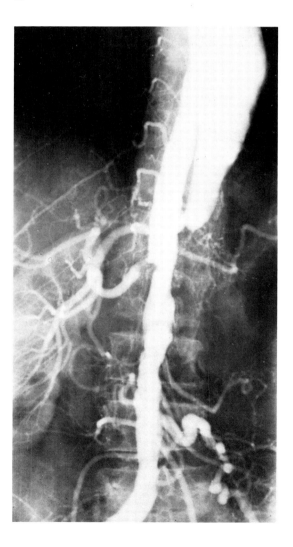

these grafts occur as a result of defective healing,
deterioration and dilatation of the arterial implant,
or degenerative changes in the host artery. (There
was an incidence of 8.5 percent of such complications in a series of 630 patients studied at Duke
University Medical Center [30].) The most common problem is occlusion of a graft or an endar-
terectomized segment (Fig. 10-21). Degenerative
changes in the host artery include formation of an
aneurysm at or near the suture lines, recurrence of
intimal atheromatosis, and stenosis of host arteries
at anastomotic sites. Defective healing and infection result in disruption of the anastomosis, rupture and retroperitoneal leaking (Fig. 10-22), formation of false aneurysms (Fig. 10-23), fistula,
sinuses, and occlusion of the graft.

The most life-threatening complication is the
development of a secondary aortoenteric fistula,
which carries a 90 percent mortality rate (Fig. 10-

Fig. 10-19. Chronic unsuspected dissection of the abdominal aorta. Stenotic right renal artery and superior
mesenteric artery arise from one lumen, the celiac axis
from the other. The left renal artery and common iliac
artery are occluded.

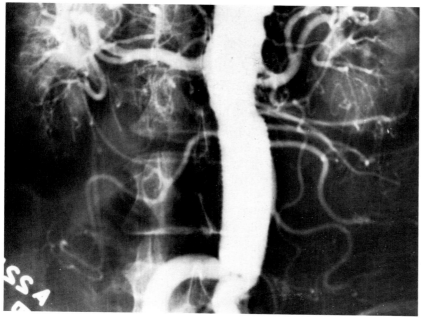

Fig. 10-20. Well-functioning aortoiliac Dacron graft. Proximal anastomosis is below the renal arteries. Note the characteristic corrugated appearance. Because the graft is not attached to the femoral artery, a femoral artery approach is quite safe.

Fig. 10-21.
A. Occluded abdominal bi-femoral aortic graft. Acute ischemic changes both lower extremities.
B. Abdominal aortic graft and right limb of the graft opened following 24 hours of treatment with urokinase. Left limb opened and then reoccluded due to chronic occlusion and poor run-off of left lower extremity. Femoral-femoral and left femoral-popliteal graft reestablished flow to the left side.

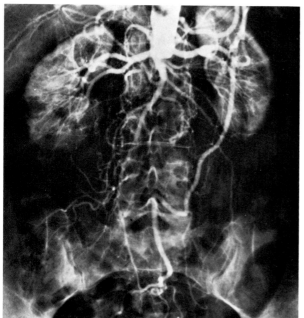

A

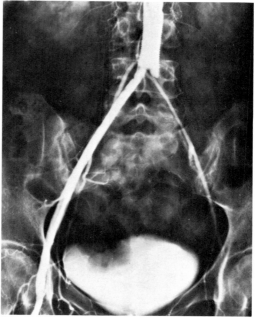

B

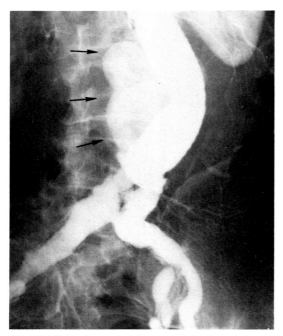

Fig. 10-22. Leaking aortic bypass graft. There is a collection of contrast medium (*arrows*) outside of the graft lumen. The leak started at the distal anastomosis.

Fig. 10-23. False aneurysm (*arrow*) at the proximal anastomosis of the aortic bypass graft (surgically proved).

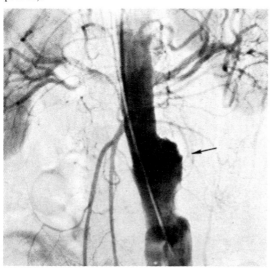

24). Patients with such a fistula may have signs of infection or abdominal pain, but the most significant and consistent finding is gastrointestinal bleeding of varying degrees of intensity. The imaging modalities are helpful in determining the presence and type of graft complication present [14, 19, 21, 22, 25]. One must be aware of the type of graft inserted and the axial appearance of the normally functioning graft [14]. Graft occlusion, hemorrhage, false aneurysm, and circumferential periprosthetic fluid collections (Fig. 10-25) may be detected. The presence of gas in these fluid collections signifies an infection, a finding best determined by CT or MRI. If no gas is present in the periprosthetic collection, but fever and leukocytosis favor infection, direct percutaneous needling may be required to prove its presence.

In those patients with intermittent minor episodes of gastrointestinal (GI) bleeding, in whom an aortoenteric fistula must always be considered, CT or MRI may confirm its presence by demonstrating periprosthetic fluid collections and gas. The CT study should be performed with adequate quantities of orally ingested contrast agent in order not to confuse these collections with bowel content. Negative results do not exclude an aortoenteric fistula. In those patients with acute hemorrhage into the bowel, an unenhanced and then a dynamic enhanced CT study (without oral contrast agent) may show the high-density blood extravasating into the bowel lumen. At this stage, however, most patients are too ill to be undergoing diagnostic steps, and they should be rushed to the operating room.

Angiography may or may not show extravasation at the fistula site; it may show aneurysm at the site of anastomosis. In the absence of imaging findings, barium studies may be helpful by showing signs of a mass eroding the duodenum or other segments of the bowel (see Fig. 10-24B). The fistula may occur between the aorta and the inferior vena cava.

The angiographic approach to studying patients with aortic grafts depends on the available vessels. Care must be used in puncturing the graft not to disrupt its pseudointimal lining with resulting thrombosis. A single wall puncture and floppy guidewire prevents this complication. A femoral approach is used if the abdominal aortic graft is anastomosed to or proximal to the iliac vessels. If an infected proximal graft is suspected, a translum-

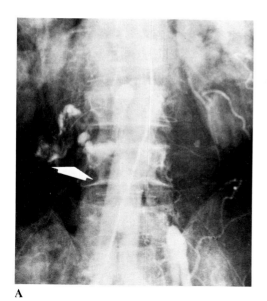

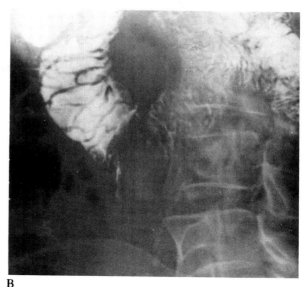

A   B

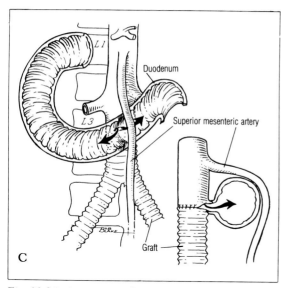

C

Fig. 10-24. Aortoenteric fistula.
A. Extravasation of contrast medium through a fistula between the proximal anastomosis of an aortic graft and the duodenum (*arrow*). The vessel in the left pelvis has filled retrograde from the left branch of the aortofemoral bypass graft.
B. Typical filling defect in the third portion of the duodenum in a patient with an aortic graft duodenal fistula.
C. Line drawing showing anatomic arrangement.

bar approach is contraindicated. The axillary approach is frequently used.

MISCELLANEOUS CONDITIONS

Miscellaneous causes for aortic narrowing include rare conditions such as arteritis [24], neurofibromatosis [20], and retroperitoneal fibrosis.

Arteritis

Arteritis may be found in children, and it is considered by some to be the leading cause of abdominal coarctation [24] (Fig. 10-26). Although types of arteritis (syphilitic, giant cell, polychondritis, and those types associated with Reiter's syndrome, rheumatoid arthritis, and rheumatic fever) lead to the development of aneurysms rather than stenosis, they usually involve the ascending aorta.

Takayasu's arteritis, a panarteritis occurring predominantly in young women, involves both the thoracic and the abdominal aorta and their branches as well as the pulmonary artery. Although aneurysms of the great vessels may form, the typical findings are those of longer areas of narrowing of the aorta sometimes with prestenotic dilatation (see Fig. 18-34). There is a high incidence of occlusion of the brachiocephalic vessels and stenosis of the renal arteries. Early in the course of the disease, there may be nonspecific symptoms and signs such as weakness, arthralgia, and chest and abdominal pain. Occlusive changes occur in the vessels later in the course of the dis-

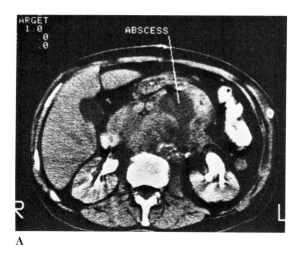

A

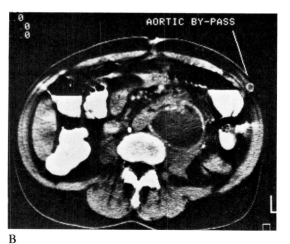

B

Fig. 10-25. CT scan shows infected abdominal aortic graft.
A. Large retroperitoneal fluid collection surrounding the graft.
B. Large abdominal aortic aneurysm distally in the aorta. Note left axillo-femoral bypass graft.

ease, and the symptom complex is then one of ischemia involving the different organs and limbs.

Takayasu's arteritis is the only form with a stenosing aortitis that involves the aorta both above and below the diaphragm.

Neurofibromatosis

In neurofibromatosis abundant fibrous adventitial tissue, thickening, sometimes atrophy of the media, and well-differentiated neural tissue may cause vascular abnormalities [20]. Long, smooth-bordered stenosis and small aneurysmal outpouchings can occur (Fig. 10-27). Although the renal arteries are most frequently involved, the aorta, pulmonary arteries, and other visceral vessels can also be affected.

Mycotic Aneurysms

Mycotic aneurysms (see Fig. 8-20) are secondary to an infectious process of the aortic wall. They are usually saccular and rounded in appearance. There is a previous history of infection and rapid progression of findings. Freedom from atherosclerosis in contiguous areas may provide a clue to the diagnosis. These aneurysms are prone to rupture early and must be surgically corrected as soon as they are suspected.

Trauma

Traumatic injury due to rapid deceleration involves the abdominal aorta less often than the thoracic aorta. Transection of the aorta with intimal damage, false aneurysm formation (Fig. 10-28), rupture, and aortic occlusion can, however, occur

Fig. 10-26. Segmental stenosis of the abdominal aorta (*open arrow*) at the level of the renal (*closed arrows*) and superior mesenteric arteries in a 2-year-old boy. The probable diagnosis is arteritis. (From I. Johnsrude and R. Lester. Abdominal Visceral Arteriography as a Guide to the Surgeon. In *Monographs in the Surgical Sciences*, Vol. 4, No. 2. Baltimore: Williams & Wilkins, 1967. Reproduced with permission of the Williams & Wilkins Company.)

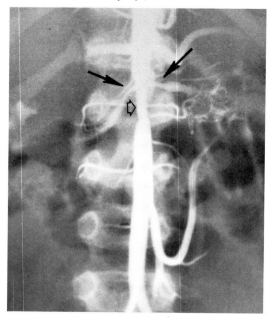

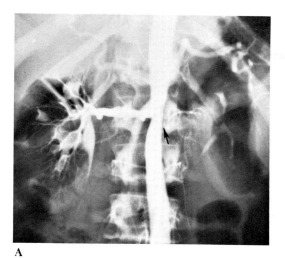

A

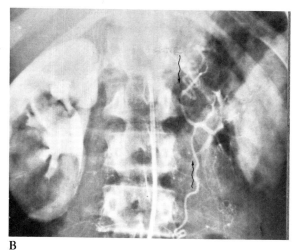

B

Fig. 10-27.

A. Abdominal aortogram in a 6-year-old child with neurofibromatosis, showing smooth narrowing of the abdominal aorta, saccular aneurysmal outpouchings of the renal artery on the right, and almost total occlusion of the left renal artery (*arrow*).

B. A delayed film shows the intrarenal vessels filling through capsular and ureteral collateral complexes (*arrows*).

Fig. 10-28. Lateral projection thoracoabdominal aortogram. There is a false aneurysm (*arrow*) of the anterior wall of the aorta at the level of the diaphragm. The patient had suffered a recent automobile accident.

at or below the diaphragm. Piercing injuries may cause intimal damage, false aneurysm formation (Fig. 10-29), hemorrhage, and arteriovenous fistulas.

Abdominal aortography should be followed in rapid succession by pelvic arteriography and selective studies of any suspicious organ systems. Always consider the potential for temporary or permanent therapeutic blockade of bleeding sites. An IA-DSA may provide rapid "real-time" angiographic evaluation in a cooperative patient, providing the field of the image amplifier is large enough to provide adequate coverage.

Embolus

An embolus may cause sudden occlusion of the abdominal aorta, paraplegia, shock, and death. Sources of the emboli may be clots from the ventricular wall in a patient with a previous myocardial infarct (Fig. 10-30), clots lying within aneurysms higher in the aorta, clots or tumor within the left atrium, or paradoxical emboli arising within the venous system and traversing a patent foramen ovale.

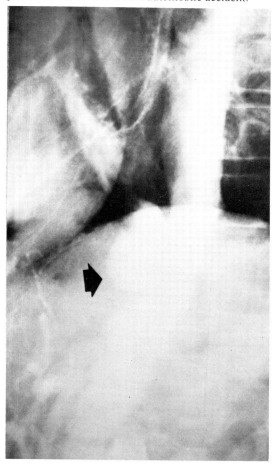

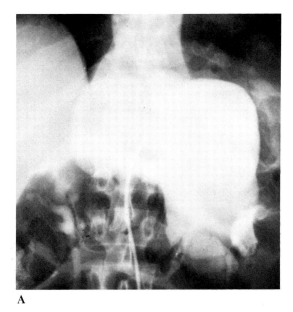

A

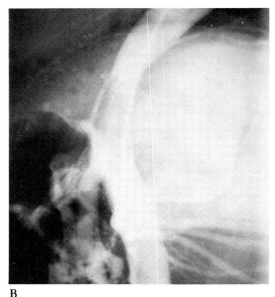

B

Fig. 10-29. Gunshot wound to the aorta.
A. Selective injection into a false aneurysm which includes the entire lesser sac.
B. Lateral projection abdominal aortogram shows marked anterior displacement of the aorta by the false aneurysm.

Retroperitoneal Tumors

Retroperitoneal tumors are mesodermal, neural, lymphatic, or embryonal in origin and are often insidious and slowly growing. These lesions are best studied by a combination of imaging modalities and percutaneous biopsy. Angiography is rarely needed except when interventional methods are required. These include selective arterial chemotherapy or selective embolization for control of bleeding, pain, or decreasing the bulk of the tumor (Fig. 10-31).

Interventional Procedures in the Abdominal Aorta

PERCUTANEOUS TRANSLUMINAL ANGIOPLASTY

Patients with atherosclerotic focal concentric aortic lesions below the level of the renal arteries may be successfully dilated [6, 7, 16, 29] (Fig. 10-32). More diffuse lesions or chronically occluded vessels are best corrected surgically. Eccentric lesions may not respond as well to this method.

The approach used depends on the location of the lesion. If the lesion is well above the aortic bifurcation, with normal caliber common iliac arteries, a single balloon with diameter measuring 1 cm, 1.2 cm, 1.5 cm, or even 2 cm may be used (Fig. 10-33). The diameter of the balloon should equal the diameter of the aorta measured just

above the stenosis. It is important to remember that wall tension is proportional to the diameter of the vessel or chosen balloon and that lower pressures are required to inflate these large balloons. Also, the wall of the larger arteries rupture at lower pressures. Careful attention to the complaints of pain by the patient preclude severe overstretching of the vessel wall and warn of impending rupture. Intraarterial pressures measured proximal and distal to the stenosis document the severity of the gradient. The main purpose of this procedure is alleviation of the pressure gradient and not an angiographically pleasing return of diameters to normal caliber.

If the proximal common iliac arteries as well as the distal abdominal aorta are involved with significant stenosis, two balloon catheters are introduced, one through each femoral artery, with a combined diameter not exceeding the caliber of the immediately adjacent normal aorta. Simultaneous dilatation of the balloons prevents the inadvertent lateral displacement and subsequent occlusion of one iliac artery by atherosclerotic debris from the other vessel.

Combined lesions may be successfully dilated.

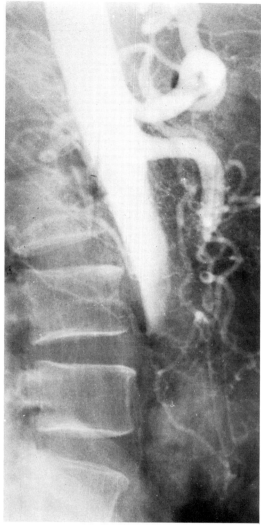

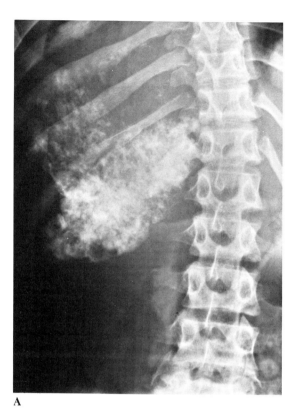

A

Fig. 10-30. Abrupt occlusion of the abdominal aorta and super mesenteric artery by large emboli arising from the left ventricle. The patient had a previous myocardial infarct.

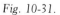

Fig. 10-31.
A. Large osteogenic sarcoma in a 12-year-old girl involving lower ribs, diaphragm, and retroperitoneal structures.
B. Selective chemotherapy of inferior phrenic and intercostal arteries (*arrows*) on multiple occasions followed by major surgical excision. The artery of Adamkiewicz, which supplies the spine, arose at a higher dorsal level on the left.

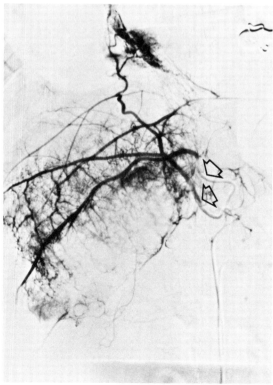

B

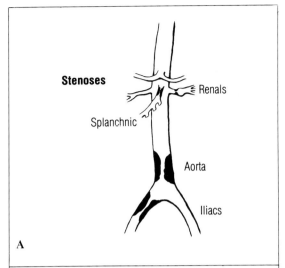

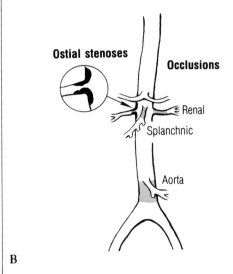

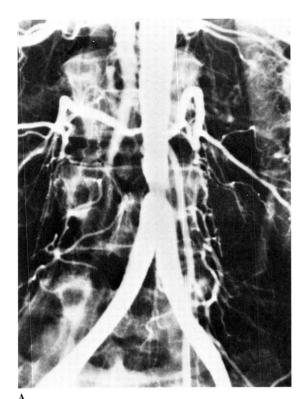

A

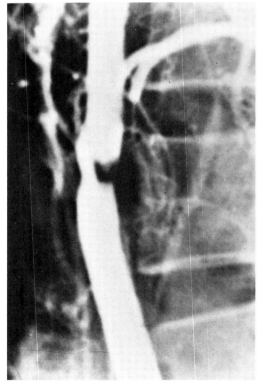

B

Fig. 10-32.

A. Indications for percutaneous transluminal angioplasty (PTA) of stenotic abdominal aorta and major branches.

B. Lesions in which to avoid PTA include occlusion of the aorta, renal, and mesenteric arteries, and ostial stenosis of the renal arteries. Acute thromboembolism may be treated by thrombolytic or clot aspiration techniques (see Chap. 7).

Fig. 10-33. Percutaneous transluminal angioplasty of focal stenosis of the distal abdominal aorta. Single 1.2-cm diameter balloon successfully dilated the lesion.

A and B. Preangioplasty aortogram demonstrates focal stenosis.

C. Lateral projection of dilated balloon.

D and E. IA-DSA post-PTA shows normal caliber of aorta.

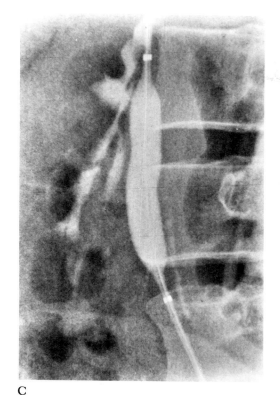

C

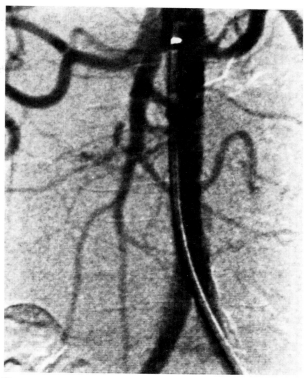

D

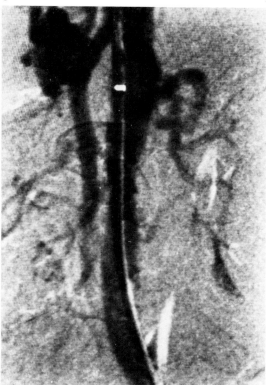

E

Figure 10-34 shows a patient with renal artery stenosis and stenoses of the distal aorta and iliac vessels. The renal artery was dilated first, followed by simultaneous bilateral balloon dilatation of the iliacs and distal aorta.

Aortic narrowing caused by chronic changes due to arteritis, neurofibromatosis, retroperitoneal fibrosis, radiation fibrosis, or stenosis due to dense circumferential fibrotic sclerosis of anastomoses with Dacron grafts are much more difficult to dilate. Multiple repeated attempts at different sittings may be necessary in order to improve the gradient [6, 7, 26].

For effective dilatation of a vessel, elastic and compliant muscular tissues, such as those in the media and adventitia of an artery, are required. The surrounding tough adventitial layer contains the disrupted inner walls of the vessel postdilatation and prevents rupture. These anatomic features are no longer present or are limited and are circumferentially replaced with scar tissue in postoperative grafts. Similarly, a burned-out arteritis may be replaced with dense fibrous collagenous tissue. Successful dilatation has, however, been achieved with Takayasu's arteritis [6].

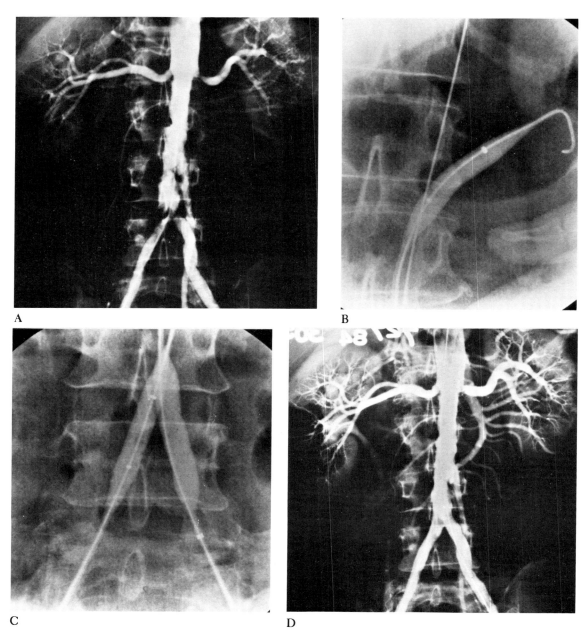

A

B

C

D

Fig. 10-34. Percutaneous transluminal angioplasty of the distal aorta, left common iliac artery, and the left renal artery during the same procedure. Double balloon technique.

THROMBOLYSIS

Review Chapter 7 for technical details of performing thrombolysis, indications, contraindications, and precautions. Figure 10-21 demonstrates successful lysis of a recently thrombosed abdominal aortic bypass graft, and Figure 10-35 shows lysis of a thrombosed aorta using high-dose selective intraarterial urokinase (4000 IU/minute).

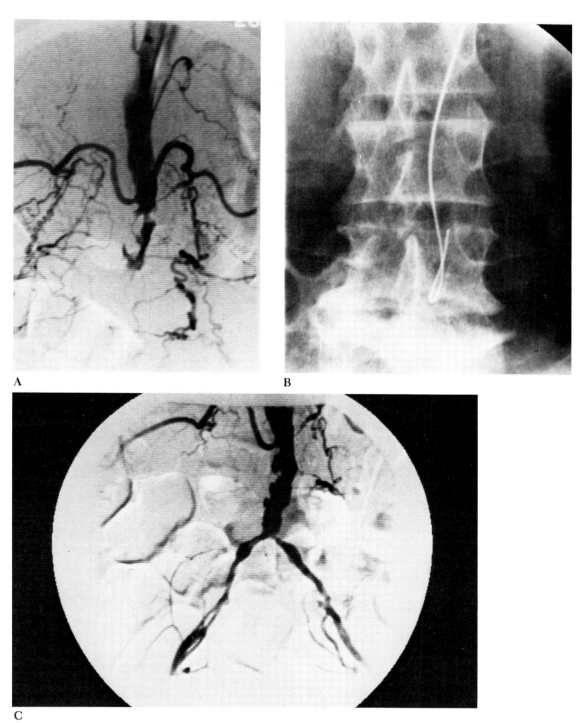

Fig. 10-35.

A. Acute total occlusion of distal abdominal aorta in an elderly patient with multisystem disease.

B. Guidewire advanced through soft clot using axillary approach.

C. Total lysis of clot following 4 hours of urokinase therapy. Subsequent therapy of stenotic vessels awaited improvement in patient's critical condition.

THERAPEUTIC EMBOLIZATION

There are a number of indications for embolizing intraabdominal and retroperitoneal structures. Selected organ systems (kidney, adrenal, GI tract, liver, and pancreas) are discussed in subsequent chapters.

Review Chapter 5 for indications, techniques, therapeutic embolic agents and their delivery systems, and precautions in performing these studies. Generally, selective catheterization of branch vessels is required for purposes of embolizing retroperitoneal bleeding sites, AVMs or AV fistulas or aneurysms, and large symptomatic, nonresectable bone or soft tissue tumors. Different embolic agents are used depending upon availability, the desired permanence of an occlusion, and ease of selective placement of a catheter of required dimension.

Lumbar arteries contribute to a variety of retroperitoneal bone and soft tissue tumors. Decreasing the vascular supply to the tumor impedes tumor growth, facilitating subsequent surgery [28]. Bone tumors cause pain by compression of periosteal nerve fibers. Although not curative, embolizing the peripheral branches of major feeding vessels to these lesions with tiny particulate material (Ivalon), and their more proximal larger branches with small coils, can prove palliative. It is important to review the vascular supply to the lesion and avoid injecting major feeding vessels to the spine (artery of Adamkiewicz). The procedure is made less laborious and requires less contrast agent if it is carefully monitored with "real-time" IA-DSA techniques.

EMBOLIZATION IN ABDOMINAL AORTIC ANEURYSMS

There are a number of high-risk patients with abdominal aneurysms in whom aneurysmal resection cannot be undertaken. In these patients, axillofemoral bypass procedures are performed to transmit blood to the lower extremities. The external or, preferably, common iliac arteries are surgically occluded following grafting, thereby stimulating retrograde occlusion of the aortic aneurysm by thrombus up to a level of the next major aortic branch (the renal arteries). When the iliacs cannot be surgically occluded, the aneurysm remains open and is subject to rupture. Under these circumstances, transcatheter therapeutic blockade

can be accomplished using a number of permanent occlusive agents [5, 15]. Because tissue adhesive agents polymerize rapidly on contact with the vascular system, they can be easily delivered through a small coaxial catheter system (3 French inner catheter through a 6.5 French outer catheter), advanced through an axillary approach [15]. The bucrylate may be opacified without delaying polymerization time by adding tantalum powder (1 g tantalum to 1 ml bucrylate). This provides a focal occlusion at the site of introduction of the adhesive. More complete occlusion of peripheral vessels can be accomplished by delaying polymerization time by injection of Ethiodol or Pantopaque mixed with the bucrylate (3 parts bucrylate to 1 part Pantopaque). However, bucrylate is becoming increasingly more difficult to obtain and other embolization methods must be used. This includes introducing a number of coils through the catheter. To prevent the coils from embolizing the nontarget, more peripheral areas, a preliminary large coil can be introduced. This acts as a baffle to trap the subsequent coils [5].

Selective intraarterial chemotherapy may also be employed for treating certain tumors. Higher concentrations of tumorocidal drugs may be used by this technique than by systemic chemotherapeutic regimens with less systemic toxicity. Improved control of primary tumors can be achieved by this means, particularly when combined with surgery (see Fig. 10-31) [9, 10].

References

1. Ampaaro, E., et al. Magnetic resonance imaging of aortic disease: Preliminary results. *A.J.R.* 143: 1203, 1984.
2. Ampaaro, E., et al. Comparison of magnetic resonance imaging and ultrasonography in the evaluation of abdominal aortic aneurysms. *Radiology* 154:451, 1985.
3. Brewster, D., et al. Angiography in the management of aneurysms of the abdominal aorta: Its value and safety. *N. Engl. J. Med.* 292:823, 1975.
4. Brodey, P., Doppman, J., and Bisaccio, L. An unusual complication of aortography with the pigtail catheter. *Radiology* 110:711, 1974.
5. Carrasco, H., and Parry, C. Transcatheter embolization of abdominal aortic aneurysm. *A.J.R.* 138:729, 1982.
6. Castaneda-Zuniga, W., et al. Nonsurgical treatment of Takayasu's disease. *Cardiovasc. Intervent. Radiol.* 4:245, 1981.
7. Castaneda-Zuniga, W., et al. Transluminal dilata-

tion of coarctation of the abdominal aorta: Experimental study in dogs. *Radiology* 143:693, 1982.

8. Chisolm, A., and Sprayregen, S. Angiographic manifestations of ruptured abdominal aortic aneurysms. *Am. J. Roentgenol.* 127:679, 1976.

9. Chuang, V. Angiographic contributions to the management of advanced cancer. *A.J.R.* 142:385, 1984.

10. Chuang, V., Wallace, S., and Benjamin, R. The therapy of osteosarcoma by intra-arterial Cisplatinum and limb preservation. *Cardiovasc. Intervent. Radiol.* 4:229, 1981.

11. Cronenwett, J., and Garret, H. Arteriographic measurement of the abdominal aorta, iliac and femoral arteries with atherosclerotic occlusive disease. *Radiology* 148:389, 1983.

12. Davis, P., and Hoffman, J. Intra-arterial digital subtraction angiography. Evaluation in 150 patients. *Radiology* 148:9, 1983.

13. Forman, J., Kurzweg, F., and Broadway, R. Aneurysms of the aorta: A review. *Ann. Surg.* 165:557, 1967.

14. Godwin, J., and Korobkin, M. Acute disease of the aorta. Diagnosis by computed tomography and ultrasonography. *Radiol. Clin. North Am.* 21:3:551, 1983.

15. Goldman, M., et al. Transcatheter embolization with bucrylate (in 100 patients). *Radiography* 2:340, 1982.

16. Heeney, D., et al. Transluminal angioplasty of the abdominal aorta. Reports of six cases in women. *Radiology* 148:81, 1983.

17. Herfkens, R., Higgins, C., and Hricak, H. Nuclear magnetic imaging of atherosclerotic disease. *Radiology* 148:161, 1983.

18. Higgins, C., et al. Multiple magnetic resonance imaging of the heart and major vessels. Studies in normal volunteers. *A.J.R.* 142:661, 1984.

19. Hilton, S., Megibow, A., and Naidich, D. Computed tomography of the post-operative abdominal aorta. *Radiology* 145:403, 1982.

20. Itzchak, Y., et al. Angiographic features of arterial lesions in neurofibromatosis. *Am. J. Roentgenol.* 122:643, 1974.

21. Justich, E., Amparo, E., and Hricak, H. Infected aortoiliac femoral grafts. Magnetic resonance imaging. *Radiology* 154:133, 1985.

22. Kam, J., Patel, S., and Ward, R. Computed tomography of the aortic and aorto-ilio femoral graft. *J. Comput. Assist. Tomogr.* 6:293, 1982.

23. Kukora, J., Rushton, F., and Granston, P. New computed tomographic signs of aortoenteric fistulae. *Arch. Surg.* 119:1073, 1984.

24. Lande, A. Takayasu's arteritis and congenital coarctation of the descending thoracic and abdominal aorta: A critical review. *Am. J. Roentgenol.* 122:643, 1974.

25. Mark, A., Moss, A., and Lusby, R. CT evaluation of abdominal aortic surgery. *Radiology* 145:409, 1982.

26. Martin, E. C., Diamond, N., and Casarella, W. Percutaneous transluminal angioplasty in non-atherosclerotic disease. *Radiology* 135:27, 1980.

27. Rosen, R., et al. Evaluation of aorto-iliac occlusive disease by intravenous digital subtraction angiography. *Radiology* 148:7, 1983.

28. Soo, C., et al. Lumbar artery embolization in cancer patients. *Radiology* 145:655, 1982.

29. Tegtmeyer, C. J., et al. Percutaneous transluminal angioplasty in the region of the aortic bifurcation: The 2 balloon technique with results and long-term follow-up study. *Radiology* 157:661, 1985.

30. Thompson, W., Jackson, D., and Johnsrude, I. Aortoenteric and paraprosthetic enteric fistulas: Radiologic findings. *Am. J. Roentgenol.* 127:53, 1976.

Arteriography
of the Kidneys

Indications

1. Space-occupying lesions
   a. Solitary or multiple cysts
   b. Malignant tumors
      (1) Renal cell carcinoma
      (2) Pelvic carcinoma
      (3) Other tumors (including metastatic, capsular)
   c. Benign tumors
   d. Pseudotumors
      (1) Intrarenal cortical rests
      (2) Renal lipomatosis and hydronephrosis
   e. Suspected abscesses
2. Renovascular hypertension
   a. Atherosclerosis
   b. Fibromuscular dysplasia
   c. Arterial thrombus or embolus
   d. Arteritides (e.g., polyarteritis nodosa)
   e. Arteriovenous fistula
   f. Aneurysms
   g. Renal vein thrombosis
   h. Unilateral pyelonephritis
   i. Unilateral hydronephrosis
   j. Perinephric lesions (hemorrhage, abscess, perinephritis)
3. Renal trauma
4. Exclusion of medical diseases in a surgical candidate
   a. Pyelonephritis
   b. Glomerulonephritis
   c. Nephrosclerosis
   d. Bilateral hydronephrosis
   e. Bilateral polycystic disease
   f. Renal ectopia, dysgenesis, agenesis, fusion malformations
5. Evaluation of potential renal donors
6. Follow-up study of renal transplants
   a. Rejection
   b. Acute tubular necrosis (ATN)
   c. Renal artery stenosis
7. Intravascular therapeutic procedures
   a. Percutaneous transluminal angioplasty (PTA)
   b. Therapeutic vascular occlusion

Approaches

1. The percutaneous femoral approach is the preferred approach. Using the femoral approach ipsilateral to the side of a suspected lesion often facilitates selective catheterization.
2. The axillary approach should be used if the femoral approach is unavailable.

Catheters

ABDOMINAL AORTOGRAM

In abdominal aortography (see Fig. 10-1) the catheter diameter should not exceed that of the catheter to be used subsequently for selective studies. The most commonly used catheter is a 5 French pigtail catheter with multiple sideholes. It may be advanced over a 145-cm 0.035-inch (0.89 mm) or 0.038-inch (0.97 mm) guidewire with a flexible curved tip. When the sideholes are placed opposite the renal arteries, there is a preferential delivery of contrast medium to the renal arteries. Less contrast media seems to be required for aortic injection, and fewer overlying vessels obscure renal arterial detail. Another catheter which is useful is a 5 French ring catheter with both end- and sideholes. This also preferentially delivers contrast medium to the renal arteries (Fig. 11-1). Renal arteries of substantially different levels, however, may not be adequately seen with a ring catheter. Catheter exchange is more difficult with the ring catheter than with a straight catheter, because the guidewire may exit through a sidehole or may not negotiate the coils. This difficulty can be overcome by straightening the coils and by withdrawing the catheter into the more narrow iliac artery.

SELECTIVE ARTERIOGRAMS

The reader should review the section on the principles of selective arteriography in Chapter 3. The catheter material of choice is polyurethane or polyethylene, and the curve that is chosen should correspond to the angle made by the renal artery with the aorta. The catheter curves that are shown in

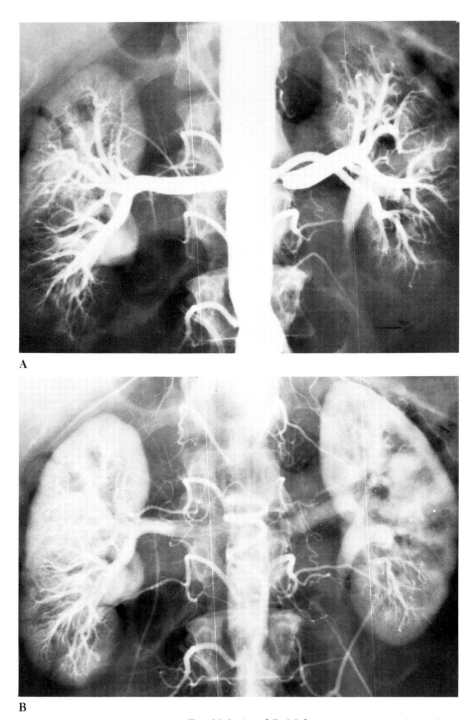

Fig. 11-1. A and B. Midstream aortogram using a ring catheter. There is stenosis of the left renal artery. The renal vessels are clearly outlined without overlying visceral vessels.

Figure 12-1 are generally satisfactory. The catheter is exchanged in the low thoracic aorta and is withdrawn slowly along its anterolateral wall. The catheter tip shifts abruptly as it enters the renal artery usually at the L1 to L2 level. When using the Mikaelsson catheter, advance the tip to the aortic arch and reform the curve (see Fig. 19-3). By advancing a very flexible guidewire approximately 6 to 8 cm beyond the catheter tip, the catheter can be brought down to the distal aorta, avoiding entry into unwanted side branches. Remove the guidewire, and the renal artery is selected by advancing the catheter to the L1 or L2 level.

Contrast Agents, Projections, and Radiographic Programming

Details concerning contrast agents, projections, and radiographic programming in arteriography of the kidneys are given in Table 11-1.

ANATOMIC CONSIDERATIONS

There is a single renal artery supplying each kidney in the majority of people (70%), arising usually at the L1 to L2 level [21]. The right renal artery is slightly more anterior than the left; a right posterior oblique (RPO) projection usually brings their origins into profile (see Chap. 10). Accessory renal arteries, which represent persistent embryonic mesonephric arteries lying along the route of ascent of the adult kidney, are more frequent in low-lying kidneys. They can arise anywhere from the iliac arteries up to the low thoracic aorta. Recognition of these accessory arteries is particularly important in renal donors in whom normal anatomy is desirable for surgical renal transplants. Lack of opacification of these arteries on selective studies may lead to misdiagnosis of a normal structure as a renal infarct or an avascular tumor (Fig. 11-2).

A normal renal arteriogram (Fig. 11-3) may show a number of small extrarenal branches arising from the renal artery before it enters the kidney. These branches consist of the inferior adrenal artery, coursing superiorly to the adrenal gland; capsular branches, which are closely applied to the outer margins of the kidney; and pelvoureteric branches. Sometimes gonadal vessels and the inferior phrenic artery may also arise from this segment of the renal artery. The main renal artery divides into anterior and posterior branches, which

in turn branch into segmental arteries. Interlobar vessels arise from these segmental arteries, course along the septa of Bertin to the junction of the medulla and cortex, and end by arching over the bases of the pyramids as the arcuate arteries. The arcuate arteries run parallel to the renal cortex, where they perpendicularly give off intralobular branches into the cortex; these branches are rarely seen as distinct vessels except by magnification studies. The posterior branch of the main renal artery is the smaller of the two branches; it is more likely to supply the upper pole; and when viewed on the anteroposterior projection, it does not form the border of the lateral portion of the kidney. The larger anterior branch is more lateral in location and, therefore, does form the border.

On the arteriogram, there is an orderly progression of opacification of progressively smaller arteries, which eventually blends gradually into the nephrogram. The nephrogram phase of the arteriogram (Fig. 11-3B), which lasts between 4 and 10 seconds after the beginning of the injection, represents the collection of contrast medium within the glomeruli, tubules, capillaries, and small veins. The renal cortical tissue is more densely stained and is well differentiated from the renal medulla. The even thickness (7 to 10 mm) of the renal cortex and the homogeneous blush of cortical tissue in the septa of Bertin are normal characteristics. The renal veins opacify in 10 to 12 seconds following the injection.

The demonstration of collateral flow is an important function of renal arteriography [54]. Collaterals are usually extrarenal in origin and bring blood from a source outside the kidney to the compromised renal circulation. There are three major networks arising from the main renal artery that take part in collateral flow: the pericapsular, perihilar, and periureteric branches. These vessels communicate with branches arising away from the renal artery, namely, the phrenic, intercostal, lumbar, adrenal, gonadal, and ureteric arteries. In addition, ureteric vessels communicate directly with the hypogastric arteries (see Fig. 10-27). Collateral flow is stimulated through some or all of these vessels if there is obstruction to the main renal artery proximal to the origin of these vessel complexes.

Capsular arteries can also supply the intrarenal circulation by means of perforating branches that communicate directly within intrarenal arcuate ar-

Table 11-1. Technical specifications in arteriography of the kidneys[a]

Arteriographic procedure	Contrast agent			Total films	Total time (sec)	Radiographic program[d] (films/sec)	Projections
	Density	Volume (ml/inj)	Rate (ml/sec)				
Adult							
Aortogram (standard)							AP. Obliques are optional. RPO is most likely to show origin of both renal arteries in profile
Straight or pigtail catheter	M, Nl	40–50	25	12	12	2/sec for 3 sec; 1/sec for 3 sec; 1 every other sec for 6 sec	
Ring catheter	M, Nl	35–40	25	12	12		
Alternate procedure (with rapid flow)	M, Nl	40–50	25	12	11	3/sec for 2 sec; 1/sec for 3 sec; 1 every other sec for 6 sec	
Selective catheterization							
Single renal artery	L	10–12[c]	6	12	12	3/sec for 2 sec; 1/sec for 2 sec; 1 every other sec for 8 sec	Supine 45 degrees oblique with involved side up shows kidney en face; involved side down shows it in profile
Accessory renal artery	L	Smaller doses (proportional to vessel size)					
Child[b]		Varies with body weight					
Aortogram							
Infants	L	1.0–1.5 ml/kg	Total within 1–1½ sec	12	8	3/sec for 2 sec; 2/sec for 2 sec; 1 every other sec for 4 sec	
Others	M, Nl						
Selective catheterization	L	2–10 ml (depends on size of vessel)	Total within 1–1½ sec	12	8		

[a]For IA-DSA studies, use half concentration of contrast agent but same volume and injection rates. Use nonionic contrast agents if renal function is compromised.

[b]Amount of contrast agent varies with body weight in children.

[c]This dosage can be doubled or tripled if a large hypervascular lesion is present, or it can be halved if there is a hypoplastic kidney.

[d]Start exposures 0.4 sec after start of injection.

M = medium density contrast agent; L = low density contrast agent; Nl = Nonionic contrast agent; (see Appendix 3).

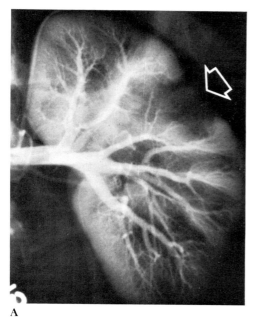

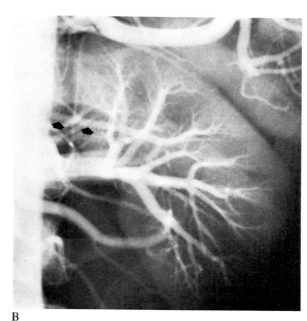

A   B

Fig. 11-2.

A. Selective left renal arteriography showing avascular area in the midlateral portion of the kidney (*arrow*).

B. This area is supplied by an accessory renal artery arising from the aorta (*arrows*).

Fig. 11-3. Normal renal arteriogram (see text for details).

A. Arterial phase. 10 ml of low density contrast agent was selectively injected by a pressure injector in 1½ seconds. Focal-spot size is 0.3 mm; magnification is ×2.

B. A nephrogram phase lasts up to 10 seconds after the beginning of the injection, and the veins fill several seconds later.

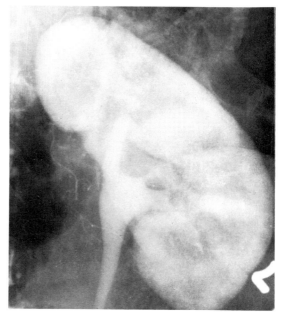

A   B

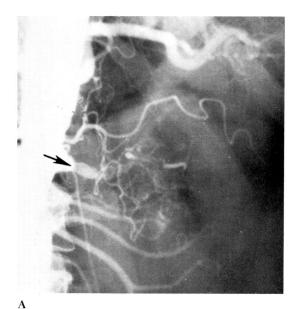

A

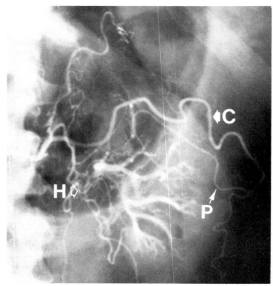

B

Fig. 11-4. Renal collaterals.
A. Aortogram showing almost total occlusion of the left main renal artery (*arrow*) due to atherosclerosis. The middle adrenal and capsular arteries are prominent.
B. Selective injection of the middle adrenal artery and the capsular complex shows that the capsular branches (C) and perihilar complexes (H) fill the renal artery distal to the stenosis. There is a perforating artery (P) arising from the capsular complex and entering the kidney through the periphery of its midportion.

teries (Fig. 11-4). Collaterals can form within the kidney from one obstructed interlobar branch to another by means of a sinus or pericaliceal collateral network of spiral vessels (Fig. 11-5; see Fig. 11-34). These collaterals communicate between interlobar and arcuate branches and are also thought to join with the vasa recta, thus providing blood to the juxtaglomerular circulation of the kidney. These collateral spiral vessels should not be mistaken for an angioma.

General Technical Considerations in Renal Angiography

A review of preliminary films prior to the study may reveal important information, such as calcium in a renal mass or curvilinear calcium in an aneurysm. The intravenous pyelogram should also be studied, because it may show pyelocaliceal defects of epithelial tumors or distortion and mass effect of renal cell carcinomas.

In many patients a computed tomography (CT) examination precedes renal arteriography. Computed tomography is a sensitive examination for an adrenal lesion, which may be the cause of hypertension. When intravenous contrast material is used, CT is able to detect all but the smallest renal mass lesions. Care must be taken to avoid performing high-volume contrast studies on consecutive

days, however, as this increases the chance of contrast-induced renal failure.

Selective renal arteriography in multiple projections with well-coned films is essential for good detail. In a supine patient, a 45-degree oblique projection with the side of interest raised brings the kidney en face; when the side of interest is down, the kidney is seen on end. At least 4 or 5 kV should be added to the radiographic technique in order to penetrate the greater density of tissue with the latter projection. The angiographer should make sure that the catheter is filled with undiluted contrast medium prior to the injection. The arterial, nephrogram, and venous phases of the circulation should be carefully studied; the lesion may not be apparent until late in the series. Magnification studies and pharmacoangiography can sometimes be useful (see Fig. 4-1).

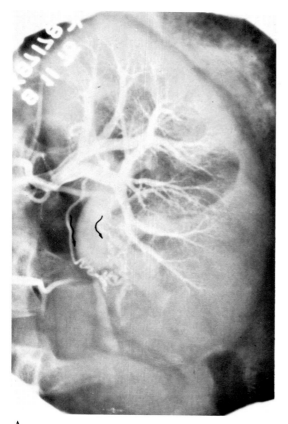

A

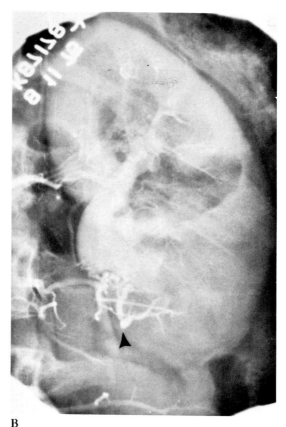

B

Fig. 11-5.
A. Intrarenal spiral collaterals and extrarenal perihilar renal collaterals (*arrows*). Previous surgical occlusion of an aberrant vessel causing ureteropelvic junction obstruction resulted in an inferior pole renal infarct and subsequent hypertension.
B. Intrarenal collaterals fill the interlobar and arcuate branches of the occluded segment (*arrowhead*).

Selective catheterization should be performed with care, particularly if there is stenosis in the proximal third of the renal artery or if the catheter tip is near a plaque, because there is danger of infarction. Side holes are not needed in selective renal artery catheters because only a small dose of contrast agent is required; because side holes add the hazard of clot formation, which can subsequently embolize, they should not be used (see Figs. 3-37, 3-38). Overinjecting in a wedge position not only can endanger the kidney but also can cause artifacts of interpretation (Fig. 11-6).

An abdominal aortogram is often useful as a guide to renal anatomy and as an assessment of the main renal arteries prior to selective catheterization. If a small lesion is suspected and no renal artery stenosis is anticipated, however, a selective study performed prior to the aortogram ensures that the vessels are not obscured by contrast-filled calices.

Diagnostic Approach and Angiographic Findings for Renal Masses

SEQUENCE OF DIAGNOSIS

The diagnostic approach for renal masses should be performed by the angiographer in the following sequence:

1. Intravenous pyelogram (IVP). A plain film of the abdomen and a retrograde pyelogram, if the collecting system is not well seen, should be included.
2. Renal ultrasound. If the lesion satisfies the cri-

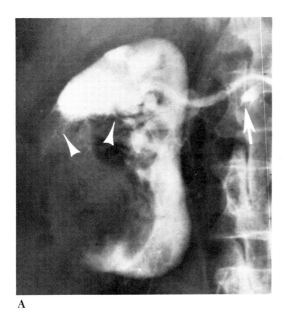

A

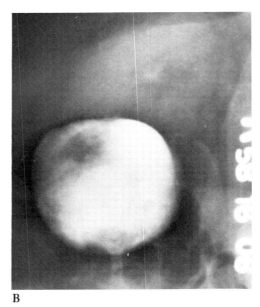

B

Fig. 11-6. Artifact of overinjection and complication of arterial dissection.

A. Lower pole segmental branch is dissected (*arrow*). Overinjection in the remaining branch shows dense focal areas of staining and poor margination of the avascular renal mass, suggesting neoplasm (*arrowheads*).

B. Benign nature of lesion proved by cyst puncture.

teria of a benign simple cyst, the examination may be stopped; however, if atypical features are present, additional studies, such as CT, angiography, or cyst puncture are needed.

3. Computed tomography. CT is useful for detecting, characterizing, and staging renal mass lesions. In some cases, such as cyst or angiomyolipoma, CT can make a benign diagnosis, and further evaluation is not needed. When a solid mass lesion, suspected of being an adenocarcinoma, is present, CT also serves as a staging examination [52].

4. Angiography. Angiography supplements CT in the staging of renal masses suspected of being primary renal adenocarcinoma. Selective venography may be needed to precisely define the extent of venous extension. Arteriography provides a vascular "road map" for the surgeon, as well as assesses the degree of vascularity of the tumor. In many patients, both venous and arterial evaluation may be obtained with a single injection in the inferior vena cava and digital examination of the arteries.

TECHNICAL FACTORS

1. Prior to the study, prepare for an extensive workup, which includes aortography, selective renal arteriograms in multiple projections, opacification of the renal vein, selective retroperitoneal arteriography (adrenals, lumbars),

selective celiac axis arteriography, and inferior vena cavography. Reserve any therapeutic attempts for another day, because therapeutic renovascular occlusion following a diagnostic study with large doses of contrast agent may induce renal failure.

2. If the tumor has questionable neovascularity, pharmacoangiography may be helpful [3] (see Fig. 4-1). Inject 15 to 20 ml of contrast agent slowly (3 or 4 ml per second) immediately following intraarterial injection of 5 to 10 μg of epinephrine. (One milligram per ampule equals 1,000 μg; place 1 mg in 10 ml of saline, remove 1 ml of this, and dilute it to 10 ml. Each milliliter now contains 10 μg.) The films should be taken slowly over a long period; 12 films over a period of 20 seconds is usually adequate.

3. In angiography of a known tumor, look carefully for the full extent of malignancy (Figs. 11-7, 11-8) including venous extension and arterial supply. The contralateral kidney can usually be assessed on the abdominal aortogram.

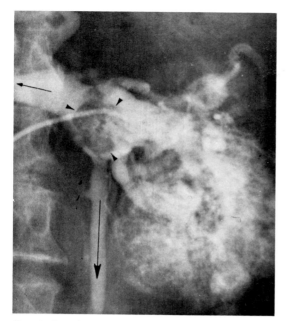

Fig. 11-7. A large hypervascular malignant tumor of the left kidney is seen on the venous phase of a high-dose left renal artery injection. There are numerous collateral veins and a large tumor thrombus (*arrowheads*) lying within the left renal vein (*small arrow*). There is retrograde flow down the testicular vein (*large arrow*). The tumor is a renal adenocarcinoma.

ARTERIOGRAPHIC FINDINGS FOR SPACE-OCCUPYING PROCESSES

Primary Renal Tumors

ADENOCARCINOMA (CLEAR CELL, HYPERNE-PHROMA) (Figs. 11-7, 11-8, 11-9). Typical findings that are seen in 65 to 85 percent of patients with these tumors are hypervascularity with large feeding vessels displacing segmental arteries, and neovascularity with irregularity of arterial walls, vascular lakes, arteriovenous shunting, and vessels showing lack of purposeful direction [16]. There is usually a tumor stain, and there may be perivascu-

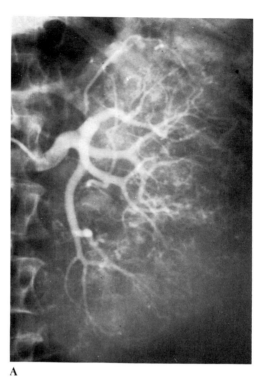

A

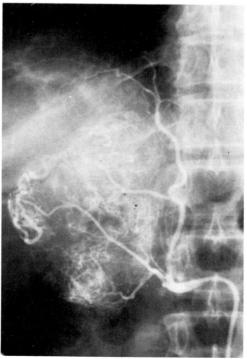

B

Fig. 11-8. Renal adenocarcinoma diffusely involving the left kidney with metastases to the opposite adrenal gland. Previous right nephrectomy was performed for hypernephroma.
A. Selective left renal arteriogram shows tumor neovascularity and large lakes of contrast medium.
B. Right adrenal arteriogram.

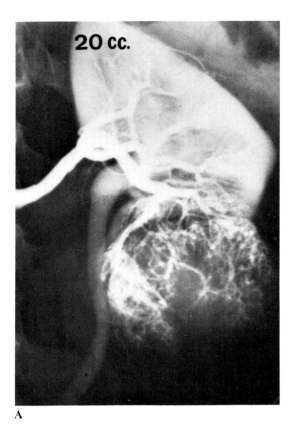

A

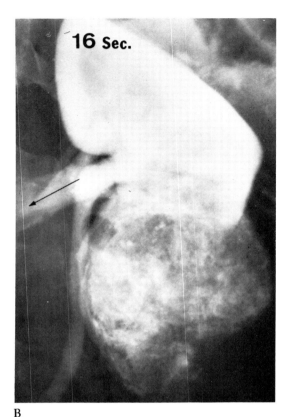

B

Fig. 11-9.
A. High-dose injection of kidney with a renal mass.
B. The renal vein is clearly outlined and is involved with tumor (*arrow*).

lar segmental areas of "cuffing" or narrowing. The renal vein may be occluded by thrombosis as well as by tumor. Sometimes neovascularity can be seen in the tumor along the course of the renal vein. Collateral venous channels do not necessarily mean an occluded renal vein, because extra renal veins do drain a tumor that has a parasitic blood supply.

Less often, these tumors may be hypovascular (15 to 35 percent). Hypovascular tumors show only vascular displacement, perivascular cuffing or occlusion, an ill-defined border, and sometimes small collections of increased vessels or neovascularity (Fig. 11-10). There is no arteriovenous shunting. The tumor may lie in the base of an otherwise benign-appearing cyst, or there may be cystic degeneration of a hypovascular tumor (Fig. 11-11).

EMBRYONAL CELL CARCINOMA (WILMS' TUMOR) [33]. Angiography has not been used as extensively in evaluating renal masses in the pediatric population as it has in adults. Although controversy exists as to the role of angiography in pediatric patients,

important information may be obtained, including not only the diagnosis of tumor but also a definition of its extent. Angiography can determine patency of the renal vein and impingement on the inferior vena cava (Fig. 11-12). Demonstration of the presence of bilateral tumors and evaluation of spread to other organs are also important (Fig. 11-13).

Although 90 percent of these tumors occur in patients under age 5, and the majority of patients with Wilms' tumor are below 3 years of age, the tumor can occur in the older age group as well. The differential diagnosis between Wilms' tumor and neuroblastoma is important and is sometimes difficult even with angiography. Arteriography may show surprisingly few changes, although this is unusual (Fig. 11-14). Often the findings are displaced intrarenal vessels, poor demarcation of normal from abnormal renal parenchyma, only slight hypervascularity, and varying degrees of tumor

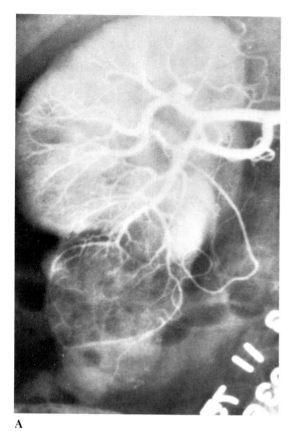

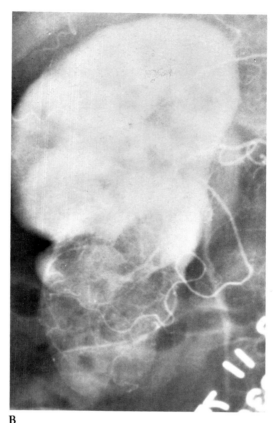

A

B

Fig. 11-10. Hypovascular adenocarcinoma of the lower pole of the right kidney.
A. Arterial phase.
B. Nephrogram phase. There is poor demarcation of tumor from the remaining kidney. There is only minimal neovascularity. A fairly homogeneous blush is seen throughout the tumor in the nephrogram phase.

neovascularity. This neovascularity is most prominent in the late arterial, early capillary phase, and there is relative lack of tumor stain. Large tumors displace adjacent normal vessels.

Epithelial Tumors

Epithelial tumors (squamous cell and transitional cell) [37] are hypovascular and are best studied by pyelograms. Occasionally they show prominent pelviureteric feeding arteries in a fine, reticular neovascularity but without arteriovenous shunting. Vascular encasement may also be present (Figs. 11-15, 11-16). These tumors are sometimes difficult to differentiate from inflammatory renal masses.

Other Malignant Lesions

Rarely tumors may arise from the connective, fatty, lymphoid, neural, and vascular tissues of the parenchyma, pelvis, or renal capsule.

Benign Tumors

ANGIOMYOLIPOMAS. Angiomyolipomas (hamartomas) are tumors composed of blood vessels, smooth muscle, and fatty tissue. They may be solitary and asymptomatic in young people. When they are a part of the spectrum of tuberous sclerosis, they are multiple, often bilateral, and are found in other systems. The solitary forms may be hypervascular, are more prone to hemorrhage and infarction, and may be indistinguishable angiographically from clear cell carcinomas (Fig. 11-17). The presence of macroscopic fat on CT strongly suggests an angiomyolipoma; however, the radiographic appearance, either by CT or angiography, depends upon the relative amounts of the muscular, vascular, and fatty tissues in the tumor. Those tumors associated with tuberous

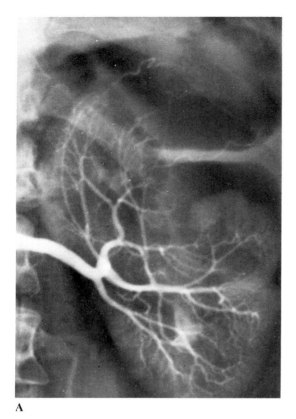

A

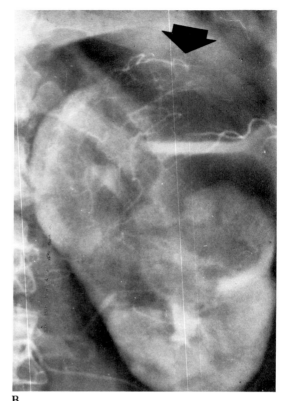

B

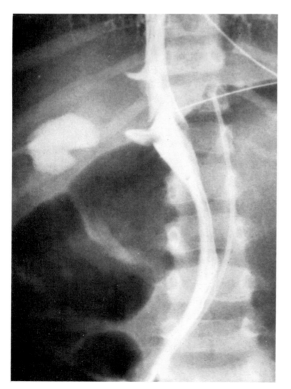

Fig. 11-11.
A. Cystic malignant tumor of the left kidney.
B. Minimal neovascularity is shown (*arrow*) over the
   surface of the cystic lesion.

sclerosis have multiple aneurysms or aneurysmal
dilatations of the interlobar and arcuate arteries in
addition to the hypervascularity of the tumor. Mi-
crocysts have also been described throughout the
rest of the kidney.

ADENOMAS. Adenomas may be homogeneously
hypervascular, hypovascular, or avascular. Surgery
is usually required to determine the precise diagnosis [43] (Fig. 11-18).

Metastatic Lesions
Lesions metastatic to the kidney usually reflect the
vascularity of the primary tumor. They are often
small and may be difficult to detect angiographically, particularly if the metastatic deposit lies in
the periphery of the kidney. Often perivascular en-

Fig. 11-12. Wilms' tumor. The inferior vena cava is
displaced by the mass.

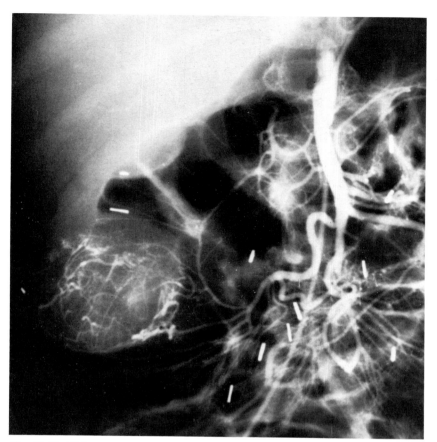

Fig. 11-13. Wilms' tumor metastatic to the mesentery. Superior mesenteric arteriogram shows a hypervascular mass.

casement due to periarterial lymphatic tumor involvement is observed (Fig. 11-19).

Benign Cysts

Benign renal cysts are avascular, sharply demarcated, smoothly marginated, space-occupying lesions. These characteristics are best seen on the nephrographic phase of the examination. The arteries are smoothly stretched and curved by the cyst and show no neovascularity (Figs. 11-20, 11-21). It is difficult to exclude malignancy on the basis of arteriography alone, and CT or cyst puncture is often needed [53]. If there is calcium in the rim of the cyst, there is a 20 percent chance of underlying malignancy (Fig. 11-22).

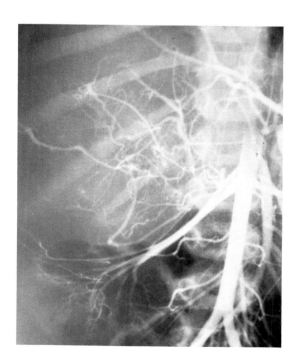

Fig. 11-14. Wilms' tumor of the right kidney upper pole showing tumor neovascularity.

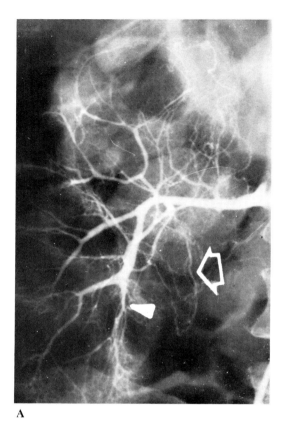

A

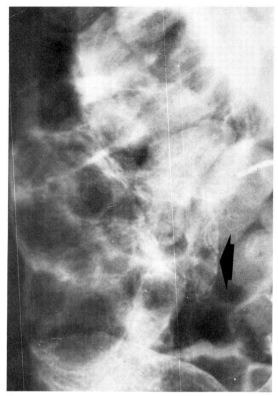

B

Fig. 11-15. Poorly vascularized transitional cell carcinoma of the kidney.
A. Arterial phase. Prominent pelviureteric branches and fine small vessel neovascularity are present diffusely through the pelvis (*arrow*). There is irregularity of the vessels due to periarterial cuffing (*arrowhead*).
B. Nephrogram phase. Avascular cystic structures represent hydronephrotic calices due to caliceal obstruction. Arrow points to prominent capillary network in the tumor in the renal hilus.

Polycystic Renal Disease

Polycystic renal disease is bilateral and may be accompanied by cystic involvement of the liver. Excretory urography, ultrasound, or CT is usually adequate to define the extent of disease. If arteriography is performed, smooth stretching of the arteries around cysts of varying sizes is seen. On the parenchymal phase, there is a characteristic irregular mottled appearance that is thought to be caused by multiple compressed small veins in the kidney. In addition, the margin of the renal cortex is irregular, with multiple smooth avascular concavities marring the otherwise smooth surface of the renal margin (Fig. 11-23). This appearance contrasts with that seen in hydronephrosis, in which the cortical margins are smooth (Fig. 11-24).

Multicystic Dysplasia

A multicystic dysplastic kidney is a collection of cysts but with no functioning renal tissue. The ipsilateral renal vessels are absent (Fig. 11-25), and the ureter is atretic.

Hydronephrosis

In hydronephrosis (Fig. 11-24) the kidneys have avascular, urine-filled sacs in place of the normal pelvis and calices. The margins of the dilated calices are smooth, as is the margin of the kidney; this appearance is best seen late in the nephrogram phase. As in all vessels feeding organs with reduced function and circulatory requirements, the main renal arterial diameter secondarily becomes smaller than normal. Typically the origin of the renal artery from the aorta is of normal width, with a rapid, tapered reduction in size. This appearance

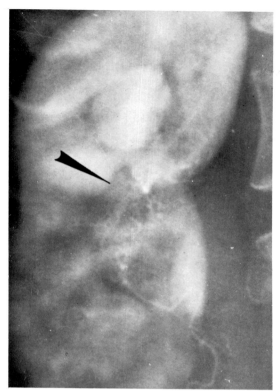

Fig. 11-16. Small collection of fine vessels (*arrowhead*) in a right-sided transitional cell carcinoma. Note obstruction of the upper pole calices.

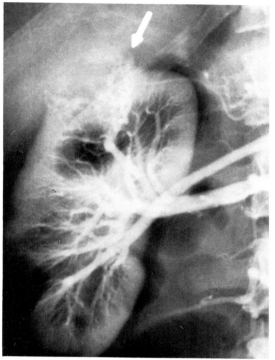

Fig. 11-17. Solitary hamartoma (*arrow*). (See text for details.) Tortuous, bizarre-appearing hypervascularity made it difficult to differentiate this tumor from a hypernephroma.

contrasts with that seen in a congenitally hypoplastic kidney, in which the renal artery is of small diameter throughout its entire length.

Pseudotumor

A pseudotumor is an overgrowth of normal parenchymal tissue that simulates a tumor roentgenologically. Histologically, however, it consists of normal renal parenchyma. It is thought to be a local overgrowth of normal renal substance occurring through compensatory hypertrophy in response to focal or diffuse disturbance of function or as a result of a maldevelopment. It can follow infection, infarction, obstruction, trauma, or maldevelopment. Often it appears to be an infolding of a column of Bertin (Fig. 11-26). A pseudotumor may present roentgenologically as a discrete mass or a segmental enlargement of the kidney which may be located within the renal substance or may extend beyond the renal outline. Pyelocaliceal defects may be apparent on urography, but on the

nephrogram phase of the IVP and on angiography, the "lesion" is represented by a homogeneous blush that fills and empties concomitantly with filling and emptying of the remaining normal renal cortical tissue.

Subacute and Chronic Infection

In subacute and chronic infection [26, 49] a hyperemic neovascular pattern with vessel encasement may be present, much as is seen in malignant neoplasms. In addition, the vessels respond to epinephrine in a fashion similar to that seen in tumors. Although the vascular hyperemic pattern is more of a reticular pattern and is more likely to surround the periphery of the lesion than to permeate it throughout, it may be difficult or impossible to differentiate the hyperemic neovascularity of inflammation from that of tumor. If this distinction cannot be made by CT or percutaneous biopsy, surgery may be required. The following types of infection may occur:

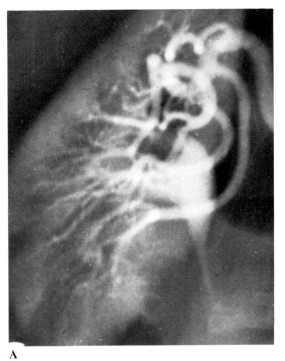

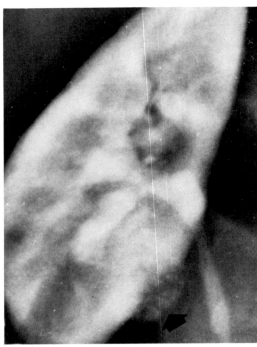

A

B

Fig. 11-18.
A. Renal cortical adenoma.
B. Note the diffuse vascularity (*arrow*) throughout the tumor. This diagnosis should be substantiated by surgery.

Fig. 11-19. A and B. Metastases to the right kidney from a primary carcinoma in the lung. There is periarterial invasion of the hilar vessels.

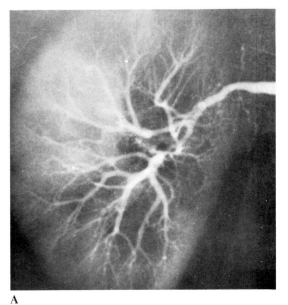

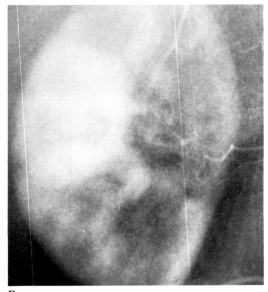

A

B

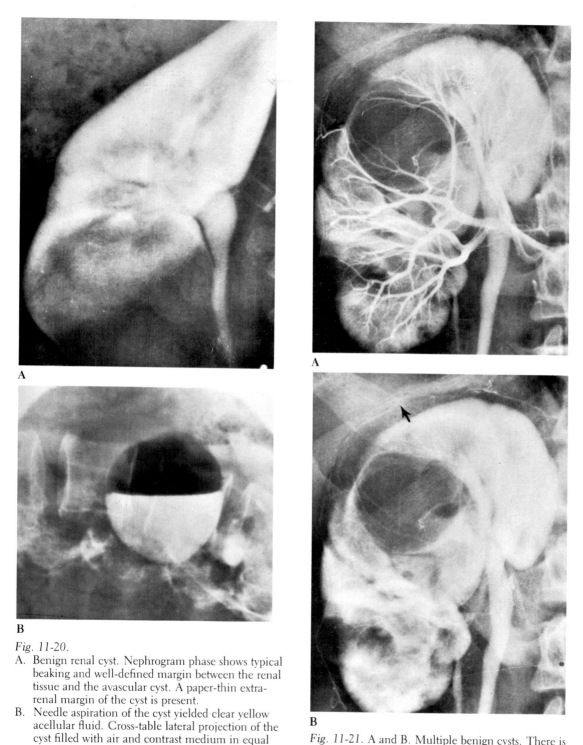

Fig. 11-20.

A. Benign renal cyst. Nephrogram phase shows typical beaking and well-defined margin between the renal tissue and the avascular cyst. A paper-thin extra-renal margin of the cyst is present.

B. Needle aspiration of the cyst yielded clear yellow acellular fluid. Cross-table lateral projection of the cyst filled with air and contrast medium in equal parts shows smooth internal margins, indicating its benign nature.

Fig. 11-21. A and B. Multiple benign cysts. There is smooth displacement of intrarenal vessels (*arrow*) around the cysts. Prominent capsular arteries are noted around the upper pole.

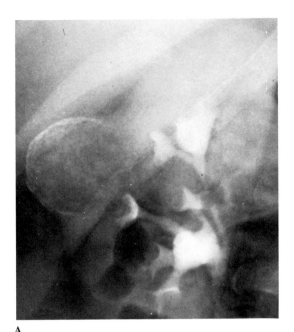

A

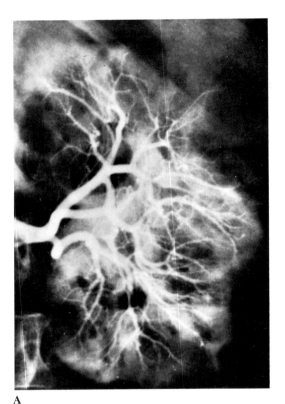

A

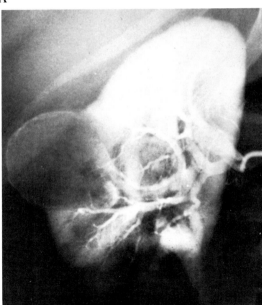

B

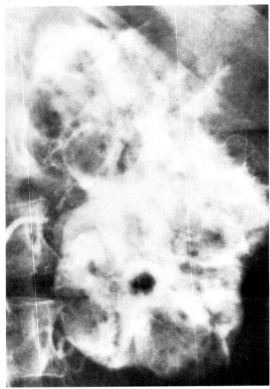

B

Fig. 11-22.
A. Calcified renal cyst on intravenous pyelogram.
B. Benign appearance on arteriogram. Needle aspirate was bloody and chocolate brown in color. Despite negative cytology, malignancy was encountered at surgery.

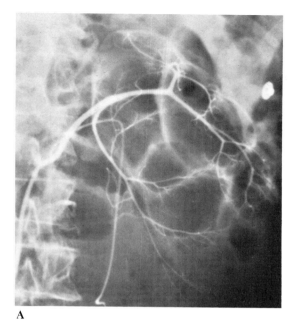

A

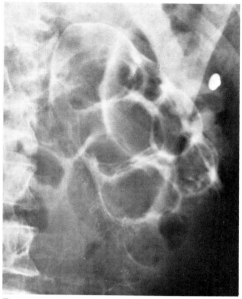

B

Fig. 11-24. A and B. Hydronephrosis. There is a very thin cortex surrounding massively dilated calices. The smooth margin of this kidney distinguishes this lesion from multiple cysts of polycystic disease. The main renal artery is hypoplastic due to decreased renal function. There is smooth displacement of intrarenal vessels over dilated calices.

1. Renal abscess (Fig. 11-27). A renal abscess often shows up as a hyperemic mass, sometimes with a well-defined hypovascular area that represents the necrotic center. The inflammatory process causes the normally sharp margin of the renal parenchyma to blend in with surrounding perinephric tissues.
2. Pyonephrosis (Fig. 11-28). In pyonephrosis the hydronephrotic sac margins and the margin of the renal cortex tend to blend in with the surrounding tissues, and the sharp demarcation from normal nephrogram and surrounding tissue is lost. Varying degrees of hypervascularity and neovascularity resulting from hyperemia

---

Fig. 11-23.
A. Adult form of polycystic renal disease in a hypertensive middle-aged patient with a positive family history.
B. The irregular cortex and multiple avascular radiolucencies seen on the nephrogram are characteristic and indicate a large number of cortical and medullary cysts.

may be seen. The vascularity seen here, particularly in the caliceal structures, is indistinguishable from that seen in epithelial tumors.
3. Xanthogranulomatous pyelonephritis. This condition is indistinguishable angiographically from pyonephrosis and advanced cases of transitional cell carcinoma. Some of the avascular areas represent granulomas rather than dilated sacs (Fig. 11-29).

DIAGNOSTIC PROCEDURES. A patient with a renal space-occupying process should be initially examined by urography (including nephrotomography). Radioisotope studies can substantiate a questionable area on the IVP as being normal renal parenchyma or can point the way to further studies. Ultrasound is most useful in confirming the benign features of a cystic lesion detected by urography. Computed tomography does an excellent job of defining renal mass lesions, and cyst puncture is not often required.

TECHNIQUES OF NEEDLE ASPIRATION. With the patient prone, sterilely prepare the skin overlying the cyst. If fluoroscopy is used, the kidney can be opacified with intravenous contrast material.

Marcaine is used to infiltrate the skin and subcutaneous tissues. A variety of needles may be used, but a 20- or 22-gauge 15-cm needle suffices for most cases. As the needle enters the cyst, there

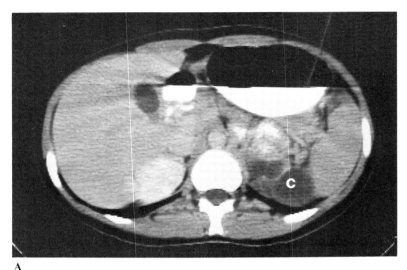

A

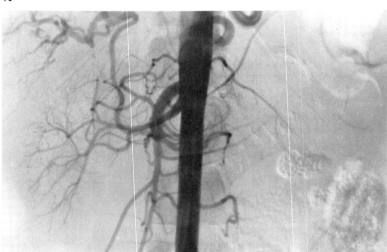

B

Fig. 11-25. Multicystic dysplastic kidney.
A. CT demonstrates a collection of cysts in the left renal fossa (C).
B. Aortography demonstrates a normal right renal artery but complete absence of the left renal artery.

is often a sudden decrease in resistance. Gentle aspiration usually results in fluid for analysis.

When ultrasound is used as the guiding modality, a second window to the lesion is often helpful. With this technique the most direct path is used for the needle aspiration. The second ultrasound window allows visual confirmation of the needle tip within the lesion.

Benign cysts yield a clear, straw-colored aspirate with a low fat, protein, and lactic dehydrogenase (LDH) content and a slightly elevated glucose level. No abnormal cells are evident on microscopy. Cystic or necrotic tumors and neoplasm associated with a cyst yield a bloody or murky aspirate with a high fat and protein content and normal LDH and glucose levels. Tumor cells may or may not be seen. Inflammatory cysts yield a murky or bloody aspirate with mildly elevated fat and protein content, a glucose level slightly lower than that of blood, and a markedly elevated LDH content. Malignant cells are not present. If contrast media are injected and radiographs in multiple projections demonstrate irregular walls or if fluid contents are suspicious, surgical exploration is generally required. Contraindications to punc-

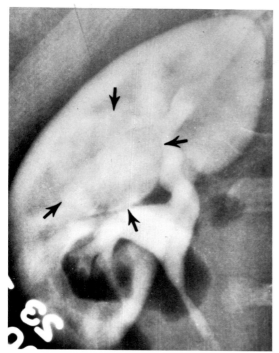

Fig. 11-26. Pseudotumor. Nephrogram of a selective arteriogram shows a homogeneous blush which fills and empties concomitant with the remaining normal cortical tissue. There was mild displacement of vessels over this area on the arteriographic phase, with no neovascularity.

turing a cyst include a neurovascular or hematologic abnormality that may cause bleeding, or a suspected echinococcal cyst.

With the advent of CT and ultrasound, renal cysts are often sufficiently well characterized that percutaneous aspiration is seldom needed. If clear yellow or straw-colored fluid is obtained, further laboratory analysis is probably not necessary; however, a positive cytology or fat stain correlates best with the presence of malignancy.

Complications of needle aspiration include renal lacerations, entry into aneurysms, renal colic due to blood clots entering the collecting system, and infection of the cyst.

Sometimes the needle is positioned at the

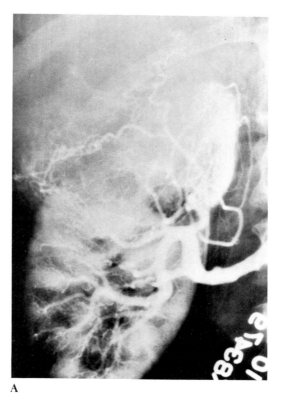

A

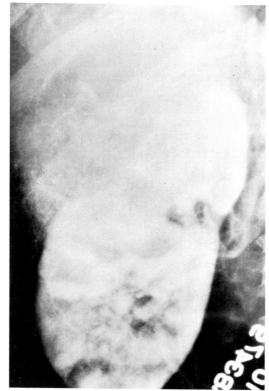

B

Fig. 11-27.
A. Renal abscess. Neovascularity and a predominant supply from the capsular arteries suggest tumor. The mass was "complex" on ultrasound.
B. It was indistinguishable arteriographically from a cystic malignancy.

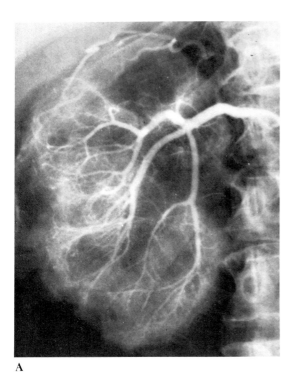

A

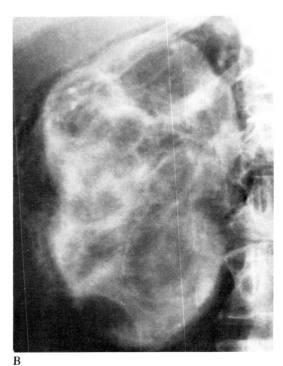

B

Fig. 11-28. A and B. Pyonephrosis. The vessels are splayed around dilated calices. There is a fine neovascularity scattered throughout, and a poor definition between the renal cortex and surrounding tissues, indicating a perinephric component.

boundary of the benign cyst and the adjacent normal parenchyma. Clear fluid is obtained, but the injection is diffuse and poorly marginated. If this occurs, remove the needle and repuncture. Patients with symptomatic cysts require draining and sclerosing the cyst walls to prevent reaccumulation of fluid. This may be accomplished by injecting into the cyst small quantities of iophendylate (Pantopaque) (6 ml if the volume of the cyst is over 100 ml, 3 ml if it is under 100 ml). Better results are obtained by percutaneously introducing a 4 or 5 French catheter with side holes into the most dependent portion of the cyst and removing its contents. If there is no bloody return, 5 to 10 ml absolute ethanol may be introduced for a period of 20 minutes and then subsequently aspirated.

Angiography of Primary Renal Vascular Disease and Renal Vascular Hypertension

Hypertension is defined as a persistent systemic diastolic pressure over 90 mm Hg. It affects 10 to 15 percent of the American population and occurs at any age, with the highest incidence in persons over age 40. The cause of primary hypertension is unknown; this includes the vast majority of hypertensive patients. In as many as 5 percent of patients, the hypertension has a known cause and the patients are, therefore, potentially curable. In such cases, the hypertension may be a result of renal vascular disease, renal parenchymal or perirenal disease, or functioning tumors of the kidney or adrenal gland [11]. Renal vascular hypertension should be suspected if the patient is at either age extreme (under age 25 or over age 50), if there is a sudden onset or a rapid acceleration of hypertension, if there is malignant hypertension, or if hypertension has developed after trauma. An abdominal bruit in a hypertensive patient under age 50 may point to a stenotic renal vascular lesion. In patients above this age, atherosclerosis is more widespread and the finding is, therefore, less significant.

Angiography is the only preoperative means of precisely demonstrating the location, type, and severity of renal vascular lesions. Vessel stenosis or

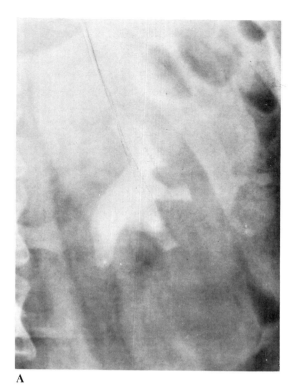

A

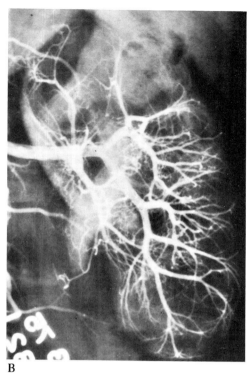

B

Fig. 11-29. Xanthogranulomatous pyelonephritis.
A. Film from intravenous pyelogram shows staghorn
   calculus and poor renal function in a large kidney,
   with a suggestion of a lower pole mass.
B and C. Arteriogram shows intrarenal branches
   splayed over large, dilated calices and granulomata
   with a fine reticular neovascularity both in the pelvis and scattered throughout the renal parenchyma.
   This vascular response to chronic inflammation is
   indistinguishable from the lesions seen in Figure
   11-16 (transitional cell carcinoma).

occlusion, aneurysms, and short circuiting due to
abnormal arteriovenous communications decrease
renal artery pulse pressure and renal blood flow,
which in turn stimulate vasopressor precursor (renin) secretions by the juxtaglomerular apparatus
lying distal to the involved segment. Tumors compress renal parenchyma or (rarely) actively secrete
these vasopressors. The renin released into the renal venous system may be assayed by obtaining
differential renal vein blood samples at the time of
the arteriogram. If renin samples ipsilateral to the
renal vascular lesion are 1½ times or more over
the other side, the lesion is very likely causing
the hypertension, and it should be amenable to
correction. Refinements of this technique include
superselective renal vein catheterization [39], stress

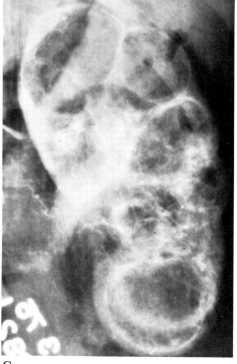

C

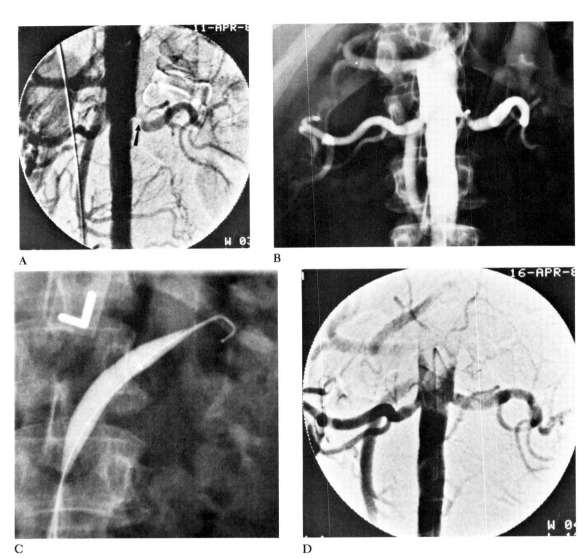

A

B

C

D

Fig. 11-30. Renovascular hypertension. A 58-year-old woman with hypertension difficult to control on medication.

A. IV-DSA demonstrates severe left renal artery stenosis. There was a gradient of 3:1 renin values on the left side compared to the right.

B. Abdominal aortogram confirms severe renal artery stenosis and provides accurate measurement for choice of balloon catheter diameter. There is also mild stenosis of the right renal artery.

C. Renal artery dilatation using an 8-mm-diameter balloon.

D. Post-PTA IA-DSA aortogram demonstrating successfully dilated left renal artery. Blood pressure dropped to near normal limits soon after PTA.

positioning (with the patient upright for 30 minutes), or the administration of an enzyme conversion inhibitor (captopril 25 mg PO) 30 to 60 minutes prior to collection. Spurious results may be obtained if diuretics or a low-salt diet have been used immediately prior to the study, or if the patient has malignant hypertension.

SCREENING METHODS

Diagnostic studies used as screening methods include the following:

1. Intravenous pyelogram. This has been abandoned due to poor sensitivity.
2. Radioisotope renogram.

3. Peripheral vein renin. This is elevated in patients with renovascular hypertension.
4. Intravenous digital subtraction arteriogram (IV-DSA). This has replaced the hypertensive urogram in many institutions, because it images the renal arteries and is easily performed on an outpatient basis [10].

Digital Subtraction Angiography

The application of digital subtraction techniques has had a major impact on the investigation of suspected renovascular hypertension. When performed with intravenous contrast injection (IV-DSA), imaging of the renal arteries becomes a relatively noninvasive procedure that may be performed as an outpatient procedure. Diagnostic studies are obtained on most patients, but patient motion or poor cardiac output with dilution of the contrast bolus degrades the images [20].

The IV-DSA may be performed with either a peripheral or central contrast injection. When a peripheral route is chosen, a large bore needle (16 gauge) or short catheter is placed in a superficial vein in the antecubital fossa, and 10 to 15 ml of contrast material (Renografin 60) is injected for 3 or 4 seconds. If a central route is chosen, selective renal vein samples for renin evaluation may be procured during the same examination (Fig. 11-30).

The initial run is centered over the expected position (L2) of the renal arteries. In some patients, both renal arteries are well seen and the examination can be stopped. In most patients, however, the origin of one of the renal arteries is obscured (often by the superior mesenteric artery), and an additional run is needed. An oblique projection is chosen to get a better look at the area in question.

Because most commercially available units have a 9-inch field of view, an additional run may be needed to evaluate both renal arteries. This is particularly true when an accessory renal artery is present. On the other hand, increased spatial resolution may be obtained if 6- or 4-inch fields are used to cone in on equivocal areas.

Most patients studied with IV-DSA require two or three runs to examine the main renal arteries. Branch renal arteries are inconsistently studied, as they are often out of the field of view. The smaller size of the branch vessels also makes them more difficult to examine due to the decreased spatial resolution of the digital systems.

Plain radiographs or nephrotomograms may be obtained to look for parenchymal abnormalities after the digital examination has been completed.

When performed with an intraarterial contrast injection (IA-DSA), the contrast load is reduced to approximately one-third of that needed for a conventional arteriogram [22]. This is particularly helpful in patients with preexisting azotemia in whom a large contrast load is likely to exacerbate renal failure. The IA-DSA also usually produces better images than IV-DSA because the contrast bolus is more concentrated over the area of interest. The disadvantage of IA-DSA is the necessity of an arterial puncture.

CONVENTIONAL ANGIOGRAPHY

Angiography should outline all vessels to both kidneys, usually in more than one projection (anteroposterior and right posterior oblique). Midstream aortography performed through a catheter with multiple side holes that has been introduced percutaneously from the femoral approach ensures that all vessels supplying the kidney are seen. Although renal arteries usually arise singly at the L1 to L2 level, accessory arteries may occur at any level from the low thoracic aorta to the iliac vessels. Early rapid sequential filling of vessels by rapidly administered contrast medium provides information about the renal arteries as they arise from the aorta, and films later in the series depict intrarenal vascularity and integrity of the nephrogram. Selective magnification studies may provide additional information in otherwise occult lesions. Pharmacoangiography may give information regarding the significance of a located lesion [12].

The angiographic hallmark of a significant area of stenosis is the presence of collateral vessels. The most common collaterals are peripelvic, pericapsular, and periureteric; other arteries involved include the lumbars, phrenics, adrenals, gonadals, and intercostals. Collaterals can also arise from within the kidney from one segmental branch to the next [24]. It is important to demonstrate the degree of stenosis; at least 50 percent and probably 80 percent stenosis must be present to be hemodynamically significant. Other findings that may be significant include a decrease in the size of the kidney (at least 1½ cm smaller), a delay in the circulation time, and poststenotic dilatation of the artery.

The pitfalls of angiography of the kidneys must

be avoided. They include a finding of differential kidney size due to a double collecting system and not to a renal arterial or parenchymal abnormality, and nonopacification of an accessory artery or a segmental renal branch due to catheter placement, which may mimic a renal infarct. Overlapping of vessel origins and intrarenal branches may hide stenoses or aneurysms. Selective overfilling of a renal artery can stain tissue and simulate vascular tumor blush. Preferential overfilling and delayed emptying of the vessels to one of the kidneys, suggesting pathology, may be caused by catheter position. Selective catheter tips can cause renal arterial spasm (see Fig. 4-7). Transient "stationary arterial waves" can mimic pathologic abnormalities (see Fig. 11-42). Iatrogenic artifacts such as dissection of an artery (see Fig. 11-6) and intrarenal embolization (see Fig. 3-38) can occur.

ANGIOGRAPHIC FINDINGS

The angiographic findings in hypertension stem from the involvement of the kidneys by primary vascular disease, parenchymal disease, or perirenal disease.

Prerenal Vascular Disease

The findings in prerenal vascular disease include:

1. Aortic atherosclerosis, with plaques obstructing the renal artery origin. Aortic aneurysm can cause extrinsic pressure of renal arteries.
2. Aortic dissection (see Fig. 10-19).
3. Aortic coarctation, either within the thorax or in the abdomen (see Fig. 10-26).
4. Aortic occlusion above the renal arteries, which may occur as a result of thrombosis and embolus.
5. Aortitis (Takayasu's disease has a 75 to 80 percent incidence of hypertension) (see Fig. 18-34).
6. Neurofibromatosis, which can cause narrowing of the thoracic and abdominal aorta or the main renal arteries due to intimal and medial proliferation, or to intramural neurofibromatous nodules (see Fig. 10-27).

Primary Renal Artery Lesions

ATHEROSCLEROSIS. Atherosclerosis occurs predominantly in persons over 45 years of age, with a higher incidence in males than in females (2:1). There is an increased incidence in those with hy-

perlipidemia and in those who are diabetic. The lesion, which is usually in the proximal third of the artery, varies in severity from small plaques to complete occlusion (see Figs. 11-1, 11-4, 11-30, 11-31). Usually the lesion is localized, and it is often eccentric but may be concentric in nature. It is bilateral in 30 to 50 percent of patients. Atherosclerotic lesions may also occur intrarenally, although they are much more frequent in the main renal artery. Lesions may progress to complete thrombosis and subsequent infarction of the kidney.

FIBROMUSCULAR DYSPLASIA. Fibromuscular dysplasia is found in patients in the younger age group, with a mean age of 35 years. It is more frequent in females, with a ratio of 3:1. It is more often seen in the middle and distal third of the main renal arteries, and it has a higher incidence of branch stenosis than that seen in atherosclerosis. The disease is bilateral in 40 percent of patients. It is sometimes acompanied by renal artery and intracranial aneurysms. The vessels of multiple systems may be involved (brachiocephalic, splanchnic, iliacs). The cause of this disease is unknown, but it is developmental and can be progressive in nature. The different forms of fibromuscular dysplasia are described in Chapter 8. The characteristic "string of beads" appearance seen in Figure 11-32 is caused by medial fibroplasia with aneurysm. A concentric focal area of narrowing due to medial fibromuscular hyperplasia is seen in Figure 11-33. A tubular focal form of narrowing of the intrarenal branches is seen in Figure 11-34. These lesions can be complicated by thrombosis and dissection. Medial fibroplasia, with or without aneurysms, is the most common variety of this disease.

FIBROUS OR MUSCULAR BANDS. Fibrous or muscular bands may occlude the renal artery at its origin from the aorta. These bands can arise from the crux of the diaphragm or from muscular strands arising from the psoas muscle (Fig. 11-35).

EMBOLI. Emboli are often bilateral. The underlying disease is usually cardiac. Filling defects and sharp cutoffs are usually observed at bifurcations, and absent collaterals are observed with a peripheral infarct.

DISSECTION. Dissection usually occurs in patients with cystic medial necrosis of the aorta. It can also arise within an aneurysm; it may occur in an area of fibromuscular dysplasia; or it may be iatrogenic. Arteriographically, intimal flaps,

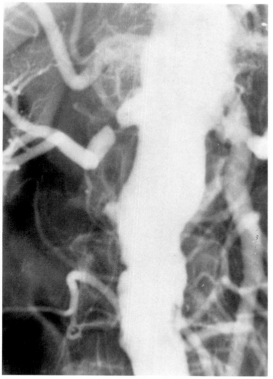

A

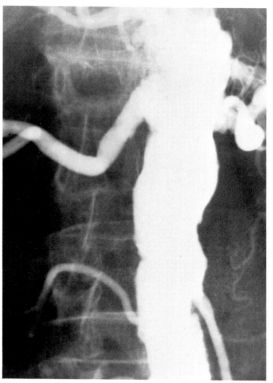

B

Fig. 11-31. Atherosclerosis.
A. A high-grade right renal artery stenosis as well as extensive changes of atherosclerosis are seen.
B. Percutaneous transluminal angioplasty has eliminated the renal artery stenosis.

Fig. 11-32. Fibromuscular dysplasia.
A. Selective right renal arteriogram reveals typical beaded appearance of fibromuscular dysplasia.
B. After angioplasty the renal artery stenosis has been obliterated and the patient became normotensive.

smooth areas of narrowing, and opacification of false lumina with delayed emptying may be observed.

RENAL ARTERY ANEURYSM. Renal artery aneurysm [44] (Figs. 11-36, 11-37) is caused by a weakening of the arterial wall, with degeneration of elastic tissue. It may be congenital, degenerative, traumatic, or inflammatory (mycotic), but most frequently it is atherosclerotic in origin. Aneurysms can be associated with fibromuscular dys-

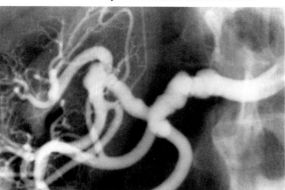

A

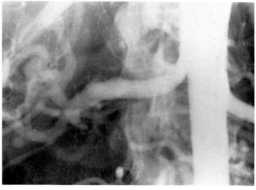

B

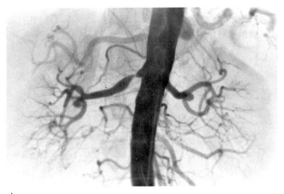

A

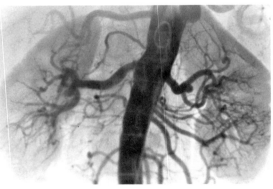

B

Fig. 11-33. Fibromuscular dyplasia.
A. The concentric smooth narrowing of the right renal artery without other significant changes of athero-sclerosis indicates fibromuscular dysplasia in this hypertensive middle-aged woman. Note the aneu-rysm of the left and right renal arteries at their bifurcations.
B. After angioplasty the stenosis is relieved and the pa-tient is normotensive.

Fig. 11-34. Fibromuscular dyplasia with intrarenal branch stenosis (*arrowhead*). Intrarenal spiral collaterals communicate between the segmental and interlobar branches.

plasia or can occur on a small vessel level subse-quent to arteritis (e.g., polyarteritis nodosa, necrotizing angiitis). True aneurysms have some component of the arterial wall present and are most commonly saccular in configuration but may be fusiform. False aneurysms have periadventitial nonarterial components forming the aneurysm wall; they are often impossible to differentiate an-giographically from true aneurysms. Aneurysms in younger patients are usually congenital in nature or are a result of fibromuscular hyperplasia. They may occur subsequent to trauma. Approximately

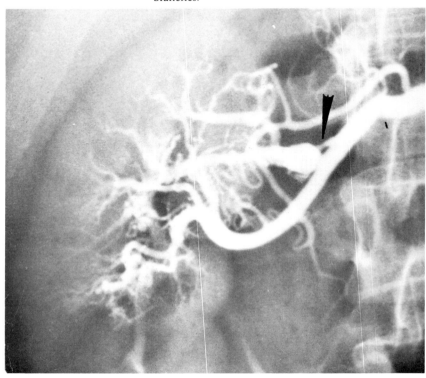

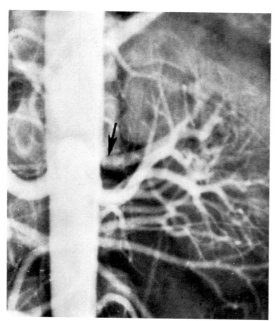

Fig. 11-35. Proximal renal artery stenosis due to a fibrous band in a 24-year-old man with hypertension. There is proximal compression of the artery (*arrow*) under the band. Renin levels were elevated on this side. Hypertension was relieved following surgical lysis of the band.

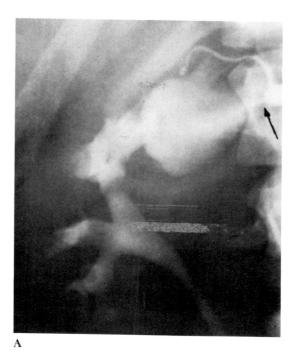

A

half are located proximal to the first bifurcation and the remainder in a renal artery branch. They are multiple in less than 10 percent of patients. Twenty-five to 50 percent of aneurysms have calcium in their walls. A high percentage of patients with renal artery aneurysms develop hypertension, and 75 percent of these patients show improvement after surgery. The hypertension may be caused by renal ischemia subsequent to the aneurysm, thrombosis, embolization, dissection, or slow flow distal to the aneurysm. In one reported series of aneurysms, only 6 percent ruptured [44]. Angiograms may show segmental delay in filling and washout of vessels beyond the aneurysm, narrowing of the diameter of vessels distal to the aneurysm, and segmental decrease in intensity of the nephrographic phase. The angiographer should try to identify the aneurysm neck and should always exclude disease in the remaining kidney. The renal veins should be evaluated for increased renin secretion.

RENAL ARTERIOVENOUS FISTULAS. Renal arteriovenous fistulas [23, 29] cause hypertension due to renal ischemia distal to the fistula. If the fistula is

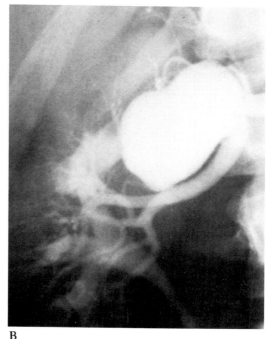

B

Fig. 11-36.
A. Large renal artery aneurysm with a jet of contrast medium (*arrow*) extruding through a markedly stenotic neck and a large collateral vessel indicating significant delay in flow.
B. This massive aneurysm displaces vessels and could conceivably be mistaken for a cyst by ultrasound.

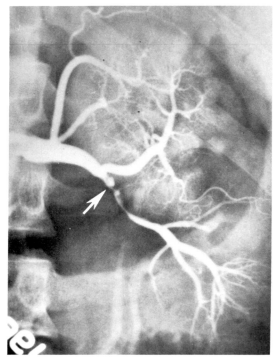

Fig. 11-37. Small mycotic aneurysm (*arrow*) in an accessory left renal artery caused by an infected embolus in a patient with subacute bacterial endocarditis. Segmental arterial narrowing and peripheral pruning due to emboli are present.

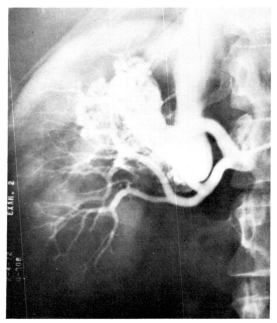

Fig. 11-38. Congenital renal arteriovenous malformation. There is a large feeding artery, a collection of multiple tortuous intrarenal arteries and veins without a mass effect, and premature filling of the renal vein and inferior vena cava. There is a striking lack of filling of vessels peripheral to the arteriovenous malformation, indicating short circuiting. This condition can cause hypertension.

large, high output failure may result. Decreased renal circulation time and increased oxygen saturation in the renal veins are evident. There may be painless hematuria and a continuous bruit over the upper abdomen and flank. Congenital forms vary from small asymptomatic hemangiomas with little or no premature venous shunting to large fistulas between the artery and vein (Fig. 11-38). Tortuous, enlarged, coiled, serpiginous, dilated vessels without mass effect and with varying degrees of premature venous filling (well before the usual 10 to 12 seconds) are best seen with selective studies. Acquired forms of fistulas occur following rupture of arterial aneurysms, trauma (e.g., penetrating, blunt, surgical, postneedle biopsy), and tumor erosion of veins. Angiographically, large feeding arteries and rapidly filling, dilated draining veins are observed.

TRAUMA. Trauma to the renal vessels can cause avulsion, disruption of the vessel wall, extrinsic compression from intrarenal or perirenal hematoma, thrombosis, false aneurysm formation, arteriovenous fistula, renal infarction, and parenchymal laceration (Figs. 11-39, 11-40).

RENAL VEIN THROMBOSIS. Occasionally renal vein thrombosis causes renovascular hypertension subsequent to renal damage, with varying degrees of renal infarction (see Fig. 21-9). Arteriographic findings in an acute or relatively acute episode of renal vein thrombosis show a generally enlarged kidney, with attenuated, stretched vessels, a delay in the nephrogram, a thickened renal cortex, and faint or absent venous filling or filling of collateral channels.

Parenchymal Disease

Many renal parenchymal lesions may lead to hypertension. These lesions include pyelonephritis, glomerulonephritis, microangiopathic hemolytic anemia, collagen diseases (polyarteritis nodosa, scleroderma), polycystic renal disease, solitary renal cysts, tumors, and hydronephrosis.

CHRONIC RENAL PARENCHYMAL DISEASE. There is a spectrum of angiographic findings present in

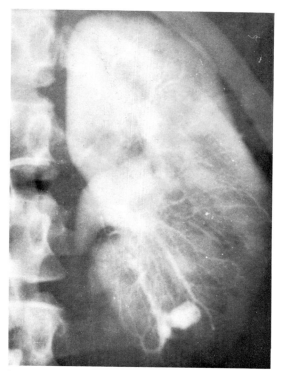

Fig. 11-39. Traumatic renal contusion with false aneurysm. Hematuria and flank pain occurred as a result of a kick in the back.

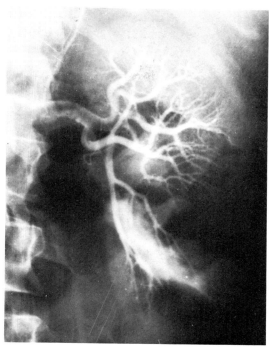

Fig. 11-40. Fractured left kidney 2 weeks after an automobile accident.

chronic renal parenchymal disease [18, 19]. Absolute differences do not occur between the major pathologic entities, but a review of some of the features may help the physician to lean toward one or another of the disease processes.

In pyelonephritis, the disease is usually focal in nature (Fig. 11-41). Asymmetric involvement and nonuniformity within the same kidney are also evident. It is often difficult to visualize small peripheral interlobar or arcuate arteries, which may be tortuous or pruned in appearance. The nephrogram is nonhomogeneous as a result of multiple cortical scars. Often the scars involve the upper or the lower pole of the kidney preferentially.

In chronic glomerulonephritis (Fig. 11-42), the lesion is bilateral and is generally uniform. There is often an abrupt decrease in the arterial caliber of the more peripheral vessels, with varying degrees of cortical atrophy. There is reduced opacification of the smaller vessels, and the nephrogram is homogeneous and the cortical margins smooth. At the end stage of glomerulonephritis the cortex may be more lucent than the medulla during the nephrogram phase, and the extrarenal capsular

branches are often more prominent than normal. Other findings include slow flow, a delayed nephrogram, poor opacification of the renal veins, and poor definition between the cortex and the medulla.

In nephrosclerosis (Fig. 11-43), characteristic histologic changes occur in patients with hypertension of long duration. Early in the course of the disease, intimal thickening of interlobar and arcuate arteries and disruption of internal elastic lamina and medial thickening occur. A necrotizing arteriolitis with fibrinoid degeneration is seen in the more malignant forms of the disease. Tortuosity, stenosis, occlusion of small vessels with ultimate cortical ischemia, and atrophy occur. A wide range of angiographic abnormalities is seen in nephrosclerosis, depending on the stage of the disease. Early in its course arteriograms may be normal. Pruning of peripheral vessels, tortuosity involving particularly the arcuate and interlobar arteries, and minor irregularities of the small vessels may occur. In the more malignant phase of the disease, the interlobar and arcuate arteries become extremely tortuous, with a gnarled appear-

288

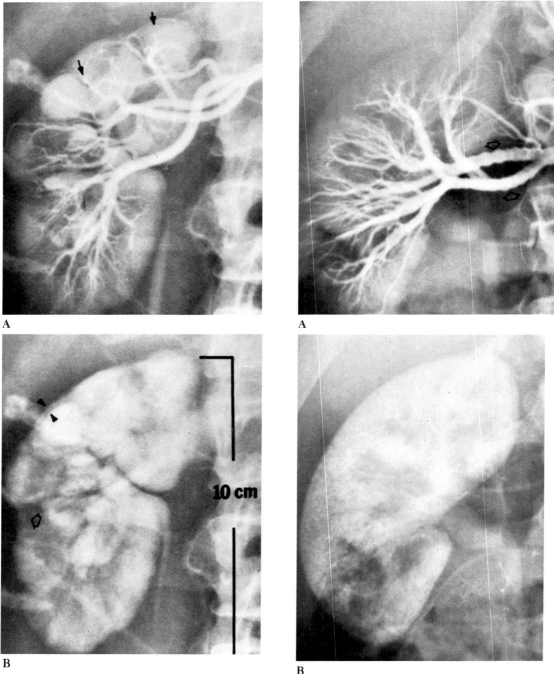

Fig. 11-41. Chronic pyelonephritis of the right kidney.
A. Arterial phase shows occlusion of some of the interlobar and arcuate arteries of the upper pole (*arrows*).
B. Nephrogram. The kidney is smaller than normal and has multiple irregular cortical scars (*open arrow*). There are dilated calices and a thinned cortex (*arrowheads*).

Fig. 11-42. A and B. Glomerulonephritis. Arrows point to "stationary arterial waves" (these are of no angiographic significance). Bilateral slow filling of vessels was encountered, as well as a gentle pruning of the distal interlobar and arcuate arteries, homogeneous filling of the cortex, and poor demarcation of the corticomedullary junction. (See Fig. 4-7 for the more severe form of the disease.)

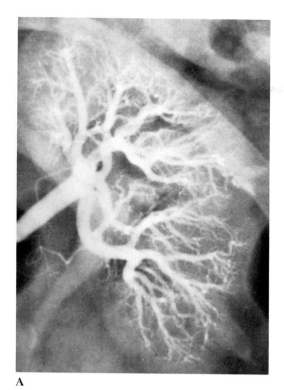

A

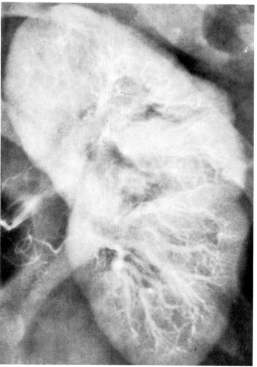

B

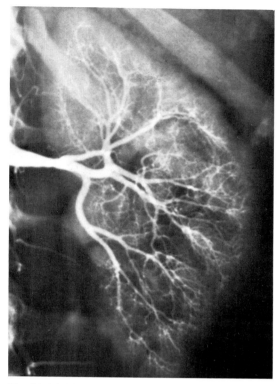

Fig. 11-44. Microangiopathic hemolytic anemia in a 17-year-old girl who developed malignant hypertension following an abortion. There is rapid tapering of the main renal artery and diminished caliber of the inter-lobar arteries and arcuate arteries. There is poor definition of peripheral arterial walls and poor cortical perfusion. This is a bilateral disease. At autopsy the changes were at the arteriolar and small vessel levels.

ance and markedly delayed flow. The cortex is poorly opacified, and the corticomedullary junction is poorly defined. The appearance of the disease is usually bilateral, but it may be unilateral in patients with unilateral renal artery stenosis. In these patients, the stenotic lesion protects the intrarenal vessels from the ravages of the elevated pressure.

In certain patients with rapidly developing malignant hypertension, hemolytic anemia with red cell fragmentation occurs together with a fibri-

Fig. 11-43. Nephrosclerosis.
A. There is poor filling of the arcuate arteries, tortuosity and dilatation of the interlobar branches, and a delay in circulation time. The cortex is poorly filled.
B. Nephrogram phase. Arterial filling persists 7 seconds after the injection.

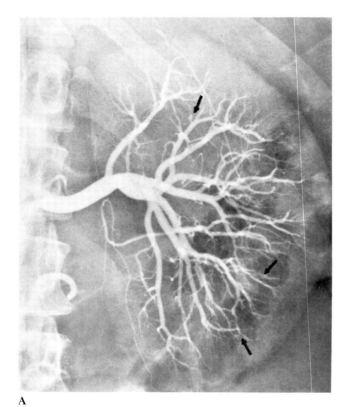

A

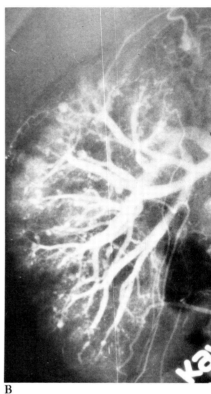

B

Fig. 11-45. Polyarteritis nodosa in two separate patients.
A. Mild form of the disease. There is an irregular margin with focal aneurysmal dilatation of several of the interlobar branches (*arrows*). Scattered areas of small vessel stenosis and occlusion due to intimal thickening occur as healing progresses.
B. A more flagrant form of the disease, which proved fatal in another patient with florid aneurysm formation.

noid necrosis of small vessel walls and resultant thrombotic microangiopathy. This condition, known as microangiopathic hemolytic anemia, accompanies other disease states as well, including eclampsia, preeclampsia, acute or chronic renal failure, disseminated carcinoma, and thrombotic thrombocytopenic purpura [17] (Fig. 11-44).

POLYARTERITIS NODOSA. Polyarteritis nodosa [4] is a disease of unknown cause involving many systems. The basic arterial abnormality is fibrinoid necrosis that results in aneurysmal dilatation, arterial wall irregularity, vascular stenosis, and occlusion of the small vessels within the kidney. These changes are usually restricted to the arcuate artery and the interlobar and segmental vessels. Angiographic findings of a minor degree of disease are seen in Figure 11-45A, and those of extensive disease in another patient are shown in Figure 11-45B. Although these findings are considered pathognomonic, similar findings can be seen in patients with necrotizing angiitis from other causes [9].

Hypertension Following Renal Transplants

There are many causes for failure of a renal allograft including rejection, infection, and stenosis or occlusion of the transplant renal artery. In many cases, detection and treatment of a renal artery stenosis can preserve an otherwise viable transplant kidney. Angiography, using either digital or conventional imaging, is essential.

The large contrast loads required with IV-DSA make this technique less desirable. Furthermore, because most renal transplants are placed in the pelvis, the overlying bones further impair the images.

The most reliable technique for examining the

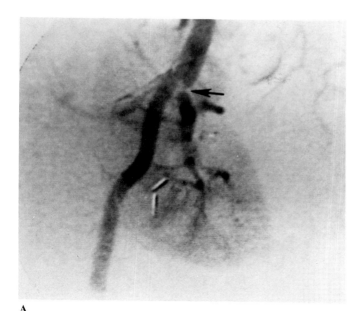

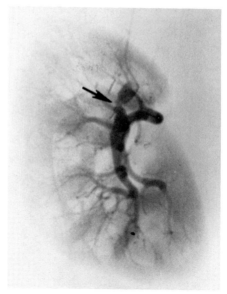

A

B

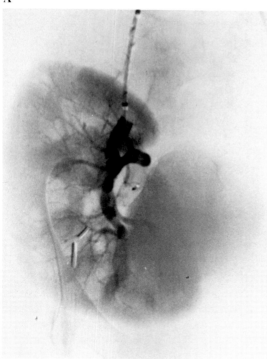

C

Fig. 11-46.
A. Intravenous digital examination reveals a high-grade stenosis in the transplant renal artery (*arrow*).
B. A significant stenosis is confirmed (*arrow*) with a selective conventional arteriogram.
C. There was an excellent result from percutaneous transluminal angioplasty.

patients with suspected transplant renal artery stenosis is conventional arteriography (Figs. 11-46B and C, 11-47). Selective injection of the feeding vessel can be used to reduce the contrast load. Furthermore, this same catheter can be used to initiate transluminal angioplasty if an arterial stenosis is found. Depending on room design, a combination of these techniques, particularly IA-DSA and conventional arteriography, may be most effective [36A].

Hypertension following renal transplants can occur as a result of graft rejection or acute tubular necrosis. Selective studies of the transplant artery with subtraction magnification techniques help to outline the renal parenchymal changes seen in graft rejection [14]. In renal rejection, nonspecific small vessel abnormalities can occur. There may be poor definition and scarring of the cortex. There may also be a delayed nephrogram, stretching and separation of the intrarenal branches, irregularities of the arterial wall of interlobar arteries, and progressive failure of opacification of intralobular and arcuate arteries and of interlobar arteries, either in a segmental or diffuse fashion (see Figs. 11-46, 11-47).

Perirenal Disease
Perirenal disease causes hypertension by extrinsic compression [35]. Underlying causes are perirenal

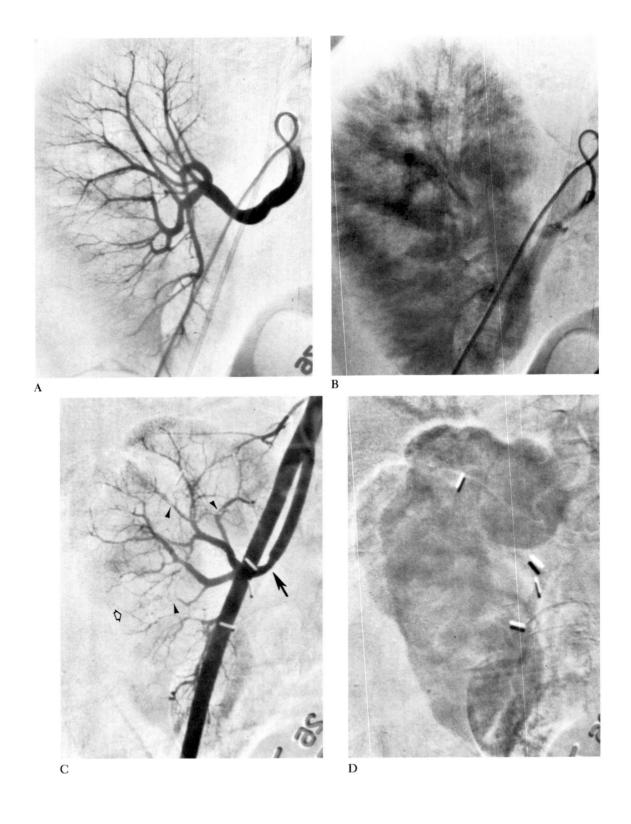

A

B

C

D

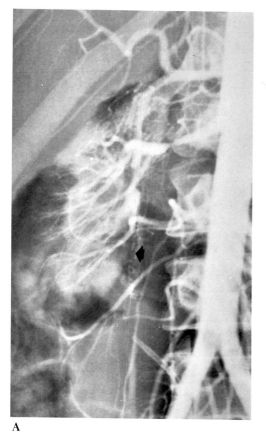

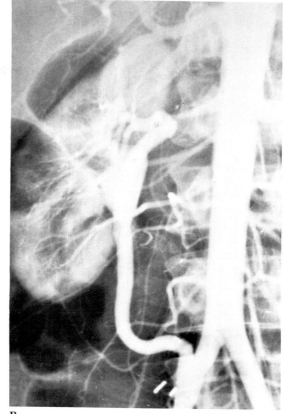

A   B

Fig. 11-48.
A. Right renal artery stenosis due to fibromuscular hyperplasia. Note the ureteric collaterals (*arrow*).
B. Postoperative bypass autogenous vein graft. The blood pressure has returned to normal. The kidney has enlarged, and the collaterals have now disappeared.

Fig. 11-47. Renal angiography in transplant rejection.
A. Subtraction film showing acute rejection of renal transplant.
B. There are multiple radiating lucent cortical defects with a palisading effect, indicating poor cortical perfusion. A biopsy showed numerous hyaline deposits in the interlobular branches.
C and D. Renal transplant, with severe hypertension and chronic rejection occurring 2 years posttransplant in another patient.
C. Arterial phase shows mild arterial stenosis at anastomotic site (*closed arrow*). There is slow circulation into the kidney, as well as multiple irregularities along the interlobar branches (*arrowheads*) with occlusion of some of the arcuate and interlobar branches (*open arrow*).
D. There is poor definition of the corticomedullary junction and cortical scars.

hematomas, retroperitoneal fibrosis, perirenal tumors, and perirenal chronic infection.

Hypertension in Children

A definable cause for hypertension in the child [6] can be found in 65 to 80 percent of cases. The spectrum of diseases causing secondary hypertension in children is different from that in adults. Chronic inflammatory renal disease (such as pyelonephritis), renal and adrenal tumors, and developmental renal abnormalities have a relatively higher incidence in children. The vascular lesions include fibromuscular dysplasia, neurofibromatosis (rarely), arteritis, and lesions associated with rubella and idiopathic hypercalcemia.

Surgery and Renovascular Hypertension

The types of corrective surgery include bypass procedures (Fig. 11-48), patch grafts, and nephrectomy. With the bypass procedures, autologous vein and prosthetic grafts are introduced, or splenic or iliac artery anastomoses are performed.

Nephrectomy is performed when there is a significant parenchymal lesion causing hypertension, partial infarction of the kidney, or failure of percutaneous transluminal angiography or of a graft. Failure to improve the hypertension may be a result of improper selection of the patient for intervention; for example, there may have been essential hypertension together with a fortuitously uncovered renal artery lesion, or an unrecognized nephrosclerosis or bilateral disease. Graft failure may be caused by a complication at the time of surgery or by the grafting material. The angiographer must be prepared to evaluate these factors. Stenosis or occlusion of the graft may be caused by fibrosis of one or all of the layers of the venous bypass material. Dilatation of the graft, as well as frank false aneurysm formation or fistulization, may occur.

EVALUATION OF POTENTIAL RENAL DONORS

Renal transplantation has become a common procedure performed at most major medical centers in the United States. Allografts from living, related donors survive longer than kidneys obtained from cadavers; however, it is essential to examine the donor to assess the potential kidney transplant and to assure that the remaining kidney is capable of providing adequate renal function.

A variety of radiographic techniques have been used for this purpose including excretory urography, radionuclide renography, digital subtraction angiography (both intravenous and intraarterial), and conventional angiography. The examinations used in each institution vary with the equipment available and the experience of the radiologists and renal transplant team; however, arteriography, either conventional or digital, is the only method of defining the kidney's vascular supply and is essential to surgical planning.

For years, conventional aortography has been used to define the number, location, and size of the renal arteries. An oblique projection is often needed to separate branches of the superior mesenteric artery from accessory renal arteries. Sometimes selective injection of renal arteries is necessary.

More recently, digital angiography has been used to evaluate potential renal donors. The IV-DSA has the advantage of not requiring an arterial puncture but is limited by poorer spatial resolu-

tion. In our review this resulted in missing 12 percent of the accessory renal arteries [44A]. The vessels not detected by IV-DSA, however, were small and usually not clinically significant. Whenever an IV-DSA examination is equivocal, conventional arteriography should be performed for clarification.

The use of IA-DSA results in improved images compared with IV-DSA but still preserves the advantages of digital imaging. The decreased contrast load and faster examination time make this an attractive alternative. In equivocal cases, conventional arteriography can easily be performed as the catheter is already in the arterial system.

PERCUTANEOUS TRANSLUMINAL ANGIOPLASTY

The technical aspects of percutaneous transluminal angioplasty (PTA) have been discussed in detail in Chapter 6. In this section those aspects peculiar to the renal arteries are addressed.

Indications

In attempting to improve regional blood flow, one must consider alternative approaches as well as the risk of no therapy. This is a difficult task because long-term follow-up of patients treated with newer modalities or improved technology is not always available; thus, each patient and specific problem must have the therapy most likely to produce a beneficial result. Some guidelines may be helpful in this decision process. Indications for renal artery PTA include

1. Single, main renal artery stenosis in a patient suspected of having renovascular hypertension. It must be remembered that idiopathic hypertension and vascular disease are both common processes; thus, it is not surprising that many patients have both and yet not have renovascular hypertension. It is also possible that some patients have both renin-mediated renovascular hypertension and idiopathic or essential hypertension. Indeed, this is presumably the explanation for the improvement but not cure of some patients with technically successful PTA. Angioplasty can make a significant contribution in these patients by lowering the hypertension and making it easier to control with fewer medications.

   Renovascular hypertension (RVH) is renin-mediated so that patients with RVH should have elevated serum renin levels. The presence of RVH can be further confirmed by finding renal vein renin levels that lateralize to the side of the renal artery stenosis [48]. In general, a renin ratio of 1.5:1 is considered lateralization.

2. Bilateral main renal artery stenoses in a hypertensive patient. This situation is not uncommon and may occur with more advanced generalized atherosclerosis or with fibromuscular dysplasia, the two most common causes of RVH. These patients are more difficult to assess because either or both renal artery lesions may be the cause of elevated renin secretion and RVH. If renal vein renins lateralize, the offending arterial stenosis may be identified, but it is also possible that both renal arteries are contributing to the process.

   Some experienced interventional angiographers perform PTA on both renal arteries at the same time; however, others prefer to dilate only one renal artery at a time. In the latter circumstance, if dilation of one vessel does not relieve the hypertension, the contralateral artery may be dilated later.

3. Main renal artery stenosis of a solitary kidney or renal transplant in a patient suspected of having RVH [41]. The absence of a functioning contralateral kidney means that renal vein renins cannot be used to demonstrate lateralization. Furthermore, in case of vascular compromise or possible nephrectomy, the patient requires dialysis or renal transplantation. The patient is at risk for renal insufficiency, however, if left untreated, and PTA may be justified in these difficult patients.

4. Branch renal artery stenosis in a patient suspected of having RVH [38]. Careful angiography is usually required to detect such lesions which may lie in small, peripheral branches (see Fig. 2-4A). Furthermore, renal vein renin collections must reflect the localized nature of the vascular stenosis [55]. Appreciable step up in renal vein renin levels may only be detectable by sampling venous efflux from the same area of the kidney as the arterial stenosis.

   These patients may also present a greater technical challenge in getting a small balloon catheter across the stenosis. In some patients occlusion of the stenotic branch vessel may be the most appropriate therapy [1].

5. Main renal artery stenosis in a patient with renal insufficiency. Although renal artery PTA is usually done for relief of hypertension, approximately one-third of patients have improved renal function after PTA.

Technique

There are several aspects of renal PTA which are different from peripheral angioplasty.

1. The stenosis must be approached in an anterograde fashion.
2. The renal artery generally arises at a 90-degree angle from the aorta. In some patients, a more acute downward angle of the renal artery makes crossing the stenosis with the balloon catheter even more difficult from the groin approach. In these patients, a high brachial or axillary artery approach may be needed [45].
3. The renal arteries often undergo vasospasm which can be severe enough to cause a renal infarct or even arterial thrombosis. In many patients this is incited by the guidewire in a branch vessel. Thus, vasodilators, such as nifedipine, are often used prior to beginning the procedure, and nitroglycerine is given as an intraarterial bolus of 50 to 100 μg during the procedure [2].
4. The blood pressure may be labile in these hypertensive patients. If possible, antihypertensive medication should be stopped before PTA; however, this may not be possible in every patient. Those patients whose diastolic blood pressure is above 110 mm Hg should be controlled on short-acting antihypertensive medications.

   A rapid drop in blood pressure after PTA can usually be controlled with saline infusion. A large-gauge intravenous line should be in place prior to beginning the procedure.

Results

The results of renal PTA must be considered in terms of technical success, clinical success, and duration of success [30]. Obviously patient selection has a significant impact on the results. Patients with single, main renal artery stenoses do much better than patients with extensive severe vascular disease. Patients with fibromuscular dysplasia (see Figs. 11-32, 11-33) usually have a very

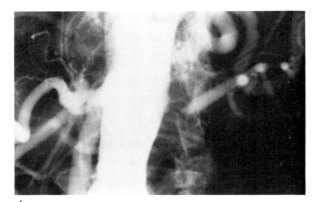

A

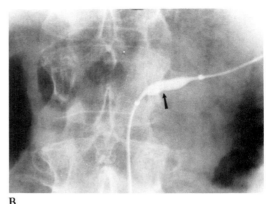

B

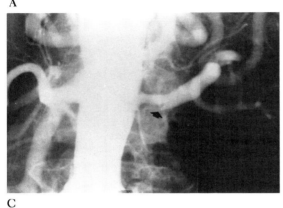

C

Fig. 11-49. Renal artery angioplasty.
A. High-grade stenosis of proximal left renal artery.
B. "Waisting" (*arrow*) of the balloon confirms the lo-
cation of the renal artery stenosis.
C. After angioplasty the stenosis has been alleviated.
Irregularity of the inferior wall (*arrow*) indicates the
expected intimal disruption.

favorable response [46]. Patients with renal artery
stenosis secondary to neurofibromatosis do poorly.

1. The technical success of crossing the stenosis
   and dilating the lesion is achieved in approximately 90 percent of cases (Figs. 11-49, 11-50,
   11-51, 11-52). Failure may be due to the inability to pass a guidewire through the narrowing or to get the balloon catheter to follow the
   guidewire. If an acute angle of the renal artery
   with the aorta is the problem, using an axillary
   approach may be successful. If the stenosis is
   very tight, a coaxial balloon catheter system
   may be used. The smaller 4.5 French coaxial
   balloon catheter passes through high-grade
   stenoses more readily than the conventional 7
   French femoral balloon catheter.
2. Among patients who have successful PTA, the
   hypertension is cured or improved in 70 to 90
   percent [32, 47]. This success rate also depends
   upon how rigorously the patient population was
   selected for PTA. Patients with lateralizing re-

nins have a higher cure rate than patients
whose renal vein renins do not lateralize [31].
Lesions involving the orifice of the renal artery
due to atheromatous plaques of the abdominal aorta often fail to respond to PTA (see Fig.
11-51) [8].
3. Because renal PTA is a relatively recent addition to the range of vascular interventional procedures, long-term follow-up is not yet available; however, patients up to 5 years after PTA
   show excellent results [40, 42, 47].

When renal artery stenoses recur they may
be due to either return of a stenosis which was
incompletely dilated or to progression of the
underlying disease process with development of
a new stenotic lesion. In either case, repeat
angioplasty may be performed with a success
rate similar to that of the initial dilation.

Complications

The complications of renal PTA include those related to angiography and those specifically due to
attempts to cross and dilate the renal artery stenosis. The most common complication is a groin
hematoma. These are seen more often after angioplasty procedures than conventional arteriography
because larger balloon catheters are used, catheters
are changed more frequently, and an anticoagulant is used during the procedure. Although it is
usually only a minor complication, dissection of
the hematoma into the pelvis or retroperitoneum

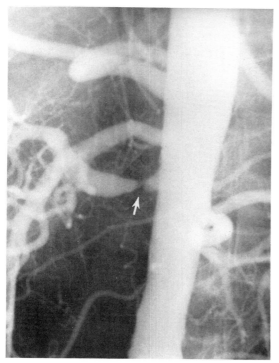

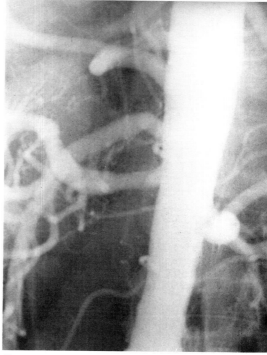

A

B

Fig. 11-50. Main renal artery stenosis.
A. Aortogram demonstrates a tight stenosis (*arrow*) of the right renal artery.
B. After percutaneous transluminal angioplasty the stenosis is alleviated.

may result in a greater blood loss than the size of the groin hematoma appears to indicate.

The other common complication is renal failure. This can be either development of acute renal failure or exacerbation of chronic renal insufficiency. In most patients this is a transient phenomenon with return of renal function by 10 days.

Complications specifically caused by the angioplasty procedure include rupture or occlusion of the renal artery, rupture of the dilating balloon, renal artery dissection, and infarction of all or a portion of the kidney. Balloon rupture is less common, as the manufacturing technology continues to improve. The primary goal when this occurs is to remove the catheter without causing vessel injury.

Laceration or rupture of the renal artery may be caused by either the guidewire or the balloon catheter. If this occurs the balloon catheter should not be removed but should be left in place and inflated to occlude the renal artery and prevent exsanguination.

Small segmental renal infarctions are probably inconsequential, but they can be minimized by careful technique and liberal use of vasodilators. Occasionally acute renal artery thrombosis complicates the dilation and threatens the kidney. This acute thrombosis often responds to thrombolytic agents such as urokinase or streptokinase.

Renal Transplant Arterial Stenosis

Percutaneous transluminal angioplasty of transplant renal artery stenosis presents two major problems not found in other patients. The route to the arterial stenosis is variable but is usually more tortuous, and the chronic immunosuppression and steroid use result in less durable tissue. Nevertheless, these lesions can be successfully dilated and renal function may be preserved.

The approach to the transplant artery depends upon the specific anatomy and type of anastomosis. End-to-side anastomoses are more easily approached via the ipsilateral femoral artery, while end-to-end anastomoses are approached from the contralateral femoral artery. The axillary artery

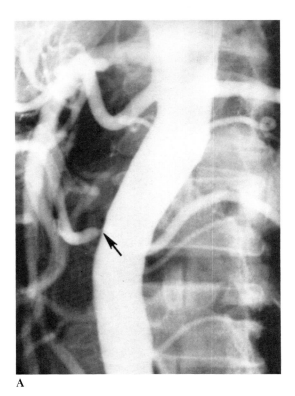

A

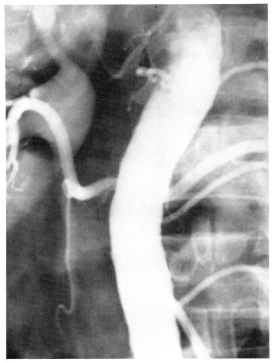

B

Fig. 11-51. Stenosis at origin of renal artery.
A. A stenosis is present at the origin of the right renal
     artery (*arrow*).
B. Although percutaneous transluminal angioplasty
     was successful in this patient, the narrowing is often
     due to atherosclerotic plaque in the aorta. These
     lesions frequently recur or fail to respond to di-
     latation.

may be entered with either type of anastomosis,
but this requires a longer, more difficult vascular
control than when the femoral artery is entered.

Heparin anticoagulation and antispasmodic
agents are equally important in treating renal
transplant artery stenosis. Added caution must be
used, however, at the site of vascular entry because
the soft tissues in patients using chronic corticosteroids may allow extensive hemorrhage and dissection along the tissue planes without detection.

The success of PTA in renal transplant artery
stenosis has improved [37A] but is still less than
the success rate expected with native renal artery
lesions. The most common causes for failure are
an inability to cross the stenosis with either the
guidewire or the balloon catheter and recurrence
of the stenosis after balloon inflation. In this latter
instance, use of a larger balloon may eliminate the
stenosis.

The application of transluminal angioplasty
techniques to the renal arteries has resulted in the
cure or improvement in renovascular hypertension
for most patients. These interventional procedures
are not without risk of significant complication and
should not be performed without surgical support

available. Although not initially attempted for
amelioration of renal failure, many patients show
significant improvement in renal function after angioplasty.

VASCULAR OCCLUSION TECHNIQUES
Methods and techniques of reduction in regional
blood flow are described in Chapter 5. They have a
limited but valuable role in the kidney.

Indications
As with renal artery dilatation, renal vascular occlusion techniques must be considered along with
alternate methods of therapy. Renal embolization
is often performed in conjunction with surgery.
Branch renal artery occlusion, however, may be
performed in an effort to eliminate the symptomatic area without surgery or to preserve as much

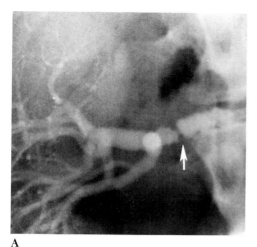

A

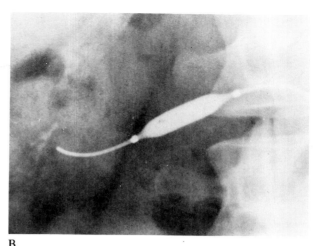

B

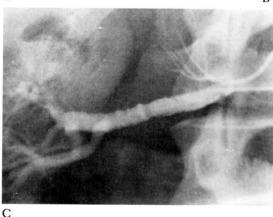

C

Fig. 11-52. Renal artery stenosis (fibromuscular dysplasia).
A. Selective right renal arteriogram reveals irregularity consistent with fibromuscular dysplasia. A high-grade stenosis (*arrow*) is also present.
B. The position of the angioplasty balloon is guided by the bony landmarks.
C. A contrast injection after angioplasty demonstrates elimination of the stenosis.

renal parenchyma as possible. Specific examples where renal artery occlusion may be beneficial include

1. Unresectable renal carcinoma. This is most commonly undertaken when there is a complicating factor, such as hematuria or intractable pain [13]. If renal collaterals are not well developed, simple embolization results in renal infarction. Although this is initially painful during the period of tissue necrosis, subsequent pain relief can be dramatic. Similarly, hematuria coming from a renal tumor can usually be

stopped. These same techniques may also be applied to metastases to the kidney from other primary tumors.

2. Presurgical reduction in tumor vascularity. Because renal adenocarcinoma is usually a hypervascular tumor, significant blood loss may occur at surgery (Fig. 11-53). Embolization of the tumor prior to operation can markedly reduce the blood loss [25]. Initial enthusiasm for the immunologic role of embolization 7 to 10 days before nephrectomy has waned [50], and renal vascular occlusion is now most commonly performed several hours to 1 day before nephrectomy.

3. Arteriovenous fistula. Localized arteriovenous communications may be occluded using transcatheter techniques [5, 28, 51] (see Fig. 5-15). The lesions can be arteriovenous fistulas, which are usually due to penetrating injury or congenital arteriovenous malformations. In the case of an arteriovenous fistula or traumatic aneurysm, occlusion of the single feeding vessel is usually therapeutic. Arteriovenous malformation or angiomatous tumors are more difficult, as the entire vascular abnormality must be eliminated. If only the supplying vessel is occluded, additional feeding arteries may be recruited.

4. Branch renal artery stenosis in a patient suspected of having renovascular hypertension. Theoretically, these lesions could be dilated with preservation of renal tissue and elimination of hypertension; however, they may be technically impossible to reach with an angio-

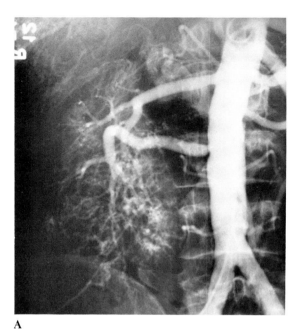

A

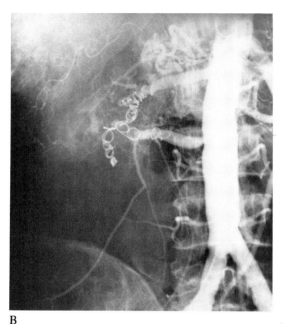

B

Fig. 11-53. Embolization of renal adenocarcinoma.
A. Two renal arteries supply the adenocarcinoma of the right kidney.
B. Embolization with Gelfoam and steel coils was performed prior to nephrectomy to reduce blood loss.

plasty balloon, and occlusion of that segment of the kidney may be therapeutic with loss of only a small portion of renal parenchyma (see Fig. 2-4).

5. Control of renal hemorrhage. Vascular occlusion techniques may be used to alleviate renal hemorrhage from a variety of causes including trauma, infection, arteriovenous fistulas, false aneurysm, renal adenocarcinoma, or metastases to the kidney [7, 13] (see Fig. 11-53).

Technique

The most common method of renal artery occlusion is with a combination of Gelfoam and steel coils. Most of these procedures are undertaken for complications of an unresectable renal malignancy, either a primary or a metastatic tumor. Gelfoam powder or small pieces of Gelfoam are injected through the catheter into the renal artery. Normal flow carries them into the tumor bed. Beware of introducing particles that are too small which may pass through arteriovenous shunts into the venous system. As more particles are injected, flow diminishes and the particles are less reliably directed into the tumor. Several steel coils are then placed in the main renal artery. These prevent backward migration of the Gelfoam into the aorta. The silk threads on the coils are thrombogenic which helps to occlude further the renal artery.

Absolute ethanol has become an attractive alter-

native to Gelfoam and coils for renal artery occlusion [13]. The ethanol denudes the endothelium resulting in complete thrombosis. Dilution of the ethanol occurs before it reaches the venous circulation so that the thrombotic process is not carried into the inferior vena cava. Ethanol should only be injected through an occlusion balloon catheter (see Fig. 5-14).

Arteriovenous fistulas are occluded with steel coils. Small particulate matter is not used as it may pass into the venous circulation and become a pulmonary embolus.

Arteriovenous malformation or angiomatous tumors are best occluded with a tissue adhesive or possibly with absolute ethanol. If the entire vascular lesion is not eliminated it may recur and develop new feeding vessels which may be even more difficult to control.

Complications

The untoward effects of these procedures include the expected results of tumor infarction and tissue necrosis. The postembolization syndrome includes flank pain, fever, and leukocytosis [27]. The gas that sometimes forms in the infarcted kidney is consistent with tissue necrosis and should not be interpreted as evidence of abscess.

The complications of embolization of the kidneys are similar to those elsewhere and are specific to the material and procedures used. The presence of an arteriovenous communication may allow particulate matter to reach the lung as an embolus. A right-to-left cardiac shunt could allow particulate matter into the arterial circulation where any organ would be at risk for embolization.

Although absolute ethanol has been used to produce excellent results with renal vascular occlusion, over injection may result in reflux into the abdominal aorta. Because ethanol is lighter than blood, it passes into anterior vessels, and occlusion of the superior mesenteric artery has been reported [34]. The use of an occlusion balloon may help to reduce the risk of this complication.

A wide variety of vascular techniques exist which may be used to accomplish either symptomatic relief or even cure a variety of renal problems. As with any interventional technique, they should be undertaken only after careful consideration of the expected gain and potential complications. When properly employed, however, symptomatic relief may be obtained without the need for surgery. When small vascular lesions are present, transcatheter occlusion techniques may eliminate the problem with sacrifice of the least amount of functioning renal parenchyma.

References

1. Bachman, D. M., et al. Selective renal artery embolization: Treatment of acute renovascular hypertension. *J.A.M.A.* 238:1534, 1977.
2. Beinart, C., et al. Arterial spasm during renal angioplasty. *Radiology* 149:97, 1983.
3. Bosniak, M. A., et al. Epinephrine-enhanced renal angiography in renal mass lesion: Is it worth performing? *Am. J. Roentgenol.* 129:647, 1977.
4. Capps, J., and Klein, R. Polyarteritis nodosa as a cause of perirenal and retroperitoneal hemorrhage. *Radiology* 94:143, 1970.
5. Castaneda-Zuniga, W. R., et al. Nonsurgical closure of large arteriovenous fistulas. *J.A.M.A.* 236:2649, 1976.
6. Chrispin, A., and Scatliff, J. Systemic hypertension in childhood: Review article. *Pediatr. Radiol.* 1:75, 1973.
7. Chuang, V. P., et al. Control of renal hemorrhage by selective arterial embolization. *A.J.R.* 125:300, 1975.

8. Cicuto, K. P., et al. Renal artery stenosis: Anatomic classification for percutaneous transluminal angioplasty. *A.J.R.* 137:599, 1981.
9. Citron, B. P., et al. Necrotizing angiitis associated with drug abuse. *N. Engl. J. Med.* 283:1003, 1970.
10. Dunnick, N. R., et al. Digital intravenous subtraction angiography for investigating renovascular hypertension: Comparison with hypertension urography. *South. Med. J.* 78:690, 1985.
11. Dunnick, N. R., and Korobkin, M. Computed tomography of the adrenal gland in hypertension. *Urol. Radiol.* 3:245, 1982.
12. Ekelund, L. Pharmacoangiography of the kidney: An overview. *Urol. Radiol.* 2:9, 1980.
13. Ekelund, L., et al. Occlusion of renal arterial tumor supply with absolute ethanol: Experience with 20 cases. *Acta Radiol. [Diagn.] (Stockh.)* 25:195, 1984.
14. Foley, W. D., et al. Arteriography of renal transplants. *Radiology* 116:271, 1975.
15. Ford, K. K., et al. Intravenous digital subtraction angiography in the preoperative evaluation of renal masses. *A.J.R.* 145:323, 1985.
16. Fritzsche, P., Andersen, C., and Cahill, P. Vascular specificity in differentiating adrenal carcinoma from renal cell carcinoma. *Radiology* 125:113, 1977.
17. Gavras, H., et al. Microangiopathic hemolytic anemia and development of the malignant phase of hypertension. *Circ. Res.* 28/29(suppl. 2):127, 1971.
18. Gill, W., and Pudvan, W. The arteriographic diagnosis of renal parenchymal diseases. *Radiology* 96:81, 1970.
19. Halperin, M. Angiography in chronic renal disease and renal failure. *Radiol. Clin. North Am.* 10:40, 1972.
20. Hillman, B. J., et al. Evaluation of potential renal donors and renal allograft recipients: Digital video subtraction angiography. *A.J.R.* 138:921, 1982.
21. Hodson, J. The lobar structure of the kidney. *Br. J. Urol.* 44:246, 1972.
22. Illescas, F. F., et al. Intra-arterial digital subtraction angiography in hypertensive azotemic patients. *A.J.R.* 143:1065, 1984.
23. Kaude, J. V., and Alexander, J. E. Congenital renal vascular malformations in childhood: Association with hypertension and detection by angiography. *Pediatr. Radiol.* 10:207, 1981.
24. Kirks, D. R., Fitz, C. R., and Korobkin, M. Intrarenal collateral circulation in the pediatric patient. *Pediatr. Radiol.* 5:154, 1977.
25. Klimberg, I., et al. Preoperative angioinfarction of localized renal cell carcinoma using absolute ethanol. *J. Urol.* 133:21, 1985.
26. Koehler, R. The roentgen diagnosis of renal inflammatory masses: Special emphasis on angiographic changes. *Radiology* 112:257, 1974.
27. Lammer, J., et al. Complications of renal tumor embolization. *Cardiovasc. Intervent. Radiol.* 8:31, 1985.
28. Lieberman, S. F., et al. Percutaneous vaso-occlu-

sion for nonmalignant renal lesions. *J. Urol.* 129:805, 1983.

29. Love, L., Moncada, R., and Lescher, A. Renal arteriovenous fistulae. *Am. J. Roentgenol.* 95:364, 1965.

30. Miller, G. A., et al. Percutaneous transluminal angiography vs. surgery for renovascular hypertension. *A.J.R.* 144:447, 1985.

31. Martin, E. C., et al. Renal angioplasty for hypertension: Predictive factors for long-term success. *A.J.R.* 137:921, 1981.

32. Martin, L. G., et al. Percutaneous angioplasty in clinical management of renovascular hypertension: Initial and long-term results. *Radiology* 155:629, 1985.

33. McDonald, P., and Hiller, H. Angiography in abdominal tumors in childhood with particular reference to neuroblastoma and Wilms' tumor. *Clin. Radiol.* 19:1, 1968.

34. Mulligan, B. D., and Espinosa, G. A. Bowel infarction: Complication of ethanol ablation of a renal tumor. *Cardiovasc. Intervent. Radiol.* 6:55, 1983.

35. Page, I. Hypertension by cellophane. *Science* 89:273, 1939.

36. Palmisa, O. Renal hamartoma (angiomyolipoma): Its angiographic appearance and response to intraarterial epinephrine. *Radiology* 102:551, 1967.

36A. Picus, D., et al. Intraarterial digital subtraction angiography of renal transplants. *A.J.R.* 145:93, 1985.

37. Rabinowitz, J., et al. Renal pelvic carcinoma: An angiographic re-evaluation. *Radiology* 102:551, 1972.

37A. Raynaud, A., et al. Percutaneous transluminal angioplasty of renal transplant arterial stenoses. *A.J.R.* 146:853, 1986.

38. Reuter, S. R., et al. Embolic control of hypertension caused by segmental renal artery stenosis. *Am. J. Roentgenol.* 127:389, 1976.

39. Schambelan, M., et al. Selective renal vein renin sampling in hypertensive patients with segmental renal lesions. *N. Engl. J. Med.* 290:1153, 1974.

40. Schwarten, D. E. Transluminal angioplasty of renal artery stenosis: 70 experiences. *A.J.R.* 135:969, 1980.

41. Sniderman, K. W., et al. Percutaneous transluminal dilatation in renal transplant arterial stenosis. *Transplantation* 30:440, 1980.

42. Sos, T. A., et al. Percutaneous transluminal renal angioplasty in renovascular hypertension due to atheroma or fibromuscular dysplasia. *N. Engl. J. Med.* 309:274, 1983.

43. Sos, T., Gray, C., and Baltaxe, H. The angiographic appearance of benign renal oxyphilic adenoma. *Am. J. Roentgenol.* 127:717, 1976.

44. Stanley, T., et al. Renal artery aneurysms: Significance of macroaneurysms exclusive of dissections and fibroplastic mural dilations. *Arch. Surg.* 110:1327, 1975.

44A. Sussman, S. K., et al. Intravenous digital subtraction angiography in the evaluation of potential renal donors. In press. 1987.

45. Tegtmeyer, C. J., Ayers, C. A., and Wellons, H. A. The axillary approach to percutaneous renal artery dilatation. *Radiology* 135:775, 1980.

46. Tegtmeyer, C. J., et al. Percutaneous transluminal angioplasty: The treatment of choice for renovascular hypertension due to fibromuscular dysplasia. *Radiology* 143:631, 1982.

47. Tegtmeyer, C. J., Kellum, C. D., and Ayers, C. Percutaneous transluminal angioplasty of the renal artery: Results and long-term follow-up. *Radiology* 153:77, 1984.

48. Thind, G. S. Role of renal venous renins in the diagnosis and management of renovascular hypertension. *J. Urol.* 134:2, 1985.

49. Viamonte, M., Jr., Roen, S., and LePage, J. Nonspecificity of abnormal vascularity in the angiographic diagnosis of malignant neoplasms. *Radiology* 106:59, 1973.

50. Wallace, S., et al. Embolization of renal carcinoma. *Radiology* 183:563, 1981.

51. Wallace, S., et al. Intrarenal arteriovenous fistulas: Transcatheter steel coil occlusion. *J. Urol.* 120:282, 1978.

52. Weyman, P. J., et al. Comparison of computed tomography and angiography in the evaluation of renal cell carcinoma. *Radiology* 137:417, 1980.

53. Weinerth, J., et al. Surgical validation of angiographic studies and renal lesions. *J. Urol.* 116:552, 1976.

54. Yune, H., and Klatte, E. Collateral circulation to an ischemic kidney. *Radiology* 119:539, 1976.

55. Yune, H. Y., et al. Measurement of renin in segmental renal veins of hypertensives. *Radiology* 146:29, 1983.

Adrenal Vascular Studies

Indications

The cross sectional imaging modalities, computed tomography (CT), ultrasound, and magnetic resonance (MR) have had a dramatic impact on adrenal angiography. Mass lesions as small as 1 cm in diameter are noninvasively imaged, and a presumptive diagnosis can be made on the basis of the clinical presentation [9, 11, 25, 30].

Arteriography is reserved for patients in whom delineation of the vascular supply of the adrenal mass is needed or when vascular intervention is contemplated. Adrenal venography remains valuable for collection of venous blood samples for hormone measurement and, occasionally, for identifying small mass lesions [5, 10, 23, 28].

Approaches

The percutaneous femoral artery and vein approaches are preferred in adrenal vascular studies.

Catheters

ARTERIAL STUDIES

1. For a flush aortogram, a Teflon end-hole catheter with multiple side holes should be used (5 French for adults; 4 or 5 French for children).
2. For semiselective studies of the inferior adrenal artery (arising from the renal arteries) and the superior adrenal branches (arising from the inferior phrenic arteries, which in turn may arise from the celiac axis), the angiographer should use a 5 French catheter with a single right angle or a double curve, or a cobra-head curved catheter with side holes and an end hole (Fig. 12-1B & C).
3. For selective catheterization of the middle adrenal branches or the inferior phrenic artery branches arising directly from the aorta, the angiographer should use a thinly tapered tip to a double-curved 5 French catheter without side holes (see Fig. 12-1A).

VENOUS STUDIES

Separate catheters with narrowed, tapered tips are required for each of the right and left adrenal veins.

1. Left adrenal vein: A catheter with a double reversed angle curve should be used. The gentle 120-degree distal curve helps to advance the 10- to 12-mm tip into the superiorly placed vein as it drains into the left renal vein (see Fig. 12-4A).
2. Right adrenal vein: A double-curved catheter should be used, with the distal curve at right angles and a tapered tip that is 6 to 10 mm in length. The second curve is 100 degrees and is located approximately 5 cm proximal to the distal curve (see Fig. 12-4B).

Contrast Agents, Projections, and Radiographic Programming

Details concerning contrast agents, projections, and radiographic programming in adrenal vascular studies are given in Table 12-1. Rapid early filming during the aortogram allows easier identification of small adrenal branches arising directly from the aorta. Delayed films allow detection of tumor stain or stain of normal adrenal cortex.

Preliminary Radiologic Studies

1. A plain film of the abdomen may show a soft tissue suprarenal mass, calcium, or metastatic involvement of bony structures. Adrenal calcification can occur in normal asymptomatic persons; it can also occur in those with Addison's disease secondary to tuberculosis, mycotic infections, hemorrhagic necrosis, trauma, or atrophy. A stippled calcification can occur throughout adrenal tumors, and a "salt and pepper" appearance of calcification can occur in patients with neuroblastoma. There is a high incidence of calcium in patients with carcinoma of the adrenal gland. Calcium is found

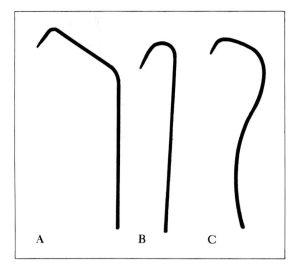

Fig. 12-1. Catheters used for adrenal arteriography.
A. Double-curved catheter with tapered tip for selective middle and inferior phrenic arteriography.
B and C. Catheters used for selective renal and celiac axis arteriograms.

in adrenal cysts, in hematomas, and rarely in adenomas and pheochromocytomas.

2. Intravenous pyelograms and nephrotomograms may outline the adrenal mass and possibly may show displacement of the kidney.

3. Ultrasonography can image the adrenal glands in most patients using either a posterior approach between ribs or an anterolateral route using the liver or spleen as a window. The left adrenal gland is often more difficult to image because of overlying bowel gas. Ultrasound is particularly valuable for differentiating cystic from solid masses.

4. The primary adrenal imaging modality has become CT [12]. The perirenal fat provides excellent contrast for adrenal imaging. Focal masses 1 cm in diameter are routinely demonstrated and smaller masses can occasionally be seen. Furthermore, characteristic features seen in some lesions, such as myelolipoma or adrenal hemorrhage may allow a definitive diagnosis.

5. Radionuclide adrenal imaging with NP-59 allows detection of hyperfunctioning adrenal cortical tumors [18, 27]. More recently meta-iodobenzyl guanidine (MIBG) has been used for hyperfunctioning medullary tumors [21]. The MIBG has the advantage of being able to detect extraadrenal pheochromocytomas.

6. Magnetic resonance imaging can display the

adrenal glands in axial as well as a variety of other planes such as coronal or sagittal. Although experience is limited, the sensitivity is similar to CT, and the signal intensity provides additional clues of the histologic nature of the lesion [25].

Special Anatomic Considerations

The average size of the normal adrenal gland is 3 to 5 cm in length, 3 to 5 cm in width at its base, and 0.4 to 0.6 cm in thickness [20]. It varies in size normally, increasing with the size and weight of the individual. The right side usually attaches loosely to the kidney, is triangular in shape, and has concave borders (see Fig. 12-2A, B). The left side is semilunar in shape and hugs the superomedial border of the upper pole of the left kidney medially (see Fig. 12-2C, D).

ARTERIAL SUPPLY

The arterial supply is variable, and multiple arteries supply each gland. The majority of the vascular supply of the adrenal gland may arise primarily from one or equally from all three of the vessels.

1. The superior adrenal arteries arise as multiple tiny branches from the inferior phrenic artery, which in turn arises from the celiac axis in 50 percent of people. The inferior phrenics arise most commonly from the aorta above the celiac axis anteriorly, either singly or as a common trunk. They can also arise below the celiac axis laterally, or from the left gastric, hepatic, superior mesenteric, renal, or gonadal arteries. The superior adrenal arteries supply the superomedial border of the gland.

2. The middle adrenal artery usually arises from the aorta between the renal arteries and the celiac axis or from the renal artery. Atypically, it can arise from the celiac axis, the superior mesenteric artery, or the inferior phrenic or lumbar artery. It supplies the anteromedial portion of the gland.

3. The inferior adrenal artery arises from the renal artery, the renal capsular artery, gonadal or ureteric vessels, and sometimes from the aorta between the renal arteries and celiac axis. It supplies the major portion of the gland, and usually the base of the gland.

Table 12-1. Technical specifications in adrenal vascular studies[a]

Vascular procedure	Contrast agent			Total films	Total time (sec)	Radiographic program		Projection
	Density	Volume (ml/inj)	Rate (ml/sec)			Films/sec	Timing	
Adult								
Aortogram	M	50	25	12	12	3/sec for 2 sec; 1/sec for 2 sec; 1 every other sec for 8 sec	Start 0.4 sec after start of injection	Anteroposterior
Renal artery	L	10	7	12	12	2/sec for 3 sec; 1/sec for 3 sec; 1 every other sec for 6 sec		
Celiac artery	M	50	8–10	16	16	2/sec for 4 sec; 1/sec for 4 sec; 1 every other sec for 8 sec		
Adrenal or inferior phrenic artery	L or L (NI)	2–8[b]	Hand	10	9	2/sec for 3 sec; 1/sec for 2 sec; 1 every other sec for 4 sec		
Selective adrenal venogram	L	2–4[b]	Hand	10	4	4/sec for 2 sec; 1/sec for 2 sec	Start at commencement of injection	
Child[c]								
Aortogram								
Infant	L	1.0–1.5 ml/kg	Total within 1.0–1.5 sec	12	8	3/sec for 2 sec; 2/sec for 2 sec; 1 every other sec for 4 sec		
Other	M							
Celiac axis	L	1.0–1.5 ml/kg	Total in 4 sec	16	12	2/sec for 4 sec; 1/sec for remainder		
Renal artery	L	2–10 ml	Total within 1.0–1.5 sec	12	8			
Adrenal or inferior phrenic artery	L or L (NI)	2–8 ml	Hand	12	8			

[a] For IA-DSA studies, use one-half concentration of contrast agent but the same volume and injection rates.
[b] Volume and rate are dependent on size of feeding artery or draining vein and size of tumor.
[c] Amount of contrast agent used in children varies with body weight.
Hand = slow hand injection; M = medium density contrast agent; L = low density contrast agent; NI = nonionic (see Appendix 3).

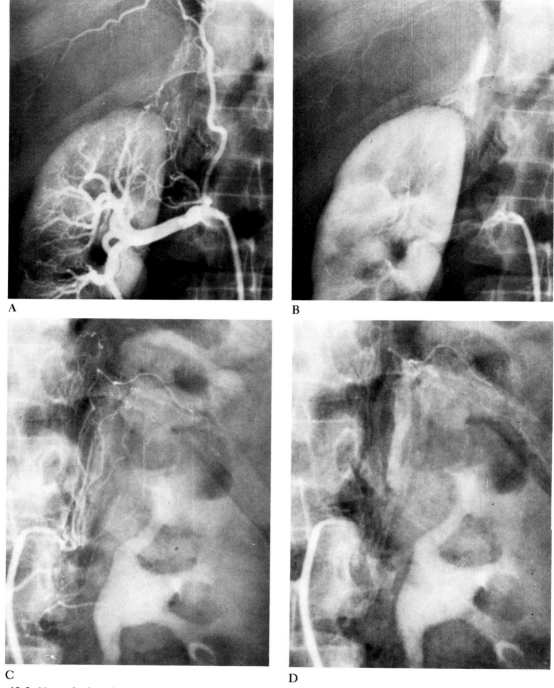

C

D

Fig. 12-2. Normal adrenal arteriograms.

A. Fortuitously, the inferior phrenic artery, middle adrenal artery, and inferior adrenal artery all arise from the right renal artery.

B. Capillary phase shows normal concave borders. The triangular shaped right adrenal gland lies superior to the right kidney.

C. Left middle adrenal arteriogram. This artery supplies the major portion of this left adrenal gland.

D. Capillary phase shows semilunar shape to the gland, which hugs the superomedial border of the upper pole of the left kidney.

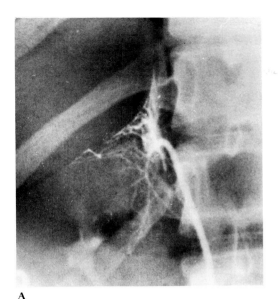

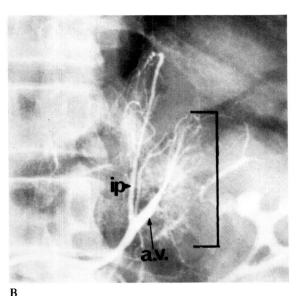

A   B

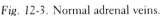

Fig. 12-3. Normal adrenal veins.
A. Right adrenal vein, arising at T11 to T12 posteromedially on the right.
B. Left adrenal vein. This vein drains in conjunction
   with the inferior phrenic vein (IP) into the left renal vein. The adrenal vein (AV) lies more laterally;
   there is a "Christmas tree" appearance to the fine
   branches of the adrenal vein. Capsular renal veins
   may also communicate.

VENOUS DRAINAGE

Venous drainage (Fig. 12-3A, B) is accomplished
through a superficial and a deep venous system.
The multiple capsular veins of the superficial system drain into various other systems, such as the
renal, phrenic, hepatic, and lumbar veins. The
deep venous system is more important to the angiographer and is more constant in position.

1. The left adrenal vein is more constant, draining
   from the left adrenal gland into the superior
   aspect of the left main renal vein. Often the left
   inferior phrenic vein and sometimes the capsular veins drain jointly with the left adrenal vein.
   When this occurs, the left adrenal vein is the
   most laterally located tributary of the three.
2. The right adrenal vein is a small vein, usually
   arising from the inferior vena cava posterolaterally at about T11 to T12, just below the hepatic vein and about 2 to 3 cm above the right

renal vein. Occasionally it arises from the right
renal vein, and sometimes in conjunction with
an accessory hepatic vein.

Special Technical Factors

ADRENAL ARTERIOGRAPHY

Because there are multiple vessels, one should always start with an aortogram, with the catheter
positioned at the T12 level (see Fig. 12-7). Rapid
films are required early in the study. The angiographer should watch closely for the origin of the
small adrenal vessels that arise from the aorta. If
there is a hypervascular tumor, the feeding vessels
may be larger than normal, and their detection
may be the only clue to pathology. A hypervascular blush may or may not be seen on films later in
the series.

Selective catheterization is usually necessary
and may require the following techniques:

1. A celiac axis arteriogram, in order to outline
   the superior adrenal arterial branches of the inferior phrenic artery.
2. Bilateral selective renal arteriograms, in order
   to opacify inferior adrenal or possibly inferior
   phrenic arteries. Both here and in the celiac
   axis, an injection of 10 to 20 μg of epinephrine
   immediately prior to the injection of contrast
   medium preferentially constricts those vessels
   not supplying the adrenal gland and directs the

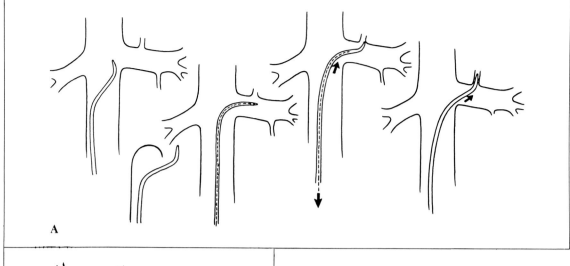

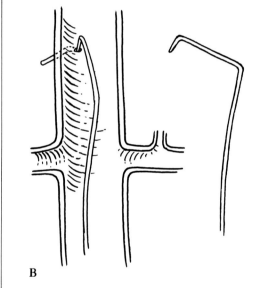

Fig. 12-4. Technique used in selective adrenal venous studies (see text for details).
A. Left adrenal vein.
B. Right adrenal vein.

ADRENAL VENOUS STUDIES

Selective adrenal venous catheterization is performed for (1) venous opacification and (2) the collection of adrenal venous effluent for hormone level determinations.

Left Adrenal Vein

A double reversed angle curved catheter should be used (Fig. 12-4A). This catheter has a gentle distal curve that forces the distal tip into the superiorly placed adrenal vein once the catheter has been placed in the left renal vein. It is also more likely to enter the more laterally placed adrenal tributary than the more medially located inferior phrenic tributary.

Place the catheter in the inferior vena cava in the usual percutaneous manner. The distal catheter shape is modified to a gentle right-angled curve by means of a Cook wire deflector or a curved stiff guidewire (do not let this guidewire protrude beyond the catheter tip). This maneuver allows selective placement of the catheter in the left renal vein. Once the guidewire has entered the renal vein orifice, advance the catheter over the wire well into the renal vein. Remove the guidewire, attach a contrast-filled syringe, and withdraw the catheter tip back to engage the adrenal vein orifice, which usually lies just lateral to the vertebral bodies. Do not confuse the intrarenal superior pole veins with the adrenal veins.

Inject only small test doses (up to 0.5 or 1.0 ml). No more than 3 to 5 ml of 60% Renografin is

contrast medium to the adrenal vessels. Under these circumstances, the injection rates should be about one-half of those listed in Table 12-1, although the total volume should remain the same.

3. Small vessel selective catheterization (e.g., middle adrenal artery or possibly the inferior phrenic artery arising from the aorta).

required per injection. Injection into the adrenal vein is usually accompanied by a transient slight discomfort in the flank. Watch carefully for extravasation or for persistent or increasing flank pain, because these signs may indicate intraadrenal hematoma and possibly subsequent infarct [2]. Bilateral adrenal infarction may induce adrenal hypofunction.

Right Adrenal Vein
The direction of the origin of the right adrenal vein as it drains into the inferior vena cava is usually cephalad (Fig. 12-4B). Advance the catheter to the right atrium over a guidewire. Following removal of the wire, fill the attached syringe and catheter with contrast agent, and slowly withdraw the catheter tip down the inferior vena cava with the catheter tip in the right posterolateral position. Repetitively inject small quantities of contrast medium (up to 0.5 ml). At the T11 or T12 level, the catheter hesitates and then inserts into the right adrenal vein. This vein is a small and delicate vessel and must be treated accordingly. Sometimes only 1 ml of contrast agent is required for opacification studies. Larger amounts of 3 to 5 ml may be required when a hypervascular tumor is present. The most frequent error of right adrenal catheterization is mistaken catheterization of a small accessory right hepatic vein (Fig. 12-5).

Problems
The most common problems that occur with venous opacification are as follows:

1. Overenthusiastic injection of contrast agent, with resulting intraparenchymal hematoma.
2. Mistaking the right accessory hepatic vein for a right adrenal vein.
3. Catheterization of adrenal veins is more difficult in patients with previous nephrectomy due to distortion of the normal anatomy.
4. Removal of venous blood for hormone determinations is often difficult and tedious due to the small size of the vein. The use of small diameter catheter tips and the drip method of collection using hydrostatic pressure (catheter hub below the level of the patient) may be more successful than active suctioning of the venous blood. Systemic heparinization prevents clotting of the catheter.

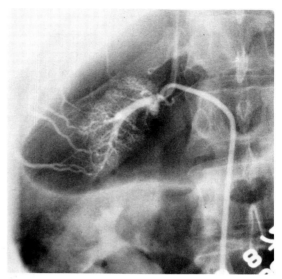

Fig. 12-5. Accessory hepatic vein (this should not be mistaken for the adrenal vein). The contour ends at the liver edge. Contrast refluxes into other hepatic veins. The hepatic vein enters more laterally or anterolaterally from the inferior vena cava than the right adrenal vein, and it has a less acute angulation from the inferior vena cava. There was no patient discomfort during this injection, in contrast to adrenal venous injections. Compare with Figure 12-3A.

5. A hypertensive crisis can occur with adrenal phlebography in pheochromocytomas, but this situation is rare.

Preferential Catheter Studies for Adrenal Lesions

Adrenal lesions for which angiography is useful are

1. Functioning tumors
   a. Pheochromocytomas. Both arteriography and venography may provide valuable information. The angiographic studies provide precise anatomic information which may be useful in planning the surgical approach. Although most pheochromocytomas can be identified by CT, occasionally small tumors missed by CT can be detected with arteriography. If a metabolically active tumor eludes CT and/or radionuclide (MIBG) detection, venous samples collected for cate-

cholamine measurement may localize the tumor [1, 5, 24].

b. Hyperfunctioning cortical adenomas. These tumors may cause Conn's syndrome, Cushing's syndrome, masculinization, or feminization. The hormonally active nature of tumors detected by CT can be confirmed and small tumors (missed by CT) can be localized by venous studies. This is most often useful in demonstrating small, aldosterone secreting adenomas. Selective gonadal venous catheterization may also be required to differentiate masculinizing or feminizing tumors of the adrenal gland from those of the gonad. Arteriography is rarely needed with cortical adenomas. Selective venous sampling from the inferior petrosal sinuses and measurement of adrenocorticotropic hormone (ACTH) levels provide documentation of an ACTH secreting pituitary adenoma (Cushing's disease) (Fig. 12-6). This may distinguish patients with a pituitary adenoma from those with an ectopic source of ACTH such as a bronchial tumor [14]. Arteriography is unnecessary.

c. Cortical hyperplasia. Adrenal venous sampling is most useful to confirm the bilateral nature of the excess hormone elaboration and exclude a unilateral process [10].

d. Adrenocarcinoma. These tumors may elaborate a variety of hormones and cause the same clinical presentation as benign adrenal adenomas. Cushing's syndrome is the most common clinical manifestation of adrenocortical carcinoma [7]. Arteriography provides important anatomic information to define the extent of the tumor and the nature of its vascular supply. Occasionally very large upper abdominal masses may distort adjacent organs to such an extent that it may be difficult to determine the tissue of origin of the tumor [11]. By defining the vascular supply, the type of tumor may be revealed [15]. Any large adrenal mass is suspicious for a primary adrenocortical carcinoma. These tumors may also extend into the vein and grow into the inferior vena cava [8]. Arteriography may reveal the arterial supply to the venous extension of the tumor; however, venography is needed to precisely de-

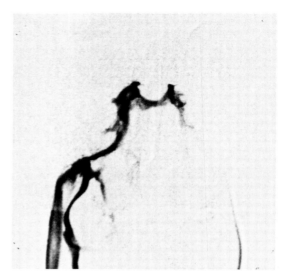

Fig. 12-6. Simultaneous bilateral inferior petrosal venous sampling for ACTH in a patient with normal adrenal glands suffering from Cushing's syndrome. A catheter is advanced from each femoral vein up to the jugular bulb and positioned anteromedially to engage the inferior petrosal vein. Digital venograms confirm correct positioning. Venous samples are obtained in search for a gradient of ACTH. A small side hole 1 mm from the tip of the catheter ensures withdrawal of blood.

fine the extent of the tumor growth within the vein. This precise delineation is essential to surgical planning [17].

2. Nonfunctioning adrenal lesions. The same angiographic definition is needed for nonfunctioning adrenal carcinomas as functioning carcinomas. Angiography is rarely needed for adrenal metastases or benign masses.

Special Precautions

Pheochromocytomas release pressor substances, which cause paroxysms of hypermetabolism together with biochemical abnormalities. This condition may occur spontaneously and is often transient. Glucagon and histamine usually stimulate these tumors to hypersecrete; they cause an elevation in blood pressure and may be used as a provocative test. Angiography (including arteriography and venous studies) can provoke a hypertensive crisis [26]. The radiographic diagnostic provocative tests may be used during the study [21]. If the pressure is elevated but no tumor is seen, an aggressive diagnostic approach is indicated, because a lesion may be present. These hypertensive crises are dangerous, and the angiographer must take certain precautions in order to preclude complications arising from them.

1. Prior to the study check for elevated vanillylmandelic acid and abnormal catecholamine levels.
   a. If norepinephrine levels are higher than normal (above 50 μg), an extraadrenal tumor may be present. These tumors occur in 10 percent of all patients with pheochromocytomas. Because pheochromocytomas (as well as neuroblastomas and ganglioneuromas) arise from chromaffin cells (pheochromocytes), knowledge of their possible location throughout the sympathetic system can be helpful in planning studies. The search for their location is often extensive and requires careful angiography of the supraclavicular area (see Fig. 12-8), the thoracic aorta, the abdominal aorta, and the pelvic vessels in addition to the suprarenal areas. Subtraction techniques may prove helpful. If the tumor is not detected by these means, 5-ml blood samples should be drawn from the veins of the pelvis, kidneys, and adrenals and from the inferior vena cava, the superior vena cava, the azygos veins, and the innominate veins for plasma catecholamine determinations. Both the patient and the angiographer should be prepared for a comprehensive examination, which may be divided into two consecutive studies.
   b. Primary elevation of serum epinephrine levels (above 25 μg) indicates that the location of the tumor is more likely in the adrenal glands. The tumors may be multiple and bilateral (10 percent of patients). If there is a family history of pheochromocytomas (particularly when they are associated with other endocrine tumors such as medullary carcinoma of the thyroid and hyperparathyroidism), they are usually bilateral. Ten percent of pheochromocytomas are malignant, and metastatic extension must be considered.
   c. If the patient has a labile blood pressure, stabilize his condition with an alpha-adrenergic blocker such as phenoxybenz-

amine hydrochloride (Dibenzyline), 10 mg given 4 times a day, for 4 to 10 days prior to the procedure.
   d. Sedate the patient heavily prior to the study.
2. During the study, a peripheral vein should be kept open at all times with an intravenous solution of 5% dextrose and water administered through a large-bore needle. Monitor pressures closely (with a physiologic monitoring unit if possible). A rise in intraaortic pressure during or immediately following the aortogram increases the likelihood that a tumor is present, and if it is not immediately demonstrated, further selective studies are required. Antihypertensive agents must be immediately available for intravenous administration; cautious administration of these drugs should be started if the pressure rises higher than 20 mm Hg systolic above the resting pressure. Phentolamine (Regitine) is a potent antiadrenergic drug that should be given intravenously in the event of a hypertensive crisis. Five mg mixed with 1 ml of sterile saline solution is injected rapidly in adults; a smaller dose (1 mg) is given in children.

Sodium nitroprusside is another antihypertensive agent that is potent and rapid-acting, and its effect ends almost immediately when the intravenous infusion of the drug is stopped. The hypotensive effect of sodium nitroprusside is augmented by ganglionic blocking agents. With this drug, hypotension is induced by peripheral vasodilatation as a result of direct action on blood vessels, independent of autonomic innervation. This drug should not be used unless there are adequate facilities for monitoring blood pressure, because it requires precise measurements of dosage rate. Tachyarrhythmias may develop during the hypertensive crisis, which can be controlled with small intravenous doses of lidocaine (50 to 100 mg).

Angiographic Findings

PHEOCHROMOCYTOMAS

Pheochromocytomas are often hypervascular tumors (Figs. 12-7, 12-8). Although the aortogram usually shows some clue as to the presence of the tumor (e.g., hypertrophied feeding artery, angiographic hypervascular blush on later films), in many patients selective studies are required for

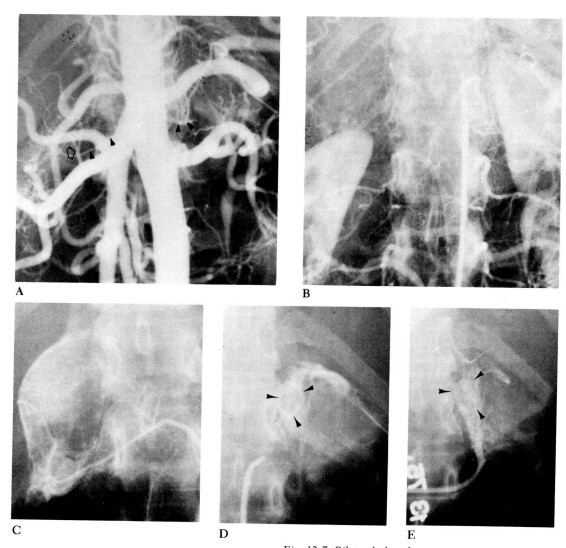

Fig. 12-7. Bilateral pheochromocytoma.

A. Abdominal aortogram. In the early phase on the right, a prominent inferior adrenal artery (from the right renal artery—*open arrow*) and middle adrenal artery (from the abdominal aorta just above the renal artery—*arrowheads*) are seen. A prominent left middle adrenal artery is also present (*arrowheads*).

B. Late phase aortogram. Very vague and nondiagnostic vascularity is present in the right suprarenal area.

C. Selective right middle adrenal arteriogram, showing obvious hypervascular tumor.

D. Left middle adrenal arteriogram, late phase, shows a 1-cm tumor (*arrowheads*) in the left adrenal gland.

E. Left adrenal venogram confirms small tumor (*arrowheads*) displacing the intraadrenal venous radicles.

diagnosis [4, 6]. These tumors are usually hypervascular and may show a dense accumulation of contrast medium in the capillary bed [3]. The vascularity is variable and is usually more prominent in the periphery of the tumor; it is sometimes faint and barely perceptible. Faint accumulation of contrast medium may be the only clue to the presence of the tumor.

Pheochromocytomas may be cystic, with small displaced vessels being the only vascular abnormality; occasionally they are densely staining, with marked neovascularity and "pooling" of contrast agent. It is difficult to determine malignant degeneration by the angiographic features alone; how-

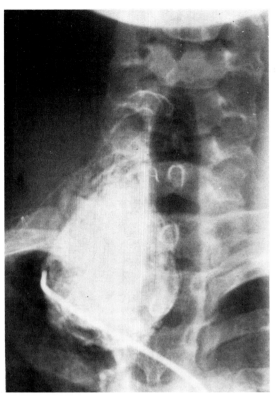

Fig. 12-8. Hypervascular functioning right su-praclavicular paraganglioma in a hypertensive patient with multiple similar tumors in the abdomen who presented with elevated norepinephrine levels.

ever, invasion of surrounding structures or metastatic deposits indicate malignancy.

The multiple endocrine neoplasia syndromes are familial disorders in which hyperplasia or tumor involve more than one endocrine gland [29]. Two types of this syndrome involve the adrenal glands. In Sipple's syndrome (multiple endocrine neoplasia type II) pheochromocytoma is associated with medullary carcinoma of the thyroid and parathyroid hyperplasia or adenoma. Multiple endocrine neoplasia type III includes not only pheochromocytoma and medullary thyroid carcinoma, but also mucosal neuromas, a marfanoid habitus and intestinal ganglioneuromatasis. In both of these syndromes, the pheochromocytomas are most often bilateral but not extraadrenal [13].

CORTICAL ADENOMAS
The fact that an adenoma is functioning does not influence its arteriographic appearance but does influence the diagnostic approach. If the tumor is functioning, the venous approach is stressed, because with this approach one not only can see angiographic abnormalities but also can withdraw venous effluent for subsequent analysis of hormonal substances. Tumors cause displacement of veins, and a comma-shaped draping of veins is often seen around a small tumor (Figs. 12-9, 12-10). If the tumor is vascular there is a proliferation of veins surrounding the gland; these veins may fill on retrograde injection. In functioning adrenal adenomas, there is often atrophy of the opposing gland (Fig. 12-10B); this is a helpful differential point in determining whether the vascular displacement is caused by a tumor or whether it is caused by a hyperplastic nodule.

Aldosteronism
In aldosteronism [28, 31], the patient presents clinically with systemic diastolic hypertension, suppressed plasma renin activity, increased peripheral venous aldosterone levels, and lowered serum potassium levels. It can be caused by cortical adrenal adenomas, adrenal hyperplasia or, rarely, by adrenal carcinoma. Because surgical removal is indicated for the adenoma and medical treatment for hyperplasia, it is important to distinguish between these two most common causes for hyperaldosteronism.

ALDOSTERONE-PRODUCING ADENOMAS. Eighty-five percent of patients with primary aldosteronism have an underlying adenoma. The adenomas are usually unilateral and small (often 1–2 cm in diameter). Rarely can they be identified by arteriograms, and only two-thirds can be detected by venograms. The typical angiographic appearance is that of displacement and distortion of the small adrenal venous radicles by the mass (see Figs. 12-9A, B). The findings are often subtle.

ADRENAL HYPERPLASIA. Adrenal hyperplasia may also cause aldosteronism (in 15 percent of cases). The hyperplasia may be diffuse where the glands are generally enlarged, with spreading of the fine venous radicles and a convexity of the borders of the glands. A nodular hyperplasia may be present, and the individual nodules are indistinguishable venographically from adenomas (Fig. 12-11). The nodules are usually smaller than adenomas, multiple, and often bilateral, and there is a relative increase in the size of the remainder of

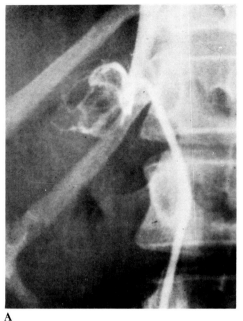

A

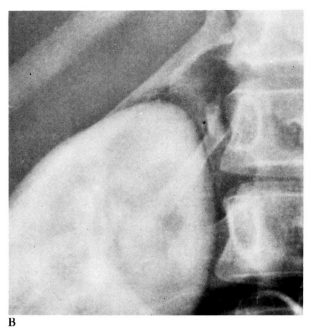

B

Fig. 12-9. Adenoma of the right adrenal gland, causing aldosteronism.

A. Right adrenal venogram shows obvious displacement of the adrenal venous radicals around the tumor.

B. Arteriogram on the same patient, showing relative radiolucency in the capillary phase of the selective adrenal arteriogram. The arterial study is not as convincing as the venogram.

Fig. 12-10. Left adrenal adenoma, causing Cushing's disease and atrophy of the right adrenal gland.

A. Left adrenal venogram shows dense staining of contrast medium (pooling) in a vein (*arrow*) surrounding the adenoma.

B. Delayed subtraction film of the right renal arteriogram shows an atrophic right adrenal gland.

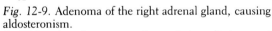

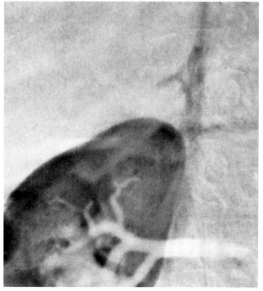

A   **B**

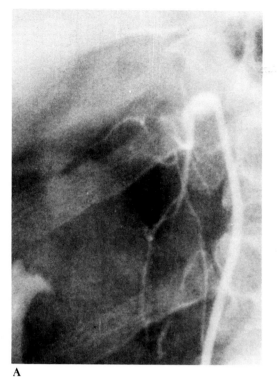

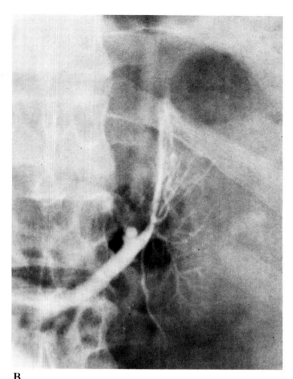

A   **B**

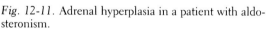

Fig. 12-11. Adrenal hyperplasia in a patient with aldo-
steronism.
A. Right adrenal venogram shows enlarged adrenal
    veins with displacement of adrenal venous radicles
    with a hyperplastic nodule superolaterally.
B. Diffusely enlarged left adrenal gland. Aldosterone
    levels were elevated bilaterally but were more severe
    on the left.

the adrenal glands. This appearance contrasts with
that of functioning adenomas, in which the remaining gland tissue atrophies.

Adrenal venous blood samples showing elevated
aldosterone levels usually lateralize the lesion, despite normal venograms.

Cushing's Syndrome
Cushing's syndrome may be caused by adrenal
adenoma, adrenal hyperplasia, or by carcinoma.
Sometimes the glands are normal in size. Rarely,
pituitary tumors or extraadrenal tumors (with ectopic ACTH production) may cause Cushing's
syndrome; these tumors can be differentiated clinically. Whether the Cushing's syndrome is caused
by an adenoma or by adrenal hyperplasia can also
be differentiated clinically (prior to angiography),

because dexamethasone suppresses the hyperplasia
but not the adenoma. Some cases of nodular
hyperplasia, however, do not suppress. Adrenal
adenomas causing Cushing's syndrome are of varying sizes. The arteriographic picture depends on
the pathology of the tumor and the extent of cystic
degeneration present. If the tumor is large, there is
displacement of the surrounding vessels. If it is
solid, there is often hypervascularity with large
feeding vessels and large prematurely filling veins.
Adrenal tumors are usually well demarcated. If the
tumor is cystic, only signs of displacement of vessels and kidney displacement may be seen. If the
adenoma is both cystic and small, it may go undetected by arteriography. It is important to study
both sides because in a functioning adenoma, the
atrophic opposite gland is usually demonstrable.

Adrenal hyperplasia may occur; usually clinical
manifestations suffice for the diagnosis. If the
radiologist's help is asked, the hyperplasia is best
studied by venography. The glands bilaterally are
larger than normal, both in mediolateral and
cephalocaudad measurements, and the lateral borders are convex. The veins are separated and may
be enlarged.

The venograms of nodular hyperplasia may show vessels displaced by small nodules (less than 2 cm) bilaterally, as well as bilateral gland enlargement. This appearance contrasts with that seen in adenomas, in which the tumor is usually larger and is unilateral, and the opposite gland is either normal in size or atrophic [22]. If the veins of only one side can be entered, the unilateral venogram and cortisol levels may still be helpful. If the cortisol level is elevated and no tumor is seen, the patient likely has a bilateral hyperplastic process, in which case the other side is also elevated. If the cortisol level is low or normal and no tumor is seen, the other side must then have the adenoma.

Adrenogenital Syndrome

Hypersecretion of testosterone or (less frequently) estrogens may occur by functioning tumors, which may be benign or malignant. Such hypersecretion may also occur with adrenal hyperplasia. Arteriography may be used to define the extent of the usually hypervascular malignant tumors. Venous studies are most helpful in the benign lesions, both for venography and for collection of blood for hormonal assay [16].

MALIGNANT TUMORS

Malignant tumors may show varying degrees of hypervascularity and neovascularity. They usually show tumor vessels with irregular margins, pooling, and an excessive capillary blush, often with extraadrenal feeding vessels (Fig. 12-12). Venographically, there may be encasement and invasion of veins, displacement, and occlusion of veins. These tumors frequently metastasize to the liver, bone, and lymph nodes and sometimes to the chest. Adrenal carcinomas frequently have calcification scattered throughout the parenchyma [11], and approximately 75 percent of them are hormonally active. They can destroy adrenal function and cause Addison's disease.

Neuroblastomas, which are usually seen in early childhood, are found in the adrenal area in 50 percent of cases. They often calcify. They cause displacement of surrounding organs, metastasize early, and although hypervascular, they usually do not require angiography for diagnosis. Neuroblastomas are often obvious on plain films of the abdomen and intravenous pyelograms by the time they are detected clinically.

Metastatic disease from other organs to the adre-

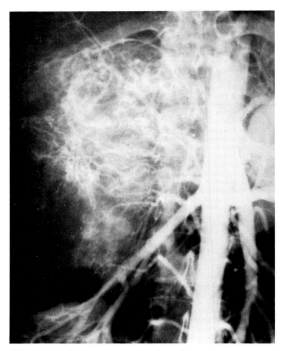

Fig. 12-12. Malignant right adrenal tumor in a patient with adrenogenital syndrome. There is marked neovascularity with prominent inferior middle and superior adrenal arteries.

Fig. 12-13. Metastatic tumor to the right adrenal gland in a patient with known carcinoma of the lung. The prominent inferior adrenal artery arising from an accessory renal artery shows tumor neovascularity, indicating a malignant process.

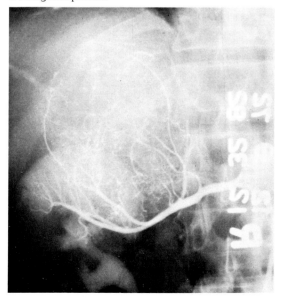

nals occurs frequently. The vascularity of the primary lesion is often reflected in the malignant adrenal metastatic deposit [19] (Fig. 12-13).

ADRENAL CYSTS

These benign, nonfunctioning adrenal cortical masses are rare; they are found most frequently in the fifth and sixth decades. They show curvilinear calcification in approximately 15 percent of cases and are often caused by hemorrhage into a normal gland or into an adenoma or other tumor. Adrenal cysts are always avascular and show characteristic displacement of vessels around a smooth, avascular mass.

References

1. Agee, O. F., Kaude, J., and Lepasoon, J. Preoperative localization of pheochromocytoma. *Acta Radiol. [Diagn.] (Stockh.)* 14:545, 1973.
2. Bayliss, R. I. S., Edwards, O. M., and Starer, F. Complications of adrenal venography. *Br. J. Radiol.* 43:531, 1970.
3. Beckmann, C. F., Levin, D. C., and Phillips, D. A. Angiography of nonfunctioning pheochromocytomas of the adrenal gland. *Radiology* 124:53, 1977.
4. Boijsen, E., et al. Angiography of pheochromocytoma. *Am. J. Roentgenol.* 98:225, 1966.
5. Cho, K. J. Current role of angiography in the evaluation of adrenal disease causing hypertension. *Urol. Radiol.* 3:249, 1982.
6. Christenson, R., et al. Arteriographic manifestations of pheochromocytoma. *Am. J. Roentgenol.* 126:567, 1976.
7. Didolkar, M. S., et al. Natural history of adrenal cortical carcinoma: A clinicopathologic study of 42 patients. *Cancer* 47:2153, 1981.
8. Dunnick, N. R., Doppman, J. L., and Geelhoed, G. W. Intravenous extension of endocrine tumors. *A.J.R.* 135:471, 1980.
9. Dunnick, N. R., et al. Localization of functional adrenal tumors by computed tomography and venous sampling. *Radiology* 142:429, 1982.
10. Dunnick, N. R., et al. Preoperative diagnosis and localization of aldosteronomas by measurement of corticosteroids in adrenal venous blood. *Radiology* 133:331, 1979.
11. Dunnick, N. R., et al. CT appearance of adrenal cortical carcinoma. *J. Comput. Assist. Tomogr.* 6:978, 1982.
12. Dunnick, N. R., and Korobkin, M. Computed tomography of the adrenal gland in hypertension. *Urol. Radiol.* 3:245, 1982.
13. Ekelund, L., and Hoevels, J. Adrenal angiography

in Sipple's syndrome. *Acta Radiol. [Diagn.] (Stockh.)* 20:637, 1979.
14. Findling, J. W., et al. Selective venous sampling for ACTH in Cushing's syndrome. *Ann. Intern. Med.* 94:647, 1981.
15. Fritzsche, P., Andersen, C., and Cahil, P. Vascular specificity in differentiating adrenal carcinoma from renal cell carcinoma. *Radiology* 125:113, 1977.
16. Gabrilove, J. L., Nicolis, G. L., and Mitty, H. A. Virilizing adrenocortical adenoma studied by selective adrenal venography. *Am. J. Obstet. Gynecol.* 125:180, 1976.
17. Geelhoed, G. W., Dunnick, N. R., and Doppman, J. L. Management of intravenous extensions of endocrine tumors and prognosis after surgical treatment. *Am. J. Surg.* 139:844, 1980.
18. Gross, M. D., Thompson, N. W., and Beierwaltes, W. H. Scintigraphic approach to the localization of adrenal lesions causing hypertension. *Urol. Radiol.* 3:241, 1982.
19. Hoevels, J., and Ekelund, L. Angiographic findings in adrenal masses. *Acta. Radiol. [Diagn.] (Stockh.)* 20:337, 1979.
20. Kahn, P. Selective angiography of the adrenal glands. *Am. J. Roentgenol.* 101:739, 1967.
21. McEwan, A. J., et al. Radioiodobenzylguanidine for the scintigraphic location and therapy of adrenergic tumors. *Semin. Nucl. Med.* XV:132, 1985.
22. Mitty, H., Gabrilove, J., and Nicolis, G. Nontumorous adrenal hyperfunction: problems in angiographic-clinical correlation. *Radiology* 122:89, 1977.
23. Nicolis, G. L., et al. Percutaneous adrenal venography: A clinical study of 50 patients. *Ann. Intern. Med.* 76:899, 1972.
24. Palubinskas, A. J., Roizen, M. F., and Conte, F. A. Localization of functioning pheochromocytomas by venous sampling and radioenzymatic analysis. *Radiology* 136:495, 1980.
25. Reinig, J. W., et al. Distinction between adrenal adenomas and metastases using MR imaging. *J. Comput. Assist. Tomogr.* 9:898, 1985.
26. Rossi, P. Techniques, usefulness and hazards of arteriography in pheochromocytoma: Review of 99 cases. *J.A M.A.* 205:547, 1968.
27. Sarkar, S., et al. A new and superior adrenal scanning agent: NP-59. *J. Nucl. Med.* 16:1038, 1975.
28. Scoggins, B.A., et al. Preoperative lateralization of aldosterone-producing tumors in primary aldosteronism. *Ann. Intern. Med.* 76:891, 1972.
29. Voorhees, M. L. Disorders of the adrenal medulla and multiple endocrine adenomatoses. *Ped. Clin. North Am.* 26:209, 1979.
30. Yeh, H. C. Sonography of the adrenal glands: Normal glands and small masses. *A.J.R.* 135:1167, 1980.
31. Yune, H., et al. Radiology and primary aldosteronism. *Am. J. Roentgenol.* 127:761, 1976.

Splanchnic Angiography

Indications

The indications for angiography of the gastrointestinal tract and its accessory organs are being modified, and in part displaced, by the continuing improvement in technology and experience of computed tomography, ultrasonography, and now, in addition, magnetic resonance imaging. Angiography still has a role in evaluating the following:

1. Primary vascular lesions
   a. Obstruction or stenosis
      (1) Atherosclerosis
      (2) Median arcuate ligament of the diaphragm
      (3) Thrombosis
      (4) Embolus
      (5) Fibromuscular dysplasia
      (6) Dissecting vessels
   b. Anomalies and congenital variations
      (1) Congenital stenosis or arterial agenesis
      (2) Arteriovenous malformations
      (3) Replaced right and/or left hepatic arteries
   c. Acquired arteriovenous fistulas and angiodysplasias
   d. Aneurysms
   e. Trauma—thrombosis, rupture, dissection, extravasation, embolus, hematoma, false aneurysms, arteriovenous fistula
2. Lesions of accessory organs (pancreas, liver, spleen, gallbladder)
   a. Space-occupying lesions
      (1) Tumors
         (a) Benign
         (b) Malignant—primary or metastatic
      (2) Cysts, pseudocysts
   b. Inflammatory lesions; abscess, pancreatitis
   c. Trauma—laceration, rupture, hematoma, hemorrhage
3. Lesions of gastrointestinal tract (stomach, small bowel, colon)
   a. Acute and chronic bleeding
   b. Benign and malignant tumors
4. Evaluation of the portal system
5. Catheter placement for:
   a. Treatment of gastrointestinal bleeding
   b. Chemotherapy infusion for malignancy
6. Selective venous catheterization for hormone evaluation

Approaches

1. The percutaneous femoral artery approach is preferable when feasible.
2. The percutaneous left axillary artery approach affords easy selective entry into either the celiac axis or the superior mesenteric arteries, but it has a higher local complication rate to the axillary artery (Fig. 13-1) and may be technically more difficult in patients with elongation and tortuosity of the aorta.
3. The percutaneous basilic vein, femoral vein, or right internal jugular vein approaches are used for hepatic vein wedge pressure measurement and angiography (see Chap. 21).
4. Percutaneous organ puncture is used in the following situations (see Chap. 23):
   a. Splenic puncture, for evaluating splenic vein, portal vein, and splenic pulp pressures.
   b. Transhepatic puncture for:
      (1) Evaluating the pancreatic venous bed, both angiographically and for hormone assay [52]; gastric and esophageal varices.
      (2) Occluding bleeding varices and measuring pressures [91, 105].
5. Umbilical vein cutdown is used for evaluating portal vein pressures and angiography [49].

Catheters

The following catheters may be used with the femoral artery approach:

1. For the celiac axis and superior mesenteric artery, use a 5, 6, or 6.5 French 65-cm polyethylene or polyurethane catheter. One or two side holes just proximal to the tip help reduce catheter recoil and limit the possibility of a "jetstream" subintimal injection.
   a. For a vessel arising at an acute angle, use a

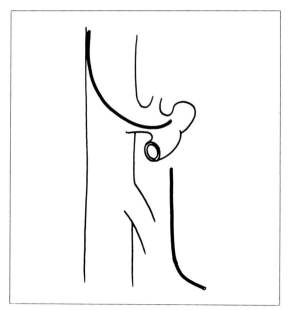

Fig. 13-1. Catheter shape for selective celiac and mesenteric arteriography from the axillary approach. An added curve 1 cm from the distal tip directed to the right or left can be formed for superselective hepatic or splenic artery catheter placement respectively.

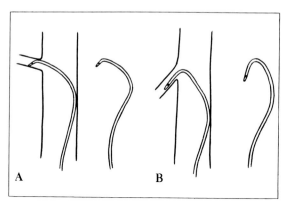

Fig. 13-2. Catheter shapes for celiac and superior mesenteric artery injections.
A. Cobra-head catheter tip.
B. Primary curve of 45 degrees ("celiac hook" or "renal double hook").

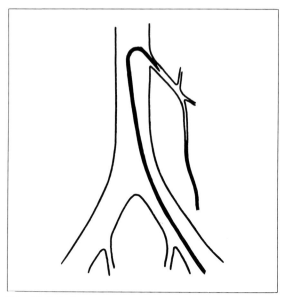

Fig. 13-3. Inferior mesenteric artery catheter. There is a sharp angulation to the catheter tip. The left femoral approach may facilitate catheter placement in the absence of significant atherosclerotic elongation and tortuosity.

curved distal tip with 45-degree-angle primary curve that is approximately 2 cm proximal to the tip (Fig. 13-2B).

b. For a 90-degree or obtuse-angle vessel takeoff, use a cobra-head catheter tip (Fig. 13-2A).

2. For the inferior mesenteric artery, use a 5 or 6 French 65-cm polyethylene end-hole catheter with a 45-degree primary curve that is approximately 1.0 to 1.5 cm proximal to the tip. Side holes are optional (Fig. 13-3). Alternately, use a 5F or 6F polyethylene end-hole catheter with a Mikaelsson curve (see Fig. 13-7C). This catheter may also be used for the celiac axis and superior mesenteric artery.

3. For superselective studies of the hepatic artery, splenic artery, gastroduodenal artery, left gastric artery, and dorsal pancreatic artery, use

a. A specific preshaped 65-cm polyethylene 5, 6, or 6.5 French catheter designed by Rosch (Fig. 13-4). A catheter deflector[1] may be required to temporarily shape a primary curve that is capable of entering the origin of the celiac axis [90].

[1]Manufactured by Cook, Inc., Box 489, Bloomington, IN 47401.

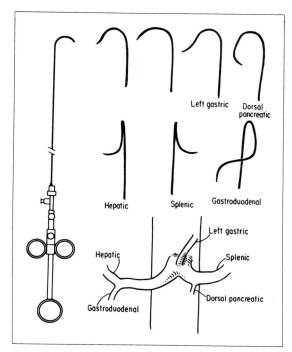

Fig. 13-4. Multiple preformed curves for selective and superselective catheterization of branches of the celiac axis. These various shapes straighten out when inserted in the abdominal aorta; the curve must be restored in the abdominal aorta at or just above the level of the origin of the celiac axis by means of an external catheter manipulator.

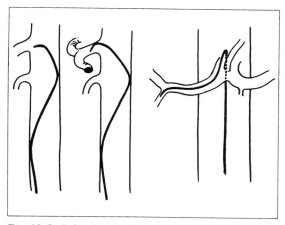

Fig. 13-5. Cobra-head catheter formulated by Judkins, with a short, obtuse-angled primary curve 1 cm or less from the tip. A gentle, sweeping secondary curve helps to force this catheter beyond the primary curve into the selected vessel once its origin has been engaged.

Fig. 13-6. Exaggerated cobra shape ("Waltman loop"). The maneuvers shown here allow the catheter tip to be placed deep within the hepatic, gastroduodenal, splenic, and left gastric branches (see text for details).

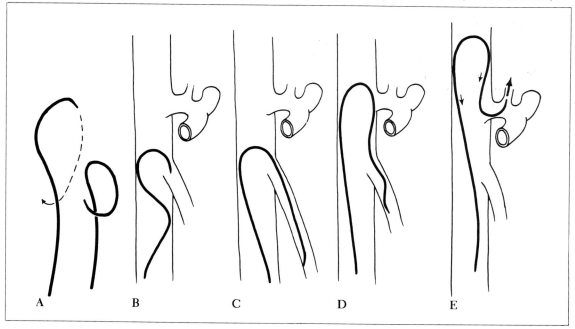

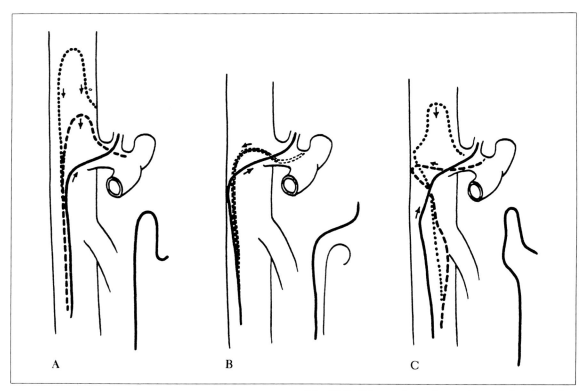

A   B   C

b. A cobra-head 5, 6, or 6.5 French polyethylene or polyurethane end-hole catheter without side holes (Fig. 13-5).

c. An exaggerated curve of a cobra-head catheter ("Waltman loop") [108] (Fig. 13-6). The curve should be formed on a polyurethane catheter immediately prior to the catheterization procedure. Place a forming wire in the catheter tip, shape as desired, and immerse the tip in boiling sterile water for 2 to 3 minutes. Both the shape and softness of the catheter induced by recent boiling facili-

Fig. 13-7. Other catheter shapes that may be adapted for superselective arteriography (e.g., the left gastric artery).

A. Reversed curve splanchnic catheter [22]. The secondary curve can be elongated (from 3 to 8 cm) to accommodate an elongated or sharply angulated celiac trunk.

B. Left adrenal vein catheter. The stiff end of the guidewire or an external manipulator must be used to advance the catheter tip well into the celiac axis. The wire is then removed and the catheter withdrawn in order to engage its tip into the left gastric artery. The catheter can be advanced deep into the vessel over a leading guidewire. This technique may also be used for selective placement in other small and large branches of the abdominal and thoracic aorta.

C. Mikaelsson curve.

tate superselective catheter placement. Engage the catheter tip into the origin of the superior mesenteric artery or celiac axis and advance it well into the artery. When the secondary curve is reached, continued advancement in the aorta causes the catheter to withdraw from the selected vessel, giving a new curve to the catheter with an exaggerated shape as it lies within the aorta. Rotating the catheter so that the tip faces anteriorly now engages the catheter tip in the celiac axis. With this new shape, withdrawing the catheter advances it more deeply into the selective branches. This technique is particularly helpful for left gastric artery catheterization. This maneuver may also be performed with other initial catheter shapes (e.g., renal double curve) and may be achieved in other locations such as over the aortic bifurcation.

d. In difficult cases in which the takeoff angle of the celiac axis is acute, catheter shapes designed for other areas may be helpful. The Simmons No. 1 or 2 curved catheter (Fig. 13-7A), which is used in brachiocephalic angiography, can be manipulated into the celiac axis and subsequently into the splenic, hepatic, or gastric artery. The curved tip, which is straightened when first introduced into the abdominal aorta, should be advanced to the aortic arch. Here the tip may be directed caudad and anteriorly and slowly pulled down to engage the celiac axis. One should take care not to form a knot in the catheter during manipulations in the arch. The catheter used for left adrenal vein catheterization can be advanced into the left gastric artery over a fixed curve guidewire or a catheter manipulator, as described previously (Fig. 13-7B). Another helpful catheter is the Mikaelsson curve (Fig. 13-7C).

A detailed, technical review of the many catheter manipulations that may be performed to achieve successful superselective catheterization of splanchnic branches was published by Chuang in 1983 [22]. He describes in great detail a variety of helpful maneuvers (similar to those described here) used successfully to catheterize the hepatic artery in 1000 patients.

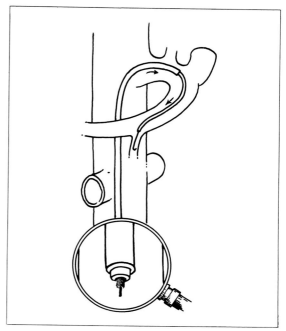

Fig. 13-8. Coaxial catheter system, containing three components: (1) a thin-walled 6 French (2-mm outer diameter) catheter with minimal tapering of the tip, which has a primary curve capable of entering the splanchnic vessel origin; (2) an inner 4 French (1.33-mm outer diameter) Teflon catheter; and (3) a guidewire with a fine, flexible, curved tip and a movable inner core.

e. An Eisenberg coaxial catheter system[2] (Fig. 13-8). There are three components to this system:
(1) A thin-walled 6 French catheter with minimal tapering of the catheter tip, which has a primary curve capable of entering the origin of the splanchnic vessel.
(2) An inner 4 French Teflon catheter, which has tensile strength and offers minimal friction.
(3) A finely made inner guidewire with a curved tip and smoothly movable inner core. When the outer catheter engages the vessel origin, the inner components are advanced to its tip. The intraluminal guidewire is advanced initially, followed in sequence by the inner Teflon catheter

[2]Manufactured by International Catheter Corp., 2040 Millburn Ave., Maplewood, NJ 07040; Electro Catheter Corp., Rahway, NJ 07065.

and then the outer catheter, first to secondary and then to third order branches. The inner guidewire and Teflon catheter together act as a leader over which the larger catheter may be advanced into the superselective position; they are removed prior to the injection of contrast medium.

4. For superselective catheterization of mesenteric branches, use a 5, 6, or 6.5 French soft polyethylene catheter with a 100-degree primary curve that is angled to the right (for colic branches) or to the left (for ileal or jejunal branches). This curve lies approximately 10 to 15 mm proximal to the tip. A secondary curve with a 45-degree angle lies 6 cm proximal to the distal (primary) curve (Fig. 13-9). The catheter is advanced over a guidewire that has been previously wedged deep in an ileal branch. After the wire is removed, the catheter tip is gradually withdrawn to the target vessel.

5. An open-ended guidewire[3] that may be used for superselective catheterization contains a steerable, removable 0.016-inch J-tipped core which facilitates entry into small peripheral branches. Once in place the core is removed and an injection may be done through the guidewire itself. Depending on the size of the wire (0.035 inch or 0.038 inch) and the viscosity and temperature of the contrast medium, up to 4 ml/second (manufacturer's specifications) may be injected. (This wire may also be used for infusion of vasopressors or injection of small, 0.1–0.3 mm, particles for embolization.)

6. For selective celiac artery and superior and inferior mesenteric artery catheterization from the axillary approach, use a 5, 6, or 6.5 French catheter with a single, gentle distal curve (see Fig. 13-1).

7. For hepatic venous wedge pressure measurements, an end-hole catheter with no side holes is necessary for obtaining accurate wedge pressure measurements. Any catheter material may be used. From the basilic, axillary, or internal jugular venous approach, a 5, 6, or 6.5 French catheter with a single, gentle distal curve passes easily through the right atrium to engage the

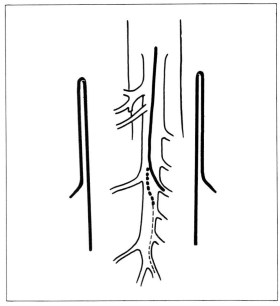

Fig. 13-9. Catheter for selective placement in branches of the superior mesenteric artery.

hepatic vein. Balloon catheters (e.g., a Swan Ganz catheter) may also be used [75]. From the femoral venous approach, a straight 5 or 6 French polyethylene catheter without side holes is advanced over a curved deflector or a fixed curve wire. A Simmons II or III catheter, shaped in the right atrium, may also be used from the femoral route. Once shaped, the tip easily engages the hepatic veins, and continued withdrawal of the catheter at the groin advances the tip deeper into the hepatic vein until a wedged position is achieved.

8. For portal venous cannulation (transhepatic), use of 30 cm or 45 cm sharply beveled 18-gauge needle with snugly fitting overlying Teflon sleeve (see Figs. 23-2, 23-3).

Contrast Agents, Projections, and Radiographic Programming

Details concerning contrast agents, projections, and radiographic programming are given in Tables 13-1, 13-2, and 13-3. Large doses of contrast medium and prolonged film timing are often required to opacify the portal venous system adequately. Contrast doses may be significantly reduced and film timing shortened by the use of digital vascular imaging systems [36, 37].

---

[3] Manufactured by USCI Division of C. R. Bard Inc., Billerica, MA 01821.

Table 13-1. Technical specifications in splanchnic angiography in the adult (arterial)[a]

Location of angiographic procedure	Contrast agent			Total films	Total time (sec)	Radiographic program		Projections
	Density	Volume (ml/inj)	Rate (ml/sec)			Films/sec	Timing	
Celiac axis	M	60	8–10	20	26	2/sec for 4 sec; 1/sec for 2 sec; 1 every other sec for 20 sec	Start films 0.4 sec after start of injection	AP RPO may show head or tail of pancreas better
Splenic artery	M	70	5	20	30	1/sec for 10 sec; 1 every other sec for 20 sec		
Hepatic artery Standard	M	40	5–8	16	18	2/sec for 4 sec; 1/sec for 2 sec; 1 every other sec for 12 sec	Start films 0.4 sec after start of injection	
For metastatic disease	M	65[c]	3 for 10 sec; 7 for 5 sec				Start films after 10 sec[c]	
Gastroduodenal artery	L	30[d]	5	16	18	2/sec for 4 sec; 1/sec for 2 sec; 1 every other sec for 12 sec	Start films 0.4 sec after start of injection	
Dorsal pancreatic artery	L or (NI)	30[d]	4	16	18			
Superior mesenteric artery For portal system[b]	M	64+	8	20	34	1/sec for 6 sec; 1 every other sec for 28 sec		
Other	M	64+	8	20	26	2/sec for 4 sec; 1/sec for 2 sec; 1 every other sec for 20 sec		
Inferior mesenteric artery	M	15–25	4–5	20	26	2/sec for 4 sec; 1/sec for 2 sec; 1 every other sec for 20 sec		

[a]For IA-DSA studies, use one-half concentration of contrast agent and one-half to two-thirds the volume with the same injection rates.
[b]For primary study of the portal system, immediately precede the contrast injection with an intraarterial vasodilator (tolazoline, 37 mg injected slowly over 1 minute) through the same catheter.
[c]Looking for small metastases.
[d]Catheter must not be wedged.
Note: M = medium density contrast agent; L = low density contrast agent; NI = nonionic contrast agent (see Appendix 3).

Table 13-2. Technical specifications in splanchnic angiography in the adult (venous)

Angiographic procedure	Contrast agent			Total films	Total time (sec)	Radiographic program		Projections
	Density	Volume (ml/inj)	Rate (ml/sec)			Films/sec	Timing	
Hepatic vein wedge	L	8	2	12	8	2/sec for 4 sec; 1/sec for 4 sec	Start films 0.4 sec after start of injections	AP
Splenic pulp	M	60	10	20	16	2/sec for 4 sec; 1/sec for 12 sec		AP: include lower thorax and upper abdomen in mid respiration
DSA (21-gauge needle)	30%	16	4	30 (frame)	15	2/sec		
Transhepatic portal venogram	M	60	10	20	16	2/sec for 4 sec; 1/sec for 12 sec		

Note: M = medium density contrast agent; L = low density contrast agent (see Appendix 3).

Table 13-3. Technical specifications in splanchnic angiography in the child[a]

Location of angiographic procedure	Contrast agent[b]			Total films	Total time (sec)	Radiographic program		Projections
	Density	Volume (ml)	Rate (ml/sec)			Films/sec	Timing	
Celiac axis and superior mesenteric artery								
Infant	L or NI	1.0–1.2 ml/kg	Total within 5 sec	16	19	3/sec for 2 sec; 1/sec for 3 sec; 1 every other sec for 14 sec	Start films 0.4 sec after start of injection	AP
Other	M or NI							
Inferior mesenteric artery								
Infant	L or NI	5–20 ml	Total within 5 sec	16	19	3/sec for 2 sec; 1/sec for 3 sec; 1 every other sec for 14 sec		AP
Other	M or NI							

[a] For IA-DSA studies, use one-half concentration of contrast agent and two-thirds to the same volume with the same injection rates.
[b] Amount of contrast agent varies with body weight in children.
Note: M = medium density contrast agent; L = low density contrast agent; NI = nonionic contrast agent (see Appendix 3).

Anatomic Considerations

THE CELIAC AXIS

The celiac axis supplies the liver, gallbladder, stomach, proximal duodenum, pancreas, and spleen (Fig. 13-10) [63, 69, 73, 96]. It arises anteriorly from the aorta at the level of the twelfth vertebra. A common trunk gives rise to three major vessels: the common hepatic, splenic, and left gastric arteries. The dorsal pancreatic artery may form a fourth branch.

The Liver

As the common hepatic artery branches to the right from the celiac axis, it gives off the gastroduodenal artery and continues on as the hepatic artery proper. This artery in turn divides into three major intrahepatic branches—the right, middle, and left hepatic arteries. The right branch supplies the right lobe; the middle branch supplies the medial segment of the left lobe; the left branch supplies the lateral segment of the left lobe. There are multiple anomalies of the origins of vessels to the liver (summarized in Fig. 13-11). Although there are small anastomoses between the intrahepatic branches which may enlarge in occlusive disease, hepatic arteries should be considered as end arteries, because their occlusion may result in hepatic necrosis. The hepatic parenchymal phase is usually homogeneous but may be mottled.

The Gallbladder

The cystic arteries arise from the right, left, or common hepatic arteries. Normally, a thin, well-defined gallbladder wall is clearly seen late in the capillary phase of celiac axis arteriography.

The Stomach

The left gastric artery arises early from the anterior superior margin of the celiac axis [101]. Special catheter shapes and maneuvers are required to enter this vessel selectively (see Figs. 13-4 through 13-8). Selective left gastric catheterization is important in detecting and treating bleeding sites from the gastric fundus, the gastroesophageal junction, and the lesser curvature of the stomach. Small portions of the gastric fundus are sometimes supplied by an often overlooked, tiny gastroesophageal branch of the left inferior phrenic artery. The inferior phrenic artery may arise just proximal to the left gastric artery but within the celiac axis, or just above the celiac axis directly from the aorta. Branches from the left gastric artery course along the lesser curvature of the stomach to anastomose with those of the usually smaller right gastric artery. The latter arises from the hepatic artery proper or from the left hepatic artery. The left gastric artery also richly anastomoses with short gastric branches of the splenic artery. The greater curvature of the stomach is supplied by the right and left gastroepiploic arteries. The right gastroepiploic artery is a direct continuation of the gastroduodenal artery and is an excellent landmark (try to identify it, because it indicates the position of the greater curvature of the stomach). It continues directly with the left gastroepiploic artery, which in turn arises from the splenic artery near the splenic hilus. Long, thin epiploic arteries course inferiorly along the surface of the greater omentum, having their origin from the gastroepiploic arteries.

The Pancreas

The head of the pancreas derives its major arterial supply from both the superior and inferior pancreaticoduodenal artery. Both the anterior and posterior branches of the superior pancreaticoduodenal artery wrap around the pancreatic head and proximal portions of the duodenum to continue down as an inferior pancreaticoduodenal branch (or branches) of the superior mesenteric artery. This branch acts as a very important anastomosis between the celiac axis and the superior mesenteric artery (see Fig. 13-19).

The body of the pancreas is served by the dorsal pancreatic artery; it has varied points of origin: the proximal splenic artery, the celiac axis, the hepatic artery, the gastroduodenal artery, or the superior mesenteric artery. An anomalous branch, supplying portions of the transverse colon, may arise from the dorsal pancreatic artery. The remaining body and tail of the pancreas are supplied by branches arising from the splenic artery; these include the pancreatica magna and caudal pancreatic branches. The transverse pancreatic artery runs for varying distances down the length of the pancreas and is fed by a number of smaller branches.

The Spleen

The splenic artery [63] is often coiled and tortuous and gives off pancreatic branches, short gastric branches, and the left gastroepiploic artery before

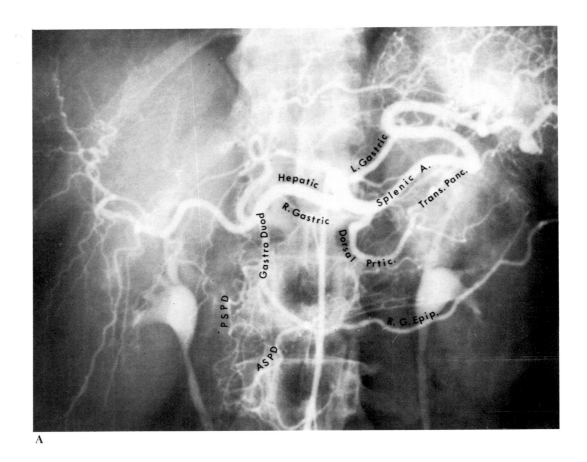

A

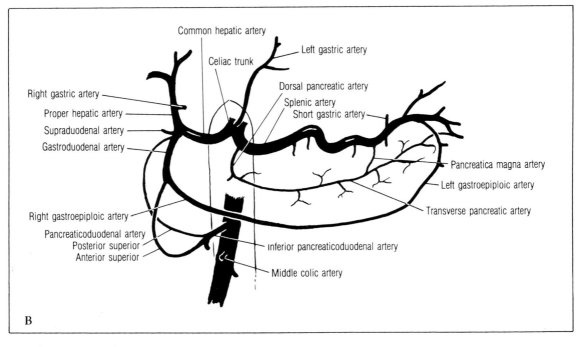

B

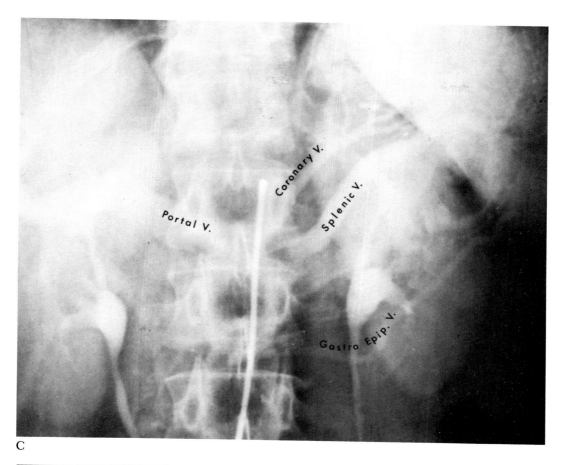

C

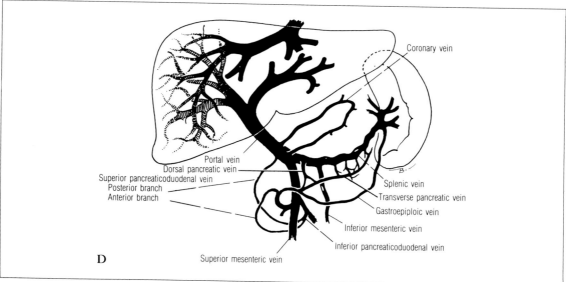

D

Fig. 13-10. Splanchnic anatomy.

A. Celiac axis arteriogram: PSPD = posterior superior pancreaticoduodenal artery, ASPD = anterior superior pancreaticoduodenal artery.

B. Line drawing of celiac arteriogram and pancreatic arteries.

C. Venous phase of the same study.

D. Portal and hepatic venous anatomy.

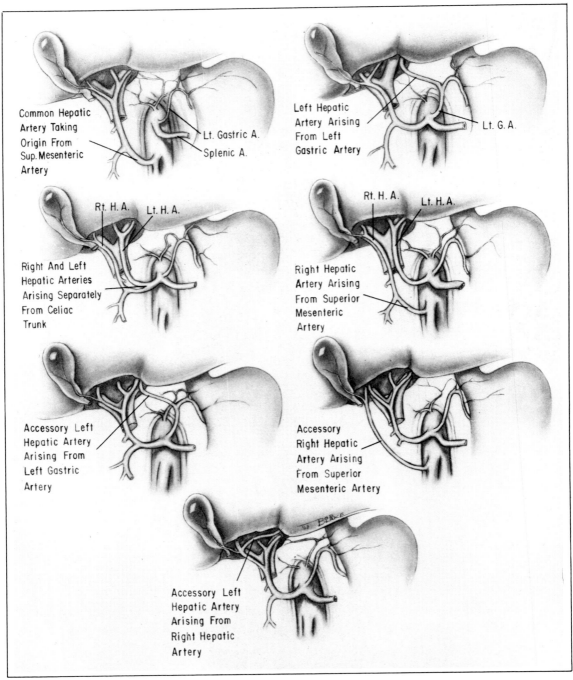

Fig. 13-11. Anomalies of the origins of branches to the liver, stomach, duodenum, and spleen. (From I. Johnsrude and R. Lester, Abdominal Visceral Arteriography as a Guide to the Surgeon. In *Monographs of Surgical Sciences*, Vol. 4, No. 2. Baltimore: Williams & Wilkins, 1967. Reproduced with permission of the Williams & Wilkins Company.)

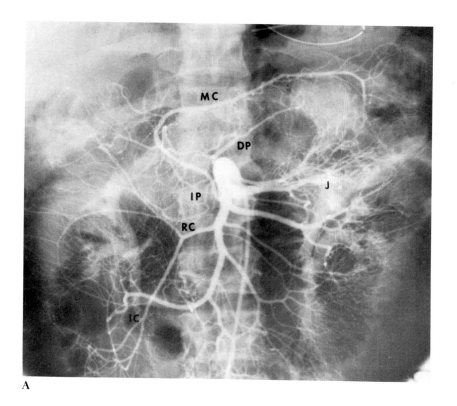

A

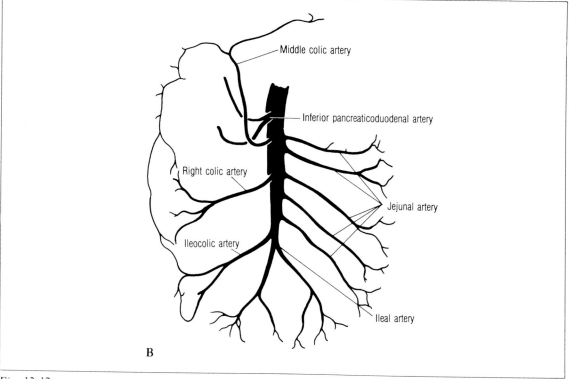

Middle colic artery

Inferior pancreaticoduodenal artery

Right colic artery

Jejunal artery

Ileocolic artery

Ileal artery

B

Fig. 13-12.

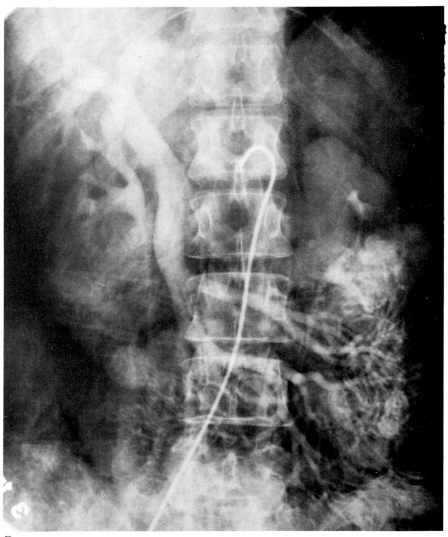

C

terminating in varying numbers of polar branches within the hilus of the spleen. A polar branch may arise proximal to the hilus.

THE SUPERIOR MESENTERIC ARTERY

The superior mesenteric artery supplies portions of the head of the pancreas, the duodenum, the jejunum, the ileum, and the colon to the level of the splenic juncture (Fig. 13-12). It arises at a point 1 to 20 mm below the celiac axis on the anterior surface of the aorta. To the right it gives off in sequence the inferior pancreaticoduodenal artery and the middle colic, right colic, and ileocolic arteries. On the left, a variable number of jejunal and ileal branches supply the respective portions of

Fig. 13-12.

A. Superior mesenteric arteriogram. MC = middle colic artery; DP = dorsal pancreatic artery (arising anomalously here from the superior mesenteric artery); IP = inferior pancreaticoduodenal branches; J = jejunal branches; RC = right colic branches; IC = ileocolic branches.

B. Line drawing of branches of superior mesenteric artery anatomy.

C. Venous phase of superior mesenteric arteriogram. Sixty ml of contrast agent was injected in 6 seconds, after 37 mg of tolazoline (Priscoline) was introduced in 1 minute through the mesenteric artery catheter. The unopacified splenic vein joins the superior mesenteric vein at the top of L2.

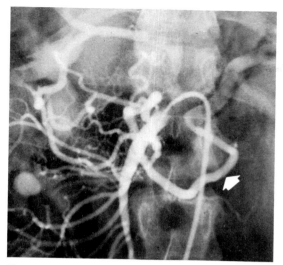

Fig. 13-13. The arc of Bühler, an embryonic vessel joining the superior mesenteric artery with the splenic artery (*arrow*).

Fig. 13-14.
A. Embryonic state. The arc of Bühler connects the celiac axis with the superior mesenteric artery.
B. Normal adult. The arc of Bühler has atrophied.
C and D. Celiacomesenteric trunk. The origins of the celiac axis and/or superior mesenteric artery have

the small bowel. The middle colic artery supplies much of the transverse colon; it divides into right and left branches to anastomose with the respective right and left colic branches. Because the left colic artery arises from the inferior mesenteric artery, these vessels form an important anastomosis (the central anastomotic channel) in obstruction of either of the mesenteric vessels or of the aorta between them (see Fig. 10-6B). A marginal artery of Drummond which derives its blood supply from the colic vessels extends along the mesenteric margin of the colon for a variable distance and is most constant in the transverse and descending colon. This artery can also form an important anastomosis in mesenteric or aortic obstructive disease. (A third, more central anastomotic channel, the arc of Riolan, is sometimes available.) Another embryonic remnant—the arc of Bühler—may be present; this is a direct vascular connection between the superior mesenteric artery and major branches of the celiac axis (Fig. 13-13). Rarely, the

not developed; and the arc of Bühler gives rise to that vessel.
E. Illustrative radiograph (lateral aortogram) demonstrating common origin of celiac axis (*small arrow*) and superior mesenteric artery (*open arrow*).

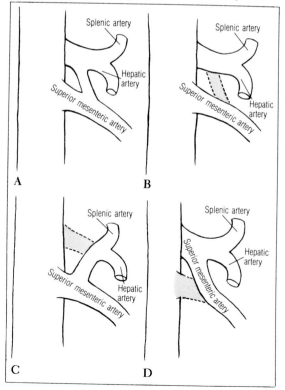

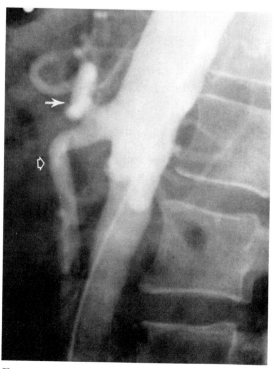

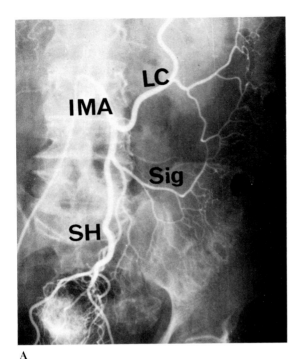

A

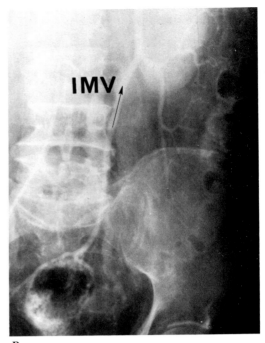

B

Fig. 13-15. Anatomy of the inferior mesenteric artery and vein.

A. IMA = inferior mesenteric artery; LC = left colic artery; Sig = sigmoid artery; SH = superior

hemorrhoidal (rectal) artery. There is a marginal artery on the mesenteric side of the descending colon.

B. IMV = inferior mesenteric vein (*arrow*).

superior mesenteric artery may be seen to arise from the same site as the celiac axis—the so-called celiacomesenteric trunk. This may be a manifestation of failure of atrophy of the arc of Bühler (Fig. 13-14).

The Inferior Mesenteric Artery

The inferior mesenteric artery (Fig. 13-15A) arises from the aorta anteriorly and to the left at the level of the third lumbar vertebra. The first major branch is the left colic artery, which has an ascending and descending division. The ascending branch of the left colic artery forms its important anastomosis with the middle colic artery. The descending branch of the left colic artery supplies the lower descending colon. The inferior mesenteric artery then gives off from one to three sigmoid branches and terminates as the superior rectal artery. Marginal branches are seen along the mesenteric side of the colon, and vasa recta course transversely around the colon. The superior rectal artery forms an important anastomosis with the middle rectal branch of the internal iliac artery. This anastomotic channel enlarges with occlusion

of the inferior mesenteric artery, the aorta below the takeoff of the inferior mesenteric artery, or the common or internal iliac arteries (see Fig. 10-6C). Three major anastomotic channels are clearly between the primary arteries of the gastrointestinal tract: the pancreaticoduodenal branches, the middle and left colic branches, and the rectal branches. Obstruction of one of these primary vessels or of the aorta or iliacs between them results in enlargement of the appropriate anastomotic channels.

The Portal and Hepatic Venous System
[30, 95] (Figs. 13-10C, D, 13-12C, 13-16)

Venous drainage of the gut, spleen, pancreas, and gallbladder enters into a common effluent, the portal vein. This vein supplies 75 percent of the total hepatic blood flow, the other 25 percent being from the hepatic artery. When the portal vein enters the liver, it branches into progressively smaller radicles which course together with hepatic arteries and bile ducts in between the hepatic lobules. They eventually terminate into minute sinusoids, which act as the common meeting place

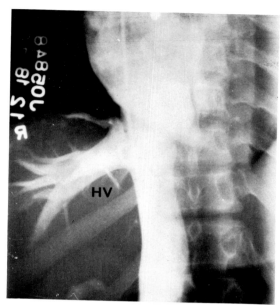

Fig. 13-16. Normal hepatic vein (HV).

of portal venous radicles and terminal ramifications of the hepatic artery, and the point of origin of the hepatic venules. The hepatic venules enter into the larger hepatic veins, which pass through the center of the hepatic lobules to eventually drain into several large hepatic venous channels, emptying into the inferior vena cava (Fig. 13-16).

The splenic vein (10 to 15 mm in diameter) arises from the splenic hilus and courses medially toward its confluens with the superior mesenteric vein to form the portal vein. Along its course it receives branches from the pancreas, the greater curvature of the stomach (short gastric veins), and the left colon and rectum (inferior mesenteric vein). The coronary vein (left gastric vein) drains into the superior margin of the splenic vein, and the gastroepiploic veins drain into its inferior margin at or near its junction with the superior mesenteric vein.

Knowledge of precise venous anatomy in this area is of considerable practical value. The veins can be selectively catheterized by a transhepatic or transjugular route, both for therapeutic obliteration of varices and for angiographic evaluation of pancreatic disease and sampling of venous blood for detecting functioning tumors [52, 91, 105].

Many venous radicles drain the small bowel and colon proximal to the level of the splenic flexure;

these radicles join to form the large superior mesenteric vein (diameter up to 10 to 15 mm). This vessel joins the splenic vein to form the portal vein at the level of the second lumbar vertebra, ventral to the inferior vena cava but behind the neck of the pancreas.

Many communications normally exist between the portal system and the systemic and pulmonary venous systems. These communications, which are rarely functional except under stress, include

1. Paraesophageal→azygos vein
2. Splenic→azygos vein
3. Portal→left gastric→left pulmonary vein
4. Gastric→renal vein
5. Splenic→renal vein
6. Mesenteric→renal vein
7. Mesenteric→gonadal vein
8. Mesenteric→retroperitoneal veins
9. Intrahepatic portal veins→hepatic veins
10. Intrahepatic portal vein→paraumbilical vein
11. Portal hemorrhoidal→systemic hemorrhoidal veins

Pharmacologic Enhancement of Studies

IMPROVEMENT OF VENOUS OPACIFICATION

Vasodilatation causes more rapid arterial flow and, therefore, prompt and dense venous opacification of the subsequently injected contrast agent [25, 26, 84, 113]. Through one limb of a Luer-Lok three-way stopcock interposed between a selectively placed catheter and a high-pressure injector, the angiographer should inject over a period of 60 seconds 1.5 ml (25 mg/ml) of tolazoline (Priscoline) diluted in 10 ml of saline solution. This solution should be flushed out of the catheter and into the vessel with an additional 3 or 4 ml of saline, followed immediately by the injection of contrast medium at a rate of 10 to 12 ml per second, with a total of up to 60 ml. Because arterial detail is lost by the injection of tolazoline, it should not be used when one is searching for tumors or arteriovenous malformations. Tolazoline should not be used in the evaluation of acute bleeding; however, it may be used to demonstrate varices in chronic low-grade gastrointestinal bleeding. Other drugs used for vasodilatation include prostaglandin E and F_2 alpha, papaverine, bradykinin, and glucagon.

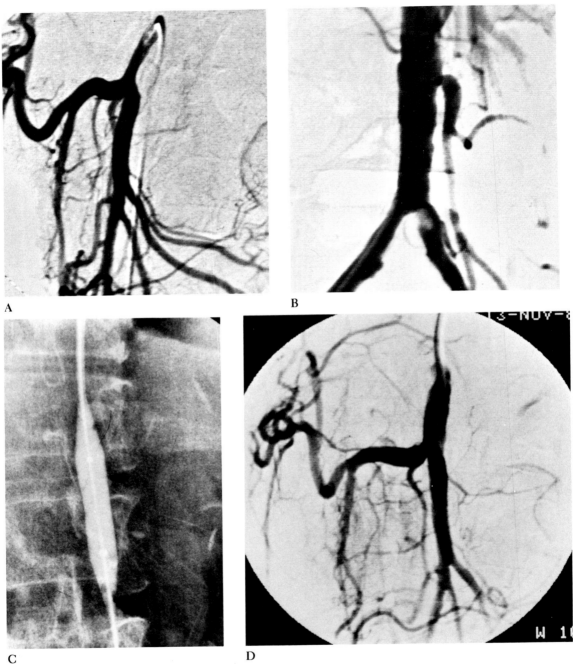

A

B

C

D

Fig. 13-17. Abdominal angina treated with percutaneous transluminal angioplasty (PTA).

A. Long tubular stenosis of the proximal superior mesenteric artery. This vessel feeds most of the gut. There was also stenosis of the celiac axis (not shown).

B. IA-DSA of the aorta also shows stenosis of the inferior mesenteric artery.

C. Stenotic segment of the superior mesenteric artery dilated with a 10-mm diameter balloon from an axillary approach.

D. Post-PTA digital angiogram shows improved diameter of the vessel.

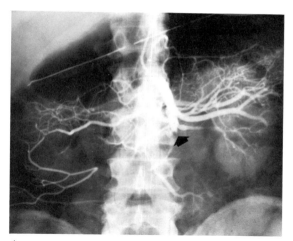

A

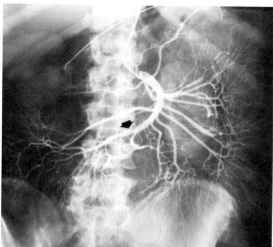

B

Fig. 13-18.

A. Acute embolus obstructing the superior mesenteric artery in a poor operative candidate. The patient had a viable bowel at this time, with some collateral flow peripherally. Chronic occlusion of the distal aorta required axillary approach.

B. The clot is beginning to lyse after bolus of intraluminal infusion of low-dose streptokinase. Total lysis of the clot was achieved after 60 hours of therapy. (Flickinger, E., et al. Local streptokinase infusion for superior mesenteric artery thromboembolism. *A.J.R.* 140:771, © by American Roentgen Ray Society, 1983.)

STUDIES OF THE PANCREAS

If superselective placement into pancreatic vessels is desired, a vasodilator (e.g., 25 mg tolazoline) should be injected slowly over a period of 1 minute directly into the catheter, followed immediately by the injection of contrast medium. If a superselective study is not possible, the surrounding major vessels should be constricted with epinephrine (10 µg) immediately prior to the injection into the celiac axis. Pancreatic vessels are less affected than the surrounding circulation, and this permits preferential flow to the pancreas. Secretin, 4 units per kilogram given intravenously, may enhance small vessel and capillary parenchymal filling.

Angiographic Findings [2, 87, 92]

PRIMARY ARTERIAL LESIONS

Major Splanchnic Vascular Narrowing or Occlusion

1. Congenital. There may be a wide spectrum ranging from mild, asymptomatic narrowing at the origin of the celiac axis to congenital absence of the celiac trunk.

2. Atherosclerosis. Atherosclerosis is the most frequent cause of narrowing and usually occurs at or near vessel origins. Marked obstruction of more than one of the three vessels (celiac artery, superior mesenteric artery, inferior mesenteric artery) is usually necessary to cause abdominal angina (see Fig. 10-8). The newer techniques of percutaneous transluminal angioplasty and clot thrombolysis may be achieved in these branches just as they are in coronary, renal, and peripheral arteries. Although less frequently applied, they may be just as successful (Figs. 13-17 and 13-18). A more detailed description of these techniques may be found in Chapters 6, 7, 8, and 11.

3. Fibrous bands. Fibrous bands from the median arcuate ligament of the diaphragm can traverse the anterior superior margin of the origin of the celiac axis (Fig. 13-19A, B, C). This condition is exaggerated during expiration. Only rarely is it symptomatic [24, 85].

4. Other causes. Other causes of narrowing include fibromuscular hyperplasia, tumors, dissecting aneurysms, and neurofibromatosis.

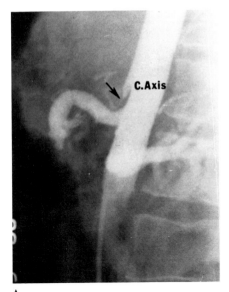

A

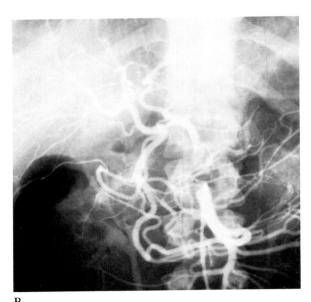

B

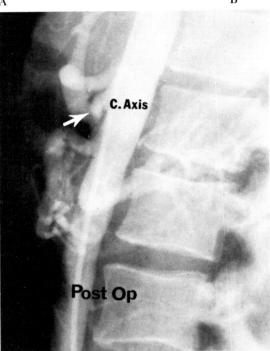

C

Fig. 13-19. Celiac axis occlusion by a fibrous band in a young male patient with postprandial pain and weight loss.
A. Lateral abdominal aortogram. Arrow points to occluded celiac axis.
B. Superior mesenteric arteriogram, showing large collaterals through the pancreaticoduodenal arcade and gastroduodenal artery.
C. Postoperative lysis of the fibrous band. The celiac axis (*arrow*) now fills in an anterograde fashion.

Splanchnic Artery Aneurysms

Aneurysms of the splanchnic arteries [27] may dissect, rupture into or outside the bowel lumen, develop arteriovenous fistulas, thrombose, or cause infarction. Whether the aneurysms are fortuitously uncovered in patients undergoing angiography for other reasons or whether they are discovered in asymptomatic patients, precise arteriographic demonstration is important. A high percentage of these aneurysms rupture. Surgical feasibility and technique may be planned on the basis of the site of the aneurysm, its patency, and the state of possible collateral circulation. Aneurysms are usually arteriosclerotic, but they may be congenital, mycotic, or traumatic in origin or may be associated with medial degeneration. The following sites of aneurysm are found:

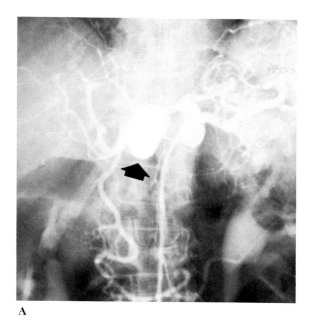

A

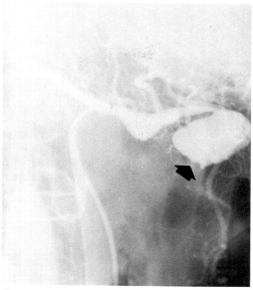

B

Fig. 13-20. Asymptomatic aneurysm of the hepatic artery (*arrows*). The aneurysm arises proximal to the gastroduodenal artery and can be excised with impunity because of the fact that collaterals can supply the liver through the pancreaticoduodenal arcade. There is also a smaller aneurysm of the celiac axis.
A. Anteroposterior view.
B. Lateral view.

1. Splenic artery aneurysm. Aneurysms of the splenic artery are the most frequent (approximately 45 percent), occurring most often in females, in whom they are prone to rupture during pregnancy (see Fig. 13-21B and C).
2. Hepatic artery aneurysm (Fig. 13-20). Aneurysms of the hepatic artery are next in frequency (15 percent), and their relationship to the remaining anastomotic channels is important when surgery is being considered. If it is proximal to the origin of the gastroduodenal artery, the aneurysm may be ligated and excised without fear of compromising hepatic viability because the liver receives its blood supply from the rich anastomosis of the pancreaticoduodenal branches. If the aneurysm is located more peripherally, hepatic end arteries are involved, and liver necrosis may follow vascular occlusion unless some form of surgical anastomosis is constructed (Fig. 13-21A).

3. Other sites. In order of decreasing frequency, other sites of aneurysm are found in the superior mesenteric artery, the celiac axis, the gastric arteries, the jejunal, ileal, and colic arteries, and the gastroduodenal and pancreaticoduodenal vessels.

TUMORS

Tumors of the Pancreas
A variety of tumors may involve the pancreas; the most common primary tumors are adenocarcinomas, cystadenocarcinomas, and functioning islet cell tumors. These tumors may be difficult to demonstrate angiographically, and their morphology and relative position within the organ govern the success of detection.

ADENOCARCINOMAS [32, 47, 66, 88]. Endoscopic retrograde pancreatography (ERP) [23, 39, 71] is the imaging modality of choice in primary ductal adenocarcinoma. In addition, computed tomography (CT) and ultrasonography have demonstrated superior ability to identify mass lesions of the pancreas as well as the presence of ductal dilatation and peripancreatic extension of disease [38, 50, 51, 54, 58, 65]. Arteriography is indicated when a pancreatic tumor is suspected but cannot be detected by other methods. It is also indicated when there is question about resectability of a known pancreatic lesion, as it may help to determine its extension locally and into surrounding

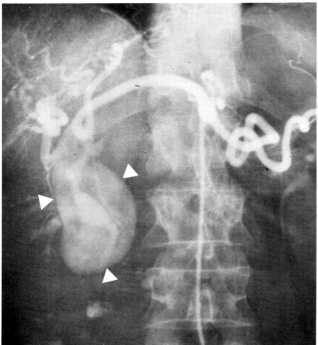

A

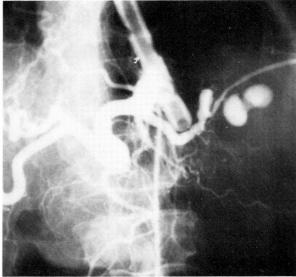

B

structures. Because of the dual blood supply of the pancreas, both the celiac axis and superior mesenteric artery must be studied, usually in both anteroposterior and right posterior oblique projections. Delayed films outlining the portal system are important, because often the first clue to disease is venous involvement or occlusion. Superselective injections into the gastroduodenal, dorsal pancreatic, or splenic arteries with magnification techniques facilitate diagnosis.

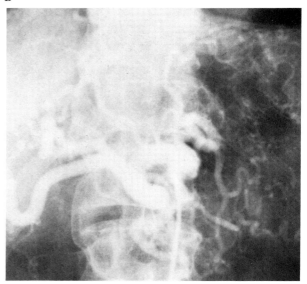

C

Fig. 13-21. False aneurysms as a result of pancreatic pseudocysts.

A. Hemorrhage from a massive false aneurysm arising from the hepatic artery distal to the gastroduodenal artery. This was a complication of a pseudocyst. The common hepatic artery is smoothly displaced superiorly by the pseudocyst, and calcium lies within the head of the pancreas. Hepatic necrosis and death followed emergency ligation.

B and C. Embolic occlusion of a bleeding false aneurysm subsequent to pseudocyst of the pancreas. B. Preembolization. C. The splenic artery occluded with gel foam emboli.

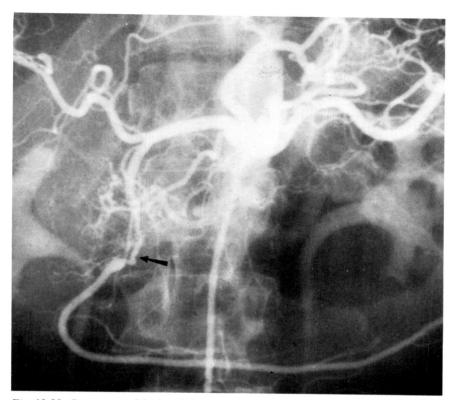

Fig. 13-22. Carcinoma of the head of the pancreas. There is invasion of the gastroduodenal artery by tumor (*arrow*). A small collection of neovascularity just above this site is also seen.

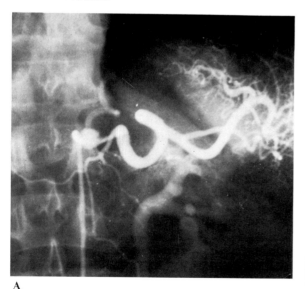

A

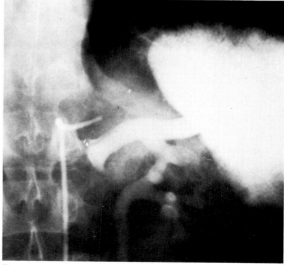

B

Fig. 13-23. Carcinoma of the body of the pancreas.
A. Invasion of the splenic artery and displacement of intrapancreatic branches.
B. Occlusion of the splenic vein.

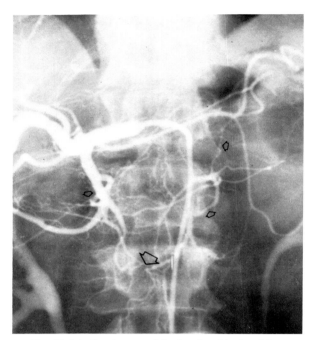

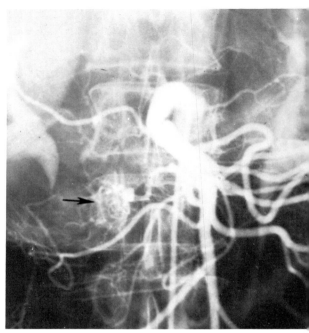

Fig. 13-24. Carcinoma of the head and body of the pancreas (common hepatic artery injection). Small vessel changes are seen, with occlusion and segmental areas of narrowing (*arrows*).

Fig. 13-25. Cystadenocarcinoma in the head of the pancreas. Superior mesenteric arteriogram shows localized neovascularity and smooth displacement of adjacent vessels by the large cystic component of the tumor (*arrow*).

Carcinoma of the pancreas is typically hypovascular. Arterial irregularity or encasement is caused by encroachment on the arterial wall, either by tumor invasion or by perivascular, tumor-engorged lymphatics. This encasement should not be confused with atheromatous plaques, which are more irregular and asymmetric, involving larger arteries closer to their aortic origin. These encased arteries present as cufflike, usually circumferential, smooth, and uniformly tapering lesions of the vessel in the vicinity of the tumor (Figs. 13-22, 13-23). There may be occlusion of small intrapancreatic vessels (Fig. 13-24) and also small collections of frank neovascularity. When the pancreatic bed is flooded with contrast medium injected superselectively, the tumor may be recognized as a hypovascular zone within the capillary parenchymal blush of the remaining normal pancreas [32]. This appearance can provide a significant point of difference from chronic pancreatitis, in which the large vessel changes may otherwise be identical, but in which there is a dense capillary stain. Tumors that lie in the head of the pancreas show vascular changes in the hepatic, gastroduodenal, dorsal, and transverse pancreatic arteries and the

vessels of the pancreaticoduodenal arcade. In tumors involving the body and tail of the pancreas, the splenic, transverse pancreatic, dorsal pancreatic, and pancreatica magna arteries may be involved. The thin, collapsible walls of the venous system allow tumor invasion and displacement early in the course of disease. Venous compression may eventually lead to occlusion and the generation of collateral channels. Vessels which may become occluded include the splenic, superior mesenteric, and left renal veins. Because irregu-

Fig. 13-26. Malignant insulin-secreting islet cell tumor.
A. Arteriogram shows hypertrophied pancreatic vessels (*arrow*).
B. Dense capillary stain of multiple pancreatic tumors (*arrowheads*) and a host of intrahepatic metastases (*white and black arrows*).

Fig. 13-27. Multiple gastrin-secreting islet cell tumors in the body and tail of the pancreas.
A. Splenic arteriogram. PM = pancreatica magna branch.
B. Capillary and venous phase showing dense capillary stain within the tumors (*arrows*).

343

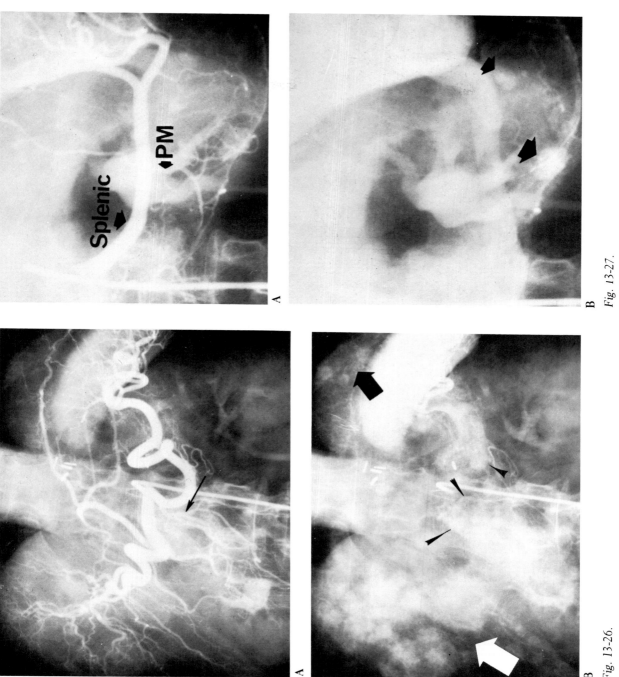

Fig. 13-27.

Fig. 13-26.

larity of the splenic veins may be caused by other conditions (e.g., previous surgery, chronic pancreatitis), this finding alone is nonspecific. When vascular changes are present they are not representative of the size of the tumor, because large lesions may have only small, localized collections of abnormal vessels. The radiographic field must include the liver so that hepatic metastases may be detected.

CYSTADENOMAS. Cystadenomas and their malignant counterparts (cystadenocarcinomas) are usually hypervascular, are often calcified, usually have a cystic component, and are frequently found in the body or tail of the pancreas (Fig. 13-25).

ISLET CELL TUMORS. Islet cell tumors of the pancreas [12, 40, 41, 62] (Figs. 13-26, 13-27; see Fig. 23-6) may be functioning or nonfunctioning. The most common functioning tumors are insulin- and gastrin-secreting tumors. Other hormones may rarely be secreted and include glucagon, secretin, serotonin, adrenocorticotropic hormone (ACTH), and melanocyte-secreting hormone. Insulin-producing tumors are suspected clinically when fasting hypoglycemia is accompanied by hyperinsulinemia. Other tumors (e.g., retroperitoneal and mediastinal mesenchymal tumors, primary tumors of the liver and adrenal glands) may cause fasting hypoglycemia but have normal blood insulin levels (see Fig. 10-28). Gastrin-secreting tumors are associated with the Zollinger-Ellison syndrome of enlarged gastric rugal folds and multiple gastric, duodenal, and jejunal ulcers. Islet cell tumors are usually single but may be multiple. Insulinomas are malignant in 10 to 20 percent of patients, and gastrinomas are malignant in over 60 percent of patients and metastasize most frequently to the liver. They vary in size, but 75 percent range from 1 to 3 cm in diameter. Usually round and circumscribed, these tumors may be found in any portion of the gland, in aberrant pancreatic tissue, or in the wall of the stomach or duodenum. Usually they lie deep within the pancreatic substance, and they have a soft consistency, making surgical detection difficult. Angiographic detection (with a success rate of approximately 65 percent) depends on the extent of capillary proliferation within the lesion. If capillary proliferation is profuse, an intense capillary stain may be detected late in the arterial phase of the study. Multiple capillary blushes may be encountered in the liver, indicating metastases. The use of superselective angiog-

raphy together with magnification and subtraction techniques yield a higher degree of detection. The increased contrast sensitivity of digital vascular systems may demonstrate tumor blushes better than conventional films, making these systems well suited to the investigation of these types of lesions.

SECONDARY TUMORS. Secondary tumors may spread to the pancreas and usually manifest vascularity similar to that of the primary tumor (e.g., hypernephroma). Peripancreatic tumors, particularly lymphomas, may invade and surround the pancreas [74].

Tumors of the Liver and Biliary System

MALIGNANT TUMORS. Primary malignant tumors are of two main types: hepatocellular (hepatoma) and bile duct carcinoma (cholangiocarcinoma). Malignancies arising from connective tissue and mesenchymal structures (e.g., hemangiosarcoma) are rarer.

The hepatoma [8, 44, 55, 77] is often richly vascularized and presents in one of three forms. The most frequent is a large solitary lesion involving one lobe (Fig. 13-28A); the second type occurs as discrete nodules of varying sizes scattered throughout the liver; the third type is a diffuse form involving the entire liver (Fig. 13-28B, C) which sometimes may be avascular. Seventy-five percent of hepatomas occur in cirrhotic livers. In the lobar form, the hepatic arteries are of larger than normal caliber and are typically tortuous, showing bizarre tumor vessels with contrast retention within the tumor and with arteriovenous shunting. Twenty-five percent of hepatomas invade and thrombose the portal venous system, and they should be considered in the differential diagnosis of portal hypertension. The intraarterial intrahepatic injection of Ethiodol [72, 115], an oily contrast medium, may prove to be useful in separating unifocal hepatoma from the multifocal variety.

Fig. 13-28.
A. Hepatoma involving the right lobe of the liver. There is marked neovascularity. Small attenuated branches supply the left lobe of the liver.
B and C. Massive hepatoma involving most of the liver. Laparotomy showed involvement of the right and left lobes of the liver. B. Selective common hepatic arteriogram prior to embolization. C. Postembolization film shows complete obliteration of all vessels to the tumor.

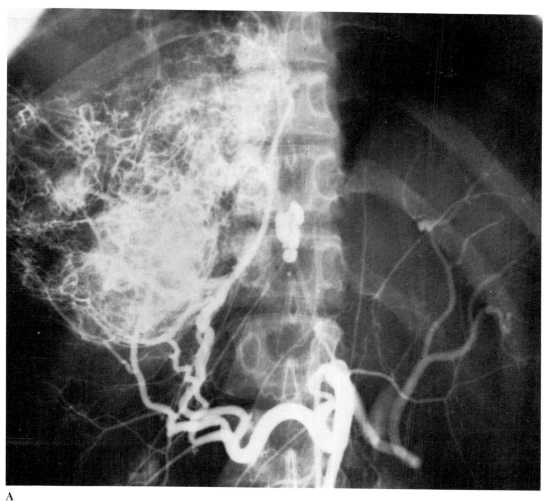

A

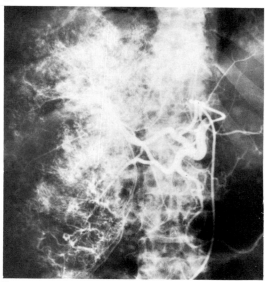

B

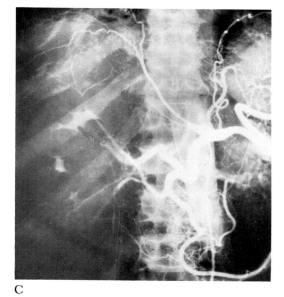

C

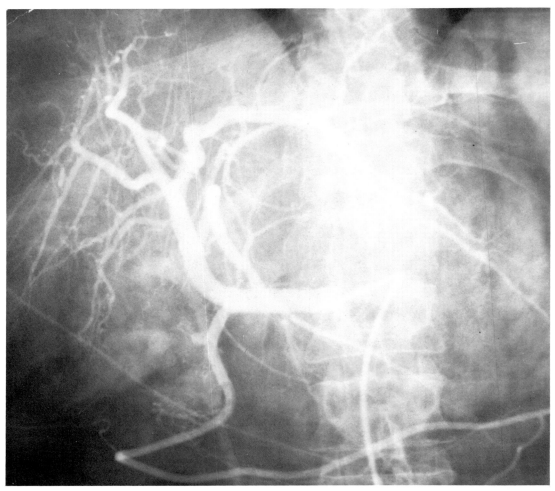

Fig. 13-29. Extensive cholangiocarcinoma of the liver. Aortography was performed to rule out abdominal aneurysm; this uncovered a large left lobe of the liver. Positive alpha-1-fetoproteins were present. There is marked displacement of the branches of the left lobe of the liver, with some periarterial invasion.

Biliary duct carcinomas [107] and tumors of the gallbladder invade and encase the cystic arteries or adjacent vascular structures (Fig. 13-29). They may also show varying degrees of fine vessel neovascularity with small, tortuous, irregular vessels. In the capillary phase, circular or branching lucent defects indicating dilated bile ducts may be observed, and invasion of portal venous radicles may be seen. Displacement of vessels occurs late in the course of the disease. These lesions are best studied via direct imaging of the biliary tree (transhepatic cholangiography or ERCP).

HEPATIC METASTASES. Hepatic metastases arise from hypervascular or hypovascular primary tumors and usually reflect the vascularity of the primary lesion. Hypervascularity with a homoge-neous capillary stain is typical in metastases from islet cell tumors of the pancreas (see Fig. 13-26), leiomyosarcomas, and carcinoid tumors of the small bowel. The most frequent tumors that metastasize to the liver arise from the gastrointestinal tract (Fig. 13-30). Metastases as small as 1 cm or less may be detected angiographically, but superselective, high-dose, magnification hepatic

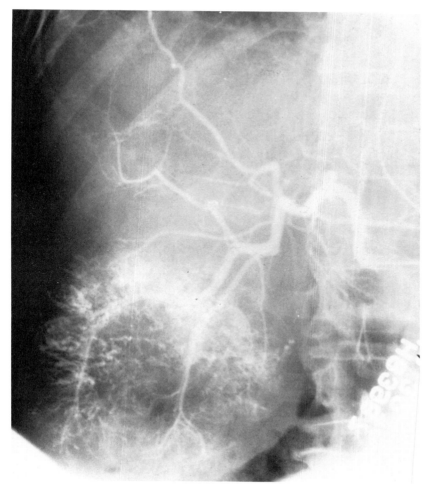

Fig. 13-30. Metastases to the liver (primary tumor in the colon).

arteriography is required in such cases. Detection of these small metastases may be important to a surgeon planning hepatic lobectomy for metastatic disease. Patency of the portal vein is important to the angiographer and must be evaluated before considering hepatic artery embolization for symptomatic metastases (e.g., carcinoid syndrome) [4, 67, 81] or other tumors (see Fig. 13-28B, C). Selective hepatic arterial chemotherapy is also performed in patients with primary and secondary hepatic tumors, allowing palliation and increased longevity. Catheters may be placed either percutaneously or at the time of surgery. Accurately outlining the arterial anatomy to the liver is impor-

tant in order to ensure maximum exposure of the chemotherapeutic agent to the liver tumor and to prevent toxicity to uninvolved normal areas. Proximal occlusion of uninvolved vessels, either by sutures at the time of surgery or coils at angiography, help to divert flow of the infusate to the tumor itself. If the percutaneous route is chosen, the chemotherapy may be given over a 2-hour period (allowing a femoral approach) but is often administered over a 2-week period. An axillary approach with a 5 French catheter allows the patient to be mobile. A headhunter curve (see Chap. 14), with its distal tip bent slightly to the right, is a helpful catheter.

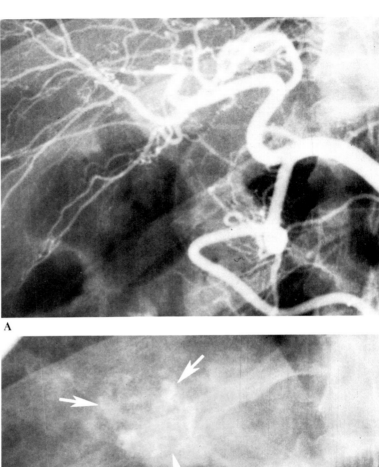

A

B

Fig. 13-31. Hepatic arteriogram showing several small hemangiomas incidentally uncovered in a young woman studied angiographically for chronic gastrointestinal bleeding.

A. Arterial phase, showing normal arteries.

B. The capillary stain persists late in the film series (*arrows*). No arteriovenous shunting is present.

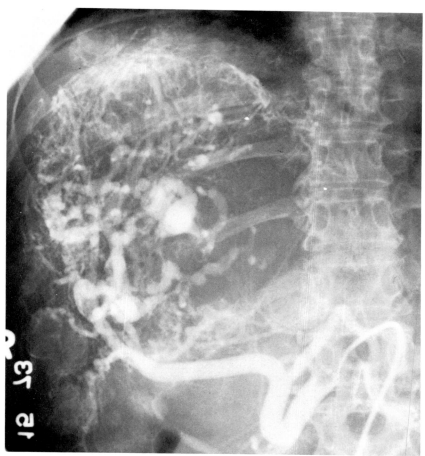

Fig. 13-32. Hemangiosarcoma. This is a very vascular tumor with a large feeding artery and many vascular pools of contrast medium. There is premature hepatic venous filling (not shown).

HEMANGIOMAS. Hepatic hemangiomas [3] are vascular, well-marginated lesions arising in the capillary phase of hepatic arteriograms and staining well into the venous phase of the study (Fig. 13-31). The feeding vessels are usually small, and the tumors are multiple and are frequently circular or semicircular in configuration. They may be associated with angiodysplasias of the colon and small bowel. Their malignant counterparts, hemangiosarcomas, have arteriovenous shunting, enlarged feeding vessels, and bizarre tumor vessels (Fig. 13-32). Hemangiomas may be seen well on ultrasound in which they present as hyperechoic masses [78, 102]. Dynamic CT scanning has demonstrated the ability to detect hemangiomas in cer-

tain instances as a particular pattern of enhancement has been described [6, 53, 56].

BENIGN TUMORS. There are several benign growths, not primarily vascular, that have fairly distinctive features. These growths should be studied in conjunction with liver scans, since unlike other space-occupying processes, they may show some radioisotope (technetium-99m–sulphur colloid) uptake [42, 48, 82].

Regenerating liver nodules occur in cirrhotic livers; they show no neovascularity but may cause vessel displacement. Characteristically, there is normal radioisotope uptake in the region of the nodule, but abnormal, spotty uptake in the area of cirrhosis (Fig. 13-33) [82].

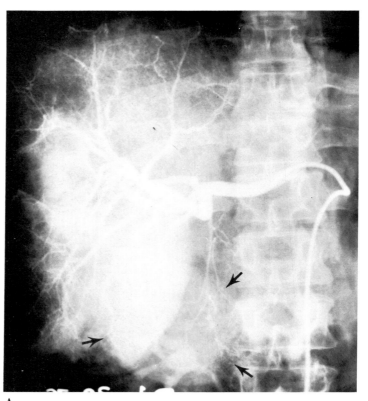

A

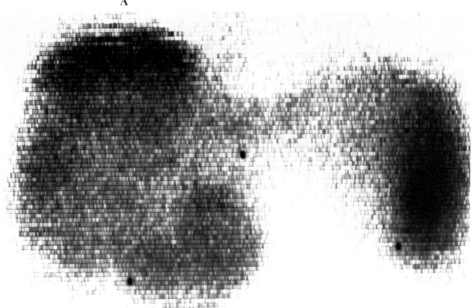

B

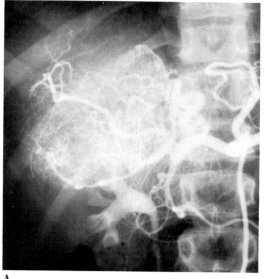 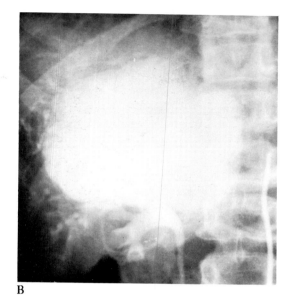

A   B

Fig. 13-34. Focal nodular hyperplasia. This is a hyper-vascular, well-marginated lesion with no arteriovenous shunting.

A. Arterial phase, showing a characteristic pattern of vessels entering the lesion from its periphery.

B. Dense capillary stain seen in the parenchymal phase of the injection. (Courtesy of Dr. L. Mazoc-chi, Wake Hospital, Raleigh, NC).

Fig. 13-33. Regenerating liver nodule in an alcoholic patient with known cirrhosis and esophageal varices.

A. Hepatic arteriogram shows a large hypovascular mass extending inferiorly and medially to the right lobe of the liver (*arrows*).

B. Technetium-99m–sulfur colloid scan, showing up-take of radioisotope in the "tumor" site.

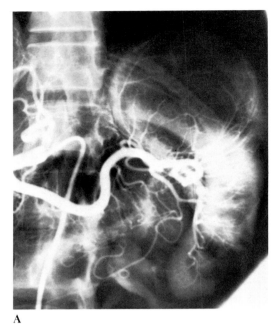

A

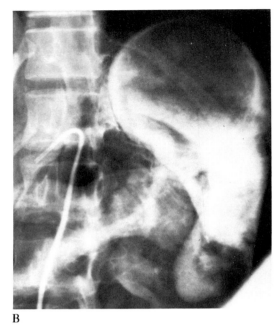

B

Fig. 13-35. Splenic cyst in an asymptomatic 43-year-old woman with no history of trauma or parasitic infection.

Focal nodular hyperplasia, like adenomas, occurs mostly in young females and is of unknown cause. It is seen in an otherwise normal liver, is well circumscribed, and may be multiple. The hepatic cells are normal, but they are clustered around bile ducts and vessels, and there is no central vein. The angiographic pattern of these lesions is similar to that of adenomas (Fig. 13-34). They are hypervascular but well marginated, and their vessels enter into them from the periphery of the tumor. There is a tumor stain in the parenchymal phase. There is usually no tumor neovascularity, arteriovenous shunting, or venous occlusion. These lesions can necrose and cause hemorrhage.

Adenomas are usually solitary, are larger than focal nodular hyperplasia, are encapsulated, and have normal hepatic cells that bear no relationship to ducts or vessels.

Tumors of the Spleen [35]

Benign cysts (either congenital or acquired as a result of trauma or parasites) are avascular and fairly well marginated, and they smoothly displace the intrasplenic branches (Fig. 13-35). It is difficult to differentiate benign from malignant solid tumors. Hemangiomas mimic the appearance of those seen in the liver. Hamartomas, as elsewhere, may show hypervascularity and neovascularity and have a propensity to arterial aneurysmal deformities. Malignant lesions, such as sarcomas and lymphomas, are often hypovascular (Fig. 13-36), but others can also show vascular findings of malignancy (arterial encasement or neovascularity with pooling and arteriovenous shunting, tumor stain in the capillary phase).

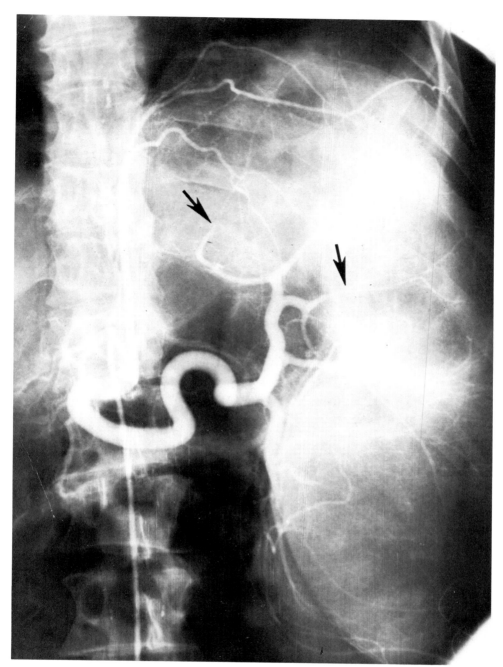

Fig. 13-36. Gross splenomegaly due to a fibrosarcoma of the spleen. The tumor is hypovascular and smoothly displaces the intrasplenic branches. There is also arterial encasement (*arrows*).

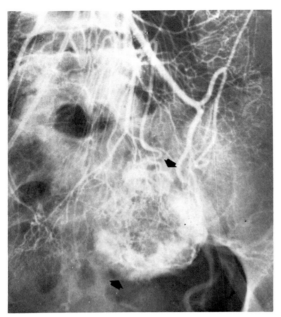

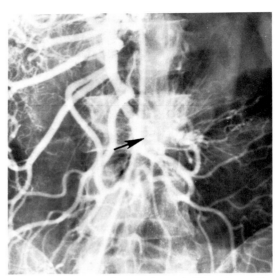

Fig. 13-38. Carcinoid tumor (*arrow*). There is a stellate pattern of the mesenteric arterial arcade. Arterial irregularity is caused by perivascular tumor extension.

Fig. 13-37. Leiomyosarcoma. Hypervascularity and neovascularity (*arrows*) are seen in a tumor involving the ileum. (Courtesy of Dr. J. Scatliff, University of North Carolina Memorial Hospital, Chapel Hill, NC.)

Tumors of the Small Bowel
[11, 29, 46, 60, 83]
Leiomyomas and leiomyosarcomas are usually vascular, well-marginated tumors with early and dense contrast accumulation and early venous filling (Fig. 13-37). Carcinoids show a stellate pattern of the terminal mesenteric arterial arcade, which represents the retracted, thickened, and foreshortened mesentery in the region of the tumor (Fig. 13-38). A perivascular tumor extension may be seen to cause an irregularity to the arterial lumen. There is poor contrast accumulation and no evidence of premature venous filling. Epinephrine (10 µg) injected immediately prior to the contrast medium may outline a dense capillary stain in the tumor. Sarcomas and lymphomas are typically hypovascular tumors, whether they are in the small bowel or in the mesentery. Adenocarcinomas are usually not hypervascular, but if large they show arterial displacement and segmental premature venous filling.

Tumors of the Colon
Malignant tumors of the colon are relatively hypovascular, but typical tumor vessels can be seen in some. Feeding vessels to the involved area are differentially prominent, and venous drainage is more rapid. Because tumors of the colon are best studied by barium examinations, angiography has little place in their evaluation. The same can be said for chronic ulcerative disease of the colon and small bowel, although there has been a revival of angiographic interest in this area [34].

INFLAMMATORY AND DEGENERATIVE DISEASES
Inflammatory Diseases of the Pancreas
PSEUDOCYSTS (Figs. 13-21, 13-39, 13-40) [57]. The cystic nature of these lesions and their rapidly changing size make ultrasound and CT the diagnostic procedures of choice; however, secondary effects on surrounding vessels sometimes make angiography necessary. Arteriographically, pseudocysts present as cystic avascular lesions, with smoothly displaced arteries around the structure. They may show localized areas of inflammatory neovascularity and splenic venous occlusion. False aneurysms can develop within the inflammatory mass, which may cause exsanguinating hemorrhage (see Fig. 13-21A, B, C). When these are encountered, they may be occluded by embolizing with Ivalon, coils, or tissue adhesives. The pseudocysts vary in size from several centimeters to very large proportions and can arise from any portion of the pancreas. They can extend in all directions to impinge on adjacent abdominal structures.

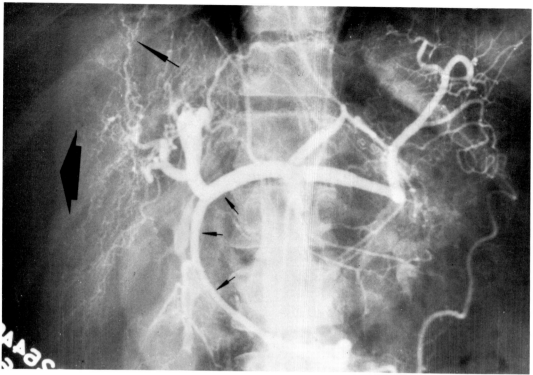

Fig. 13-39. Pseudocyst in the head of the pancreas of a patient with severe cirrhosis and ascites (*large arrow*). There is smooth displacement of intrapancreatic branches as well as the splenic, hepatic, and gas-troduodenal arteries (*small arrows*). Prominent proximal branches and tortuous distal intrahepatic branches (*top arrow*) indicate cirrhosis. The liver edge is displaced medially by the ascites.

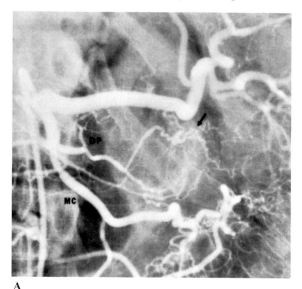

A

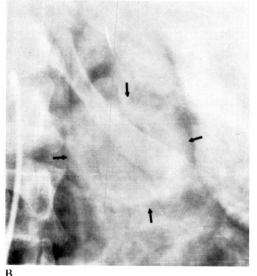

B

Fig. 13-40. Small pseudocyst in the tail of the pancreas.

A. Arteriogram. An anomalous middle colic (MC) branch arises from the splenic artery. The dorsal pancreatic (DP) branch supplies tortuous inflam-matory arteries (*arrow*) around the periphery of the pseudocyst.

B. The capillary phase shows a thick-walled cystic structure (*arrows*).

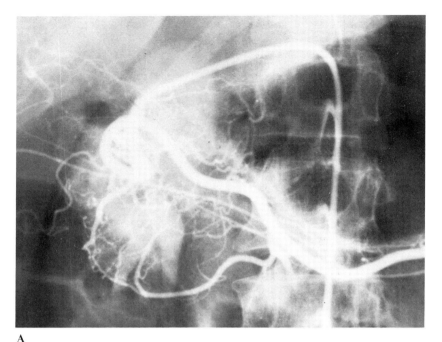

A

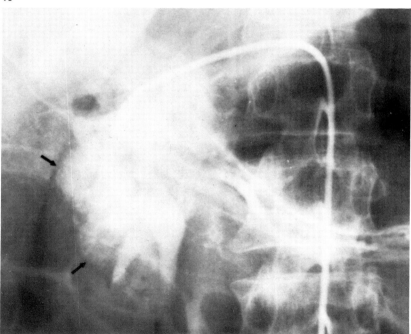

B

Fig. 13-41. Chronic pancreatitis (gastroduodenal arteriogram).
A. Vessels are displaced around a localized mass in the
head of the pancreas.

B. Hypervascular stain in the capillary phase (*arrows*)
(this is not seen in carcinoma of the pancreas in
which there is a differential decrease in capillary
stain). Localized chronic pancreatitis was found at
surgery.

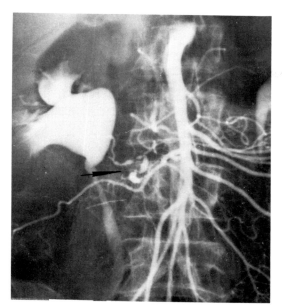

Fig. 13-42. Chronic pancreatitis. Superior mesenteric artery injection shows small aneurysms (*arrow*) and vessel irregularity in the pancreaticoduodenal branches.

PANCREATITIS. This entity, as in pancreatic neoplasms, is best studied by ultrasound, CT, and ERCP. Pancreatitis may be difficult to differentiate angiographically from pancreatic neoplasia (Figs. 13-41, 13-42) [1, 89, 110]. Some differential points may be helpful. The vascular pattern varies from normal in milder forms of pancreatitis to localized hypervascularity in the subacute forms, to serpiginous pancreatic arterial irregularity and venous deformity or occlusion in the chronic forms. The chronic form may be difficult to differentiate from cancer. In tumor, the vascular changes are more striking, are localized to the area of the tumor, and often involve vessels of adjacent structures. In chronic pancreatitis, on the other hand, only the intrapancreatic vessels are involved, and the process is prone to involve diffusely the entire pancreas. Superselective flooding of the pancreatic bed with contrast medium (even up to as much as 50 ml in a nonwedged position) outlines a hyperemic parenchyma in pancreatitis but a hypovascular section in the capillary phase in carcinoma. Small aneurysms of the intrapancreatic arteries are fairly characteristic of chronic pancreatitis (Fig. 13-42) [110].

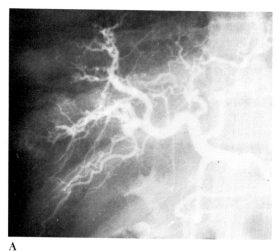

A

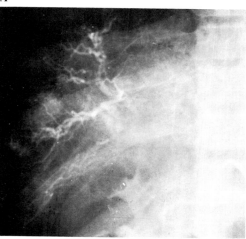

B

Fig. 13-43. Postnecrotic cirrhosis.
A. Early arterial phase, showing prominent hepatic arteries proximally and marked tortuosity of the peripheral branches.
B. Late arterial phase, with localized areas of hypervascularity which likely represent regenerating nodules. No radioisotope uptake occurred on liver scan. No alpha-1-fetoproteins were present, which suggests that there was no primary hepatic tumor.

Inflammatory Diseases of the Liver and Biliary System

Diffuse intrahepatic arterial stretching is a nonspecific sign of an enlarged liver. It may be caused by failure of the right side of the heart or by intrinsic liver disease such as fatty degeneration. In contrast to space-occupying lesions, there is usually a normal homogeneous or sometimes mottled, generalized parenchymal stain during the hepatogram phase.

In chronic cirrhosis with a small, scarred liver, the central hepatic arteries have a comparatively large caliber. The more peripheral parenchymal vessels are all involved and show a tortuous, spiraled appearance (Figs. 13-39, 13-43).

Regenerating liver nodules can occur and may be confused with malignancy. Hypervascularity with localized tortuous vessels often occurs, but there is usually no arteriovenous shunting (Fig. 13-43). Alternately, diffuse stretching of attenuated hepatic arteries and a normal parenchyma may be seen in regenerating liver (see Fig. 13-33). The radioisotope liver scan is helpful, because it typically shows a "hot" lesion rather than the "cold" lesion of a tumor. Patients with primary tumors of the liver usually have elevated levels of alpha fetoproteins, while those patients with regenerating nodules do not [82].

Localized intrahepatic smooth displacement of vessels may occur in hepatic cysts, chronic hematomas (see Fig. 13-48), and abscesses. Abscesses (e.g., amebic, hydatid) often have a hyperemic margin. During the hepatogram phase, the hypovascular lesion contrasts with the homogeneous stain of the surrounding normal parenchyma. Subhepatic and subphrenic abscesses may also have the same hyperemic margins (Fig. 13-44) [28, 76].

In cholecystitis the cystic arteries may be hypertrophied, and a thickened gallbladder wall with a hyperemic stain may be observed (Fig. 13-45).

Peliosis (hemorrhagic area, purpura) hepatis is a rare but sometimes fatal cause of bleeding which presents a characteristic angiographic appearance. The liver is studded with scattered extravasated collections of contrast medium, localized within the hemorrhagic cysts. These cysts can rupture and cause intraperitoneal hemorrhage and intrahepatic hematoma. Peliosis hepatis is thought to be caused by localized hepatic parenchymal necrosis with

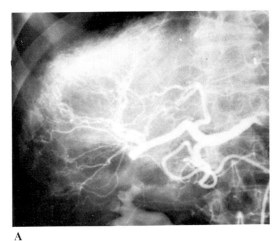

A

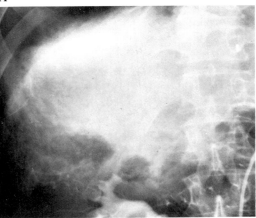

B

Fig. 13-44. Subphrenic abscess. There is a hyperemic margin surrounding the abscess.
A. Arterial phase.
B. Parenchymal phase.

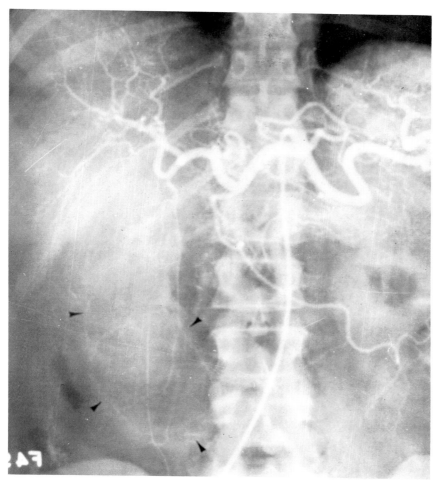

Fig. 13-45. Empyema of the gallbladder. Prominent cystic arteries supply a hyperemic, thick-walled gallbladder (*arrows*).

subsequent connection of these necrotic areas to sinusoids. It is known to occur in patients using anabolic androgenic agents and also in those using contraceptive pills. These lesions can regress following withdrawal of medications but can continue on to form hepatic angiosarcoma [80, 109] (Fig. 13-46).

Inflammatory Diseases of the Spleen
Nonspecific enlargement of the spleen (e.g., as a result of hepatic disease, blood dyscrasias, splenic vein occlusion, or systemic infections) results in an enlarged splenic artery and splenic branches, usually without undue stretching. The splenic vein is often poorly visualized following arterial injection.

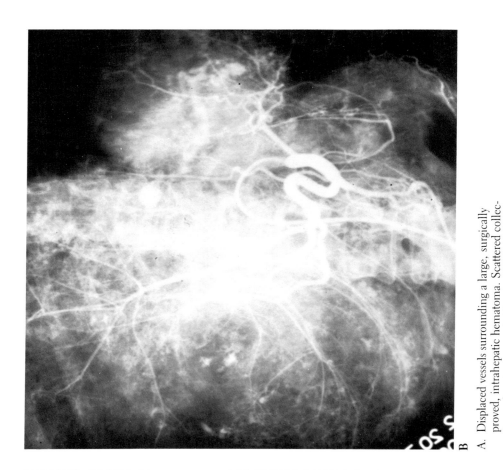

Fig. 13-46. Peliosis hepatis progressing to hemangiosarcoma. Two operative procedures were performed on this young female patient, who entered the hospital with abdominal pain and a drop in hematocrit. The patient used contraceptive pills, which were thought to cause fibrinoid degeneration of vessels and subsequent hemorrhagic areas. These areas can rupture and bleed.

A. Displaced vessels surrounding a large, surgically proved, intrahepatic hematoma. Scattered collections of contrast agent (with purpuric spaces) are evident. No tumor was seen on microscopy.

B. Repeat arteriogram taken several months later shows rapid progression. Angiosarcoma was identified at the second operative procedure.

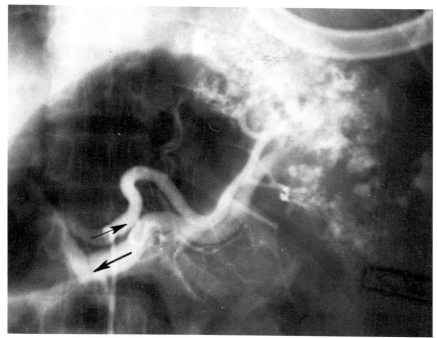

Fig. 13-47. A selective splenic arteriogram showing splenic trauma. Multifocal points of extravasation of contrast medium and premature filling of the splenic vein are seen. Splenic artery (*upper arrow*). Splenic vein (*lower arrow*).

BLUNT TRAUMA

The spleen is the most vulnerable intraabdominal organ to blunt trauma [10, 64, 97]. The following angiographic findings may also be found in trauma involving other organs (Figs. 13-47, 13-48): extravasation of contrast medium (often multifocal and seen best in the late arterial and capillary phases of arteriography); subcapsular or intrasplenic avascular spaces representing hematoma; splenic laceration with loss of intact margin; and premature venous filling. The spleen may be displaced away from the diaphragm or abdominal wall by hematoma; however, splenic displacement away from the diaphragm is not a reliable finding by itself, because the spleen may normally be situated in this position. Most of these patients must undergo surgery. Patients may be stabilized, however, by temporarily occluding major feeding vessels with a coaxially introduced Fogarty balloon catheter, or by injecting other embolic agents (Gelfoam, coils; see Chap. 5).

PORTAL HYPERTENSION

Description

The total amount of blood passing through the liver is one-quarter of the cardiac output. Approximately 25 percent of this blood enters through the higher pressure arterial system, and the remainder through the lower pressure (approximately 10 mm Hg) portal system. At the central meeting point of these vascular systems (the sinusoids), the pressure is 4 to 8 mm Hg. The blood leaves the liver through hepatic veins (pressure of 3 to 6 mm Hg) and enters into the lower pressure inferior vena cava (2 to 5 mm Hg).[+] An increase in resistance to this normal sequence of events causes altered hemodynamics in all vascular systems [20, 79, 106]. These altered hemodynamics are reflected by enlargement of the portal vein branches (particularly in the esophageal and gastric regions), stagnation of flow, and alternate methods of drainage, with retrograde flow through the normally closed communications to the systemic venous system. Occasionally even the communications between the portal and the pulmonary venous systems may open, with a resulting decrease in systemic oxygenation. Portal venous flow directed away from the liver is termed *hepatofugal flow*; that directed toward the liver is known as *hepatopetal flow*. With

[+]1 mm Hg = 1.32 cm H$_2$O.

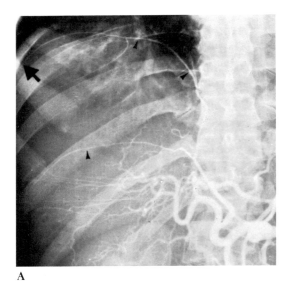

A

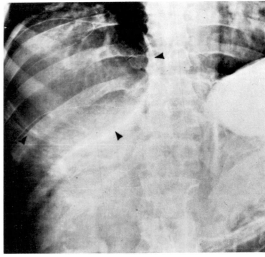

B

Fig. 13-48. Large intrahepatic hematoma (the patient was in an automobile accident 4 months previously).
A. Early arterial phase with arterial displacement (*arrows*).
B. Wall of hematoma (*arrows*).

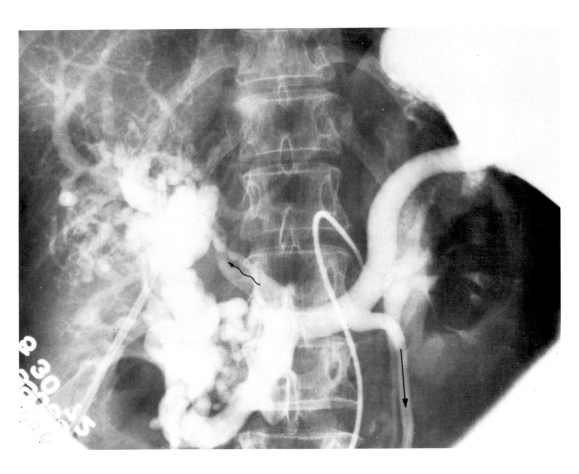

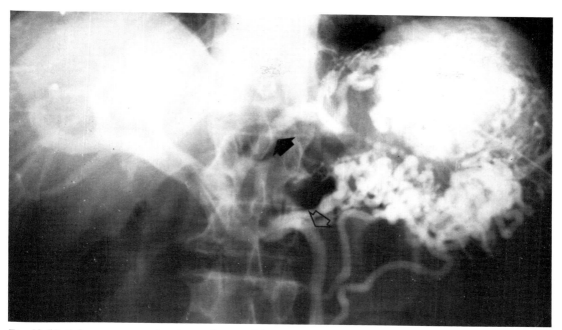

Fig. 13-50. Splenoportogram showing occlusion of the splenic vein from chronic pancreatitis. Hepatopetal flow is present, since large collaterals bypass the area of obstruction and travel toward the liver. Coronary vein (*black arrow*). Inferior mesenteric vein (*open arrow*). (From I. Johnsrude and R. Lester, Abdominal Visceral Arteriography as a Guide to the Surgeon. In *Monographs of Surgical Sciences*, Vol. 4, No. 2. Baltimore: Williams & Wilkins, 1967. Reproduced with permission of the Williams & Wilkins Company.)

decreased portal flow to the liver, the hepatic arterial system must compensate by increasing the flow, and the hepatic arteries are, therefore, often enlarged and tortuous. Decreased outflow from the hepatic veins requires a compensatory increase in hepatic fluid return through lymphatic channels. Much of this increased return is in a central direction toward the liver hilus and the cisterna chyli, with a resulting increase in pressure and volume in the thoracic duct.

As portal pressure increases and flow through the portal vein diminishes, there is a gradual decrease in the size of the portal vein, which may eventually occlude entirely. Moreover, the venous outflow from the liver may be so impaired that

Fig. 13-49. Obstruction of the portal vein due to metastases to the porta hepatis from carcinoma of the colon. The obstruction (*wavy arrow*) is bypassed by large collaterals. There is hepatofugal flow down the inferior mesenteric vein (*straight arrow*). This is the venous phase of a splenic arteriogram.

hepatic blood leaves the liver by retrograde flow through the portal vein (see Fig. 13-54). Portal hypertension may be present when the normally available portal systemic shunts are functioning well and varices do not develop. When these spontaneous shunts are not sufficient to prevent varices subsequent episodes of hemorrhage occur; surgically created shunts may then be required for adequate decompression. Shunts can be created at the portacaval level (end-to-side shunt, side-to-side shunt), at the splenic vein level (splenorenal shunt, distal splenorenal [Warren] shunt), or at the mesenteric vein caval level (end-to-side mesocaval shunt, **H** shunt). Knowledge of these shunts is important because the angiographer may have to determine their patency.

Causes of Portal Hypertension
1. Prehepatic causes.
   a. Portal vein thrombosis or splenic vein thrombosis (due to tumor, pancreatitis, abscess, other infections, or trauma, or spontaneous in onset) (Figs. 13-49, 13-50).
   b. Hyperdynamic states such as arteriovenous malformation or arteriovenous fistula.
2. Intrahepatic cirrhosis (Figs. 13-51, 13-52, 13-53, 13-54). Intrahepatic cirrhosis (Laennec's cirrhosis, biliary cirrhosis, hemochromatosis, chronic congestive cirrhosis) is the

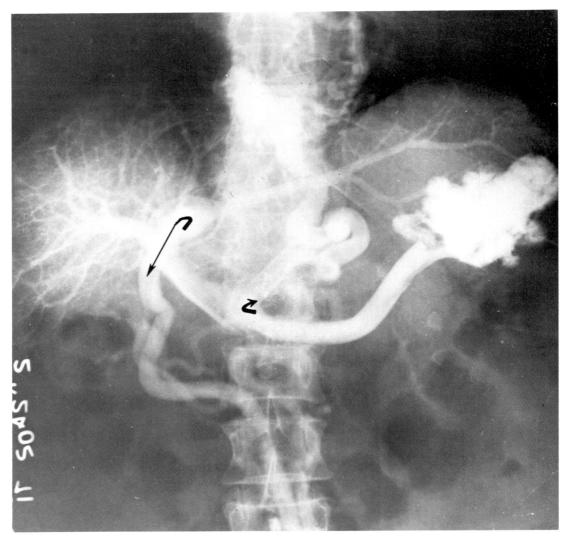

Fig. 13-51. Cirrhosis (splenoportogram). There is portal hypertension with hepatofugal flow directing blood away from the liver through a large coronary vein (*lower arrow*) and then to gastric and esophageal varices. A large umbilical vein descends to a caput medusae (*upper arrow*).

cause of 90 percent of cases of portal hypertension. It causes obstruction to the venous outflow of the liver by a fibrotic reaction that initially involves the hepatic veins. Schistosomiasis causes an intrahepatic but presinusoidal obstruction; there is subsequent increase in resistance to the portal venous flow.

3. Posthepatic obstruction. Because the hepatic veins are the outflow tract of the liver, disease here (or beyond, such as in the high inferior vena cava or right atrium) causes back pressure effects on the portal venous system. Thrombosis of the hepatic veins (Budd-Chiari syndrome; Fig. 13-55), congenital bands obstructing the hepatic vein or the inferior vena cava,

tumors, and constrictive pericarditis can also cause portal hypertension.

Angiographic Radiologic Evaluation of the Portal System

SPLENOPORTOGRAM. A splenoportogram (see Figs. 13-50, 13-51) is a direct percutaneous splenic pulp needle puncture. The advantages of this technique are that it shows more dense opacification of the venous system and that direct splenic pulp pressure measurements are available. The disadvantage is that it is more traumatic, particularly with a friable spleen, bleeding diathesis, or underlying ascites. The safety of this technique may be increased by the use of digital vascular imaging systems, smaller needles, and smaller contrast loads [15] (Fig. 13-52). False-positive occlusions (due to hemodynamic pressure and flow changes) may occur. A full description of technique of performance and other particulars is found in Chapter 23.

INDIRECT PORTOGRAPHY (see Figs. 13-49, 13-53). Indirect portography (venous phase of the arteriogram) often requires vasodilators (e.g., tolazoline) to enhance portal venous opacification. Some radiologists, however, are reluctant to use these agents in patients with histories of upper gastrointestinal bleeding. This technique is less dangerous than direct portography, and pathology may be detected in the arteriographic phase of the study in the gut, liver, spleen, and pancreas. Disadvantages of this technique are the inability to measure portal pressures directly and the fact that

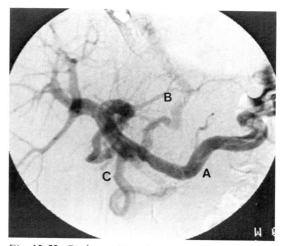

Fig. 13-52. Cirrhosis. Digital splenoportogram using a 21-gauge, thin-wall needle injecting 30% meglumine diatrizoate at 4 ml/sec (16 ml total).
A. Splenic vein.
B. Hepatofugal flow in a large coronary vein.
C. Hepatofugal flow in a recanalized paraumbilical vein.

Fig. 13-53. Cirrhosis and previous splenectomy. Venous phase of superior mesenteric arteriogram shows diminutive portal vein (*arrow*), retrograde flow into massive gastric varices, and spontaneous shunting through a gastrorenal anastomosis (*curved arrow*) into the inferior vena cava (*open arrow*).

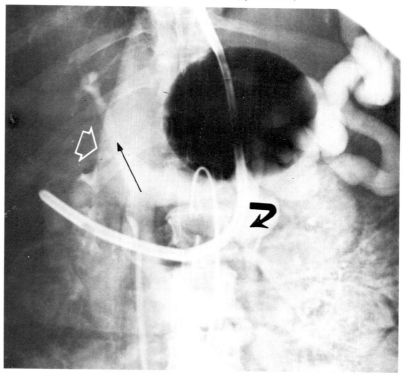

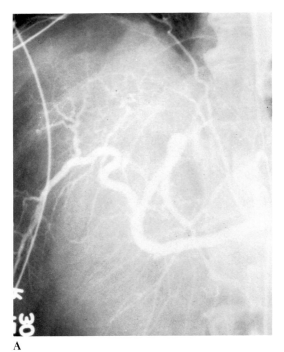

A

Fig. 13-54. Severe cirrhosis.
A. Hepatic arteriogram, showing prominent proximal vessels and tortuous intrahepatic branches.

Fig. 13-55. Hepatic vein thrombosis (Budd-Chiari syndrome). This young patient had paroxysmal nocturnal hemoglobinuria as the underlying cause for hepatic vein thrombosis. Hepatomegaly, ascites, and abdominal pain were the presenting symptoms. A spidery network of veins replaces the normal structures (compare with Fig. 13-16).

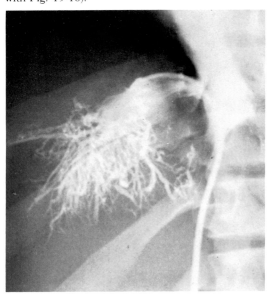

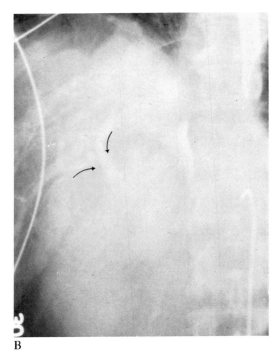

B

B. Retrograde flow through the portal veins (*arrows*) (see text, p. 368).

the contrast agent in the venous phase is often too dilute to outline the venous system clearly. The use of digital vascular imaging systems with increased contrast sensitivity may yield earlier and denser opacification of the portal venous system following the selective intraarterial administration of contrast agents (Fig. 13-56). This may be achieved without the use of vasodilators. Additionally, the use of the newer nonionic and lower osmolarity ionic contrast agents, which undergo less in-vivo dilution, may enhance portal venous visualization with either conventional or digital systems.

HEPATIC VENOUS STUDIES (Figs. 13-57, 13-58). Hepatic venous studies (wedge pressure measurements and contrast injections) [106] are performed to exclude hepatic venous occlusive disease and to help evaluate the severity of portal hypertension. The wedge position of the catheter in a small hepatic venule measures a pressure relative to that of the communicating sinusoids; the normal pressure is between 3 and 11 mm Hg. This pressure measurement includes not only that within the sinusoid but also the intraabdominal pressure. Because ascites, heart failure, and other conditions

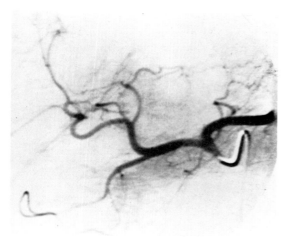

A

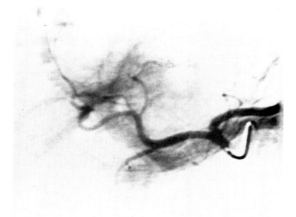

B

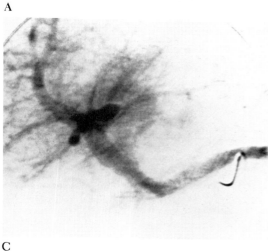

C

Fig. 13-56. Digital indirect arterioportography. Preoperative "roadmap" for surgical placement of a chemotherapy infusion pump (metastatic colon cancer). Thirty percent meglumine diatrizoate injected at 5 ml/sec for 6 seconds (total 30 ml).

A. Early arterial phase. Conventional anatomy is demonstrated.

B. Late arterial phase. Filling of portal vein is already identified.

C. Midvenous phase. Dense opacification of the portal vein has occurred.

Fig. 13-58. Hepatic wedge injection in a patient with severe cirrhosis. There is retrograde flow into the portal vein (PV), and a mottled nonhomogeneous stain in the liver parenchyma. The corrected sinusoidal pressure is 21 mm Hg.

Fig. 13-57. Hepatic venous wedge pressures (see text for details). An approach from the antecubital vein is preferable; the internal jugular vein and the femoral vein are alternate routes.

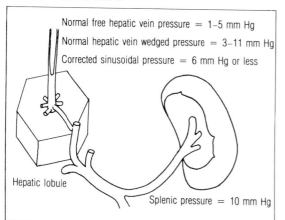

Normal free hepatic vein pressure = 1–5 mm Hg

Normal hepatic vein wedged pressure = 3–11 mm Hg

Corrected sinusoidal pressure = 6 mm Hg or less

Hepatic lobule

Splenic pressure = 10 mm Hg

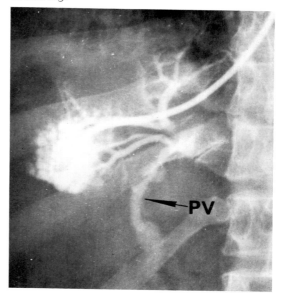

PV

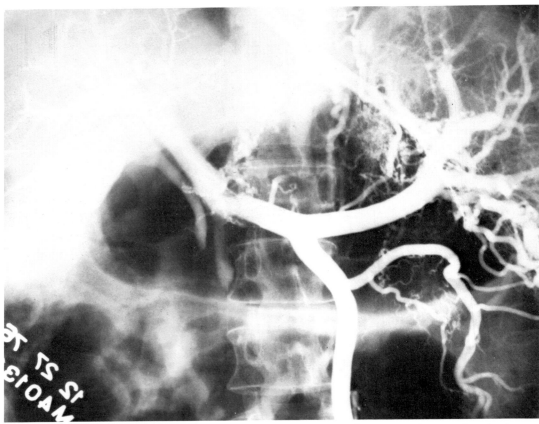

Fig. 13-59. Transhepatic portal vein catheterization
(see Chap. 23).

can influence this pressure, an accurate measurement of true sinusoidal pressure is obtained by subtracting from the wedge pressure that pressure measured with the catheter lying free within the hepatic vein. Thus hepatic wedge pressure (normally 3 to 11 mm Hg) minus free hepatic vein pressure (normally 1 to 6 mm Hg) equals corrected sinusoidal pressure (normally 1 to 5 mm Hg).

If sinusoidal pressure is elevated due to increased resistance at sinusoidal or postsinusoidal level (as in cirrhosis), this elevation can be accurately measured. Three grades of elevation are recognized: mild elevation of corrected sinusoidal pressure (6 to 10 mm Hg); moderate elevation (10 to 18 mm Hg); and severe elevation (19 mm Hg or higher). Because no pressures can be transmitted to the sinusoids in presinusoidal obstruction or portal vein thrombosis, hepatic venous wedge pressures are normal or subnormal in these conditions.

A controlled injection of contrast medium into the hepatic venous wedge catheter normally shows anterograde flow into the hepatic vein and some retrograde flow into the portal veins, which rapidly clears. In hepatic or prehepatic disease, there are varying degrees of severity of retrograde flow into the portal venous system, with slow clearing of contrast medium. In addition, the homogeneous hepatic parenchymal stain seen in the normal person may be replaced by a marked nonhomogeneous mottled stain in persons with severe cirrhosis (Fig. 13-58). A better appreciation of the intrahepatic venous communications may be obtained by using a balloon catheter (No. 7 French Swan Ganz catheter). This catheter can be positioned more proximally in the hepatic vein, and larger doses of contrast medium can be administered.

PERCUTANEOUS TRANSHEPATIC CATHETERIZATION (Fig. 13-59). This type of catheterization is not performed unless other maneuvers have proved unsuccessful and the patient is a poor surgical candidate. It is used for percutaneous transhepatic therapeutic embolization of bleeding varices. Pa-

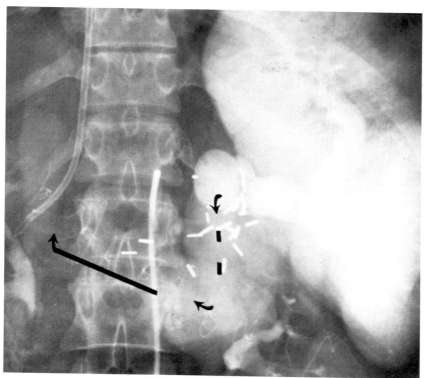

Fig. 13-60. Patent Warren shunt (distal splenic vein to renal vein). The selective splenic arteriogram floods the spleen with contrast medium, which eventually drains through the splenic vein, through the anastomosis into the renal vein (*short arrows*), and then to the inferior vena cava (*long arrow*).

tients with a bleeding diathesis or large amounts of ascites present a greater risk. The approach is described in Chapter 23.

TRANSJUGULAR VEIN APPROACH. The transjugular vein approach, described by Rosch, may be used to evaluate the portal venous system, the hepatic venous system, and the biliary system and may also be used to obtain liver biopsies. The approach is described in Chapter 23.

PARAUMBILICAL VEIN CATHETERIZATION. This type of catheterization may be of value when the transhepatic technique is contraindicated. It requires a surgical incision in the supraumbilical area for cannulation of the paraumbilical vein [49, 59].

SURGICAL APPROACH. Portal hemodynamics and anatomy can be evaluated at laparotomy; however, this method suffers the grave disadvantage of inadequate preoperative planning. A minilaparotomy may be performed in the angiographic suite.

One of the jejunal portal venous radicals are selectively entered with a 5 F catheter and advanced to the splenic vein under fluoroscopic control. The catheter tip can be manipulated and positioned both for purposes of portal venography and embolic therapy of subsequently opacified varices.

Evaluation of a Patient
with Portal Hypertension
Patients with recurrent episodes of gastrointestinal bleeding in the past and known varices need evaluation preparatory to a shunt procedure. First, total panhepatic angiography should be performed. This study includes arteriography to exclude lesions such as tumors and arteriovenous malformations; visualization of the venous phase of selective splanchnic vessel arteries to outline the status of the portal venous anatomy; and hepatic venous wedge pressure measurements. If the portal vein is patent and a Warren decompression shunt or a splenorenal shunt is anticipated, the left renal vein should also be outlined. The Warren shunt is an anastomosis of the distal splenic vein to the left renal vein, leaving the spleen intact (Fig. 13-60).

The gastric varices are also ligated. In the spleno-renal shunt, the spleen is sacrificed and the anastomosis is between the proximal splenic vein and the left renal vein. If the splenic vein or the portal vein or both are occluded, the position and diameter of the superior mesenteric vein should be clearly outlined, because this vessel may be used in a mesocaval or **H** shunt (a graft between the superior mesenteric vein and the inferior vena cava) (Fig. 13-61).

If the patient is bleeding acutely from the gastrointestinal tract and has known varices, the angiographer should modify the study in the following ways:

1. Determine the source of bleeding (whether or not it is variceal; see the following section).
2. Determine the pathologic venous anatomy only if it is expedient to do so.
3. Direct one's energies toward slowing or stopping the bleeding (selective arterial catheterization and vasoconstrictive infusion or embolization of the bleeding artery if the bleeding is nonvariceal). Superior mesenteric arterial infusion with vasoconstrictive medication may be performed if the bleeding is variceal in origin. There is evidence, however, that when vasopressin is administered intravenously, in similar doses as when used intraarterially, it is just as effective as when the intraarterial route is used; similar responses may be seen in portal pressures, mesenteric flow, and cardiac output [5, 17, 21, 104]. The intraarterial route of vasopressin administration may, therefore, be rarely necessary for variceal bleeding. If the patient's condition prevents surgical intervention of variceal bleeding and there is no response to intravascular vasoconstrictive medications, one may employ transhepatic portal venous embolization. This is considerably more invasive, however, than endoscopic transesophageal sclerosis, which when performed by an experienced endoscopist, is equally effective.

SPONTANEOUS INTRAABDOMINAL BLEEDING

Arteriography plays an important role in detecting the site of bleeding and, under certain circumstances, in therapy for bleeding. The latter is accomplished by intraarterial injection of vasoconstrictor medications or occlusion of feeding vessels.

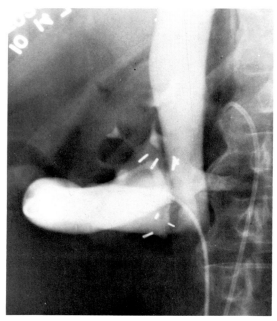

Fig. 13-61. Patent **H** shunt between the superior mesenteric vein and the inferior vena cava. The catheter is introduced from the inferior vena cava directly into the shunt.

Bleeding Outside of the Gastrointestinal Tract

When bleeding occurs outside the lumen of the gastrointestinal tract [61], the clinical manifestation may be sudden collapse due to shock, or there may be a progressive weakness with loss of hematocrit. If the bleeding is into a confined space and is relatively acute, there is pain of varying severity. Abdominal aortography followed by expeditious, appropriate selective arteriography usually defines the cause of the bleeding, which includes the following: leaking aortic or iliac artery aneurysm or anastomosis of aortic graft; dissecting aortic aneurysm; leaking visceral artery aneurysm; delayed rupture of the spleen, liver, or kidney following trauma; bleeding from hypervascular tumor or arteriovenous malformation, peliosis hepatis or hepatic adenoma. If clinically appropriate, bleeding may be stopped in selected high surgical risk patients by catheterization embolization techniques (see Chap. 5).

Gastrointestinal Bleeding

Gastrointestinal bleeding [5, 9, 18, 19, 33, 43, 68, 86, 94, 111] may arise from lesions of the gastroin-

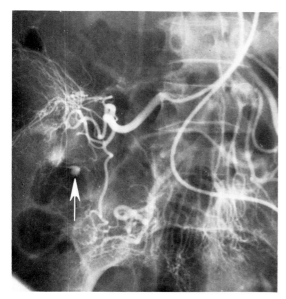

Fig. 13-62. Bleeding cecal diverticulum. The catheter is in the ileocolic artery. There is extravasation of contrast medium in a localized collection within the diverticulum (*arrow*). The patient responded well to treatment with vasopressin.

testinal tract or, rarely, from vessels of the accessory organs (e.g., hepatic artery aneurysm causing hematobilia; false aneurysm in a communicating pancreatic pseudocyst). The bleeding may be acute or chronic. Acute bleeding may be mucosal (gastritis), venous (varices), or arterial (Mallory-Weiss tears, ulcers, diverticula, aneurysms, arteriovenous malformations, hemangiomas, or tumors).

Acute bleeding may arise from the upper or lower gastrointestinal tract. It should be handled in the following manner:

1. If feasible, endoscopy should be performed prior to angiography in patients with upper gastrointestinal bleeding. A nasopharyngeal bleeding source and blood dyscrasias must be excluded.
2. The patient should have a nuclear medicine, radionuclide bleeding study with either technetium-99m–sulphur colloid or technetium-99m-labeled red blood cells. While angiography may detect bleeding rates of 1 ml/minute or greater, radionuclide studies may detect bleeding of 0.1 ml/minute to 0.2 ml/minute. In the face of a negative radionuclide study, detection of an acute bleeding site on an angiogram would be unlikely and angiography should be postponed [16, 70, 100, 114].

3. The abdomen must be free of barium. The patient should be actively bleeding at the time of the study. A positive nasogastric aspirate differentiates upper from lower gastrointestinal bleeding. The patient should have lost at least two units of blood in the past 24 hours. Supportive treatment of the patient should be instituted in the angiographic room. An intravenous line for measuring central venous pressure should be introduced. A Foley catheter may be placed to record urine output and to decompress the bladder so as not to obscure pelvic sources of bleeding.
4. All possible bleeding arteries should be adequately opacified. If upper gastrointestinal bleeding is proved, confine the study to the stomach, duodenum, and lower esophagus and search for varices. The left gastric artery and the small gastroesophageal branches from the inferior phrenic artery may arise proximal to the tip of the catheter and escape opacification. Fill the stomach (or colon) with air prior to the contrast injection. This may be accomplished with a nasogastric tube or with gas-releasing granules such as those used for double contrast upper GI studies. Gaseous distension should be monitored fluoroscopically. Generally 400 to 500 cc of air are sufficient. Include the lower esophagus in the celiac injection. If there is rectal bleeding and a negative nasogastric aspirate, perform superior mesenteric and then inferior mesenteric angiography. Empty the contrast filled bladder so as not to obscure the rectosigmoid. (Ask the patient to urinate if a Foley catheter has not been placed.) Pay close attention to the cecum and right colon. Two injections each in the superior and inferior mesenteric arteries may be needed to visualize the upper and lower portions of the bowel. Use adequate doses of medium-density contrast agent (e.g., 50 to 60 ml per injection in the superior mesenteric artery), and prolong the films to 25 to 30 seconds. Beware of pyelograms, and beware of bony structures that may overlie and obscure points of extravasation. In all cases, perform an abdominal aortogram if selective studies fail to outline the bleeding source; rarely, anomalous feeding branches or unsuspected aortoenteric fistulas are thus uncovered (see Fig. 10-24). Digital vascular imaging systems employing newer, larger (at least 12

in.) image intensifiers may prove to be very useful in that, with their inherent increased contrast sensitivity, they may potentially identify sites of bleeding usually missed with conventional filming.

5. If the bleeding site is confined (e.g., diverticulum; Fig. 13-62), extravasation of small amounts of contrast medium can easily be detected. On the other hand, fairly extensive bleeding over a large surface area may be difficult to define (e.g., gastritis; Fig. 13-63). The bleeding may be sporadic—it may temporarily cease, and repeat injections in the same artery occasionally can uncover an otherwise hidden bleeding site.

6. If varices are suspected, they may be seen on the venous phase of the arteriogram. As a result of dilution of contrast medium in the venous system, extravasation of contrast medium from bleeding varices is not usually seen. Even if varices are seen, be sure to search for an active arterial bleeding site (e.g., gastritis, Mallory-Weiss tear [Fig. 13-64], stress ulcer). The two conditions are associated in more than 20 percent of upper gastrointestinal bleeding. If extravariceal causes are excluded, direct transhepatic portal venous evaluation and treatment for severe bleeding may be undertaken if the patient is too ill for surgery and other methods fail.

Common causes of failure to detect arterial bleeding sites are as follows:

1. Bleeding has stopped (the usual cause).
2. Large bleeding surface area.
3. Variceal bleeding—dilution of contrast medium in the venous phase prevents adequate visualization. The varices may not be detected by the indirect arteriographic route.
4. Bleeding artery is not selectively opacified (e.g., left gastric artery; Fig. 13-65).
5. Not enough contrast injection.
6. Bleeding site is off the film, or films were not extended over a sufficiently long period. For detecting varices, at least 25 to 30 seconds is required.
7. Unfavorable anatomy. The inferior mesenteric artery is often difficult to cannulate, particularly in older patients (see Fig. 13-3). Celiac

Fig. 13-63. Capillary phase of celiac axis arteriogram in a cirrhotic patient with known varices diffusely bleeding from multiple gastric erosions (*arrow*). There is poorly localized extravasation of contrast medium. The patient responded well to treatment with vasopressin in the celiac axis.

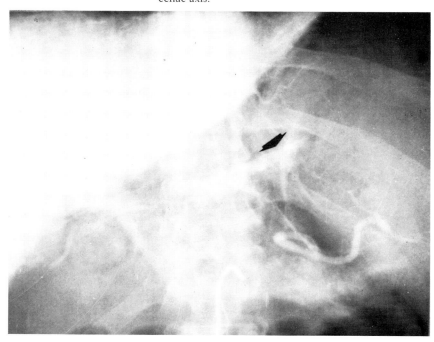

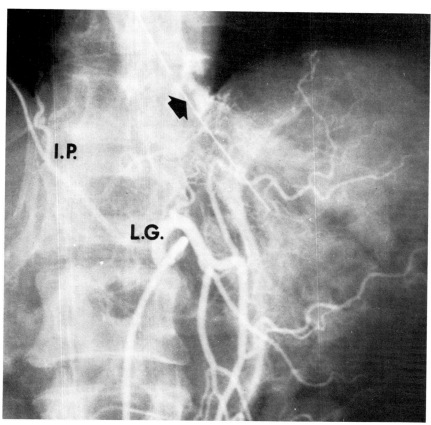

Fig. 13-64. Left gastric arteriogram showing a Mallory-Weiss tear of the distal esophagus in a patient with severe hemorrhage following an episode of vomiting. There is extravasation at the esophagogastric junction (*arrow*). The patient responded well to vasopressin infusion. LG = left gastric artery; IP = inferior phrenic artery.

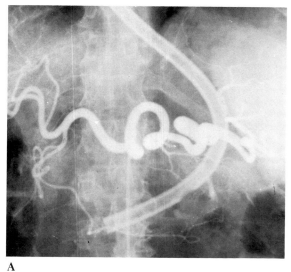

A

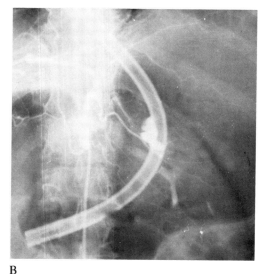

B

Fig. 13-65. Upper gastrointestinal bleeding.
A. Celiac axis angiogram shows no bleeding site.

B. Anomalous origin of the left gastric artery (and a replaced left hepatic artery) from the aorta. The bleeding site is now obvious.

stenosis, anomalies, aortic aneurysm, and tortuous iliacs or occluded femorals are frequent.

8. Rapid deterioration of the patient's condition on the radiographic table.

Intraarterial catheter treatment may be used for gastrointestinal bleeding. This treatment is accomplished by constricting bleeding vessels by means of intraarterial infusion of vasoconstricting drugs or by occluding the bleeding vessels.

VASOCONSTRICTIVE INTRAARTERIAL THERAPY [5, 7, 93, 111]. This therapy has the most satisfactory results in treating gastric bleeding sites, particularly erosive gastritis (80 percent success rate); bleeding diverticula (up to 95 percent success rate); and bleeding varices (55 to 95 percent success rate). It can be helpful in controlling bleeding from other areas, but with a lower rate of success. It has also been used in treating severe bleeding from ulcerative colitis [19]. The angiographer should observe the following steps of treatment:

1. Place the catheter tip as close to the site of hemorrhage as possible. Always search for more than one site of bleeding. Remember that bright red blood from the rectum can arise from a large upper gastrointestinal hemorrhage. Duodenal bleeding may propagate blood rapidly anterograde down the bowel, and the nasogastric aspirate may be clear.

2. If the patient has esophageal or gastric varices (proved by previous upper gastrointestinal series, endoscopy, or the venous phase of a splanchnic arteriogram) and has no extravasation of contrast medium to suggest active arterial bleeding, you may assume that the varices are causing the bleeding.

   If intravenous vasoconstrictors are ineffective, and if transhepatic or transesophageal sclerotherapy is not considered place the catheter in the superior mesenteric artery and infuse with vasoconstrictive medications. The portal pressure may be reduced by as much as 50 percent by this technique. Meticulous catheter care during infusion is essential. There may be leaking at the puncture site, and clots may form around the catheter both at the puncture site and around and within the catheter tip in the selective vessel. Occlusion of vessels must be avoided. The position of the catheter tip should be checked with contrast injections if there is

suspicion of catheter displacement or if there is failure of response to treatment. Important equipment and techniques to include are a one-way valve to prevent backup of blood into the catheter tip; a slow-speed, accurate automatic injector constantly injecting either a vasopressor or (if bleeding has stopped) saline solution; accurate measurements of drug dosage; and adequate external fixation of the catheter.

A commonly used vasoconstrictive medication is vasopressin (Pitressin) [9]. In addition to its constrictive action on blood vessels, this posterior pituitary extract acts directly on the smooth muscle of the bowel and is catabolized predominantly in the liver. Vasopressin can cause abdominal cramps, antidiuresis, vascular overloading due to diversion of blood from the splanchnic area into the general circulation, pulmonary edema, bradycardia and reduction in cardiac output (due to constriction of coronary arteries), transient blood pressure elevation, and portal venous system thrombosis; therefore, one must watch the dosage carefully. The vasoactive effect continues for approximately 30 minutes following discontinuance of the drug. It has no deleterious effect on the liver.

Vasopressin may be used in (1) the superior mesenteric artery, to control portal hypertension during bleeding (also during surgery), and (2) a superselective vessel, to control arterial bleeding (Fig. 13-66). If superselective catheterization is not possible, place the catheter in the major feeding vessel more proximally. Although the dose of vasopressin varies from 0.1 to 0.4 IU per minute injected directly into the vessel supplying the bleeding site, the *minimum* dose necessary for stopping bleeding should be used. Vascular response should be measured by angiographic demonstration of vascular constriction and absence of extravasation. A repeat arteriogram should be performed after 30 minutes of infusion of 0.2 IU per minute with the drug. If the response is good, continued infusion with the same or a smaller dose should be instituted while the patient is clinically monitored. If the bleeding has not stopped, increase the dosage to 0.3 or even 0.4 IU per minute. If the bleeding does not stop with this dosage administered for another 30 minutes, consider other options (these may include embolization if the vascular anatomy and the target organ are amenable). Do not compromise the patient's ca-

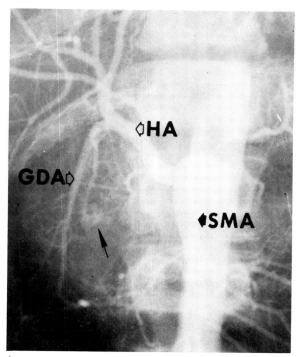

A

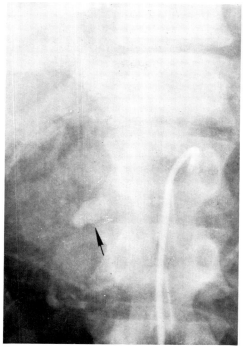

B

Fig. 13-66. Response to vasopressin in a bleeding duodenal ulcer.

A. Superior mesenteric arteriogram, showing anomalous hepatic artery (HA) origin from the superior mesenteric artery (SMA), and bleeding (*arrow*) arising from the supraduodenal branch of the gastroduodenal artery (GDA).

B. Extravasation at site of ulcer (*arrow*).

C. Arteriogram after selective gastroduodenal artery infusion with vasopressin for 30 minutes. The vessels are narrowed and there is no extravasation. The infusion was continued for an additional 12 hours, and then the dose was gradually diminished over 24 hours.

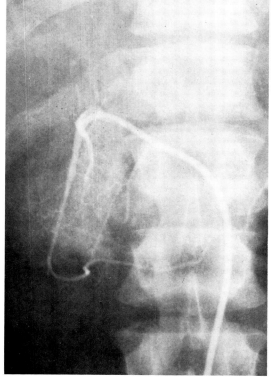

C

pacity to undergo surgery with prolonged ineffectual treatment. When bleeding stops in patients with actively bleeding nonvariceal sites, the effective dose of vasopressin should be continued for 24 hours. If control of bleeding persists, halve the dose for another 12 hours. After this, the catheter can be left in place and kept open by saline infusions for an additional 24 hours in case bleeding resumes. If necessary, the catheter may be left in place for several days.

Epinephrine [93], another vasoconstrictive drug, has not been as helpful as vasopressin and currently is not in general use.

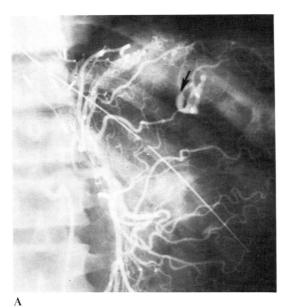

A

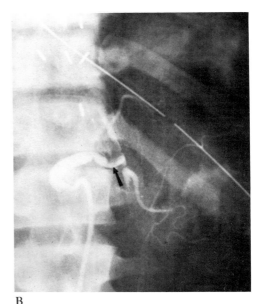

B

Fig. 13-67.

A. Selective left gastric arteriogram, showing bleeding within the gastric fundus (*arrow*). There was no response to vasopressin.

B. Left gastric artery embolized with autogenous clot (*arrow*) mixed with aminocaproic acid (see text for details).

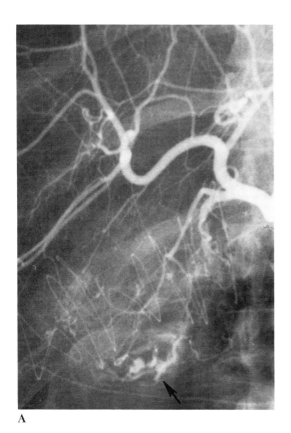

A

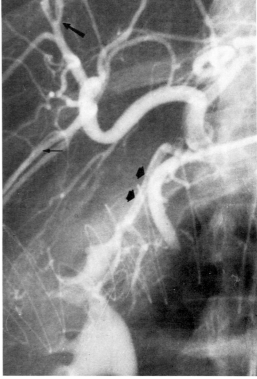

B

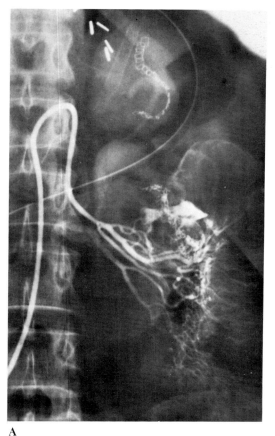

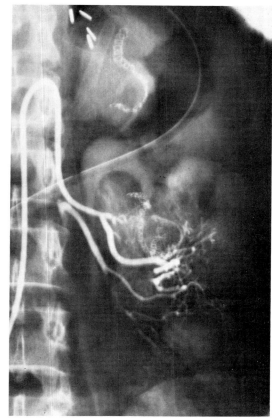

A   B

Fig. 13-69.
A. Bleeding from anastomosis of gastrojejunostomy.
B. Embolized mesenteric (jejunal) branch with Gelfoam.

SELECTIVE ARTERIAL OCCLUSION [14, 33, 45, 86, 103]. This technique is used early in the course of treatment if the bleeding arises from easily catheterized branches of the left gastric artery or the gastroduodenal artery. Occlusion accom-

---

Fig. 13-68. Postoperative upper gastrointestinal bleeding following extensive surgery for carcinoma of the hepatic flexure invading the duodenum.
A. Celiac axis arteriogram shows surgically occluded gastroduodenal artery and bleeding site (*arrow*) supplied by the posterior branch of the superior pancreaticoduodenal artery.
B. Postembolization film. The bleeding artery was occluded with autogenous clot, and no further bleeding occurred (*thick arrows*). There are small emboli in the peripheral hepatic artery branches (*thin arrows*). There were no sequelae to the hepatic artery emboli, possibly because of rapid lysis of the embolic material and their small size.

plishes cessation of hemorrhage without compromising the well-collateralized circulation of the stomach or adjacent structures. The short gastric branches of the splenic artery (supplying the greater curve) cannot be selectively catheterized and are best treated with vasoconstrictive methods. In all other areas (e.g., colon, small bowel), vessel occlusion is performed only when all other measures fail and the patient is a poor candidate for surgery. The catheter must be placed well within the superselective vessel and as close to the bleeding site as possible, and the emboli must be introduced slowly to prevent reflux into nontarget arteries (Figs. 13-67, 13-68, 13-69, 13-70; see Fig. 5-5). Infarction of viable structures must be avoided at all costs. Catheter occlusive techniques include the following:

1. Injection of autologous clot. Remove 10 ml of blood and allow it to clot. Inject the clot slowly and carefully into the catheter. Although not

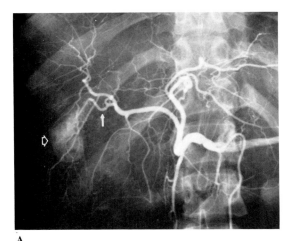

A

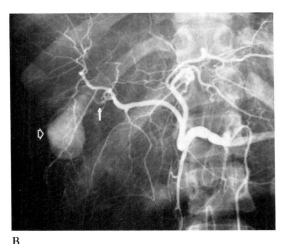

B

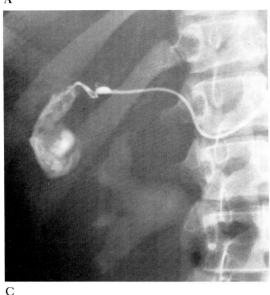

C

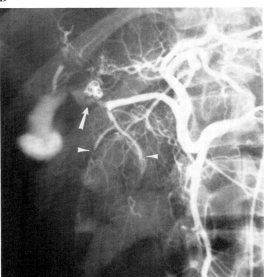

D

Fig. 13-70.
A and B. Filling of aneurysm (*open arrow*) and bidirectional flow in main feeding branch (*small arrow*).
C. Cannulation of main feeder for Ivalon injection.
D. Coils (*arrow*) placed in right hepatic artery. Some Ivalon has refluxed into the cystic artery (*arrowheads*).

usually necessary, the clot may be extruded into the bleeding vessel by following the clot with a guidewire. A more firm clot can be made by mixing 1 ml (250 mg) of aminocaproic acid (Amicar) with 9 ml of blood. The temporary duration of the clot occludes the bleeding vessel without compromising circulation and makes this the preferred method of occluding bleeding vessels in the gastrointestinal tract.

2. Gelfoam in larger particulate form (2 to 3 mm pieces) may be mixed with blood and contrast agent and carefully extruded into the bleeding vessel. This material may be used if it is difficult to form a clot with the patient's blood.

This, like autologous clot, ultimately recanalizes and allows reperfusion of the occluded vessel. It, therefore, is a preferred occluding agent when temporary occlusion only is desired.

3. Ivalon sponge, a polyvinyl alcohol, is inert and easily compressible [103]. If it is wetted in saline, then compressed, dried, and gas sterilized, small pellets may be cut and pre-

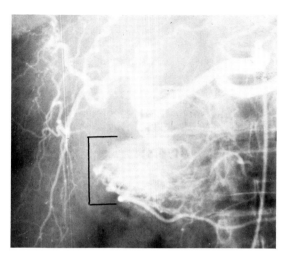

Fig. 13-71. Large arteriovenous malformation of the duodenum. The patient had recurrent episodes of upper gastrointestinal bleeding.

Fig. 13-72. Arteriovenous malformation of the cecum (*open arrow*) in a young woman with recurrent rectal bleeding. Prominent arterial branch (*straight arrow*) and premature venous return (*curved arrow*).

pared for embolic purposes. When introduced into the bloodstream, the Ivalon pellets swell, resume their original size, become invaded by fibrocytes, and completely occlude the vessel. Ivalon can also be obtained in particles of various size from 150 to 1000 μm (see Chap. 5). Slow extrusion of emboli with a guidewire from the superselectively placed catheter tip prevents reflux of emboli to nontarget vessels. This technique may be used when permanent occlusion of vessels is required, such as with a bleeding false aneurysm in a pseudocyst.

4. Tissue adhesives (cyanoacrylate) may be used. This substance forms a firm permanent adhesive immediately on contact with blood. Its use requires skill and experience [31, 112].

5. Balloon catheters may be used. A 2 or 3

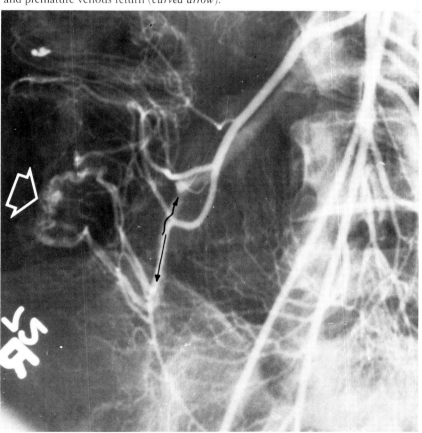

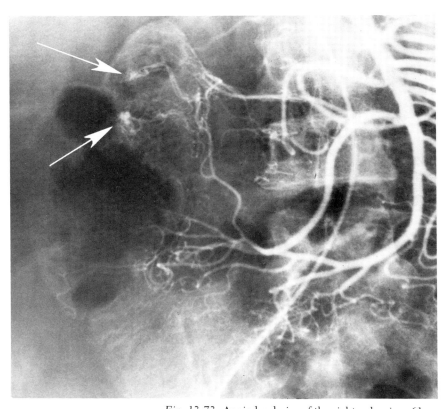

Fig. 13-73. Angiodysplasias of the right colon in a 61-year-old woman with recurrent episodes of rectal bleeding. Superior mesenteric arteriogram shows two tuftlike collections of contrast medium (*arrows*) and prominent early draining veins in the hepatic flexure.

French Fogarty catheter may be introduced into a 7 or 8 French thin-walled catheter placed selectively into the bleeding vessel. As an alternative, 5, 6, or 7 French double lumen balloon-tipped catheters are now available.[5] Temporary occlusion of the artery can be accomplished by inflating the balloon tip. This catheter may also be used to prevent reflux of embolic material, by temporarily inflating the balloon during the embolization. Additional details concerning occluding devices (e.g., steel coils and chemical sclerosing agents) are given in Chapter 5.

If bleeding is chronic or recurrent and low grade, the likely underlying cause is tumor, inflammation, arteriovenous malformation, or telangiectasia [13, 98]. This situation is not an emergency, and angiography should be performed after the use of more conventional techniques (i.e., endoscopy, upper gastrointestinal series, small-bowel series, barium enema). Thorough selective and superselective studies may be necessary; even then, the chances of finding the lesion in our experience has been only 30 percent. Angiographic findings reflect those of the primary lesion; for example, a large feeding artery and prematurely filling large drainage vein of an arteriovenous malformation (Figs. 13-71, 13-72), a small vascular tuft or densely staining vein of vascular ectasia (Fig. 13-73), tumor neovascularity, or periarterial cuffing of a primary bowel tumor (see Figs. 13-37, 13-38).

Either chronic or acute gastrointestinal bleeding in patients with abdominal aortic grafts may be an ominous finding, because aortoenteric fistulas at anastomotic sites (aortoduodenal proximally, ileoenteric or femoral-enteric at lower sites) can result in exsanguinating hemorrhages, which can occur weeks to years after surgery. Extravasation is a late finding in the acutely ill patient. More subtle findings include false aneurysm at the anastomotic site. There may be no angiographic clue of this potentially lethal condition, but barium studies of the gastrointestinal tract may define a corrugated extrinsic defect at the site of the problem (see Chap. 10).

MESENTERIC ISCHEMIA

Mesenteric ischemia [99] may be occlusive, resulting from conditions such as atheromatous disease, dissection, or mesenteric emboli; however, it is most frequently nonocclusive and is associated with a low-flow syndrome. This condition occurs in patients with low cardiac output due to cardiogenic or hemorrhagic shock, cardiac arrhythmias, and congestive heart failure. Digitalis has been implicated as a cause of nonocclusive mesenteric ischemia. Clinically, the patient presents with abdominal pain, usually without rebound tenderness, and nonspecific distension of the bowel, with gas noted on the flat film of the abdomen. This condition may progress on to complete bowel infarction and death.

The angiographic pattern, best seen on selective superior mesenteric artery studies, shows varying degrees of arterial narrowing. Multiple short segmental constrictions at the origin of branches may be either focal in nature or tapered. There is often reduced filling of the finer arterial branches, with poor visualization of the arcades and intramural vessels. This reduced filling may be localized to one segment of the bowel or may be generalized throughout the circulation. These findings are caused by vasospasm; if it is reversed by a test dose of an intraarterial vasodilator (e.g., papaverine, 45 mg given over a period of 15 minutes), prolonged intraarterial treatment of 3 mg per minute of papaverine for a number of hours may obviate the problem. This treatment is effective only if the patient's underlying shock has responded to therapy; if the condition is irreversible, bowel infarction usually ensues.

Arterial irregularities, vasospasm, and poor peripheral vascular filling may occur in patients being treated with vasopressors and may be seen as an artifact from catheter manipulations. It is usually not difficult to differentiate these findings from the fixed vascular irregularities due to periarterial encasement of tumor.

Pitfalls of Splanchnic Angiography

1. Pathologic conditions may be missed due to the following factors:
   a. The presence of unrecognized anomalous vascular origins (e.g., a hepatic tumor supplied primarily from the right hepatic branch replaced from the superior mesenteric artery).
   b. The contrast agent may be delivered beyond the vessel supplying the lesion (e.g., beyond a bleeding left gastric artery).
   c. The venous phase may be missed due to insufficient films and/or length of film timing (e.g., varices may not be seen).
   d. The area of interest may be off the film (e.g., bleeding from a hiatus hernia or a high-lying splenic flexure).
2. The catheter may whip out of the selective position in the celiac axis or superior mesenteric artery during injection of contrast medium. Choose the catheter curve carefully, and, if necessary, add side holes to the distal tip. Monitor fluoroscopically the catheter response to short (1-second) injections at the proposed rate. Prevent undue catheter torque causing withdrawal of the tip from the orifice by holding the catheter firmly during catheter attachment to the injector.
3. Vascular artifacts simulating tumor invasion or primary vascular disease may be caused by spasm due to superselective catheter placement or to manipulations with guidewires. If this presents a problem in interpretation, check the same vessels on the prior aortogram.
4. Arterial and venous irregularities simulating primary vascular disease or tumor invasion may occur as a result of previous surgery.
5. Complications of superselective catheterization include arterial dissection with subsequent occlusion, and embolization of end arteries. Although potentially serious, these conditions often resolve themselves. If the patient shows progressive symptoms despite heparinization and supportive therapy, surgical intervention may be required.
6. Overdose of contrast medium superselectively through a catheter wedged in the pancreatic vessels can cause abdominal pain and elevation of serum amylase.

References

1. Aakhus, T., et al. Angiography in acute pancreatitis. *Acta Radiol.* [*Diagn.*] 8:119, 1969.

2. Abrams, H. (ed.). *Angiography* (3rd ed.). Boston: Little, Brown, 1983. Vol. 2, sections 4 and 5.

3. Abrams, R., et al. Angiographic features of cavernous hemangioma of the liver. *Radiology* 92:308, 1969.

4. Allison, D., Modlin, I. M., and Jenkins, W. J. Treatment of carcinoid liver metastases by hepatic artery embolization. *Lancet* 2:1223, 1977.

5. Athanasoulis, C., et al. Angiography, its contributions to the emergency management of gastrointestinal hemorrhage. *Radiol. Clin. North Am.* 14:265, 1976.

6. Baert, A. L., Marchal, G. J., and Wilms, G. E. Comparative study of angiography and dynamic computed tomography in liver angioma. *Radiology* 148:599, 1983.

7. Barr, J., Lakin, R., and Rosch, J. Similarity of arterial and intravenous vasopressin on portal and systemic hemodynamics. *Gastroenterology* 69:13, 1975.

8. Bass, E. The radiologic diagnosis of hepatoma with special emphasis on angiography. *S. Afr. Med. J.* 49:745, 1974.

9. Baum, S., and Nusbaum, M. The control of gastrointestinal hemorrhage by selective mesenteric arterial infusion of vasopressin. *Radiology* 98:497, 1971.

10. Boijsen, E., et al. Angiography in hepatic rupture. *Acta Radiol.* [*Diagn.*] 11:363, 1971.

11. Boijsen, E., and Reuter, S. Mesenteric angiography in evaluation of inflammatory and neoplastic diseases of the intestine. *Radiology* 87:1028, 1966.

12. Boijsen, E., and Samuelsson, L. Angiographic diagnosis of tumors arising from the pancreatic islets. *Acta Radiol.* [*Diagn.*] 10:161, 1970.

13. Boley, S. J., et al. On the nature and etiology of vascular ectasias of the colon; degenerative lesions of aging. *Gastroenterology* 72(4):650, 1977.

14. Bookstein, J., et al. Transcatheter hemostasis of gastrointestinal bleeding using modified autogenous clot. *Radiology* 113:266, 1974.

15. Braun, S. D., Newman, G. E., and Dunnick, N. R. Digital splenoportography. *A.J.R.* 144:1003, 1985.

16. Bunker, S. R., et al. Scintigraphy of gastrointestinal hemorrhage: Superiority of TC 99m–red blood cells over TC 99m sulphur colloid. *A.J.R.* 143:543, 1984.

17. Burgener, F. A., and Gutierrez, O. H. Intravenous versus superior mesenteric artery vasopressin infusion for the treatment of variceal bleeding. *Radiology* 142:769, 1982.

18. Casarella, W., et al. Rightsided colonic diverticula as a cause of acute rectal hemorrhage. *N. Engl. J. Med.* 286:450, 1972.

19. Cavaluzzi, J., Kaufman, S., and White, R., Jr. Vasopressin control of massive hemorrhage in chronic ulcerative colitis. *Am. J. Roentgenol.* 127:672, 1976.

20. Child, C. (ed.). *Portal Hypertension, As Seen by 17 Authorities* (Vol. 14 in *Major Problems in Clinical Surgery*). Philadelphia: Saunders, 1974.

21. Chojkier, M., et al. A controlled comparison of continuous intraarterial and intravenous infusions of vasopressin in hemorrhage from esophageal varices. *Gastroenterology* 77:540, 1979.

22. Chuang, V. P., et al. Superselective catheterization technique in hepatic angiography. *A.J.R.* 141:803, 1983.

23. Clouse, M., Gregg, J., and Sedgwick, C. Angiography versus pancreatography in diagnosis of carcinoma of the pancreas. *Radiology* 114:605, 1975.

24. Cornell, S. Severe stenosis of celiac axis: Analysis of patients with and without symptoms. *Radiology* 99:311, 1971.

25. Davis, L., et al. The use of prostaglandin E_1 to enhance the angiographic visualization of the splanchnic circulation. *Radiology* 114:281, 1975.

26. Dencker, H., et al. Superior mesenteric angiography and blood flow following intra-arterial injection of prostaglandin F_2 alpha. *Am. J. Roentgenol.* 125:111, 1975.

27. Deterling, R., Jr. Aneurysm of the visceral arteries. *J. Cardiovasc. Surg.* 12:309, 1974.

28. Deutsch, V., Adar, R., and Moses, M. Angiography in the diagnosis of subphrenic abscess. *Clin. Radiol.* 25:133, 1974.

29. Diamond, A., et al. Arteriography of unusual mass lesions of the mesentery. *Radiology* 110:547, 1974.

30. Doehner, G., et al. The portal venous system: Its roentgen anatomy. *Radiology* 64:675, 1955.

31. Dotter, C., Goldman, M., and Rösch, J. Instant selective arterial occlusion with isobutyl 2-cyanoacrylate. *Radiology* 114:227, 1975.

32. Eisenberg, H. Angiography of the Pancreas. In S. K. Hilal (ed.), *Small Vessel Angiography: Imaging, Morphology, Physiology, and Clinical Applications.* St. Louis: Mosby, 1972.

33. Eisenberg, H., and Steer, M. The nonoperative treatment of massive pyloroduodenal hemorrhage by autogenous clot embolization. *Surgery* 79:414, 1976.

34. Eklund, L., Brahme, F., and Hildell, J. Angiography in Crohn's disease revisited. *Am. J. Roentgenol.* 126:941, 1976.

35. Eklund, L., Göthlin, J., and Pettersson, H. Angiography in expansile lesions of the spleen. *Am. J. Roentgenol.* 125:81, 1975.

36. Flannigan, B. D., et al. Intraarterial digital subtraction angiography: Comparison with conventional hepatic arteriography. *Radiology* 148:17, 1983.

37. Foley, W. D., et al. Digital subtraction angiography of the portal venous system. *A.J.R.* 140:497, 1983.

38. Freeny, P. C., Marks, W. M., and Ball, T. J.

Impact of high resolution computed tomography of the pancreas on utilization of endoscopic retrograde cholangiopancreatography and angiography. *Radiology* 142:35, 1982.

39. Frick, M. P., et al. Accuracy of endoscopic retrograde cholangiopancreatography (ERCP) in differentiating benign and malignant pancreatic disease. *Radiology* 146:865, 1983.

40. Fujii, K., et al. Arteriography in insulinoma. *Am. J. Roentgenol.* 120:634, 1974.

41. Fulton, R., et al. Preoperative angiographic localization of insulin-producing tumors of the pancreas. *Am. J. Roentgenol.* 123:367, 1975.

42. Galloway, S., et al. Minimal deviation hepatoma: A new entity. *Am. J. Roentgenol.* 125:184, 1975.

43. Galloway, S., Casarella, W., and Shimkin, P. Vascular malformations of the right colon as cause of bleeding in patients with aortic stenosis. *Radiology* 113:11, 1974.

44. Gammill, S., et al. A comparison of scans and angiograms in selecting patients with hepatomas for hepatic lobectomy. *Am. J. Roentgenol.* 123:522, 1975.

45. Gold, R., et al. Transarterial electrocoagulation therapy of a pseudoaneurysm in the head of the pancreas. *Am. J. Roentgenol.* 125:422, 1975.

46. Goldstein, H., and Miller, M. Angiographic evaluation of carcinoid tumors of the small intestine: The value of epinephrine. *Radiology* 115:23, 1975.

47. Goldstein, H., Neiman, H., and Bookstein, J. Angiographic evaluation of pancreatic disease: A further reappraisal. *Radiology* 112:275, 1974.

48. Goldstein, H., et al. Angiographic findings in benign liver cell tumors. *Radiology* 110:339, 1974.

49. Gothlin, J., Dencker, H., and Tranberg, K. Technique and complications of transumbilical catheterization of the portal vein and its tributaries. *Am. J. Roentgenol.* 125:431, 1975.

50. Haaga, J., et al. Computed tomography of the pancreas. *Radiology* 120:589, 1976.

51. Hessel, S. J., et al. Prospective evaluation of computed tomography and ultrasound of the pancreas. *Radiology* 143:129, 1982.

52. Ingemansson, S., Lunderquist, A., and Holst, J. Selective catheterization of the pancreatic vein for radioimmunoassay in glucagon secreting carcinoma of the pancreas. *Radiology* 119:555, 1976.

53. Itai, Y., et al. Computed tomography of cavernous hemangioma of the liver. *Radiology* 137:149, 1980.

54. Jafri, S. H., et al. Comparison of CT and angiography in assessing resectability of pancreatic carcinoma. *A.J.R.* 142:525, 1984.

55. Jewell, K. Primary carcinoma of the liver: Clinical and radiologic manifestations. *Am. J. Roentgenol.* 113:84, 1971.

56. Johnson, C. M., et al. Computed tomography and angiography of cavernous hemangiomas of the liver. *Radiology* 138:115, 1981.

57. Kadell, B., and Riley, J. Major arterial involvement by pancreatic pseudocysts. *Am. J. Roentgenol.* 99:632, 1967.

58. Kamin, P. D., et al. Comparison of ultrasound and computed tomography in the detection of pancreatic malignancy. *Radiology* 139:778, 1981.

59. Kessler, R., and Zimmon, D. Umbilical vein angiography. *Radiology* 87:841, 1966.

60. Kinkhabwala, M., and Balthazer, E. J. Carcinoid tumor of the aliment tract. II. Angiographic diagnosis of small intestinal and colonic lesions. *Gastrointest. Radiol.* 3:57, 1978.

61. Koehler, P., Nelson, J., and Berenson, M. Massive extraenteric gastrointestinal bleeding; angiographic diagnosis. *Radiology* 119:41, 1976.

62. Korobkin, M. T., et al. Pitfalls in arteriography of islet cell tumors of the pancreas. *Radiology* 100:319, 1971.

63. Kupic, E. A., et al. Splenic arterial patterns; angiographic analysis and review. *Invest. Radiol.* 2:70, 1967.

64. Lepasoon, J., and Olin, T. Angiographic diagnosis of splenic lesions following blunt abdominal trauma. *Acta Radiol.* [*Diagn.*] 11:257, 1971.

65. Levin, D. C., Wilson, R. E., and Abrams, H. L. Changing role of pancreatic arteriography in the era of computed tomography. *Radiology* 136:245, 1980.

66. Lunderquist, A., et al. Angiography in carcinoma of the pancreas. *Acta Radiol.* [*Suppl.*] 235, 1965.

67. Lunderquist, A., et al. Gelfoam powder embolization of the hepatic artery in liver metastases of carcinoid tumors. *Radiology* 22:65, 1982.

68. Malt, R. Control of massive upper gastrointestinal hemorrhage. *N. Engl. J. Med.* 286:1043, 1972.

69. Michels, N. A. *Blood Supply Anatomy of the Upper Abdominal Organs.* Philadelphia: Lippincott, 1955.

70. Miskowiak, J., Nielsen, S. L., and Munck, O. Scintigraphic diagnosis of gastrointestinal bleeding with TC 99M-labeled blood-pool agents. *Radiology* 141:499, 1981.

71. Moss, A. A., et al. Combined use of computed tomography and endoscopic retrograde cholangiopancreatography in assessment of suspected pancreatic neoplasm: Blind clinical evaluation. *Radiology* 134:159, 1980.

72. Nakakuma, K., et al. Hepatocellular carcinoma and metastatic cancer detected by iodized oil. *Radiology* 154:15, 1985.

73. Nebesar, R., et al. *Celiac and Superior Mesenteric Arteries.* Boston: Little, Brown, 1969.

74. Neiman, H., et al. Angiographic features of peripancreatic malignant lymphoma. *Radiology* 115:589, 1975.

75. Novak, D., Butzow, H., and Becker, K. Hepatic occlusion venography with a balloon catheter in patients with end to side portacaval shunts. *Am. J. Roentgenol.* 127:949, 1976.

76. Novy, S., et al. Pyogenic liver abscess: Angiographic diagnosis and treatment by closed aspiration. *Am. J. Roentgenol.* 121:388, 1974.

77. Novy, S., et al. Angiographic evaluation of primary malignant hepatocellular tumors in children. *Am. J. Roentgenol.* 120:353, 1974.

78. Onodera, H., et al. Correlation of the real-time ultrasonographic appearance of hepatic hemangiomas with angiography. *Radiology*, 152:564, 1984.

79. Orlof, M. J. A symposium on progress in the treatment of portal hypertension. *Arch. Surg.* 108:269, 1974.

80. Pliskin, M. Peliosis hepatis. *Radiology* 114:29, 1975.

81. Pueyo, I. L., et al. Carcinoid syndrome treated by hepatic embolization. *A.J.R.* 131:511, 1978.

82. Rabinowitz, J., Kinkabwala, M., and Ulreich, S. Macroregenerating nodule in the cirrhotic liver: Radiologic features and differential diagnosis. *Am. J. Roentgenol.* 121:401, 1974.

83. Ramer, M., et al. Angiography in leiomyomatous neoplasms of the small bowel. *Am. J. Roentgenol.* 113:263, 1971.

84. Redman, H. Mesenteric arterial and venous blood flow changes following selective arterial injection of vasodilators. *Invest. Radiol.* 9:193, 1974.

85. Reuter, S. Accentuation of celiac compression by the median acute ligament of the diaphragm during deep expiration. *Radiology* 98:561, 1971.

86. Reuter, S., Chuang, V., and Bree, R. Selective arterial embolization for control of massive upper gastrointestinal bleeding. *Am. J. Roentgenol.* 125:119, 1975.

87. Reuter, S. R., and Redman, H. C. *Gastrointestinal Angiography* (Vol. 1 in *Monographs in Clinical Radiology*). Philadelphia: Saunders, 1972.

88. Reuter, S., et al. Differential problems in the angiographic diagnosis of carcinoma of the pancreas. *Radiology* 96:93, 1970.

89. Roe, M., and Greenough, W. Marked hypervascularity and arteriovenous shunting in acute pancreatitis. *Radiology* 113:47, 1974.

90. Rösch, J. Superselective arteriography in the diagnosis of abdominal pathology: Technical considerations. *Radiology* 92:1008, 1969.

91. Rösch, J., and Dotter, C. Retrograde pancreatic venography: An experimental study. *Radiology* 114:275, 1975.

92. Rösch, J., and Steckel, R. Selective Angiography of the Abdominal Viscera. In W. N. Hanafee (section ed.), *Selective Angiography* (Section 18 in *Golden's Diagnostic Radiology*). Baltimore: Williams & Wilkins, 1972.

93. Rösch, J., et al. Selective arterial infusions of vasoconstrictors in acute gastrointestinal bleeding. *Radiology* 99:27, 1971.

94. Rösch, J., et al. Selective arterial embolization: A new method for control of acute gastrointestinal bleeding. *Radiology* 102:303, 1972.

95. Ruzicka, F., and Rossi, P. Arterial portography: Patterns of venous flow. *Radiology* 92:777, 1969.

96. Ruzicka, F., and Rossi, P. Normal vascular anatomy of the abdominal viscera. *Radiol. Clin. North Am.* 8:3, 1970.

97. Scatliff, J., et al. The "starry night" malpighian body marginal sinus circulation in spleen trauma. *Am. J. Roentgenol.* 125:91, 1975.

98. Sheedy, P., Fulton, R., and Atwel, D. Angiographic evaluation of patients with chronic gastrointestinal bleeding. *Am. J. Roentgenol.* 123:338, 1975.

99. Siegelman, S., Sprayregen, S., and Boley, S. Angiographic diagnosis of mesenteric arterial vasoconstriction. *Radiology* 112:533, 1974.

100. Smith, R. K., Arterburn, J. G. Advantages of delayed imaging and radiographic correlation in scintigraphic localization of gastrointestinal bleeding. *Radiology* 139:471, 1981.

101. Sundgren, R. Selective angiography of the left gastric artery. *Acta Radiol.* [*Suppl.*] 299, 1970.

102. Taboury, J., et al. Cavernous hemangioma of the liver studied by ultrasound: Enhancement posterior to a hyperechoic mass as a sign of hypervascularity. *Radiology* 149:781, 1983.

103. Tadavarthy, S., et al. Therapeutic transcatheter arterial embolization. *Radiology* 112:13, 1974.

104. Valla, D., et al. Vasopressin perfusion of esophageal varices in cirrhotic patients: Cineangiographic study. *Radiology* 152:45, 1984.

105. Viamonte, M., Jr., et al. Selective catheterization of the portal vein and its tributaries. *Radiology* 114:457, 1975.

106. Viamonte, M., Jr., Warren, W., and Fomon, J. Liver panangiography in the assessment of portal hypertension in liver cirrhosis. *Radiol. Clin. North Am.* 8:147, 1970.

107. Walter, J., Bookstein, J., and Bufford, E. Newer angiographic observations in cholangiocarcinoma. *Radiology* 118:19, 1976.

108. Waltman, A., et al. Technique for left gastric artery catheterization. *Radiology* 109:732, 1973.

109. Whelan, J., Creech, J. L., and Tamburro, C. Angiographic and radionuclide characteristics of hepatic angiosarcoma found in vinyl chloride workers. *Radiology* 118:549, 1976.

110. White, A., Baum, S., and Buranasiri, S. Aneurysms secondary to pancreatitis. *Am. J. Roentgenol.* 127:393, 1976.

111. White, R., Jr., et al. Pharmacologic control of hemorrhagic gastritis: Clinical and experimental results. *Radiology* 111:549, 1974.

112. White, R., et al. Therapeutic embolization with long term occluding agents and their effects on embolized tissue. *J.A.M.A.* 237:204, 1977.

113. Widrich, W., Nordahl, D., and Robbins, A. Contrast enhancement of the mesenteric and portal veins using intra-arterial papaverine. *Am. J. Roentgenol.* 121:374, 1974.

114. Winzelberg, G. G., et al. Radionuclide localization of lower gastrointestinal hemorrhage. *Radiology* 139:465, 1981.

115. Yumoto, Y., et al. Hepatocellular carcinoma detected by iodinated oil. *Radiology* 154:19, 1985.

Aortic Arch and Brachiocephalic Angiography

Indications

1. Diagnosis of lesions of the neck, face, and scalp.
   a. Anomalies of the origin and position of the vessels.
   b. Occlusive disease: Symptomatic or asymptomatic patient with a bruit. May present clinically as transient ischemic attacks, amaurosis fugax, vertebral insufficiency, or completed stroke.
      (1) Atherosclerosis.
      (2) Thrombosis.
      (3) Emboli.
      (4) Aortic dissection.
      (5) Cephalic arterial dissection.
      (6) Fibromuscular dysplasia.
      (7) Neurovascular compression syndromes.
      (8) Arteritis (e.g., Takayasu's, giant cell, moyamoya, temporal arteritis).
      (9) Postirradiation.
   c. Aneurysms.
   d. Arteriovenous malformations and arteriovenous fistulas.
   e. Trauma.
      (1) Arteriovenous fistulas.
      (2) False aneurysms.
      (3) Vessel occlusions, lacerations, avulsions.
   f. Tumors.
      (1) Hemangiomas.
      (2) Nasopharyngeal angiofibromas.
      (3) Nonchromaffin paragangliomas (e.g., carotid body tumors, glomus vagale).
      (4) Parathyroid adenomas.
      (5) Thyroid tumors.
      (6) Secondary vascular compromise by hypopharyngeal and laryngeal tumors.
2. Diagnosis of intracranial lesions.
   a. Primary vascular lesions.
      (1) Occlusions.
      (2) Aneurysms.
      (3) Arteriovenous malformations.
   b. Trauma.
      (1) Subdural and epidural hematomas (usually by computed tomography).
      (2) Arteriovenous fistulas.
      (3) Arterial or venous occlusions.
   c. Space-occupying processes (usually by computed tomography).
      (1) Benign and malignant tumors.
      (2) Abscesses.
      (3) Hematomas.
3. Postoperative evaluation (e.g., endarterectomy, extracranial to intracranial bypasses, aneurysmectomy).
4. Interventional angiography: embolization for epistaxis, false aneurysms, traumatized vessels, arteriovenous malformations and fistulas, vascular and nonresectable tumors.
5. Percutaneous transluminal angioplasty.

Digital Subtraction Versus Conventional Angiography

Many angiographic procedures previously studied by conventional techniques are now performed by either intravenous or intraarterial digital subtraction angiography.

Intravenous digital subtraction angiography (IV-DSA) (Fig. 14-1) is reserved for the patient who is well hydrated, is cooperative, has reasonably good cardiac output and renal function, and has no contraindications for the relatively large dose of contrast agent generally required for a diagnostic study. Misregistration artifacts (due to involuntary swallowing and pulsating calcified plaques), poor opacification due to low cardiac output, arterial superimposition, and some degradation of spatial resolution are some of its limitations. Large intravenous doses of medium-density contrast agent can cause angina, congestive heart failure or orthostatic hypotension, exacerbation of renal failure, and occasional transient ischemic attacks in susceptible patients. There is a higher risk

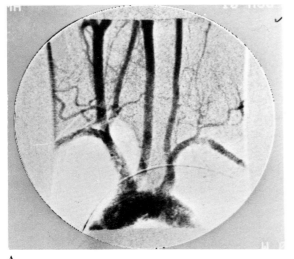

A

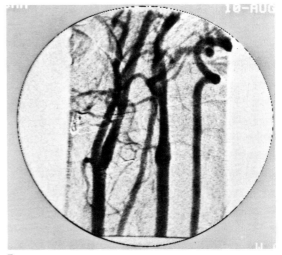

B

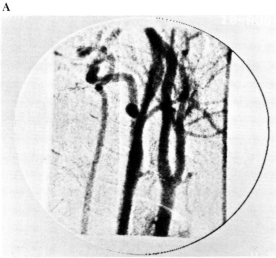

C

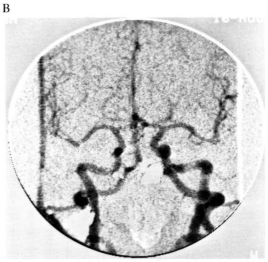

D

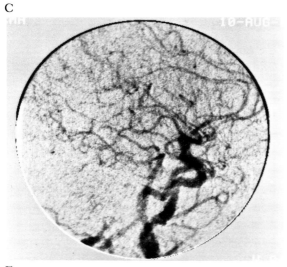

E

Fig. 14-1. IV-DSA study of brachiocephalic vessels.
A. Aortic arch in right posterior oblique (RPO) projection.
B and C. Carotid bifurcations (6-in. mode) in RPO
   and LPO projections. The margin of the cone on
   the right side of the patient extends just beyond the
   larynx; that on the left, just lateral to the intervertebral foramen. The superior margin extends up to
   reach the siphon.
D. Intracranial anteroposterior (AP) Towne projection.
E. Intracranial off-lateral view.

of allergic reactions and a greater tendency to emesis with large intravenous dosages of contrast agent. The relative lack of invasion due to the catheter being placed in the venous system rather than in the arteries allows performance of the procedure on an outpatient basis with no risk of embolization to the intracranial system. Patient selection must be controlled, keeping these limitations and advantages in mind.

IV-DSA is helpful in the following circumstances [43, 45, 61]: patients with an asymptomatic carotid bruit (particularly if scheduled for major surgery of other organ systems); patients with nonspecific neurologic symptoms possibly related to cerebrovascular insufficiency; ectatic subclavian extracranial carotid arteries presenting as pulsatile masses; postoperative conditions following procedures such as endarterectomies, aneurysm repairs, bypass grafts, or extracranial to intracranial anastomosis; status of major intracranial dural sinuses and jugular veins; differentiation of pituitary tumor from a parasellar aneurysm; follow-up of patients with aneurysms or arteriovenous malformations (AVMs) who are not surgical candidates.

Intraarterial digital subtraction angiography (IA-DSA) is more invasive than IV-DSA, for it requires intraarterial catheter placement (Fig. 14-2). Because smaller doses of contrast medium are required, smaller diameter catheters may be used. Patients may be studied on an outpatient basis, but longer periods of observation are required before discharge than for IV-DSA studies [59]. The smaller dose of contrast agent (one-third or less of the dose for conventional angiography) also provides greater safety when studying children, high-risk patients, and patients who may require evaluation of multiple systems. IA-DSA affords less spatial resolution than does conventional filming, but despite this, it provides very adequate studies in most circumstances. Contrast enhancement improves visualization of capillary blushes, making diagnosis of some neoplastic and inflammatory conditions more certain, particularly those otherwise obscured by overlying bone. The "real time" display capabilities and "road mapping" provided during catheterization are particularly valuable during interventional procedures of the head and neck, where significant alterations in flow patterns during embolization of vessels must be closely monitored.

With state-of-the-art digital equipment, most

extracranial and intracranial lesions may be studied by IA-DSA techniques [48, 56, 63]. In our laboratory, we view IA-DSA as only one of a number of angiographic recording capabilities required to sustain a sophisticated angiographic facility. Our studies use a combination of the available modalities. In a routine study for transient ischemic attacks, IA-DSA examinations of the arch and brachiocephalic origins in RPO and LPO projections are followed by selective simultaneous biplane bilateral carotid conventional film studies. The conventional studies provide optimal evaluation of the extracranial and intracranial vessels with little added contrast agent and little added risk. 105-mm spot films of the common carotid bifurcations, when considered necessary, give another dimension with little added time involved. IA-DSA of the posterior fossa with subclavian artery injections completes the study. In elderly patients or those at risk, the carotid bifurcations and intracranial vessel are also evaluated with DSA by injecting into the aortic arch or near the origin of the vessel.

Simultaneous conventional biplane filming provides the best spatial resolution of most intracranial lesions (aneurysms, AVMs, tumors, arteritis, small emboli, etc.). It is also used in those who cannot cooperate and in trauma patients. This may be supplemented with IA-DSA for evaluating capillary blushes, arteriovenous shunting, or vessels that are difficult to catheterize selectively. All patients undergoing interventional studies are monitored with IA-DSA. The initial evaluation, however, is performed with conventional magnification studies in order to provide optimal detail.

Technique

APPROACHES

1. Catheter approach
   a. Percutaneous femoral artery approach is particularly useful when multiple brachiocephalic vessels require study (e.g., intracranial aneurysms, AVMs with multiple feeders, brachiocephalic occlusive disease, superselective study of internal and external carotid artery, and subclavian branch arteriography).
   b. Percutaneous axillary artery approach is used when catheter techniques are preferred

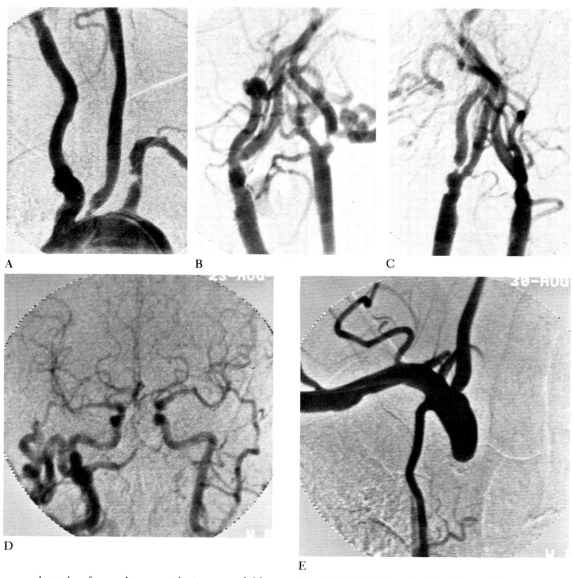

Fig. 14-2. IA-DSA study of brachiocephalic vessels.

A. Aortic arch in RPO. Occlusion of right subclavian artery at its origin. Severe stenosis of left common carotid artery at origin. Severe stenosis of left subclavian artery with no antegrade filling of either vertebral artery (see Fig. 14-47).

B and C. Bilateral RPO and LPO projections centered over carotid bifurcations. Severe bilateral carotid bifurcation disease.

D. Intracranial circulation in AP projection. Occipital branches bilaterally form collaterals with the vertebral arteries and other branches of the subclavian arteries.

E. Arteriogram of occluded right subclavian artery.

but the femoral approach is unavailable. The right axillary artery approach permits four-vessel selective studies (right vertebral artery, both carotid arteries, left subclavian artery, and catheterization of the right thyrocervical and internal mammary arteries). The left axillary approach is less satisfactory and should be used only if the right axillary artery is unavailable or if selective study of the left vertebral or left subclavian branches is necessary.

c. Carotid artery approach. Small-caliber thin-walled catheters are threaded over guidewires directly inserted into the carotid artery following low carotid artery puncture. However, the increased possibility of damage to a vital artery precludes the general acceptance of this technique by angiographers.

d. Translumbar approach is rarely necessary but is used when both axillary and femoral arteries are unavailable and IV-DSA techniques are inadequate. A traditional T12 translumbar approach (see Chap. 3) is obtained with an 18-gauge 8-in. needle covered with a 5 French thin-walled Teflon sheath. No. 5 French catheters of various configurations can be advanced through this sheath for selective studies of the brachiocephalic vessels. Alternatively, midstream aortic arch injections can be performed (using IA-DSA) through an extralong translumbar needle with its Teflon sleeve long enough to reach the aortic arch.

2. Direct vessel puncture (see Chap. 3)

Direct carotid puncture is now rarely used and should be reserved for patients where the femoral approach is difficult or impossible. It is particularly contraindicated in the following conditions: atherosclerotic plaques or tumor invasion, blood dyscrasias, hypertension, or the uncooperative patient.

a. Direct carotid artery puncture may be used in angiography of an ipsilateral intracranial space-occupying lesion. The angiographer can perform external compression of the opposite carotid artery to stimulate arterial crossover to the opposite cerebral hemisphere.

b. Puncture of the brachial artery is used particularly for retrograde flush angiography of posterior fossa lesions. The right carotid and vertebral arteries fill with a right-sided injection; the left vertebral artery fills with a left brachial artery injection.

3. Arteriotomy

Arteriotomy of the temporal artery may be performed for biopsy and angiography.

4. Cross-compression angiography

The angiographer may perform temporary manual occlusion of the carotid or subclavian artery opposite the one being injected. This maneuver often fills vessels across the circle of Willis.

5. Intravenous digital subtraction angiography

A catheter is placed in the superior vena cava

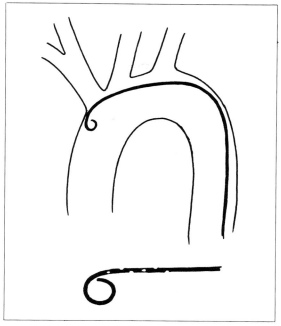

Fig. 14-3. The optimal catheter for aortic arch injection: a thin-walled "pigtail" Teflon 5 or 6 French catheter with multiple side holes.

or right atrium, preferably through an antecubital vein, but alternatively through the femoral vein.

CATHETERS

Midstream Thoracic Aortic Arch Studies
For midstream aortic arch studies, a catheter with a fairly large internal diameter is required for rapid delivery of a large dose of contrast medium. For the femoral approach, a 90- or 100-cm 5, 6, or 7 French thin-walled "pigtail" catheter with multiple side holes may be used (Fig. 14-3). Some 90-cm 5 French thin-walled catheters deliver up to 25 ml/sec of medium-density contrast agent. For the axillary approach, a 60-cm 5 French thin-walled pigtail catheter with multiple side holes is preferred. A similar catheter may be used for IV-DSA.

Selective Studies
Selective and superselective studies require a catheter with a small outside diameter so as not to obstruct critical vessels. Preformed curves are available for different needs. They vary to accommodate tortuous or anomalous vessel takeoffs and superselective vessel placement. Larger diameter

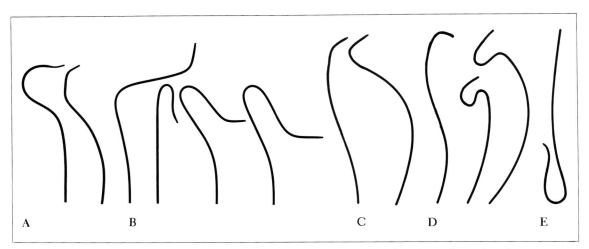

Fig. 14-4. Multiple catheter shapes for selective brachiocephalic angiography.

A. Hincks No. 3 and No. 1 shapes.
B. Simmons No. 4, 1, 2, and 3 catheter shapes. Catheters in A and B are in 4.5, 5, 6.5, and 7 French diameters and are torque-controlled.
C. Bentson-Hanaffee-Wilson catheter shapes.
D. Newton catheter shapes in non-torque-controlled 5 French diameter.
E. "Shepherd's crook" shape for the axillary approach (torque control).

(6.5 or 7 French) selective catheters may have to be used if they follow aortic arch midstream studies with large-bore catheters; also, these are easier to maneuver if tortuous arteries are present. Alternatively, the larger catheter used for midstream injection may be replaced with a smaller 5 French catheter inserted through a 7 French sheath in the groin. Coaxial 2, 2.5, 3, or 4 French catheters can be introduced through a 5, 6, or 6.5 French thin-walled tapered catheter or a 7 or 8 French non-tapered catheter for purposes of therapeutic embolization.

There is a large variety of catheter shapes. The angiographer should choose his catheters with care to obviate frequent catheter changes. However, if his initial choice meets with failure, he should not hesitate to exchange it for another. The catheters described in this section allow selective catheterization under almost all circumstances (Fig. 14-4).

FEMORAL APPROACH. With the femoral approach, the following catheters may be used:

1. Hincks 5, 6, or 6.5 French catheter. Even the smaller diameter catheters now have torque control capabilities. A No. 1 curve is used for normal carotid and subclavian artery (Figs. 14-4A, 14-5); a No. 3 curve is used for increasingly tortuous vessel takeoffs (Figs. 14-4A, 14-6).
2. Simmons 5, 6, or 6.5 French catheter is used for tortuous arteries or for carotid or subclavian arteries with unusual origins (Figs. 14-4B, 14-7, 14-8):

   a. No. 1 for a narrow aorta.
   b. No. 2 for a moderately narrow aorta.
   c. No. 3 for a wide aorta.
   d. No. 4 for an elongated aorta.

These catheters are sometimes too rigid to be advanced into superselective positions high in the carotid or subclavian arteries. Injections are then made just beyond the origins of these vessels. Often, however, they can be advanced over relatively rigid J-shaped guidewires (0.038-in., 3-mm J for 6.5 French and 0.035 3-mm J for 5 French) to higher levels in the carotid artery.

3. Bentson-Hannafee-Wilson 5 French polyethylene catheters are used for selective and superselective studies. The catheter tip is inserted into the orifice of the brachiocephalic artery, and a 0.035-in. (0.89-mm) guidewire with a tapered core is introduced and advanced to the desired level. The small diameter and flexibility of the catheter allows it to follow the guidewire easily. A No. 1 catheter shape is used for patients with normal branch origins; a No. 2 shape is used for a branch artery with

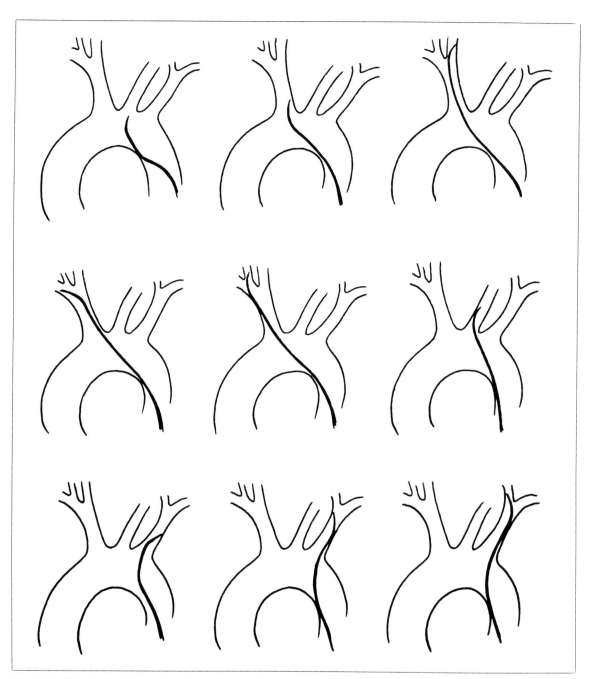

Fig. 14-5. Hincks "head hunter" catheter No. 1. This single catheter shape can catheterize all four vessels to the head and neck in patients with normal carotid and subclavian artery origins. It can be advanced deeper into the vessel with a joint forward and rotary twisting action at the catheter hub, or alternatively, over a leading tapered-core guidewire with a straight or curved tip (0.035-in. for 5 French, 0.038-in. for 6.5 French).

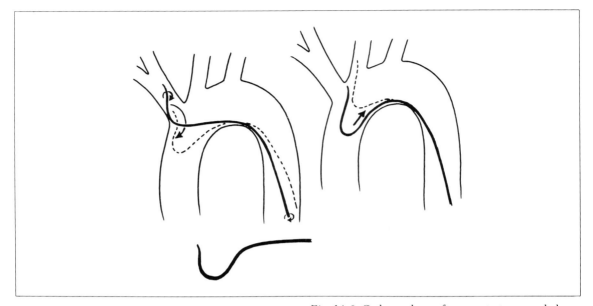

Fig. 14-6. Catheter shapes for more tortuous and elongated vessels. Hincks No. 3 catheter. To position the catheter in the left carotid position after innominate placement, advance the "knee" of the curve into the ascending aorta and slightly rotate the catheter tip counterclockwise so that it faces more anteriorly, then slowly withdraw the catheter to engage it in the left carotid orifice.

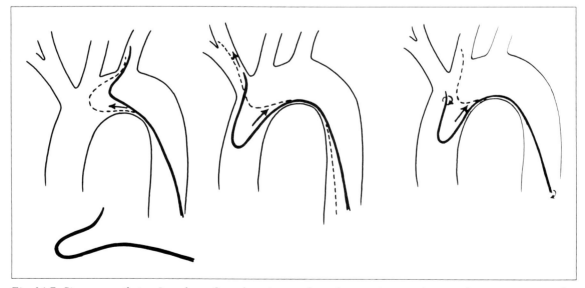

Fig. 14-7. Simmons catheter. In order to form the primary curve of the catheter, place the catheter tip in the left subclavian artery and advance the catheter. The bend of the secondary curve is then the leading point of the catheter as it enters the ascending aorta. Engage the catheter tip in the innominate artery and withdraw the catheter, thus forcing the tip higher into the common carotid or subclavian artery.

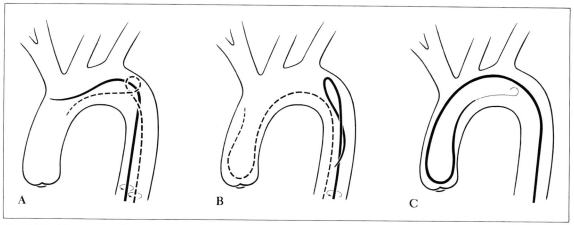

Fig. 14-8. Alternate methods of forming Simmons curve.

A and B. Place the knee of the catheter high in the aortic arch, rotate clockwise rapidly to scissor at the knee. Combine rotation with short forward thrusts. Advance the scissored catheter over the arch and rotate to open the scissored configuration. This process can be aided by a stiff guidewire tip placed just proximal to the knee.

C. Advance a flexible-tip guidewire (gentle distal curve) over the aortic valve and back up the ascending aorta to the aortic arch. Follow the guidewire with the catheter. Alternatively, form the catheter curve over the aortic bifurcation in the pelvis (see Fig. 9-1D).

through a thin-walled 5, 6, or 7 French catheter over a 0.018-in. guidewire to superselective catheter positions. A nontapered tip on an outer 7 French catheter allows a 4 French inner coaxial catheter diameter.

7. Balloon catheters. Special balloon occlusive catheters (Berenstein) have an inner lumen accommodating a 0.038-in. guidewire. The balloon provides control over the flow of contrast and emboli, and prevents reflux of emboli to nontarget areas (see Chap. 5). This system also allows a coaxial 3 French catheter to be placed superselectively for embolization purposes.

AXILLARY APPROACH. With the axillary approach, a 5, 6, 6.5, or 7 French catheter should be used. A 60-cm catheter with a "shepherd's crook" curve (Fig. 14-10) is preferred. It is important to keep the catheter diameter as small as possible to prevent complications in the small-caliber axillary artery.

CAROTID APPROACH. A 4 or 5 French polyethylene or thin-walled Teflon sheath with a preformed obtuse distal curve is used to cover the percutaneous catheter needle (inside diameter 0.037 in.). The metal needle is removed once the artery has been entered, leaving the sheath in place. The sheath can then be advanced to the desired level over a guidewire. A low carotid puncture site is required.

CONTRAST AGENTS, PROJECTIONS, AND RADIOGRAPHIC PROGRAMMING

Technical specifications for conventional arteriography in aortic arch and brachiocephalic angiog-

tortuous origin (Fig. 14-4C; see Fig. 14-9). Be careful not to dislodge atherosclerotic plaques with this maneuver.

4. Newton 5 French polyethylene catheters have multiple configurations (Fig. 14-4D). The first shape is used for children and young adults, the remainder for older patients with tortuous vessels and acutely angled takeoffs.

5. Berenstein 7 French polyurethane torque-controlled catheter with a 5 French distal 10 cm. The tip has a short "hockey stick" shape. The exquisite control provided by the 7 French shaft combined with the 5 French tapered tip allows the superselective catheterization of external carotid branches required for embolization procedures.

6. A coaxial catheter system is often needed for superselective external carotid branch angiography and embolization. A 3 or 2.5 French thin-walled Teflon catheter can be advanced

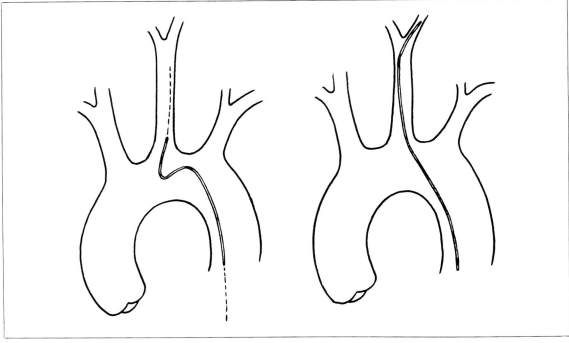

Fig. 14-9. Placement of a small diameter catheter in the brachiocephalic vessels. The tip of the catheter is engaged in the origin of the target vessel, and a guidewire with a tapered core is advanced well into the carotid artery. The guidewire acts as a leader over which the catheter may then be advanced.

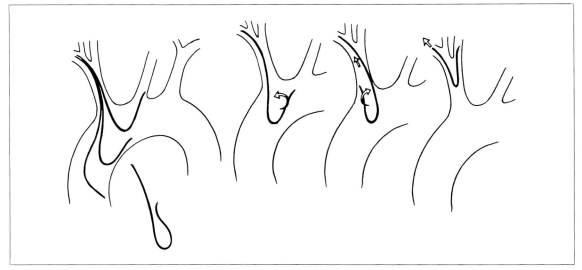

Fig. 14-10. The axillary approach, using a catheter with a "shepherd's crook" curve. The catheter straightens in the ascending aorta. Manipulate the original curve into the catheter tip and withdraw the catheter into the left carotid artery. The origin of this vessel is often close to the innominate artery, lying on the same plane or slightly anterior to it. To enter the right vertebral artery, advance the catheter into the innominate artery while maintaining the curve, rotate laterally and bypass the carotid origin, and immediately rotate medially to enter the vertebral artery.

raphy are given in Table 14-1, and for IV-DSA and IA-DSA in Table 14-2.

PROJECTIONS

Aortic Arch Angiography for
Brachiocephalic Occlusive Disease
An aluminum wedge filter may be applied to equalize radiographic density in the neck with that in the thorax and base of the skull. The following projections are used:

1. Right posterior oblique (RPO), 45 to 60 degrees. The patient's head is turned as far as possible to the right (Fig. 14-11A). This projection optimally outlines the origins of the innominate artery, the left carotid artery, and the left subclavian artery, the bifurcation of both common carotid arteries, and the origin of both vertebral arteries. The exposure field includes an area from just below the origin of the innominate artery up to the carotid siphon. The origin of the right subclavian artery is hidden behind the right common carotid artery in this projection.
2. Left posterior oblique (LPO), 45 degrees. The patient's head is turned incompletely to the left. This projection outlines the origin of the right subclavian artery and allows another view of the carotid bifurcations and the vertebral artery origins.
3. Anteroposterior (AP). The filming is centered slightly higher on the patient in order to include the sylvian point of the middle cerebral arteries intracranially (Fig. 14-11B). If automatic tabletop movements are available, the tabletop may be shifted 3 seconds after the start of the injection to include all the intracranial structures.

IV-DSA
The same RPO projection is used to study the brachiocephalic vessels as they arise in the aortic arch as in conventional angiography. Here a large mode (9 to 14 in.) is used with a 512 × 512-pixel matrix (newer machines provide a 1024 × 1024-pixel matrix). Occasionally, the LPO injection is also required to better define the origin of the right subclavian artery.

Separate injections are necessary to focus on the common carotid bifurcations, which are angled more steeply in RPO and LPO projections. If an LU arm (see Chap. 1) is available, the x-ray tube may be angled 25 degrees to the head. Try to observe the carotid bifurcation of interest as it overlies the cervical spine (to obviate motion artifacts produced from swallowing over the air-filled larynx). A smaller, 6-in. mode improves resolution of the carotid bifurcations. Try to include the carotid siphons on these projections. Occasionally an AP projection better demonstrates the bifurcations in patients with tortuous vessels. Electrocardiogram gated studies may improve the quality of these examinations, but limits the exposure rate to 2 per second.

A limited evaluation of the intracranial structures is obtained using the same matrix and mode centered over the head and an additional injection in one of three projections: 30 degrees off lateral to outline the siphon; a Townes view to better define the posterior circulation; a Waters projection to define the middle cerebral arteries [43].

Intracranial Angiography
Special care should be taken in positioning the patient's head. True frontal projections permit accurate evaluation of shift of midline vascular structures. If multiple vessels are being studied, simultaneous biplane conventional angiography helps to limit the dose of contrast agent to the brain. In order to accommodate biplane angiography on the standard 14 × 14-in. film changers, when the head is centered to the AP changer, the object-film distance is exaggerated on the lateral changer. The resulting distortion can be minimized by using a maximal focal spot size of 0.6 mm, increasing the focal spot–film distance to 60 in., and coning precisely to the area of interest. Fogging due to scattered radiation is eliminated by loading the films in alternate spaces in the changer. Alternatively, using a 0.3-mm focal spot and 40-in. distance rare earth screen film combination and carbon fiber backing to the screens, 2× magnification can be obtained on the lateral projection.

In the frontal projection, the central beam should pass 12 to 15 degrees caudad to the orbitomeatal line for studies of the anterior circulation and 30 degrees for the posterior circulation (Fig. 14-12). The former beam angle superimposes the orbital roofs on the petrous ridges; it is achieved by a combination of slight angulation of the x-ray tube and flexion of the head. These measures throw the bifurcation of the internal carotid artery

Table 14-1. Technical Specifications in Conventional Aortic Arch and Brachiocephalic Angiography

Arteriographic Procedure	Contrast Agent			Total Films	Total Time (sec)	Radiographic Programming		Projection
	Density	Volume (ml/inj)	Rate (ml/sec)			Films/Sec	Timing	
Adults								
Aortic arch	M	50	25–30	10	6	1/sec for 1 sec; 3/sec for 2 sec; 1/sec for 3 sec	Start films at the start of injection	RPO, AP, LPO
Selective studies								
Common carotid artery	L[a]	10–12	8–10	12	12	2/sec for 3 sec; 1/sec for 3 sec; 1 every 2 sec for 6 sec[b]	Start films 0.2 sec after injection	Biplane AP and lateral with alternate filming
Internal carotid artery	L[a]	10	8	12	12		Start films 0.2 sec after start of injection	Biplane, Towne (AP), and lateral with alternate filming
External carotid artery	L[a,c]	6	4	12	12			
Vertebral artery	L[a]	8	6	12	12			
Retrograde brachial injection for intracranial angiography	L[a]	Right[a] 40 Left[a] 30	20 20	12	12		Start films 1.0 sec after start of injection	Biplane AP and lateral with alternate filming
Subclavian artery	L[a]	18[d]	8	9	6	2/sec for 3 sec; 1/sec for 3 sec		AP
Innominate artery	M	20	10[e]	9	6			AP
Children[f]								
Aortic arch								
Infant	L	1.5 ml/kg	Total within 1.0–1.5 sec	10	4	4/sec for 2 sec; 1/sec for 2 sec	Same as adult	Same as adult
Other	M							
Selective studies	L[a]	2–10 ml		12	12	Same as adult	Same as adult	Same as adult

[a]Conray-60. Nonionic contrast agents may also be used.
[b]For biplane studies with alternate filming, the film timing must be doubled to accommodate the alternately empty spaces (e.g., here 4/sec for 3 sec, 2/sec for 3 sec, and 1/sec for the remainder).
[c]Nonionic contrast agents recommended.
[d]Use less if there is occlusion distal to the vertebral artery in order to prevent overdose to the posterior fossa.
[e]Catheter with side holes may be required to prevent recoil.
[f]Amount of contrast agent required in children varies with body weight.

Table 14-2. Technical Specifications in Digital Subtraction Studies of Brachiocephalic Vessels

Angiographic Procedure	Contrast Agent Density	Vol (ml/inj)	Rate (ml/sec)	Total Time[a] (sec)	Frames/sec	Digital Programming Timing	Projection/Mode[b]
IV-DSA[c]							
Aortic arch	M	30–35	25–30	12–15	2–3/sec	Start frames 3–4 sec after start of injection[d]	RPO } Large mode LPO } (9–14 in.)
Carotid bifurcation	M	30–35	25–30	12–15	2–3/sec	Start frames 3–4 sec after start of injection[d]	RPO } Magnification mode LPO } to include siphon
Intracranial	M	40–45	25–30	12–15	2–3/sec	Start frames 4–5 sec after start of injection	20 degrees off lateral (carotid siphon); Caldwell (middle cerebral); Towne (vertebrobasilar). Use 6-in. mode
IA-DSA							
Aortic arch	½ M	30	20–30	4–6	3–4 sec		Same as IV-DSA
Selective carotids	½ L[e]	8–10	8 sec	6–8	3/sec	Start frames 2–3 sec before injection	
Posterior fossa selective vertebral artery	½ L[e]	6–8	Hand injection				Towne; lateral
Subclavian artery	½ L[e]	16	8 sec	8–10	2–3/sec		Lateral

[a]Terminate series as dictated by real-time evaluation.
[b]Size of mode dictated by diameter of image intensifier. Usually there are at least two different magnification modes.
[c]Contrast agent injected in right atrium.
[d]Timing varies with estimated cardiac output and circulation time.
[e]Half-strength low-density (30%) contrast agent.
IV-DSA = intravenous digital subtraction angiography; IA-DSA = intraarterial digital subtraction angiography; M = medium-density contrast agent; L = low-density contrast agent.

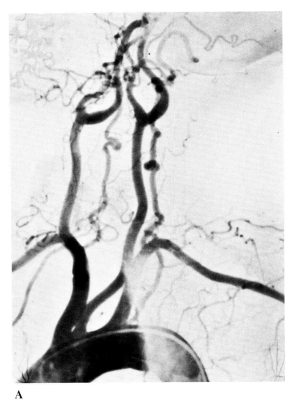

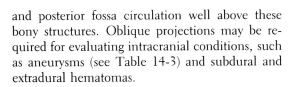

A

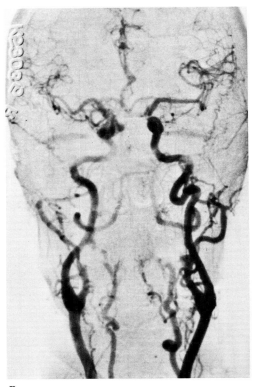

B

Fig. 14-11. Conventional brachiocephalic angiography with aortic arch injection using digital subtraction techniques with conventional filming.
A. RPO projection.
B. AP projection. Compare with IA-DSA study seen in Fig. 14-2.

and posterior fossa circulation well above these bony structures. Oblique projections may be required for evaluating intracranial conditions, such as aneurysms (see Table 14-3) and subdural and extradural hematomas.

FILMS

Subtraction techniques are often essential. The first film of any series should be made with no contrast medium in order to make a subtraction mask. The suggested film timing in conventional aortic arch studies allows (1) the initial film for a subtraction mask, (2) a full second for injection to allow contrast medium to enter the brachiocephalic vessels, (3) multiple films during the period of optimal opacification, and (4) sufficient delayed films to evaluate delayed flow phenomena such as seen in subclavian "steal."

Subtraction studies are often critical in evaluating intracranial conditions, such as capillary blushes and premature venous filling of tumors, venous angiomas, and venous occlusive disease. Here IA-DSA studies are easy to perform and may prove invaluable in making a correct diagnosis.

Anatomic Considerations

NORMAL ANATOMY

There are two important concepts when considering the anatomy of brachiocephalic vessels: functional anatomy and extracranial-intracranial communications. The concept of functional or territorial anatomy is particularly important in studying the brachiocephalic vessels, for there are a large number of potential feeding vessels, each arising from a different trunk; any of these may supply a given lesion. Each of these must be studied to give a complete angiographic picture of the pathologic process. Potentially hazardous communications of vessels outside with those within the brain may be uncovered. Some of these may not be angiographically visible except by selective or superselective contrast studies and high resolution magnification filming. It is important to know

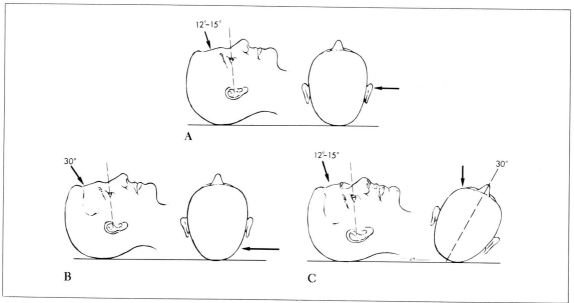

Fig. 14-12.
A. Standard projections for carotid arteriogram.
B. Standard projections for angiography of the posterior fossa.
C. Oblique projections, which are useful in evaluating intracranial aneurysms and subdural or epidural hematomas.

the regions in which these occur and the vessels that usually feed them. As with other parts of the body, instead of memorizing the traditional points of origin of many of these branches, it is more reasonable to study all possible feeding arteries to the territory [24]. Understanding these concepts is critical for the angiographer anticipating an endovascular therapeutic maneuver in order to avoid embolization to nontarget areas within the brain. Only the most basic anatomic considerations are presented here [23, 32].

THE AORTIC ARCH

There are three branches of the aortic arch. The first is the innominate artery, which usually arises to the right of the trachea but can arise more distally and to its left. The second branch is the left common carotid artery. The third branch is the left subclavian artery, which in the younger patient is in a straight line with the axis of the descending thoracic aorta. With increasing age of the patient, one finds tortuosity and elongation of the aortic arch, with subsequent changes in the angular relationships of the origin of these vessels with the

aorta, which sometimes makes selective catheterization of these branches more difficult.

THE CAROTID SYSTEM

The External Carotid System [13, 24, 25]
The external carotid artery arises anteromedially from the common carotid artery at about the level of the fourth cervical vertebra (Fig. 14-13). The superior thyroid artery comes off anteriorly at or just above the carotid bifurcation; it supplies thyroid tumors and occasionally parathyroid adenomas. Thereafter, the external carotid artery forms three major divisions: the facial-lingual, the pharyngo-occipital, and the internal maxillary. There are cross communications between the right and left sides as well as between each of these major divisions, communications with intracranial branches of the internal carotid artery, and communications with branches of the subclavian arteries (costocervical, thyrocervical, and muscular branches of the vertebral arteries).

The *facial-lingual* division of the external carotid artery generally feeds muscles and skin of the face. The lingual artery arises anteriorly, followed by the facial artery, but these two can arise as a common trunk. This trunk may have mandibular, masseteric, infraorbital, labial, nasal, and ophthalmic branches. However, these areas may instead be fed, either individually or in multiples,

Table 14-3. Angiographic Investigation of Cerebral Aneurysms

1. Study the side of greatest suspicion with biplane angiogram.
2. If this angiogram is positive, and patient's condition permits, do four-vessel angiogram to rule out additional aneurysms.
3. If this angiogram is negative, continue search until all vessels are outlined (including cross-compression AP study of the carotid artery). Also include both posterior inferior cerebellar arteries.
4. If the anterior communicating artery has an aneurysm, seen only by injecting one side, inject the normal side and use cross compression to determine presence of collateral flow for the surgeon.
5. If vascular displacement uncovers an associated hematoma, call surgeon immediately and defer further studies.
6. If aneurysm is found, do additional views to outline the aneurysm neck (using only 6 or 7 films for arterial phase) as follows:

Location	Additional Views	X-ray Tube to Orbitomeatal Line	Center X-ray Beam
1. Anterior communicating artery	Oblique 25 degrees away from injection side	Towne	3–4 cm above lateral aspect of ipsilateral superior orbital rim
2. Internal carotid bifurcation	Same as 1 or submentovertex view	Towne	Same as 1
3. Ophthalmic artery origin	Same as 2	Towne	Same as 1
4. Posterior communicating artery origin	Paraorbital oblique 55 degrees away from injection side	12 degrees cephalad	1 cm posterior to inferior portion of lateral rim of ipsilateral orbit
5. Internal carotid artery (cavernous portion)	Same as 4 or submentovertex view or Caldwell projection	Same as 4	Same as 4
6. Distal end basilar artery	Oblique 25 degrees away from or toward side of injection or submentovertex view	5 degrees cephalad 25 degrees Towne	Nasion Same as 1
7. Junction of vertebral artery and basilar artery	Oblique 15 degrees away from injection side or submentovertex view	Same as 6	Foramen magnum
8. Posterior inferior cerebellar artery	Paraorbital oblique 55 degrees away from side of injection	12 degrees cephalad	Foramen magnum
9. Anterior inferior cerebellar artery origin	AP or submentovertex view	15 degrees caudad	Nasion

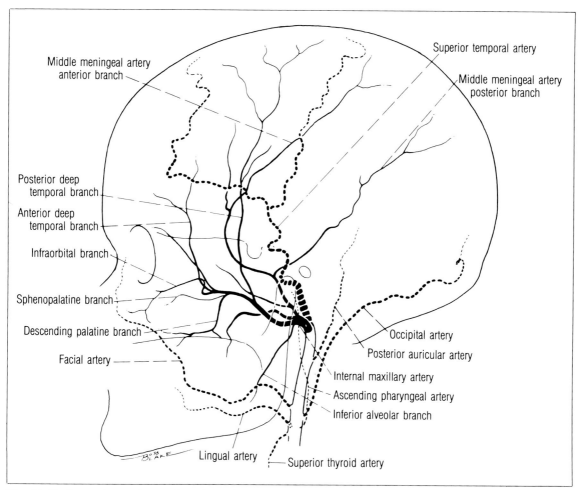

Fig. 14-13. External carotid artery branches. The internal maxillary artery and its many branches are outlined with a solid black line; all other branches are outlined with dotted lines.

from terminal branches of the internal maxillary division.

The *pharyngo-occipital* division gives rise to the occipital and ascending pharyngeal branches. The occipital artery is the first posterior branch passing posterosuperiorly, medial to the mastoid process, and supplies the stylomastoid area and the occipital and suboccipital musculocutaneous areas. Meningeal branches pass through the mastoid foramen and sometimes through other adjacent foramina. Branches of the occipital artery communicate with the thyrocervical and costocervical and vertebral muscular branches. The posterior auricular branch arises from the posterior surface

of the external carotid artery, just above the occipital artery, sometimes supplying branches to the meninges and a branch to the seventh nerve. The ascending pharyngeal artery ascends from the posterior medial surface of the external carotid artery, between the internal carotid artery and the lateral wall of the pharynx. It supplies the carotid body (and any associated tumors); its pharyngeal branch supplies angiofibromas; its tympanic branch, tumors of the tympanum or jugular fossa. The ascending pharyngeal artery also supplies meninges of the posterior fossa as well as portions of the ninth through twelfth cranial nerves. Intracranial communications with the internal carotid artery siphon can occur through meningohypophyseal trunks.

The *internal maxillary* division is the anterior terminal branch of the external carotid artery and

provides the major vascular supply to the deep facial structures, the orbit, and the infratemporal
fossa, and supplies peripheral segments of the trigeminal and oculomotor nerves. It provides many
anastomoses with, and sometimes can be the major vascular supply of, territories traditionally supplied by the lingual-facial or pharyngo-occipital
divisions. An important group of internal maxillary branches are an ascending group (middle and
accessory meningeal branches, and anterior tympanic artery) and a posterior group (pharyngeal
branch, and the artery to the foramen rotundum).
The middle meningeal artery ascends vertically
through the foramen spinosum, gives branches to
the fifth and seventh cranial nerves, and anastomoses with branches of the petrous and cavernous
portions of the internal carotid artery (be aware of
this when embolizing dural AVMs and vascular
tumors) before continuing on its course. A posterior branch of the meningeal artery courses along
the floor of the middle cranial fossa toward the
dura of the cerebellar convexity; an anterior
branch supplies the parietal and frontal dura. The
middle meningeal artery may arise from the
ophthalmic artery and rarely from the petrous portion of the internal carotid artery. Less commonly,
the ophthalmic artery arises from the middle meningeal artery, an important anatomic point in
embolization procedures if blindness is to be
avoided.

The accessory meningeal artery arises just distal
to the middle meningeal artery or occasionally
from the middle meningeal artery itself. It passes
through the foramen ovale to the dura of Meckel's
cave.

In the posterior group of the internal maxillary
artery, the pharyngeal branch supplies the upper
pharynx and tumors arising in the vicinity. The
artery of the foramen rotundum does two things. It
forms an anastomosis with branches of the internal
carotid artery. It also supplies the maxillary division of the fifth cranial nerve.

A final group of vessels arises from the pterygopalatine portion of the internal maxillary artery.
Its terminal branch, the infraorbital artery, courses
along the infraorbital groove to emerge on the face
through the inferior orbital foramen. The descending palatine artery arises in the pterygopalatine
fossa and courses anteriorly on the medial side of
the alveolar border of the hard palate. The sphenopalatine artery enters the nasal cavity through

the sphenopalatine foramen where it divides into
lateral and septal branches. There are other,
smaller pharyngeal and palatine branches.

The superficial temporal branches are the terminal branches of the external carotid artery, which
supplies the skin and scalp and provides anastomoses with other occluded vessels of the external and
internal carotid circulation.

The Internal Carotid System

ARTERIES. The internal carotid artery penetrates
the base of the skull as it leaves the bony carotid
canal; it then runs through the outer layer of the
dura mater to enter the cavernous sinus (Fig. 14-
14). Several small meningohypophyseal branches
arise from its intracavernous S-shaped segment
(the siphon). Usually these branches are not visible
(except on magnification films), but they can be
pathologically hypertrophied when they feed
tumors and AVMs in the base of the skull and
tentorium. The internal carotid artery leaves the
cavernous sinus as it passes under the anterior
clinoids to become an intradural structure. Immediately thereafter, the ophthalmic artery arises
anteriorly to supply the orbit and the meninges on
the floor of the anterior cranial fossa. Important
anastomoses occur between terminal branches of
this vessel and those of the internal maxillary artery. The posterior communicating artery passes
posteriorly to join the posterior cerebral artery, although sometimes the latter vessel arises directly
off the internal carotid artery. Just above this point,

Fig. 14-14. Intracranial vessels, showing the carotid
circulation (see text).
A. Lateral projection. 1 = internal carotid artery; 2 =
   posterior cerebral artery; 3 = anterior choroidal
   artery; 4 = ophthalmic artery; 5 = ethmoid
   branches of the ophthalmic artery. Anterior cerebral artery complex (*dotted lines*): 6 = anterior cerebral artery; 7 = frontopolar artery; 8 = pericallosal artery; 9 = callosomarginal artery. Middle
   cerebral artery branches (*solid line*): 10 = middle
   cerebral artery; 11 = orbitofrontal branches; 12 =
   frontal branches; 13 = parietal branches; 14 =
   posterior temporal branches; 15 = anterior temporal branches; ☆ = tuberculum sellae and midpoint
   of a line joining the internal occipital protuberance
   and the coronal suture.
B. AP projection. The sylvian point lies half-way between the inner surface of the skull and the roof of
   the orbit or the petrous pyramid, whichever lies
   lower.

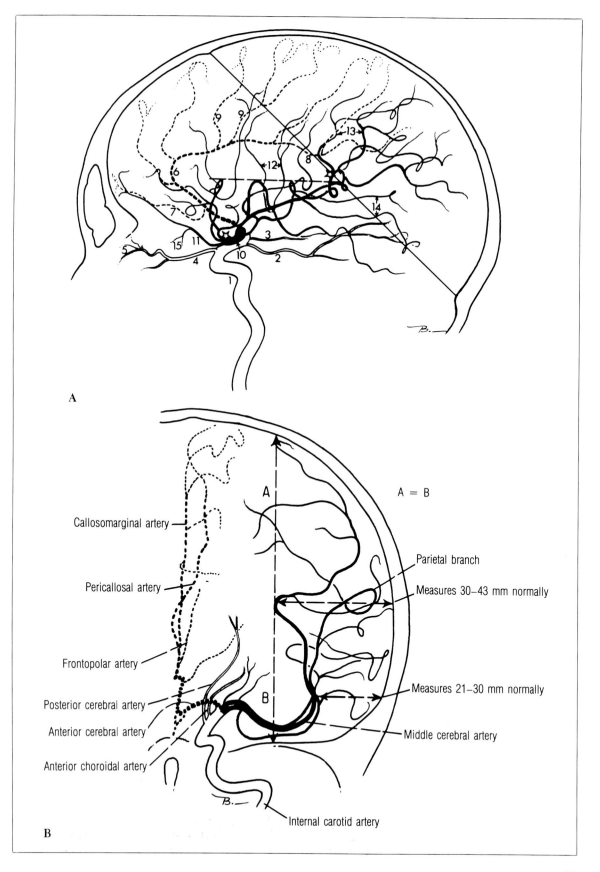

A

B

Callosomarginal artery

Pericallosal artery

Frontopolar artery

Posterior cerebral artery

Anterior cerebral artery

Anterior choroidal artery

Internal carotid artery

A = B

Parietal branch

Measures 30–43 mm normally

Measures 21–30 mm normally

Middle cerebral artery

the anterior choroidal artery courses posteriorly and laterally to enter the choroid plexus of the temporal horn.

The internal carotid artery bifurcates into anterior and middle cerebral branches. The *anterior cerebral* artery travels medially to the midline (the horizontal limb), where it is united with the opposite anterior cerebral artery by the anterior communicating artery. A tiny branch, the recurrent artery of Heubner, arises from this horizontal segment to supply portions of the basal ganglia and internal capsule. The anterior cerebral artery then ascends upward and forward to the rostrum and genu of the corpus callosum and continues posteriorly along the body of this structure as the pericallosal artery. The first major branch of the anterior cerebral artery is the frontopolar branch, which extends in the midline to the frontal pole. This branch is an important angiographic landmark because it shifts, together with the anterior cerebral artery, with frontal lobe masses. More posteriorly located space-occupying lesions shift the anterior cerebral artery alone, with the frontopolar branch remaining in the midline. The callosomarginal branch of the anterior cerebral artery extends posteriorly in the pericallosal sulcus.

The middle cerebral branch of the internal carotid artery passes laterally and horizontally, between the frontal lobe above and the temporal lobe below, to the sylvian fissure. In this horizontal segment, multiple small lenticulostriate branches extend posteriorly to supply the basal ganglia and internal capsule. Then, at a point approximately 3 cm from the inner table of the skull, the major branches of this artery turn superiorly and posteriorly. The major branches of the middle cerebral artery are divided into the frontal, anterior and posterior parietal, and anterior and posterior temporal branches. From these major branches smaller ones arise, which lie against the insula.

On the lateral projection, these small branches (sylvian vessels) are portrayed as rows of loops of small arteries, the upper margins of which correspond to the superior insular sulcus (horizontal broken line in Fig. 14-14A) while the lower margins correspond to the sylvian fissure. A line joining the inferior margins is a good landmark, indicating normal vascular relationships in the temporal lobe. This latter line should lie parallel to and within 1.5 cm of a line joining the tuberculum sella to the midpoint between the coronal

suture and the internal occipital protuberance (the two open stars in Fig. 14-14). Displacement above this line indicates temporal lobe space-occupying processes. The superior and inferior margins of this group of sylvian vessels join to form the sylvian triangle, which is another important landmark in determining vessel displacement. Major branches of the middle cerebral artery leave the sylvian fissure by curving around the operculum onto the surface of the brain. The sylvian point (as seen on the AP projection) represents the most medial and superior position of the most posterior branch of the middle cerebral complex (Fig. 14-14B). On the frontal projection it should lie 30 to 43 mm medial to the inner table of the skull, and halfway between the superior inner surface of the skull and the roof of the orbit or the petrous pyramid, whichever is lower.

VEINS OF THE ANTERIOR CIRCULATION. The venous phase of the carotid arteriogram (Fig. 14-15) is as important as the arterial, and the angiogram is incomplete without it. The superficial veins appear first, usually anteriorly and then posteriorly. If these veins appear prematurely in a localized area, this may signify tumor or AVM, or a luxury perfusion response to vascular occlusion. The veins may be occluded by thrombus or may be displaced by subdural or epidural masses such as hematoma. Approximately 8 seconds into the angiographic series the deep veins appear, again anteriorly first and then posteriorly. They fill in sequence on each side, first the septal vein (lying in the septum pellucidum) and then the thalamostriate veins (in the lateral wall of the lateral ventricle). These veins join at the venous angle (at the level of the foramen of Munroe) to form bilateral midline structures, the internal cerebral veins, which lie along the roof of the third ventricle. These vessels join to form the single midline structure, the great vein of Galen. The basilar vein of Rosenthal courses from each side around the midbrain (in company with the anterior choroidal and posterior cerebral arteries) to join the great vein of Galen at its point of origin. The vein of Galen lies under the splenium of the corpus callosum and joins the internal longitudinal sinus (inferior sagittal sinus) to form the straight sinus; before this it receives some important draining veins from the posterior fossa (see below). The straight sinus courses inferomedially to join the superior longitudinal sinus (superior sagittal sinus) at the torcula. From here the venous

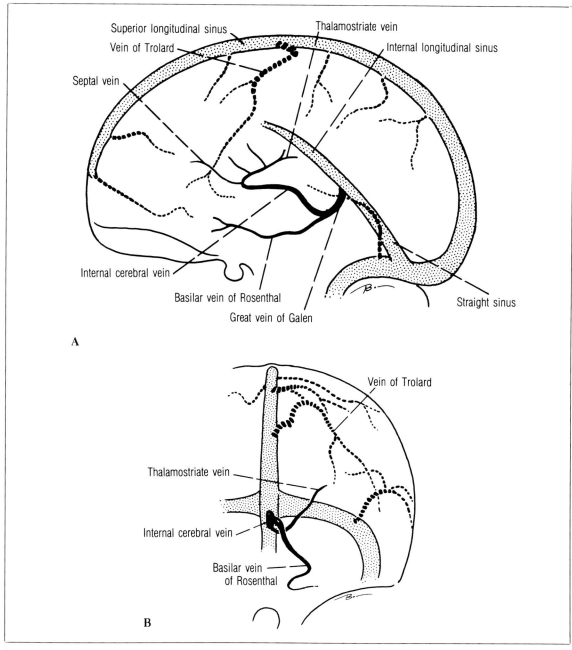

Fig. 14-15. Veins of the anterior circulation. The deep veins are shown as solid lines, the superficial veins as dotted lines, and the major sinuses as stippled gray areas. (See text for details.)
A. Lateral projection.
B. AP projection.

drainage flows into the lateral sinuses and then to the jugular vein. Displacement due to masses can be detected on frontal projections by abnormal position of the midline internal cerebral veins. Enlarged lateral ventricles are portrayed by lateral displacement of the thalamostriate veins. Inferior displacement of the basilar vein of Rosenthal is produced by tentorial herniation.

THE VERTEBRAL SYSTEM

Extracranial Arteries

The vertebral artery arises from the subclavian artery on each side and ascends in the upper six vertebral transverse foramina to penetrate the dura at the level of the foramen magnum. Multiple muscular branches arise from the cervical portion to form collaterals (in obstructive disease) with terminal branches of the external carotid artery, costocervical and thyrocervical branches of the subclavian artery, and muscular branches of the opposite vertebral artery. Radicular spinal branches also arise from this portion of the vertebral artery to join the anterior spinal artery. Just before the vertebral arteries fuse to form the basilar artery, they each give off small spinal branches that, in turn, join to course down the anterior aspect of the spinal cord (see Chap. 15). These vessels may be hypertrophied in vascular tumors and AVMs of the spine. In addition, meningeal branches arise from the distal extracranial portions of the vertebral arteries to supply portions of the dura of the posterior fossa. These branches are important considerations in evaluating tumors and AVMs of the meninges.

Posterior Fossa Arteries (Fig. 14-16)

The important vessels of the posterior fossa are briefly summarized here. The posterior inferior cerebellar artery (PICA) arises from the vertebral artery, usually above the foramen magnum. Anatomically, the PICA is intimately related to the medulla, the inferior portion of the fourth ventricle, the inferior vermis, the tonsils, and the inferior aspect of the cerebellar hemispheres. The basilar artery courses upward in a median shallow groove on the anterior surface of the pons, being separated from the clivus by a space of 1 to 2 mm. Minute pontine branches and occasionally the internal auditory artery may be outlined by magnification digital subtraction techniques. The anterior inferior cerebellar artery arises from the inferior third of the basilar artery and supplies structures in close proximity to the internal auditory meatus. Before the termination of the basilar artery, superior cerebellar branches arise on each side to course laterally around the midbrain to supply the superior surfaces of the cerebellar hemispheres. These still lie below the tentorium.

The basilar artery bifurcates terminally into two posterior cerebral arteries, which course posteriorly above the tentorium to encircle the midbrain. Branches extend out to supply the occipital poles, the medial and inferior portions of the occipital

Fig. 14-16. Branches of the vertebral artery and basilar artery (see text for details). The dotted lines indicate the infratentorial branches; the solid line indicates the supratentorial branches.
A. Lateral projection.
B. Half-axial (Towne) projection. PICA = posterior inferior cerebellar artery.

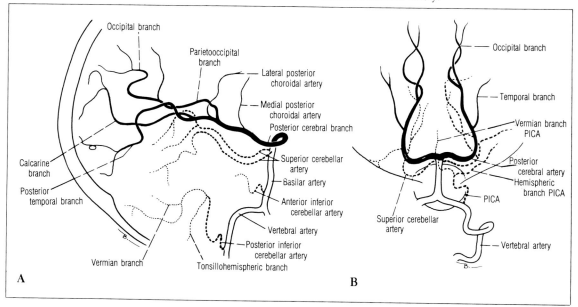

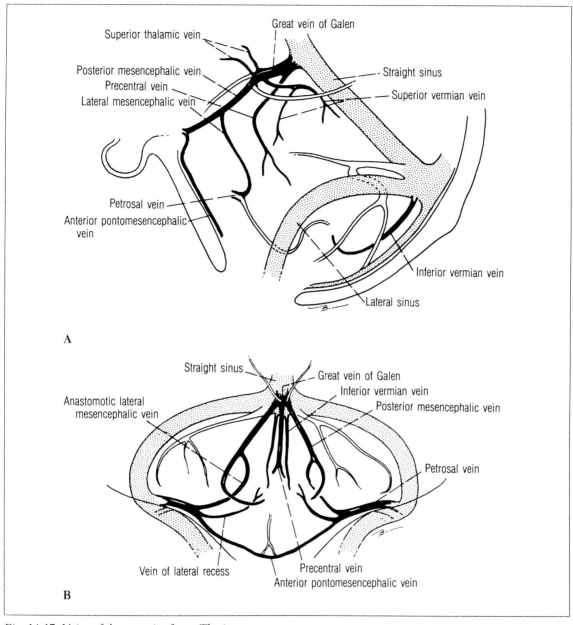

Fig. 14-17. Veins of the posterior fossa. The important branches are shown in black; the sinuses are the stippled gray areas.
A. Lateral projection.
B. Half-axial (Towne) projection.

lobes, and the inferior portions of the temporal lobes.

Venous Drainage of the Posterior Fossa
(Fig. 14-17)
Although these veins are complex and can often be outlined only by good selective vertebral subtraction studies, they are important in evaluating posterior fossa mass lesions. The following six veins are particularly helpful: The precentral cere-

bellar vein and anterior pontomesencephalic vein, which are midline structures; the superior and inferior vermian veins, which on the lateral projection outline the vermis; the posterior mesencephalic vein; and the petrosal vein. The precentral cerebellar vein (seen well in the lateral projection) flows in the midline from the fourth ventricle upward in the cleft between the upper portion of the cerebellum and the brain stem to drain into the vein of Galen. The close association of this structure to the fourth ventricle dictates its normal position, which is approximately midway between the tuberculum sella and the torcula (Twining's line). Posterior displacement from this point indicates a mass in the brain stem, whereas anterior displacement points to a mass in the cerebellum. The anterior pontomesencephalic vein, best seen on lateral projection, is a plexus of veins closely applied to the anterior surface of the brain stem. These veins drain into the superior petrosal sinus and into the posterior mesencephalic vein. The latter vein in turn courses high around the midbrain to enter the great vein of Galen. Posterior displacement of the pontomesencephalic vein indicates a mass in the clivus or the pontine subarachnoid cistern; anterior displacement means a mass in the brain stem or the cerebellum. The petrosal vein runs within the cerebellopontine angle and drains the anterior aspect of the cerebellum and pons. Its close proximity to the internal auditory meatus may be helpful in evaluating cerebellopontine angle tumors. The vermian veins outline the vermis. The superior vermian vein drains the anterior and the superior surface of the cerebellum and empties into the vein of Galen either separately or in conjunction with the precentral cerebellar vein and the posterior mesencephalic vein. The inferior vermian veins arise near the cerebellar tonsils and course cephalad in the midline on either side of the vermis, draining into the straight sinus.

COLLATERAL CIRCULATION

It is important to understand the angiographic anatomy of the collateral circulation and intracranial-extracranial communications for a number of reasons. In occlusive brachiocephalic extracranial and intracranial disease, retrograde delayed flow through collaterals to the vascular bed of an occluded vessel is recognized on delayed films in the angiographic series (Fig. 14-19). This may portray a viable vascular bed peripheral to a point of occlu-

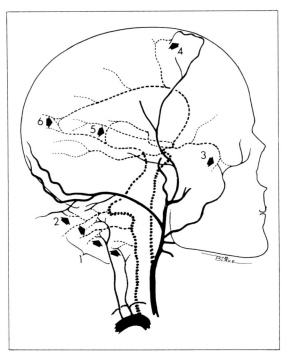

Fig. 14-18. The collateral circulation in extracranial and intracranial occlusive disease. The vertebral and carotid systems are shown as dotted lines; the external carotid and cervical branches of the subclavian artery are shown as solid lines. The cervical arterial collateral network joins the subclavian with the carotid and vertebral arteries (1, 2). The ascending cervical and deep cervical branches of the subclavian artery anastomose with muscular branches of the vertebral artery and the occipital branch of the external carotid artery. There are anastomoses between the terminal branches of the external carotid artery and the ophthalmic artery (3); there are also anastomoses between the meningeal branches of the external carotid artery through the rete mirabile to the leptomeningeal branches on the surface of the brain (4). Multiple intracranial communications occur across the circle of Willis, across the midline (anterior communicating and anterior cerebral arteries), between the anterior and posterior choroidal branches (5), and over the surface of the brain between the peripheral branches of the anterior, middle, and posterior cerebral arteries (6).

sion that is acceptable for surgical bypass procedure. All possible feeding vessels to a vascular tumor or an AVM must be carefully displayed in order to ensure complete surgical or endovascular therapy. Then, prior to definitive therapy, potential arterial feeders to nontarget areas may be ligated surgically or isolated with larger centrally positioned emboli. Unusual vascular origins sup-

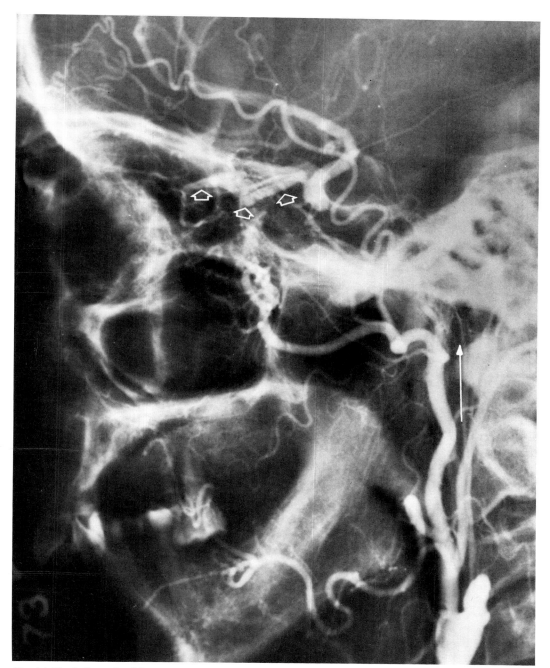

Fig. 14-19. Collaterals of the terminal branches of the external carotid artery and the ophthalmic artery (*open arrows*) supply the intracranial circulation in a patient with occlusion of the internal carotid artery near its origin. The long arrow is along the course of the ascending pharyngeal branch.

plying vital structures (e.g., ophthalmic artery from the middle meningeal artery) must be uncovered to avoid neurologic deficit in therapeutic attempts. Finally, all intracranial-extracranial communications and potential anastomoses must be carefully researched to avoid inadvertent occlusion of intracerebral nontarget areas. Keep in mind that otherwise small or invisible communications can enlarge once occlusion of proximal vessels changes the normal pressure relationships (Figs. 14-18, 14-19, 14-20).

Communications from extracranial to intracranial branches are as follows:

1. Ascending cervical and deep cervical branches of the subclavian artery to the vertebral artery (Fig. 14-20).
2. Occipital branch of the external carotid artery to muscular branches of the vertebral artery.
3. Ascending pharyngeal branch of the external carotid artery to both the vertebral and internal carotid artery (its posterior branch also supplies the ninth through twelfth facial nerves).
4. Superficial temporal artery to the ophthalmic artery (Fig. 14-19).
5. Middle meningeal artery to the ophthalmic circulation or to the internal carotid artery (its proximal portion can contribute to the seventh cranial nerve).
6. Terminal branches of the internal maxillary artery with internal carotid circulation.

Intracranial communications also occur.

1. Around the circle of Willis: across the midline by anterior communicating and midline branches of the anterior cerebral artery and from posterior to anterior through the posterior communicating arteries.
2. Anastomoses between the anterior and posterior choroidal arteries.
3. Over the surface of the brain between peripheral branches of the anterior, middle, and posterior cerebral arteries (Fig. 14-21).
4. Through the rete mirabile to the leptomeningeal arteries on the surface of the brain.

ANOMALIES

Familiarity with the numerous anomalies of the origin of the brachiocephalic vessels [16] precludes incorrect interpretations and incomplete evalua-

tion of the intracranial cerebral lesions by the catheter approach. The brachiocephalic vessels and the aortic arch are derived from eight primitive vascular arches that connect the anteriorly located truncus arteriosus with the posteriorly positioned paired aortae. Persistence of some portions of these arches and involution of others results in the normal adult configuration of vessels. Anomalies occur when there is failure of involution of some of these primitive vessels.

Normally the aorta arches to the left, a persistence of the left fourth primitive arch. If the right fourth primitive arch persists instead, it will arch to the right. If the right-sided arch with its brachiocephalic vessel origins is a mirror image of the left arch, and it descends on the right, there is a very high incidence of associated intracardiac anomalies (98%). If there is a right-sided arch with the aorta descending instead on the left, or if there is an associated anomalous left subclavian artery with the anomalous right-sided aortic arch, then

Fig. 14-20. Cervical arterial collateral network. Branches of the occipital artery anastomose with the vertebral artery (*curved arrow*), which fills in a retrograde fashion (*wavy arrow*) in a patient with complete occlusion of the left subclavian artery proximal to the vertebral artery. There is occlusion of the left middle cerebral branches (*straight arrow*) and stenosis of the internal carotid artery at the siphon.

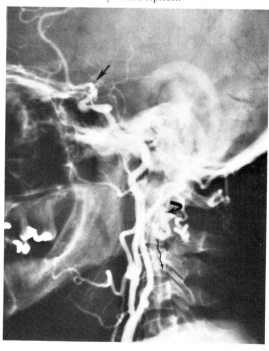

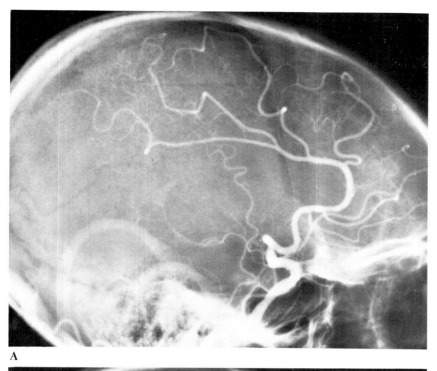

A

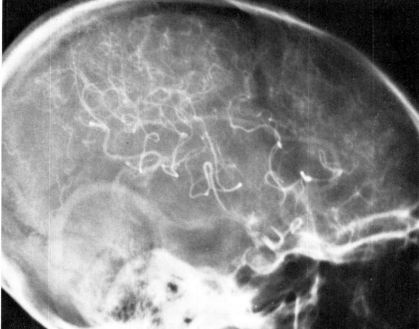

B

Fig. 14-21. Intracranial collateral.
A. Occlusion of the middle cerebral artery at its origin.
B. Delayed film shows filling of the middle cerebral group via collaterals arising from the anterior cerebral artery over the surface of the brain.

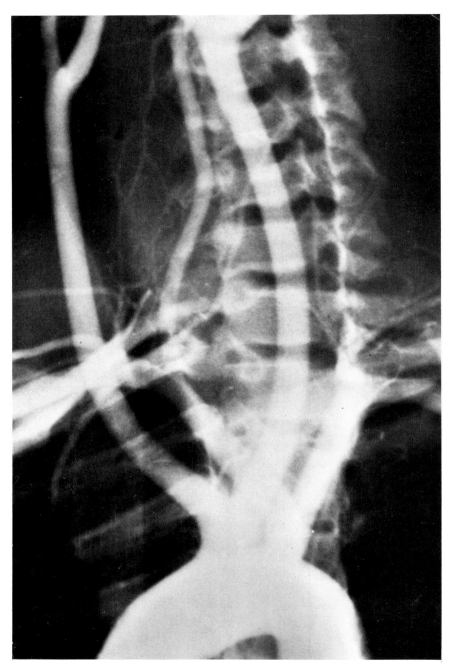

Fig. 14-22. Three common anomalies of the origin of the brachiocephalic vessels: a common origin of the left carotid artery with the innominate artery; a high origin of the innominate artery to the left of the trachea; and an anomalous origin of the right subclavian artery distal to the left subclavian artery. The left vertebral artery is traumatically occluded.

intracardiac anomalies are much less frequent. The double aortic arch reflects a persistence of both primitive arches. There are many variants of this phenomenon, with atresia between segments as well as variations in the size of the descending aorta and in the relative size of each arch. Cervical arches arise unusually high; they may be located in the thoracic outlet or may even extend up beyond the neck. Cervical arches are considered the result of persistence of the third arch rather than the fourth during embryonic development. An abnormally high position of a right- or left-sided arch is often associated with anomalous brachiocephalic branch origins.

There are a variety of anomalies of brachiocephalic vascular origins. There may be as many as six separately arising vessels from the aorta (both carotids, the subclavians, and the vertebrals) or a single common trunk, or a host of other combinations. The most commonly found anomalies are a high origin of the innominate artery (to the left of the trachea), a common origin of the left carotid artery with the innominate artery (Fig. 14-22), an anomalous origin of the right subclavian artery distal to the left subclavian artery (Fig. 14-22), and an anomalous origin of the left vertebral artery from the aorta (Fig. 14-23D). The left subclavian artery may arise anomalously in a right-sided aortic arch. Rarely, other anomalies develop: (1) the right subclavian artery arises directly from the aorta proximal or just distal to the right carotid artery; (2) a double innominate artery; (3) the right vertebral artery arises directly from the aorta; (4) the external carotid artery arises directly from the aorta (Fig. 14-23A, B, C); (5) variations in the level of the common carotid artery bifurcation; (6) a carotid trunk; (7) absence of the common carotid artery (right or left); (8) duplication of vessels; and (9) origin of the vertebral arteries from the carotid arteries. Unusual anastomoses between the carotid artery and the basilar artery can occur as a result of the presence of remnants of primitive vessels (e.g., persistent trigeminal, acoustic, or hypoglossal arteries) (Fig. 14-24).

Technical Considerations

In the large majority of patients studied for intracranial nonocclusive disease and space-occupying lesions, intraarterial catheter techniques are safely and easily performed. However, this is not as true in patients with atherosclerotic disease who are being studied for transient ischemic attacks. In such patients there is a delicate balance of intracranial collateral flow, which may be easily upset by otherwise inconsequential hemodynamic changes. Contrast agent cannot be cleared easily through stenosed vessels, which leads to longer cell contact. Nonetheless, adequate evaluation of intracranial structure sometimes is difficult without selective studies. The detail of smaller vessels is often not seen well enough if there is only an aortic arch injection. Also, high-grade stenosis of the internal carotid artery in the neck, together with the delayed flow and overlapping vessels, may lead to an erroneous diagnosis of total occlusion of the vessel. Consequently, surgical correction may be denied a potentially curable lesion.

Surgical mortality and morbidity are significantly higher in patients operated on for extracranial occlusive disease who do not have adequate evaluation of the intracranial circulation. These complications must be balanced against the possibility of complications from the angiographic procedure. Some patients can be adequately evaluated by multiple projection aortic arch digital subtraction studies alone (IV-DSA and/or IA-DSA) [43, 56]. The remaining patients require selective biplane intracranial studies in order to elucidate an obscure angiographic or clinical finding. Complicating neurologic sequelae from femoral cerebral angiography have been considerably decreased by this general approach. There is hope that they will be reduced further by use of the newer nonionic contrast agents.

The angiographer should be aware of the clinical history and pertinent findings with regard to the vascular territory of greatest concern. Noninvasive studies such as duplex scanning and periorbital Doppler ultrasonography should be reviewed. Be aware of neck bruits and decreased carotid pulse pressures. A palpable pulse may be felt in the neck (a patent external carotid artery) despite an occluded internal carotid artery. Bruits may be absent if the lesion is sufficiently severe to prevent enough flow to produce the necessary turbulence. A loud bruit may be due to an inconsequential stenosis of an external carotid artery. Check for differences in blood pressure or strength of pulse or a delay in pulse transmission between the upper extremities. Recognize a tortuous thoracic aorta or calcification in the brachiocephalic vessels on the

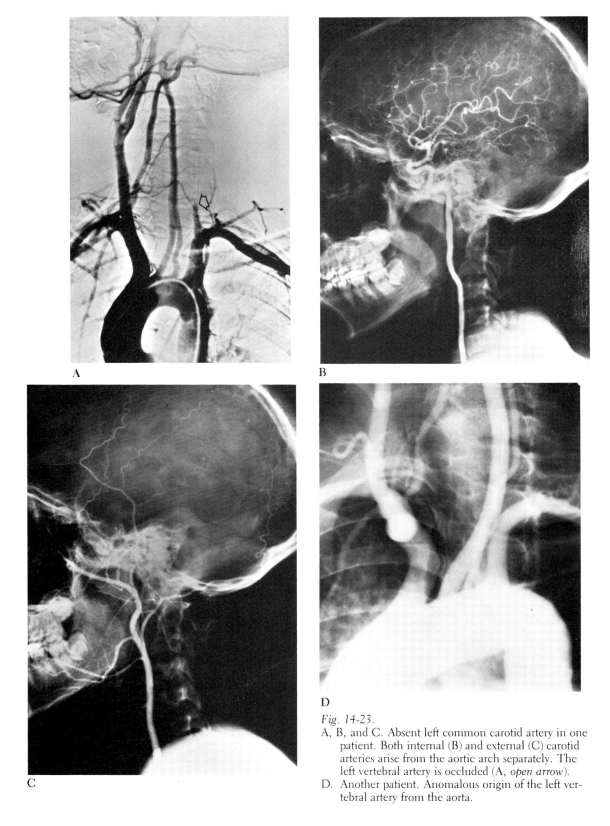

A

B

C

D

Fig. 14-23.
A, B, and C. Absent left common carotid artery in one
  patient. Both internal (B) and external (C) carotid
  arteries arise from the aortic arch separately. The
  left vertebral artery is occluded (A, *open arrow*).
D. Another patient. Anomalous origin of the left vertebral artery from the aorta.

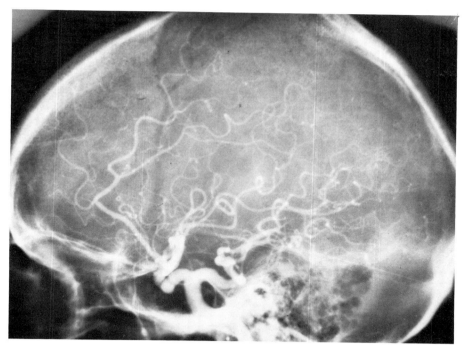

Fig. 14-24. Primitive trigeminal artery. Primitive acoustic arteries arise somewhat lower, and the primitive hypoglossal arteries arise in the cervical portion of the internal carotid artery.

chest x-ray. Exercise care in preparing the patient and performing the study. Guard against dislodging atherosclerotic plaques, and also the inadvertent embolization of blood clots into the brain.

The following points are helpful to the angiographer:

1. In those patients undergoing IV-DSA, be aware of their renal function, state of hydration, cardiac output, and ability to cooperate. If need be, use the newer nonionic contrast agents [8, 40] despite their exorbitant price. There appears to be less neurotoxicity, less discomfort, and greater patient tolerance. When used with IA-DSA, smaller quantities are required, which helps to offset their greater cost. Warn the patient not to perform a Valsalva maneuver during the procedure, for this decreases cardiac output. Swallowing is the single most common cause of motion artifact in DSA studies of the brachiocephalic branches.

2. Give the study priority in the day's work.

3. Do not contribute to hypotension by giving meperidine or other hypotensive drugs preangiographically. Atropine, 0.5 mg IM, helps to prevent vasovagal reactions. Diazepam (Valium), 10 mg PO, is usually sufficient sedation.

4. Do not prolong the procedure. The complication rate is directly proportional to the length of time the patient is on the table.

5. Heparinize those patients in whom a prolonged study is anticipated. A dose of 45 IU/kg (approximately 3000 IU in an average 70-kg adult) may be given intravenously or intraarterially immediately after insertion of the catheter into the aorta in those patients without intracranial hemorrhage or other contraindications. The heparinization helps to prevent clot formation within the catheter. In intracranial studies, repeated forceful flushing of the catheter is even more vital than in other parts of the body.

6. Simultaneous biplane studies require fewer injections, less contrast agent, and less time on the examining table than multiple single plane studies.

7. Do not advance a catheter or guidewire into a plaque-filled artery.

8. Branches of the subclavian artery (deep cervical branch of the costocervical trunk) supply the spinal cord; selective injections of even small quantities of contrast medium into these vessels have been known to cause paralysis. Small test

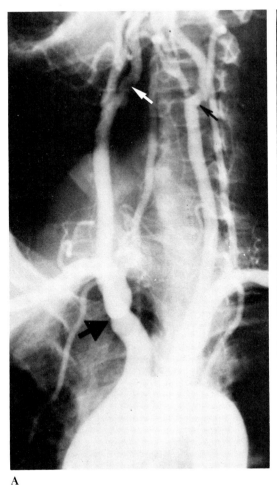 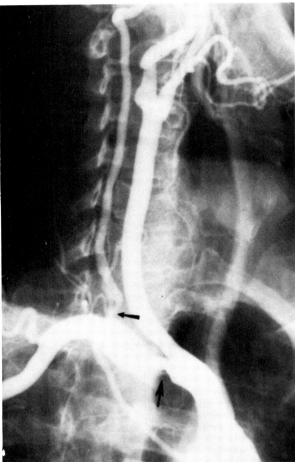

A   B

Fig. 14-25. Typical atherosclerotic plaques.

A. RPO projection. The origin of the right subclavian artery is obscured by the overlying right carotid artery (*large arrow*). There are plaques of the left carotid bifurcation and the right internal carotid origin (*small arrows*).

B. LPO projection. An innominate artery injection clearly outlines the stenotic right subclavian (*large arrow*), right vertebral (*small arrow*), and right internal carotid arteries.

injections should be used in the subclavian artery, and if unusual myoclonic contractions of the extremities occur or if undue pain is experienced, that portion of the study should be terminated immediately. If paralysis occurs after this injection, attempt an immediate exchange transfusion of spinal fluid (see Chap. 16).

9. In patients with diseased vertebral arteries, posterior fossa IA-DSA may be safely performed by injecting 30 to 43% contrast agent into the proximal subclavian artery (8 ml/sec for 20 ml), while a blood pressure cuff is inflated on the ipsilateral arm to a pressure higher than systolic.

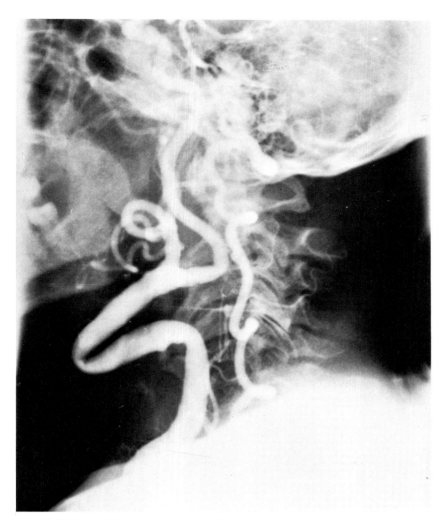

Fig. 14-26. Innominate artery injection shows marked tortuosity and elongation of both the right common carotid artery and the right vertebral artery. The patient presented with a pulsatile mass in the neck.

Angiographic Findings
[14, 15, 20, 51, 55]

ATHEROSCLEROSIS

The age range of patients with the highest frequency of atherosclerosis is in the fifth to seventh decades. Plaques, sometimes with ulcerations in their base, cause arterial stenosis of varying degrees of severity (Figs. 14-2, 14-25, 14-27). Tortuosity, elongation, and dilatation of vessels present clinically as pulsating masses. Although the cause of these masses must be recognized, they need no treatment (Fig. 14-26). Although stenosis is usually localized to the origin of brachiocephalic vessels and their major bifurcations, significant lesions can occur high in the cervical course of the internal carotid artery, at the level of the siphon and also in the intracranial vessels (Figs. 14-27, 14-28). Severe stenosis of the internal carotid artery origin may lead to delayed flow through a stringlike vessel. Its narrow appearance may be due, in part, to luminal collapse secondary to decreased flow and, in part, to layering of contrast medium on its posterior wall. Although sometimes recognized by IV-DSA, this condition often requires selective carotid angiography [34, 44].

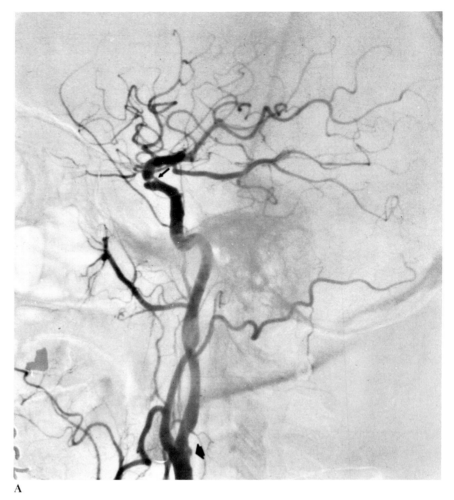

A

Fig. 14-27.
A. Conventional subtraction study of a lateral projection of a selective left carotid injection, showing severe stenosis of the left internal carotid artery at the level of the siphon (*small arrow*). There is an ulcerating plaque of the left internal carotid artery near its origin (*large arrow*).
B and C. Another patient: arch injection (B) and selective right carotid arteriogram (C). The irregular ulceration is seen best on the selective study.

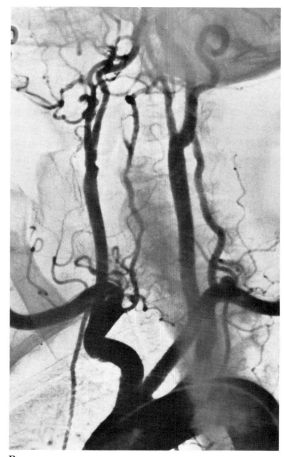

B

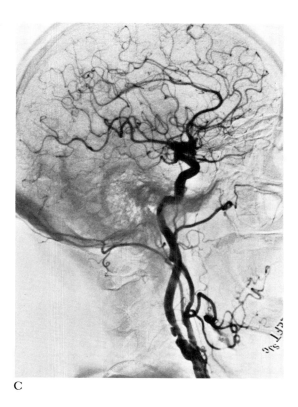

C

Complications of thrombosis and embolization can occur from stenotic plaques. If occlusive disease is seen in one area, the circulation above and below that area and the circulation in the remaining brachiocephalic vessels must be evaluated. Intracranial circulation is maintained by collateral flow following vascular occlusion; the angiographer must be aware of all the available avenues of collateral flow, for these may also, in turn, be endangered by stenosis. Surgical correction or percutaneous transluminal angioplasty may be directed toward improving this collateral flow (e.g., the external carotid artery) rather than toward correction of a hopelessly, chronically occluded internal carotid artery.

Extracranial-to-intracranial bypass procedures (occipital to basilar artery—superficial temporal artery to middle cerebral artery [Fig. 14-28]) may also be performed. Occasionally collateral flow induced by extracranial vascular occlusion may steal blood from the brain rather than supply it. A typical example of this phenomenon is the "subclavian steal" induced by subclavian stenosis of an artery proximal to the vertebral artery. Collateral flow to the involved upper extremity distal to the obstruction often includes retrograde flow down the vertebral artery; this removes blood normally destined for the posterior fossa circulation (Fig. 14-29).

Atherosclerosis often involves the common carotid bifurcations and the internal carotid arteries at their origins. The external carotid arteries may also be involved; however, this involvement is of less significance unless this artery provides an important collateral to the intracranial circulation. The vertebral arteries are often involved near their origins, as are the subclavian arteries.

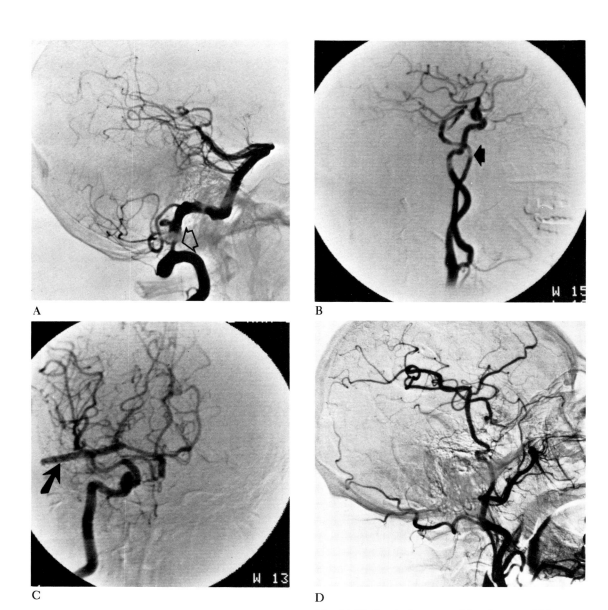

Fig. 14-28. Surgical extracranial to intracranial by-
passes.
A. Lateral projection right vertebral arteriogram shows
    severe stenosis high in the course of a dominant left
    vertebral artery.
B and C. Right occipital artery to posterior cerebral
    artery surgical bypass in lateral (B) and AP (C) pro-
    jections.
D. Temporal artery to middle cerebral artery bypass
    in another patient with occlusion of the inter-
    nal carotid artery.

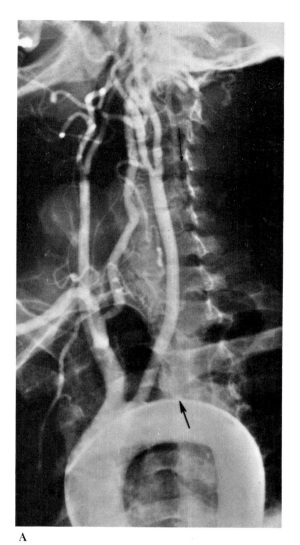

A

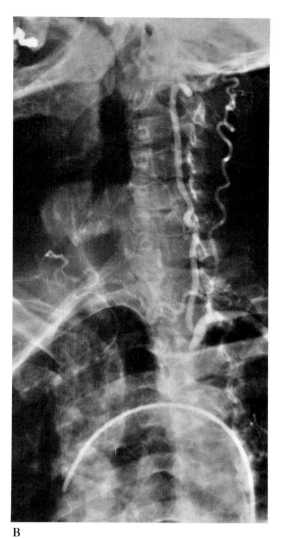

B

Fig. 14-29.
A and B. "Subclavian steal" due to occlusion of the
  left subclavian artery. Note retrograde flow down
  the left vertebral artery and other cervical branches
  on the delayed films to fill the left subclavian artery.

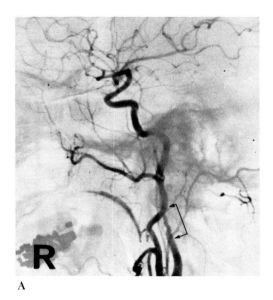

A

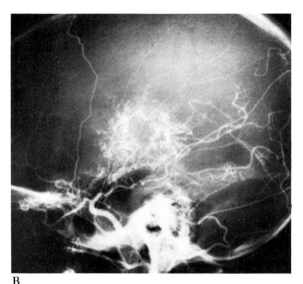

B

Fig. 14-30. Unusual conditions causing extracranial and intracranial occlusive disease.

A. Fibromuscular dysplasia of the internal carotid artery (*arrows*); conventional subtraction study of the lateral projection of a right common carotid injection. These lesions are located higher than those of atherosclerosis, and they occur in younger patients and more often in women. A similar lesion was present on the opposite side (not shown).

B. Idiopathic progressive intracranial arterial occlusion in a child. A large number of dilated, tortuous, deep cerebral perforating arteries act as collaterals. The Japanese name *moyamoya disease*, meaning "puff of smoke," describes this appearance.

OTHER DISEASES CAUSING OCCLUSION AND STENOSIS

Occlusion and stenosis of the brachiocephalic vessels may be caused by a number of diseases other than atherosclerosis [47]. Fibromuscular dysplasia (Fig. 14-30A), arteritis, trauma, and other conditions are discussed in Chapter 8. Focal dissection of the cervical or intracranial portions of the internal carotid or vertebral arteries can occur spontaneously or can be associated with fibromuscular dysplasia. They appear as false channels, tapered occlusions, or dissecting aneurysms [19]. There can be a progressive idiopathic occlusion of the distal internal carotid arteries, which also affects the arteries of the posterior fossa. The term *moyamoya* ("puff of smoke") [17] has been used to describe the characteristic appearance of the resulting plethora of tiny intracranial collaterals, which particularly involve the deep cerebral perforating arteries (Fig. 14-30B).

INTRACRANIAL BLEEDING

Intracranial bleeding may be subarachnoid, intracerebral, subdural, or epidural in location. Computed tomography (CT) scans uncover the general location and sometimes the nature of the bleeding site. Angiography is usually required to determine the underlying pathologic condition.

Subarachnoid hemorrhage may be due to aneurysms, AVMs (pial or dural), trauma, or arteritis.

Intracerebral hematomas may be due to hypertension, aneurysms, AVMs, tumors, trauma, arteritis, blood dyscrasias, or secondary to arterial embolism or to venous occlusion. Subdural or epidural bleeding usually occurs subsequent to trauma.

Computed Tomography and Angiography in Intracranial Bleeding

In patients with a *subarachnoid hemorrhage*, unenhanced CT scans may help to determine the location of bleeding, for blood in the subarachnoid spaces remains visible for approximately 5 days. If blood is seen in the subarachnoid space, a contrast enhanced CT scan need not be performed immediately, for angiography will have to be performed. An enhanced CT study need be performed only if no blood is detected.

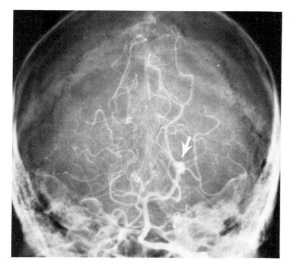

Fig. 14-31. A mycotic aneurysm (*arrow*) of the left posterior cerebral artery in a patient with subacute bacterial endocarditis. Note its more peripheral location.

CT scans help determine the location of the bleeding site by visualizing the aneurysm or other vascular abnormality, by determining the preponderance of subarachnoid collection of blood, or by pinpointing the location of an associated intracerebral hematoma. In patients with an anterior communicating artery aneurysm, the bleeding is usually in the inferior portion of the pericallosal cistern, or there is a hematoma in the septal or low frontal area. A pericallosal artery aneurysm causes a hematoma in the corpus callosum. Both a posterior communicating artery and a middle cerebral artery aneurysm cause bleeding into the sylvian fissure. A middle cerebral artery aneurysm forms hematomas in the temporal lobe; aneurysms in the posterior communicating artery bleed into the uncus or medial portions of the temporal lobe. A ruptured posterior communicating artery aneurysm or basilar artery aneurysm causes predominant hemorrhage into the interpeduncular and perimesencephalic cisterns, whereas a posterior inferior cerebellar artery (PICA) aneurysm bleeds into the fourth ventricle. In patients where multiple aneurysms are detected by angiography, CT scan sometimes will determine which one is bleeding.

The patient is usually operated on promptly once the aneurysm is uncovered if the bleeding is mild or minimal and the patient remains alert.

Emergency surgery is performed if vascular displacement suggests a large hematoma. If bleeding is moderate to severe by CT scan, and there is associated spasm of vessels seen on the angiogram, or if the patient is drowsy or confused, or has a stiff neck, surgery is delayed in order to decrease operative mortality.

An *intracerebral hematoma* located by unenhanced CT scan of the brain should be followed by contrast enhancement in an attempt to uncover an underlying tumor nodule, angioma, AVM, or large aneurysm. Angiography is sometimes deferred until the patient's condition stabilizes, unless surgical removal of the hematoma is necessary. Both primary tumors and secondary tumors (e.g., glioma, choriocarcinoma) can hemorrhage into the brain substance.

Hypertensive bleeds are most likely to occur in the following areas (in decreasing order of frequency): putamen, subcortical white matter, thalamus, pons, cerebellum.

Aneurysms

Intracranial berry aneurysms are found most frequently in patients in the fourth and fifth decades. They usually occur at points of arterial branching; the highest incidence is around the circle of Willis. Common sites are the origin of the posterior communicating artery, the junction of the anterior communicating with the anterior cerebral artery, and the proximal middle cerebral branches. Mycotic aneurysms tend to occur in the peripheral branches of major intracranial arteries (Fig. 14-31).

Aneurysms may occur virtually anywhere in the intracranial circulation [1, 26] and may be multiple in 20 percent of patients (Fig. 14-32). A patient with subarachnoid hemorrhage suspected of having an intracranial aneurysm should, therefore, have all the intracranial vessels investigated. Once an aneurysm has been located, determine its size and shape, the width of its neck and its relationship to surrounding vessels, and whether or not there is evidence of bleeding. *Bleeding aneurysms* may develop arterial spasm, which may be focal and located near the aneurysm or may involve all the arteries at the base of the brain. The spasm may be severe enough to delay filling of the aneurysm un-

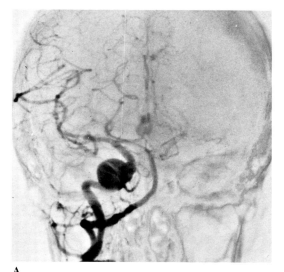

A

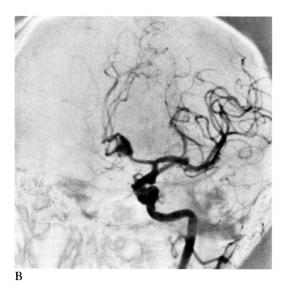

B

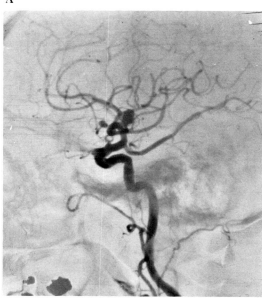

C

Fig. 14-32. Multiple intracranial berry aneurysms in the same patient.
A. A large aneurysm involving the right internal carotid artery (subtraction AP projection).
B. Three aneurysms involving the left anterior intracranial circulation: the internal carotid artery, the anterior cerebral artery, and the middle cerebral artery. These aneurysms are best seen on a subtraction film of a left carotid injection, with an oblique projection that is 30 degrees to the right.
C. A subtraction film of a lateral projection with a left carotid injection shows the same aneurysms.

til late in the angiographic series, or it may not opacify at all. A number of patients with known subarachnoid hemorrhage will not demonstrate an aneurysm on the initial angiographic study, and some will never have the cause of bleeding defined. A loculated aneurysm may mean a weakened wall and thus may point to it as the bleeding site.

Special projections may be required to evaluate the full nature of the aneurysm (Table 14-3). In addition to the standard frontal and lateral projections, intraorbital views show the middle cerebral artery well. Oblique views with the nose turned 20 to 30 degrees away from the site of injection may better define the anterior communicating artery and the trifurcation of the middle cerebral artery. Submentovertical projections give another view of internal carotid and basilar artery aneurysms. Compression of the opposite carotid or vertebral artery during selective angiography of the

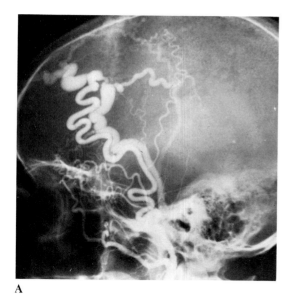

A

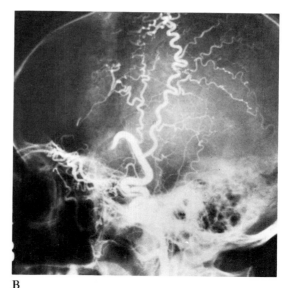

B

Fig. 14-33. Traumatic arteriovenous fistula of the scalp, resulting from an automobile accident 9 months previously.

A. Selective external carotid arteriogram taken before embolization shows a markedly hypertrophied superficial temporal artery and premature filling of a large draining temporal vein. Many other small branches of the external carotid artery are also hypertrophied.

B. Embolic occlusion with Ivalon pellets. The arteriovenous fistula was obliterated and flow diverted away from the frontal to the parietal branches of the superficial temporal artery. More emboli were then introduced.

C. Subsequent arteriogram with an exchanged catheter shows occlusion of more superficial temporal artery branches. There is now reflux of contrast agent into the internal carotid circulation with a forced contrast injection. No additional emboli can be introduced at this point for fear of intracranial complications. The patient was discharged in 24 hours.

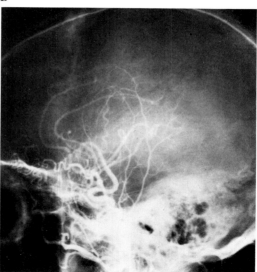

C

respective vessels helps delineate the surrounding vascular bed and determines the feasibility of the surgical occlusion of the feeding vessels.

ARTERIOVENOUS MALFORMATIONS AND FISTULAS

Arteriovenous malformations (AVMs) and arteriovenous fistulas [33] have large, tortuous feeding arteries, a racemose tangle of closely packed vessels, and prematurely draining dilated veins. The absence of a mass effect helps to distinguish them

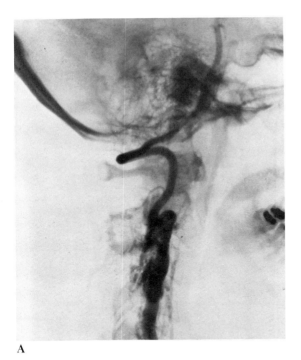

A

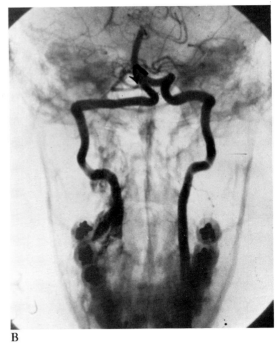

B

Fig. 14-34. Large arteriovenous communication arising from the right vertebral artery fed by multiple subclavian branches, but with normal external carotid arteries.
A. Right vertebral artery demonstrates multiple fistulas.
B. Left vertebral arteriogram shows a normal supply to the posterior fossa, but retrograde flow to the communication.

from hypervascular tumors. Vascular displacement can occur, however, when there is associated hematoma from bleeding or there is a mass of grossly dilated draining veins. Since flow through AVMs is greater and faster than normal, they require more rapid delivery of larger doses of contrast agent and more rapid film timing (3 to 4 per second). There may be many feeding branches from intracranial arteries of the anterior as well as the posterior circulation from both sides. There may also be contributions from the extracranial circulation. Therefore, selective biplane studies of multiple vessels are often required.

Arteriovenous malformations primarily involving the scalp, face, and neck are supplied largely by branches of the external carotid artery (Fig. 14-33) but also by branches of the subclavian artery (Fig. 14-34). Often they have meningeal feeding vessels

that perforate the skull (Fig. 14-35A). Large and complex calvarial AVMs can occur, with multiple bilateral feeding vessels arising from subclavian, vertebral, external, and even internal carotid terminal branches.

Intracranial AVMs are more common than those in extracranial locations and are classified on the basis of their arterial supply.

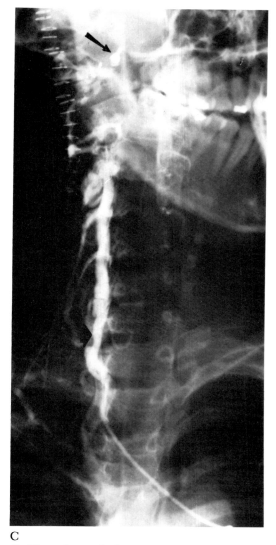

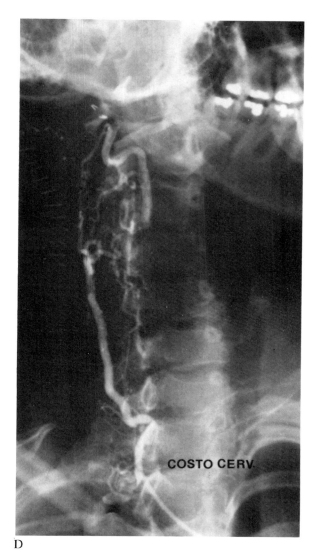

C

D

C. The right vertebral artery was sacrificed with a surgical clip high in its course (*small arrow*). All the
communications were subsequently embolized with
Ivalon and multiple coils.

D and E. Additional deep cervical branches from the
subclavian artery supplied the lesion and were embolized.

428

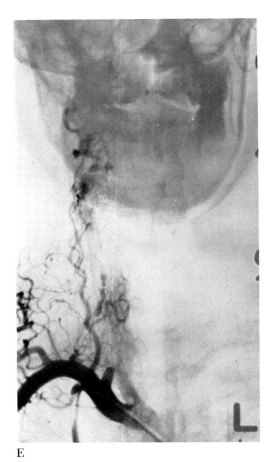

E

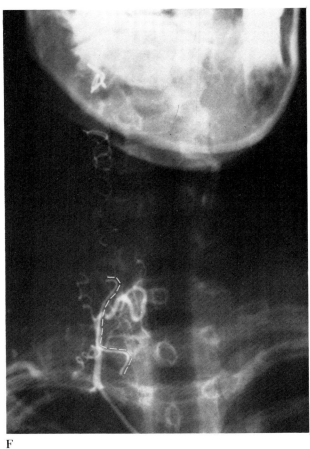

F

Fig. 14-34 (continued)
F. Final closure of communication by embolizing ascending cervical branch. Note: One of the coils
   placed in low vertebral artery is alarmingly elongated due to a mismatch of the diameter of the coil
   helix and the stenosed segment of artery (*broad arrow* in C).

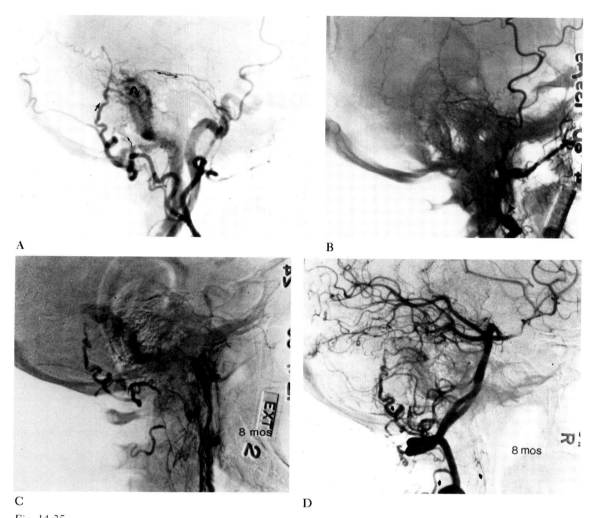

A

B

C

D

Fig. 14-35.
A. Primarily dural AVM with multiple feeders from the occipital, auricular, and meningeal branches. There is prompt filling of the sigmoid sinus (*curved arrow*), probably through the emissary vein.
B. Occlusion of major feeding vessels arising from occipital branch. Microparticles of Ivalon were used.
C, D, and E. Eight months later symptoms recurred. Ascending pharyngeal and auricular branches communicate directly with the AVM and with peripheral branches of the proximally occluded occipital artery. Note major meningeal branch arising from the ophthalmic artery.

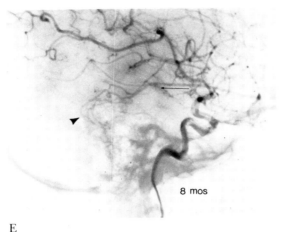

8 mos

E

Fig. 14-35 (continued)

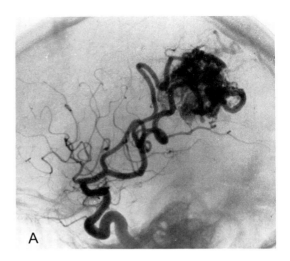

A

1. Pure pial lesions are supplied only by cerebral or cerebellar arteries (Fig. 14-36; see also Fig. 5-15). The majority are supratentorial.
2. Pure dural AVMs receive only a meningeal arterial supply (Fig. 14-37).
3. Mixed pial and dural lesions receive blood from both cerebral and meningeal arteries.

Venous angiomas are vascular malformations in which veins are the predominant vascular constituents [39, 41, 57]. The arterial phase in an angiogram may be normal or may reflect mass effect if bleeding has occurred. The venous phase demonstrates a branching collection of enlarged tortuous medullary veins that converge to form a large central channel that courses through the brain substance to end in a cortical vein, dural sinus, or (less commonly) deep venous system (Fig. 14-38).

TEMPORAL ARTERITIS

Temporal arteritis [28] is an inflammatory process involving the brachiocephalic vessels, generally with a predilection for the temporal artery. It is usually diagnosed by a biopsy of the superficial temporal artery. Microscopically, there is a giant

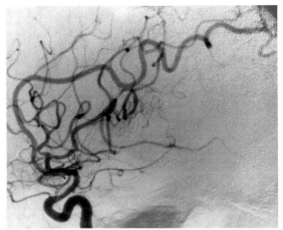

B

Fig. 14-36. A cerebral arteriovenous malformation (AVM) treated with intravascular glue (isobutyl-2-cyanoacrylate) in a 28-year-old man who had severe intracerebral hemorrhage from a parietooccipital AVM.

A. An angiogram before gluing shows the large parietal AVM; some additional portions of the AVM were filled by the posterior cerebral artery on vertebral angiography. Note the lack of filling of the anterior cerebral artery.

B. After gluing. The two main middle cerebral arteries feeding the AVM have been occluded. (Courtesy Dr. Ralph Heinz, Duke University Medical Center, Durham, NC.)

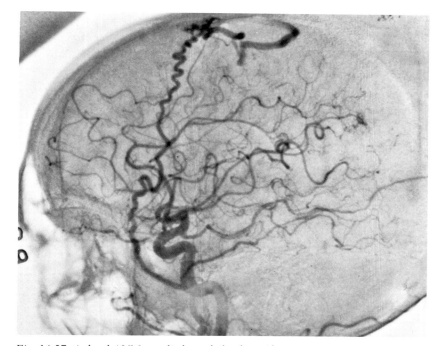

Fig. 14-37. A dural AVM supplied purely by the middle meningeal artery.

Fig. 14-38. Venous angioma (*arrows*): see text.
A. Lateral projection.
B. AP projection.

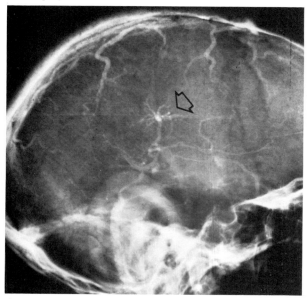

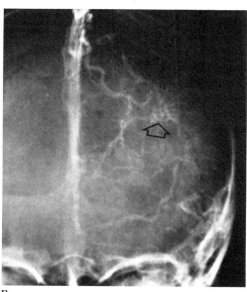

A   B

cell granulomatous reaction in the vessel wall, with resulting destruction and proliferation of cells. Since skip lesions can occur, and since the biopsy site in the proximal vessel may be free of disease, the arteriographic studies may help to determine more peripheral foci of involvement. A hand injection of 6 ml of low-density contrast agent following surgical exposure of the superficial temporal artery outlines the arteries, which, if they are involved with arteritis, show diffuse areas of irregular constriction, arterial dilatation, or obliteration of vessels (Fig. 14-39). In our experience, only those patients with gross pathologic evidence of disease at the site of the biopsy have shown convincing angiographic abnormality.

TRAUMA

Selective angiography can uncover occluded or lacerated vessels, false aneurysms and arteriovenous communications, and underlying causes of severe epistaxis (Figs. 14-40, 14-41) [42]. Subdural and epidural hematomas, cerebral contusion, and cerebral edema are common and, for the most part, are studied by means of CT scan.

TUMORS OF THE FACE AND NECK

Angiography can help to delineate the blood supply, to outline the relationship of the neoplasm to major vessels and, on occasion, to establish a specific diagnosis.

Juvenile Nasopharyngeal Angiofibromas

A nasopharyngeal angiofibroma [36] is an uncommon lesion found almost exclusively in the nasopharynx of the adolescent male. It is very vascular, is locally invasive, and can have a variable blood supply. Smaller lesions may be supplied entirely by branches of the external carotid artery (usually the internal maxillary branch); they may extend across the midline, lateral to the pterygoid fossa and posteriorly. The lesions may derive vascular supplies from dural branches of the internal carotid artery as they extend cephalad into the sphenoid sinus. Multiple projections during superselective angiography should include frontal, lateral, and mentovertical views of both internal and external vascular supplies (Fig. 14-42).

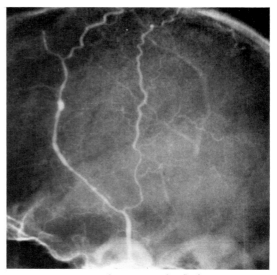

Fig. 14-39. Temporal arteritis. The findings are straightening, diffuse areas of narrowing, and arterial dilatation.

Fig. 14-40. A large false aneurysm (*short wide arrow*) involving the external carotid artery with a fistula to the external jugular vein (*long thin arrow*) in a patient who suffered a recent automobile accident.

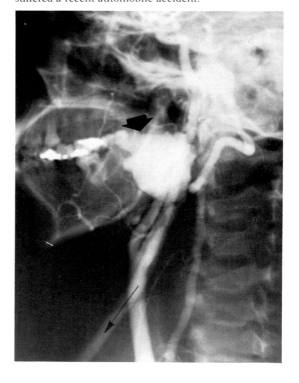

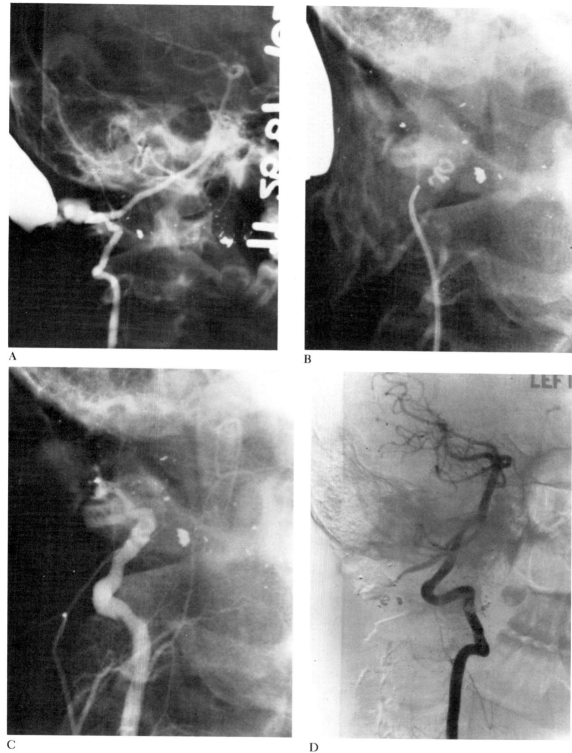

A

B

C

D

Fig. 14-41.

A. Severe bleeding from a false aneurysm in the high right vertebral artery 4 days after a gunshot wound (gloved finger controls bleeding).

B. Vessel embolized with coils distal and proximal to the lesion through a thin-walled 5 French catheter. The left vertebral artery and basilar arteries were patent and uninvolved (not shown).

C. Postembolization right vertebral artery (occluded).

D. Left vertebral artery (patent).

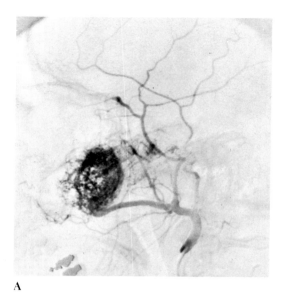

A

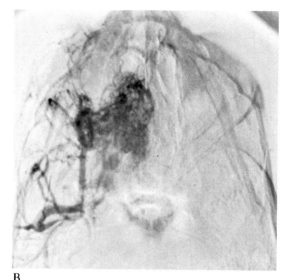

B

Chemodectomas

Chemodectomas [35] are slow-growing, hypervascular tumors of varying sizes, which in the head and neck are primarily located in the region of the carotid body (carotid body tumor), the inferior ganglion of the vagus nerve (glomus vagale tumor), the jugular bulb (glomus jugulare), and the floor of the middle ear (glomus tympanicum, which lies along the course of the tympanic branch of the glossopharyngeal nerve).

Carotid Body Tumors

Carotid body tumors are supplied primarily by the external carotid artery and often widen the angle of the common carotid bifurcation (Fig. 14-43). Other vessels, such as the thyrocervical and costocervical trunks of the subclavian artery and the vertebral muscular branches, may sometimes supply these tumors.

Glomus Vagale Tumors

Glomus vagale tumors lie more cephalad in the neck and deep to the angle of the mandible. They are supplied primarily by branches of the external carotid artery, and there is anterior displacement of both internal and external carotid arteries (Fig. 14-44).

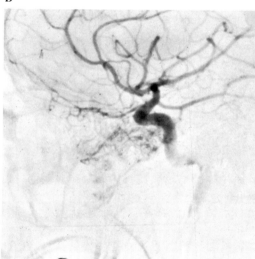

C

Fig. 14-42. Nasopharyngeal angiofibroma.
A. Lateral projection subtraction film of a selective right external carotid arteriogram. There is a hypervascular mass supplied by the internal maxillary artery.
B. Similar injection: a mentovertical view showing posterior and medial extension of the tumor.
C. Lateral projection subtraction film of a right internal carotid arteriogram showing vascular supply to the tumor from branches of the internal carotid artery.

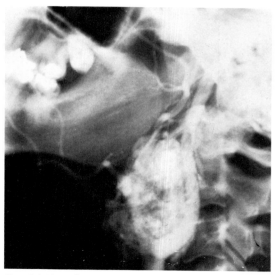

Fig. 14-43. Selective left common carotid arteriogram of a carotid body tumor. The hypervascular mass widens the angle of the bifurcation.

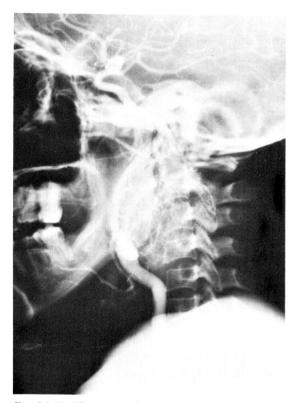

Fig. 14-44. Glomus vagale tumor of the left neck. The large, hypervascular tumor displaces the common, internal, and external carotid arteries anteriorly.

Glomus Jugulare Tumors

Glomus jugulare tumors (Fig. 14-45) are supplied primarily by the external carotid artery. Larger tumors may be supplied by branches of the internal carotid artery, the vertebral arteries, the contralateral external carotid artery, and the branches of the thyrocervical trunk. The tumors may invade and obstruct the jugular vein; this is important information for the surgeon. If the jugular vein anatomy is not well seen on the subtraction film of the venous phase of the arteriogram, a retrograde internal jugular venogram is required.

Tumors of the Glomus Tympanicum

Because of their location, glomus tympanicum tumors are clinically detected earlier than others and are usually smaller at the time of diagnosis. Selective angiographic and subtraction techniques are essential in demonstrating the small tumor stain in the petrous bone.

Other Primary Tumors

Other primary tumors of the neck and face include primary neurogenic tumors, malignant neoplasms involving the skull or scalp, and those involving the bony structures. These tumors are of varying degrees of vascularity. Sometimes the only angiographic manifestation is displacement of major branches or encasement or occlusion, with only a faint display of neovascularity or tumor stain.

Metastases

Metastatic lesions to the neck usually display the angiographic manifestations of vascularity common to the primary lesion (e.g., hypervascular metastases from a thyroid carcinoma).

Thyroid Lesions

The thyroid is supplied by the superior and inferior thyroid arteries. The superior thyroid artery arises anteriorly as the first branch of the external carotid artery. The inferior thyroid artery is the most medial branch of the thyrocervical trunk. These arteries can become hypertrophied with thyroid adenomas, diffuse goiter with thyrotoxicosis, and malignant tumors of the thyroid gland. In the benign lesions, the contours of the gland tend to be regular and well defined; in the malignant lesions, typical neovascularity and poorly defined margins are evident.

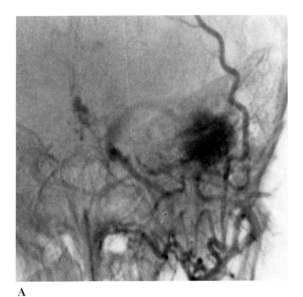

A

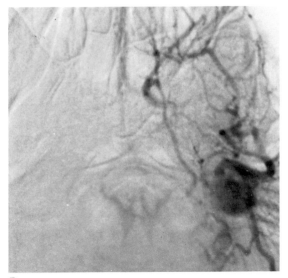

B

INTRACRANIAL LESIONS

The discussion of other specific intracranial lesions is beyond the scope of this text. The reader is referred to standard textbooks in neuroradiology [2, 32, 49].

Interventional Procedures of the Brachiocephalic Vessels

Percutaneous transluminal angioplasty may be performed on stenotic lesions of selected brachiocephalic vessels. Endovascular therapeutic embolization is helpful in a number of lesions in the extracranial brachiocephalic circulation as well as intracranially.

There is an understandable reluctance to perform brachiocephalic interventional procedures for fear of permanent neurologic damage due to inadvertent occlusion or embolization of vessels supplying vital structures. Only persons experienced with catheter techniques, familiar with vascular anatomy, technically facile with interventional methods, knowledgeable enough to choose correctly from the variety of available endovascular therapeutic methods, and alert to early clinical and angiographic signs of potential problems should perform the procedure. It is also important to be familiar with the patient's clinical presentation and alternate measures of treatment and to have a well-informed rapport with both patient and attending physicians. One must weigh the potential danger

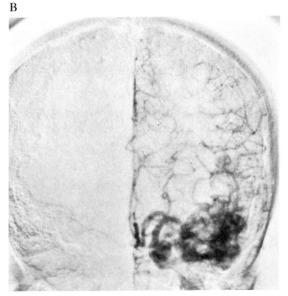

C

Fig. 14-45. Glomus jugulare tumor invading the left jugular fossa (subtraction films).
A. External carotid arteriogram (AP projection).
B. External carotid arteriogram (mentovertical view).
C. Internal carotid arteriogram (AP projection). The vascular supply is from both the internal carotid and the external carotid systems.

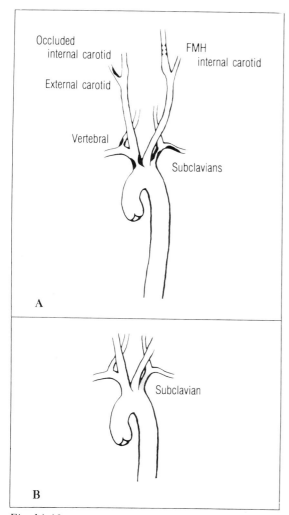

Fig. 14-46.
A. Indications for PTA of brachiocephalic vessels
   (FMH = fibromuscular hyperplasia).
B. Contraindications.

and benefit of the procedure against those of high-risk surgery or of permitting a patient to succumb to an untreated, potentially curable lesion.

PERCUTANEOUS TRANSLUMINAL ANGIOPLASTY OF BRACHIOCEPHALIC VESSELS

Indications

There are certain vessels that, under limited circumstances, may be treated by percutaneous transluminal angioplasty (PTA). They should all be symptomatically related to the involved vessel. They should be either unapproachable by surgery or of lesser risk and cost than surgery. These vessels

include stenosis of: left and right subclavian arteries (with subclavian steal or ischemic symptoms to the upper extremity) [30]; innominate artery; vertebral artery origin (concentric, nonulcerating lesion) [29, 31]; internal carotid artery (nonatherosclerotic, e.g., fibromuscular dysplasia, high in cervical course, and inaccessible to surgery) [3, 7, 46]; external carotid artery origin (when there is occlusion of the internal carotid artery or high-grade stenosis of a siphon) [7, 27]; common carotid artery (sometimes in conjunction with surgery) (Fig. 14-46).

General Methodology

Review the *general methodology* of percutaneous transluminal angioplasty in Chapter 6.

Special Preparations

Special preparations are required for PTA of brachiocephalic vessels. These are geared to preventing platelet deposition and thrombus formation, and to decreasing cerebral edema if there is inadvertent cerebral embolization. Patients should be on antiplatelet therapy for at least 2 days prior to the procedure. This includes aspirin 300 mg tid and dipyridamole 50 mg tid. Dexamethasone 10 mg IM should be administered with the preangiographic medications of diazepam 10 mg PO and atropine 0.5 mg IM. The patient must be awake and alert during the procedure in order to permit detection of earliest signs of neurologic deficit. Nifedipine 10 mg PO or SL should be available to reduce arterial spasm in certain vascular beds (e.g., external and internal carotid arteries). Intravenous low molecular weight dextran, administered slowly during the procedure, will decrease platelet aggregation. Heparin 5000 IU IV or IA should be administered through the catheter during the procedure. It should not be used during PTA of fibromuscular dysplasia lesions, for dissecting intramural lesions may be a hazard [7].

Precautions

There are important *precautions* common to all brachiocephalic PTA procedures. These include:

1. An accurate assessment of the location and length of the lesion as well as of any accompanying lesions of the other brachiocephalic vessels that may be contributing to the patient's symptoms.

2. The target lesion should be evaluated on films and lead skin markers placed for fluoroscopic monitoring, in order to save valuable time during balloon catheter placement. IA-DSA capabilities for monitoring the procedure also help in this regard.

3. Immediately prior to the procedure, the angioplasty balloon should be carefully purged of air by introducing half-strength low-density contrast medium and suctioning it with the catheter upside down. Air emboli cannot be tolerated in the brain in case of a ruptured balloon. The balloon should respond rapidly to inflation and deflation.

4. Careful manipulation of the floppy tipped guidewire through the lesion is required. The balloon catheter must never be advanced through the lesion except over a leading guidewire through the lesion.

5. With some of the vessels there should be pressure monitoring through a closed manifold system.

6. The periods of inflation should be short (5 seconds in internal and external carotid and vertebral arteries, 15–30 seconds in others).

7. The patient's neurologic status must be carefully monitored.

Subclavian Artery Stenosis

Subclavian artery stenoses may be neurologically symptomatic if found proximal to the vertebral artery, particularly if the vertebral artery is the dominant vessel and if there is stenosis of other associated brachiocephalic vessels. Embolic debris from the procedure entering the vertebral artery does not appear to be a problem [30, 31, 38], possibly because of retrograde flow down this vessel during and for several seconds after completion of the angioplasty procedure. Transluminal dilation of a stenotic right subclavian artery is potentially more risky than the left, because the immediately adjacent right carotid artery may transport debris intracranially. This has caused some interventionists to compress the right carotid artery during the dilation maneuver (to divert flow to the right subclavian peripheral vasculature) or to use a right axillary approach [62]. Lesions having impact on or across the vertebral artery origin are at risk for occluding this branch during the procedure. Irregular ulcerating plaques have a higher risk for em-

bolization, particularly to the upper extremity. Thrombosis of the vessel is a contraindication to PTA, for debris from this lesion may embolize peripherally (Fig. 14-46B).

TECHNIQUE. Prior to the procedure, measure the diameter and length of the lesion and the diameter of the adjacent normal vessel. The diameter of the selected balloon should equal that of the normal adjacent vessel. Determine the position of the stenosis in relation to the vessel origin and to that of the vertebral artery. A femoral approach is preferred. An axillary approach may also be used, but puncturing the vessel with a dampened pulse is sometimes difficult. Catheterize the origin of the subclavian artery with a 5 French, thin-walled catheter with a gentle distal curve (multipurpose) or a Hincks head-hunter curve. Gently probe the stenotic lumen with a floppy 0.035-in. guidewire tip (Benson or 15-mm J), avoiding force; when the guidewire is through the lesion, advance the 5 French catheter beyond the stenosis. Withdraw the guidewire, measure intraluminal pressures, and introduce 4000 to 5000 IU heparin through the catheter. Replace the floppy tip guidewire with a heavy-duty 185- to 220-cm long 0.038-in. guidewire, passing it well beyond the subclavian artery but allowing 100 cm of the guidewire external to the patient. Replace the 5 French diagnostic catheter with a 7 French 100-cm angioplasty balloon catheter. An angioplasty catheter with a tapered balloon is particularly useful in this area [30]. Do not force the balloon catheter through the stenotic lesion. If it does not pass easily, the lesion may have to be predilated with a Staple van Andel tapered-tip 7 French catheter. Once the balloon lies across the lesion, inflate it for periods of 15 to 30 seconds, always monitoring the patient clinically. Often only one or two dilations are necessary. Monitor the results of dilation with IA-DSA. Whereas before dilation there is no antegrade flow up the vertebral artery, once the vessel is successfully dilated, the subclavian steal is reversed, the gradient disappears, and systemic pressures are equal in both upper extremities. Usually subclavian arteries are easily dilated, but occasionally the plaques are firm and the stenosis severe, requiring multiple dilations (Figs. 14-47, 14-48, 14-49).

Innominate Artery

The same precautions are required with the innominate artery [31, 54, 62] as with the subclavian

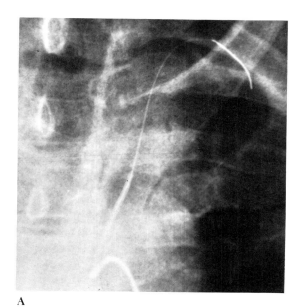

A

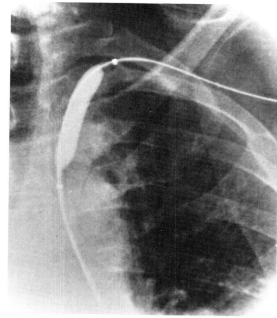

B

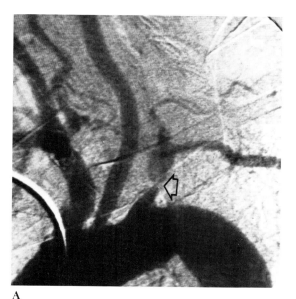

A

C

Fig. 14-47. PTA of the left subclavian stenosis seen in Fig. 14-2.
A. Steerable 0.018-in. guidewire required to bypass lesion.
B and C. Successful dilation of stenotic segment.

Fig. 14-48.
A. IV-DSA study shows severe stenosis of left subclavian artery with no antegrade filling of the left vertebral artery.
B. Conventional arteriogram better defines anatomy.
C and D. Deformity on balloon disappears, indicating successful dilation.
E. Successful dilation is confirmed by IA-DSA study, which shows antegrade flow through the left vertebral artery.

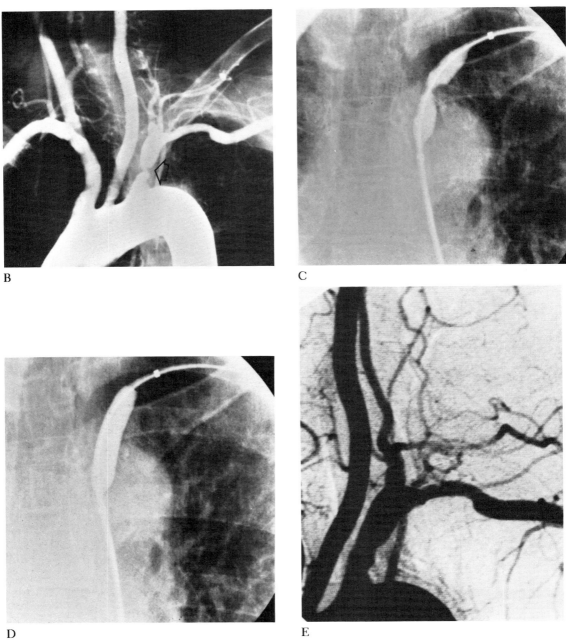

B

C

D

E

Fig. 14-48 (continued)

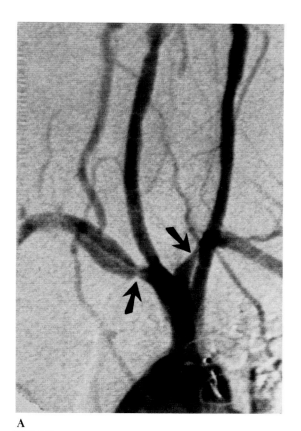

A

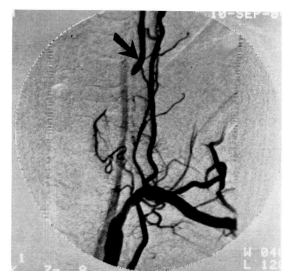

B

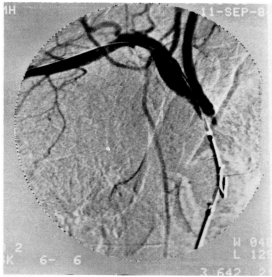

C

D

Fig. 14-49. Bilateral subclavian artery stenosis.

A. IA-DSA study of aortic arch in LPO projection shows right subclavian artery stenosis (*arrows*).

B. Selective left subclavian IA-DSA shows stenosis of the left proximal subclavian artery, occlusion of the left vertebral artery at its origin with distal portion filled by collaterals.

C. Right subclavian artery following PTA.

D. Left subclavian arteriogram following PTA. Note that the guidewire remains in the distal portion of the subclavian artery during the injection of contrast agent, with the catheter tip proximal to (and not within) the dilated segment.

artery. Only smooth concentric lesions should be considered, for there is added risk for cerebral embolization. Three methods of decreasing this risk are available: (1) Extrinsic compression of the right carotid artery during and immediately after the balloon has been deflated helps divert the flow of blood away from the carotid circulation. (2) Pass an occlusive balloon catheter up from the opposite femoral artery to lodge within the proximal right carotid artery. In the absence of neurologic response to test inflations, the angioplasty balloon catheter is next advanced over the stenotic lesion. Both balloons are then inflated for short periods (5–15 seconds) until the vessel is successfully dilated. (3) Dilate the innominate artery during operative carotid arteriotomy. By this means embolization of intravascular debris can be avoided by ensuring arterial back-bleeding at the arteriotomy site. This surgical procedure (carotid arteriotomy) is much less extensive than that required for endarterectomy or bypass procedure of the innominate artery. Similar angioplasty methods (sometimes combined with surgery) can be used for dilating the common carotid artery near its origin from the innominate artery or the aortic arch.

Vertebral Artery

Patients with vertebral basilar insufficiency (blurred vision, vertigo, ataxia, drop attacks) may be candidates for PTA of the vertebral artery. They should not have untreated concurrent carotid disease or should have continued symptoms despite prior carotid endarterectomy. The symptoms should be clearly related to the lesion. The stenotic lesions should be smooth and concentric, and should be located near the origin of the vertebral artery. The vessel distal to the stenosis should be free of disease. Marked tortuosity of the subclavian artery leading to the vertebral artery and tortuosity of the proximal vertebral artery distal to the stenosis may make successful catheterization and subsequent dilation of the vessel difficult or impossible. Surgical support should be available in case of complications.

TECHNIQUE. The same precautions are required as described for other brachiocephalic vessels. The point of stenosis is carefully monitored and marked on the skin surface with a lead marker. The vertebral artery is catheterized from a femoral approach with a 7 French Hincks head-hunter with a tapered 5 French tip. The tip is eased beyond the stenosis over a leading floppy-tipped guidewire. A straight flexible-tipped 220- or 260-cm 0.038-in. exchange guidewire replaces the initial guidewire, and the diagnostic catheter is replaced with a 100-cm 7 French 4-mm balloon angioplasty catheter with a 1-cm tip. Heparin 5000 IU is given intravenously during the procedure. Once the balloon is across the stenosis, it is dilated for 5-second intervals while the deformity of the balloon produced by the lesion and its subsequent disappearance are monitored fluoroscopically. No pressure measurements are made during the procedure, for the vessel is almost totally obstructed by the catheter. IA-DSA performed with the catheter withdrawn into the subclavian artery but a 0.028-in. guidewire still in place across the stenosis records the effectiveness of the treatment.

External Carotid Artery

Patients with occlusion of the internal carotid artery or severe stenosis of the internal carotid siphon frequently develop important collaterals from the ipsilateral external carotid branches. Also, these branches may be used to surgically bypass the occlusion (e.g., occipital artery to posterior fossa vessels, superficial temporal to middle cerebral artery [Fig. 14-28]). Stenosis of the external carotid artery at its origin jeopardizes these potential benefits and should therefore be corrected. PTA is a viable method, for there is less fear of intracerebral embolization when the internal carotid artery is occluded [7, 53].

TECHNIQUE. Methods used are similar to those for the other brachiocephalic vessels, including a lead marker on the patient's skin at the exact point of stenosis. A 7 French 100-cm long 4-mm diameter balloon catheter is advanced from the femoral artery over a 260-cm long 0.038-in. exchange guidewire previously positioned through a 5 or 6.5 French diagnostic catheter in the common carotid artery. The tip of the guidewire remains in the distal common carotid artery. The exchange guidewire is replaced with a 0.035-in. floppy-tipped steerable guidewire with a gentle curve on its end, which is advanced through the stenosis into the proximal external carotid artery to a level just proximal to the internal maxillary artery. A 5 French diameter angioplasty catheter may not be used, for it accepts only a 0.028-in. guidewire, and this catheter-guidewire combination is not sufficiently stable for advancing and manipulating the balloon catheter in the common carotid artery. A 0.016- or 0.018-in. steerable guidewire (alone or coaxially within a 0.038-in. injectable guidewire to give it body) may improve selective maneuverability. Nifedipine 10 mg SL helps prevent arterial spasm. The balloon catheter follows the guidewire, and 5-second dilations are carried out. Pressures are not measured across the stenosis due to the small size of the vessel being occluded by the catheter.

Internal Carotid Artery

Atherosclerotic plaques in the internal carotid artery usually involve the common carotid bifurcation, are often irregular, are prone to embolize, and should be managed surgically. There are, however, recent reports of successful percutaneous transluminal angioplasty of atherosclerotic stenotic lesions involving both the common carotid artery bifurcation as well as the proximal internal carotid artery in patients who are at high risk for surgery [14A, 51A]. Fibromuscular dysplasia usually involves the internal carotid artery higher in its course, often in areas inaccessible to surgery. Symptomatic patients with this condition are candidates for PTA. The procedure may be performed intraoperatively [46] or by the usual percutaneous approach [7, 31, 62].

TECHNIQUE. Technique is identical to that described above for external carotid PTA, except that a 5- or 6-mm diameter 3- or 4-cm long balloon catheter is used. Heparin is avoided due to the possibility of dissection and intramural bleeding.

THERAPEUTIC EMBOLIZATION

Indications

1. Extracranial
   a. AVMs
   b. Arteriovenous fistula
   c. Vascular neoplasms
   d. Trauma—bleeding, lacerated or transected arteries, false aneurysm
2. Intracranial
   a. AVM
   b. Arteriovenous fistula (carotid cavernous)
   c. Certain vascular tumors

Embolizing intracranial lesions should be almost solely in the realm of those neuroradiologists who have experience and sophisticated neurosurgical skill in the event of complications. The reader is referred to more comprehensive articles on this subject [9, 10, 21, 22, 52, 60].

Therapeutic embolization may be performed using standard percutaneous transluminal approaches. Occasionally the embolization may be performed jointly with the neurosurgeon placing the catheter through an arteriotomy site [9] or surgically interrupting a potentially dangerous vascular pathway prior to the procedure (Fig. 14-34). Some vascular lesions are best treated with initial embolization, making subsequent surgical removal easier and less dangerous (see Fig. 14-50) [50]. In all cases, safety during all phases of the study, superselective catheter placement, occlusion of the interstices of some lesions (not only the feeding vessel), and prevention of emboli to nontarget areas are particularly important. In more complex lesions, embolization may have to be carried out in multiple stages.

Review Chapter 5 for general principles of methodology, embolic material, and delivery systems used during percutaneous embolization. There are a number of features unique to embolization in the region of the head and neck that must be stressed regarding patient preparation, choice of embolic materials, and delivery systems [4, 5].

Patient Preparation

The risks, alternative methods of treatment, and expected results must be clearly understood by the patient. Complications such as cerebral infarction, intracranial hemorrhage, and even death must be discussed. A total angiographic evaluation of the lesion, with all possible feeding vessels and extracranial to intracranial communications, together with the vascular supply to cranial nerves, must be reviewed.

Corticosteroids (100 mg hydrocortisone IV) are given 12 hours prior to the procedure and gradually tapered over the next 72 hours to control cerebral edema and any associated inflammatory reaction encountered. Anticonvulsants are used when brain lesions are embolized. Broad spectrum antibiotics are given intravenously 4 hours before and for 2 to 3 days after the procedure to control any possible introduction of bacterial contaminants. The patient's electrocardiogram, vital signs, and neurologic status are closely monitored during the procedure; a urinary bladder indwelling catheter is positioned to prevent bladder distention and also to

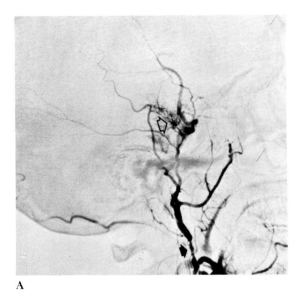

A

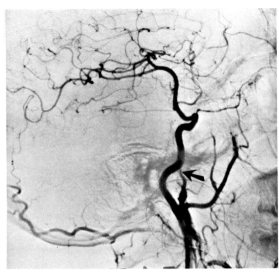

B

Fig. 14-50. Preoperative embolization of a large vascular meningioma.
A. Preembolization arteriogram. Note spasm of the distal external carotid artery (*arrow*).
B. Selective occlusion of middle meningeal artery (*arrow*) branches with Gelfoam.

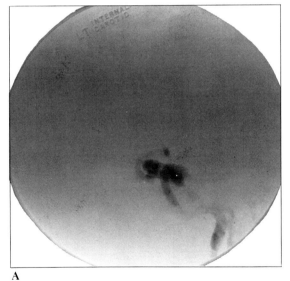

A

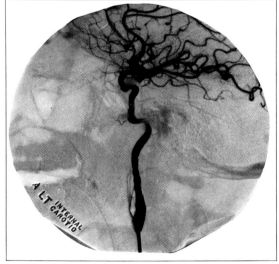

B

Fig. 14-51. An internal carotid-cavernous fistula secondary to a head injury from an auto accident treated with the Debrun detachable balloon.
A. Lateral carotid arteriogram before the balloon therapy. There is a large internal carotid-cavernous shunt with early filling of the ophthalmic vein and the superior and inferior petrosal sinus. Note the scanty anterior and middle cerebral artery perfusion.

B. After the balloon therapy, there is excellent contrast-medium filling of the intracranial circulation, without evidence of a fistula. There is slight narrowing of the internal carotid artery by the balloon which was filled with contrast material before being detached. (Courtesy Dr. Ralph Heinz, Duke University Medical Center, Durham, NC.)

monitor urinary output. Neuroleptanalgesia is induced by an anesthesiologist using fentanyl (0.002 mg/kg). Children are examined angiographically and treated under general anesthesia.

Introduce an arterial sheath with a hemostasis valve (usually 7 French but sometimes smaller) into the femoral artery puncture site, through which all catheters may be easily introduced. A catheter occluded by embolic materials or clot may be easily removed and exchanged. The sheath is sutured to the skin to prevent inadvertent withdrawal.

The sidearm in the hub allows continuous infusion of heparinized saline with a positive pressure pump that prevents clot formation between the catheter and sheath. In patients with no contraindications to anticoagulation, and in whom small branches are being catheterized, 3000 or 4000 IU of heparin may be given systemically to prevent formation of clots. Calcium channel blockers (nifedipine 10 mg PO or SL) should be given to prevent vasospasm.

Embolic Material and Delivery System
The type of embolic material used depends on the nature of the lesion under investigation, its vascular anatomy and relationship to uninvolved vessels, its flow characteristics, the accessibility of the lesion by the catheter, and whether or not permanent occlusion is desired. Thus, if the lesion is peripheral in location (e.g., intracranial) and is accessible only by microcatheter, liquid embolic materials or detachable balloons are necessary. If a larger bore catheter tip can be wedged into the target vessel of an external carotid branch, other particulate or liquid materials may be introduced. If there are large communicating vessels to the venous system present, a coil or detachable balloon is used [12, 37, 58]. If only temporary occlusion is necessary (as in epistaxis), Gelfoam is selected [18]. The embolic material also depends on the type of delivery system that can be successfully positioned for the embolization. See Tables 5-1 and 5-2.

THE EXTERNAL CAROTID ARTERY. In general, *external carotid* branches are superselectively catheterized with a coaxial catheter delivery system. A thin-walled 5 French catheter may be advanced to the orifice of the internal maxillary artery, occipital, facial, or ascending pharyngeal branches. The Berenstein catheter has a 7 French

shaft with torque control, but its distal 10 cm has a 5 French diameter with a small hockey-stick curve. This combination allows excellent external control for superselective placement of the catheter tip. A 3 French inner Teflon catheter or injectable lumen guidewire may be advanced coaxially further into the lesion through this catheter. Sometimes the tip of a standard 5 French catheter can be wedged into the target vessel for direct introduction of particulate material.

Better control of flow, and therefore more accurate positioning of the embolic material is obtained with an occlusive balloon catheter (see Fig. 5-12). The modified (Berenstein) occlusive balloon catheter has a 6 French shaft and an inner lumen that accepts a 0.038-in. guidewire, an open-ended injectable wire, and a coaxial 3 French catheter. Both liquid (bucrylate) and particulate injectables, including Ivalon and coils of varying diameter helix, may be introduced. The occlusive balloon also prevents reflux of emboli into the proximal circulation. To position the balloon catheter, the external carotid artery is first catheterized with a conventional diagnostic catheter, which is then exchanged for the balloon catheter over a 260-cm guidewire previously advanced to the proximal portion of the internal maxillary artery. The smaller, 3 French coaxial catheter can be manipulated into smaller target branches for eventual embolization with the help of an inner 0.018-in. steerable guidewire.

By inflating the balloon, the volume of subsequent embolic material required to treat the lesion can be estimated by determining how much contrast agent is required to fill the lesion.

There are certain precautions when tissue adhesive is injected into selective external carotid branches.

1. The injection should be fluoroscopically monitored. To do so requires a radiopaque adhesive. It is made radiopaque, but is otherwise unchanged, by adding tantalum (gray-colored powder; 1 gm/ml bucrylate) or tantalum oxide (white; used if near the skin surface). This combination hardens immediately on contact with blood or other ionic materials. The adhesive is made radiopaque with a longer polymerizing time (2–3 seconds) by adding Pantopaque (50% volume). This allows further penetration of vessels.

2. The flow of adhesive is limited if it is injected into a closed system beyond an inflated balloon; it penetrates further if the balloon is deflated during injection or a balloon system is not used.

3. Do not overinject into a circulation closed with an occlusive balloon. Intracranial-extracranial anastomoses may open with reflux into the brain. Overfilling the vessel may cause the catheter tip to adhere to the vessel wall. Estimate the amount needed by measuring the quantity of contrast agent required to fill the lesion with the balloon inflated.

4. Do not inject adhesive directly through an inflated balloon catheter to avoid adhesion of the tip to the vessel wall.

5. Inject through an inner coaxial catheter advanced well beyond the tip of the occlusive balloon or standard catheter. Coat the tip of the 3 French catheter with a thin layer of silicone to ease its withdrawal.

6. Precede the injection of tissue adhesive, and flush it out of the catheter system, with small controlled injections of nonionic 5% glucose. Simultaneously injecting 5% glucose through the outer balloon catheter during the injection of the bucrylate also helps prevent adhesion to the vessel wall. Withdraw the inner catheter when near the end of the bucrylate injection.

7. Allow the glue to polymerize and occlude the vessel over a period of a few seconds before deflating the balloon. Deflate the balloon slowly to avoid reflux of emboli back into circulation proximal to the catheter tip.

INTERNAL CAROTID ARTERY. Embolization of the internal carotid artery intracranial branches requires a flow-directed 2 French catheter. For arteriovenous fistulas the Debrun [10] or White [58] detachable balloon catheter is introduced (Fig. 14-51). A Kerber calibrated-leak balloon catheter [11, 21, 22] is required for depositing liquid tissue adhesive into AVMs (see Appendix 16).

VERTEBRAL ARTERY. A traumatized vertebral artery may require total embolic occlusion [6]. Embolization should be performed only if the opposite vertebral artery is patent. Detachable balloon catheters may be used [12]; however, coils are less expensive and more widely available, and require less expertise (see Fig. 14-41). Be sure to use a coil of appropriate helix diameter. One that is too small

migrates up the vessel beyond the target area; one that is too large elongates in the artery with the danger of its proximal end extruding into the parent subclavian vessel (see Fig. 14-34). If the vertebral artery has to be sacrificed, the coils or balloons should be placed on either side of the site of trauma. This prevents blood from entering it in an antegrade fashion up the vessel proximal to the lesion and also retrograde down the vertebral artery distal to the lesion. As a rule, arteriovenous fistulas are best treated with detachable balloons, usually from the arterial side, but occasionally from the venous side. By depositing the balloon into the fistulous opening, one may preserve the integrity of the vertebral artery.

References

1. Bailey, L., and Loeser, T. Intracranial aneurysms. *J.A.M.A.* 211:1993, 1971.

2. Baker, R., Raumbaugh, C., and Kido, D. Pathology of Cerebral Vessels. In H. Abrams (ed.), *Abrams' Angiography: Vascular and Interventional Radiology* (3rd ed.). Boston: Little, Brown, 1983. Pp. 271–303.

3. Belan, A., et al. Percutaneous transluminal angioplasty of fibromuscular dysplasia of the internal carotid artery. *Cardiovasc. Intervent. Radiol.* 5:79, 1982.

4. Berenstein, A., and Kricheff, I. Embolization Techniques Used in Head and Neck Pathology. In R. Bergeron, A. Osborne, and P. Som (eds.), *Head and Neck Imaging Excluding the Brain.* St. Louis: Mosby, 1984. Pp. 353–373.

5. Berenstein, A., and Kricheff, I. Catheter and material selection for transarterial embolization technical considerations. I. Catheters. II. Material. *Radiology* 132:619, 1979.

6. Bergsjordet, B., et al. Vertebral artery embolization for control of massive hemorrhage. *A.J.N.R.* 5:201, 1984.

7. Bird, C. R., and Hasso, A. Percutaneous Transluminal Angioplasty of the Carotid Artery. In W. Castaneda-Zuniga (ed.), *Transluminal Angioplasty.* New York: Thieme-Stratton, 1983. Pp. 154–161.

8. Bryan, R., et al. Neuroangiography with Iohexol. *A.J.N.R.* 4:344, 1983.

9. Cromwell, L., and Harris, A. Treatment of cerebral arteriovenous malformations: Combined neurosurgical and neuroradiologic approach. *A.J.N.R.* 4:366, 1983.

10. Debrun, G., et al. Embolization of cerebral arteriovenous malformations with bucrylate. Experience in 46 cases. *J. Neurosurg.* 56:615, 1982.

11. Debrun, G., et al. Two different calibrated leak balloons: Experimental work and applications in humans. *A.J.N.R.* 3:407, 1982.

12. Debrun, G., et al. Endovascular occlusion of verte-

bral fistulae by detachable balloons with conservation of the vertebral flow. *Radiology* 130:141, 1979.

13. Djindjian, R., and Merland, J. *Superselective Arteriography of the External Carotid Artery.* Berlin: Springer-Verlag, 1978.

14. Fields, W., et al. Joint study of extracranial arterial occlusion. V. Following surgical or nonsurgical treatment for transient cerebral attacks and cervical carotid artery lesions. *J.A.M.A.* 23:211, 1973.

14A. Frietag, J., Coke, R., and Wagemann, W. Percutaneous angioplasty of carotid artery stenosis. *Neuroradiology,* 28:126, 1986.

15. Gomensoro, J., et al. Joint study of extracranial arterial occlusion. VIII. Clinical radiographic correlation of carotid bifurcation lesions in 177 patients with transient cerebral ischemic attacks. *J.A.M.A.* 244:95, 1973.

16. Haughton, V., and Rosenbaum, A. E. The Normal and Anomalous Aortic Arch and Brachiocephalic Arteries. In T. H. Newton and D. G. Potts (eds.), *Radiology of the Skull and Brain: Angiography.* St. Louis: Mosby, 1974. Vol. 2, Book 2, p. 1145.

17. Hinshaw, D., Jr., Thompson, J., and Hasso, A. Adult arteriosclerotic moyamoya. *Radiology* 118:633, 1976.

18. Horton, J., et al. Polyvinyl alcohol foam—Gelfoam for therapeutic embolization: A synergistic mixture. *A.J.N.R.* 4:143, 1983.

19. Houser, O., et al. Spontaneous cervical cephalic arterial dissection and its residuum: Angiographic spectrum. *A.J.N.R.* 5:27, 1984.

20. Houser, O., et al. Atheromatous disease of the carotid artery: Correlation of angiographic, clinical, and surgical findings. *J. Neurosurg.* 41:321, 1974.

21. Kerber, C., Bank, W., and Manelfe, C. Control and placement of intracranial microcatheters. *A.J.N.R.* 12:157, 1980.

22. Kerber, C. W., and Heilman, C. B. New calibrated-leak microcatheters for cyanoacrylate embolization and chemotherapy. *A.J.N.R.* 6:434, 1985.

23. Kido, D., Baker, R., and Raumbaugh, C. Normal Cerebral Vascular Anatomy. In H. Abrams (ed.), *Abrams' Angiography: Vascular and Interventional Radiology* (3rd ed.). Boston: Little, Brown, 1983. Pp. 231–270.

24. Lasjaunias, P. Arteriography of the Head and Neck: Normal Functional Anatomy of the External Carotid Artery. In R. Bergeron, A. Osborne, and P. Som (eds.), *Head and Neck Imaging Excluding the Brain.* St. Louis: Mosby, 1984. Pp. 344–354.

25. Lasjaunias, P. *Craniofacial and Upper Cervical Arteries.* Baltimore: Williams & Wilkins, 1981.

26. Lin, J., and Kricheff, I. Angiographic investigation of cerebral aneurysms. *Radiology* 105:69, 1972.

27. Mirfakhraee, M., et al. External carotid angioplasty in cerebrovascular insufficiency. *Radiographics* 4:423, 1984.

28. Moncada, R., et al. Selective temporal arteriography and biopsy in giant cell arteritis. Polymyalgia rheumatica. *Am. J. Roentgenol.* 122:580, 1974.

29. Motarjeme, A. Percutaneous Transluminal Angioplasty of the Vertebral Artery. In W. Castaneda-Zuniga (ed.), *Transluminal Angioplasty.* New York: Thieme-Stratton, 1983. Pp. 200–202.

30. Motarjeme, A., et al. Percutaneous transluminal angioplasty for treatment of subclavian "steal." *Radiology* 155:611, 1985.

31. Motarjeme, A., et al. Percutaneous transluminal angioplasty of the brachiocephalic arteries. *A.J.N.R.* 3:169, 1982.

32. Newton, T. H., and Potts, D. G. *Radiology of the Skull and Brain: Angiography.* St. Louis: Mosby, 1974. Vol. 2, Books 1–4.

33. Newton, T. H., and Troost, B. Arteriovenous Malformations and Fistulas. In T. H. Newton and D. G. Potts (eds.), *Radiology of the Skull and Brain: Angiography.* St. Louis: Mosby, 1974. Vol. 2, Book 4, p. 2490.

34. Nov, A., et al. Internal carotid occlusion by DSA. "Diagnostic trap" relearned. *A.J.N.R.* 6:105, 1985.

35. Palacios, E. Chemodectomas of the head and neck. *Am. J. Roentgenol.* 110:129, 1970.

36. Patterson, C. Juvenile nasopharyngeal angiofibroma. *Otolaryngol. Clin. North Am.* 6:839, 1973.

37. Pevsner, P., and Doppman, J. Therapeutic embolization with a micro-balloon catheter system. *A.J.N.R.* 1:171, 1980.

38. Ringelstein, E., and Zeumer, H. Delayed reversal of vertebral artery blood flow following percutaneous transluminal angioplasty for subclavian "steal" syndrome. *Neuroradiology* 26:189, 1984.

39. Rothfus, W., et al. Cerebellar venous angioma: "Benign entity?" *A.J.N.R.* 5:61, 1984.

40. Sage, M., et al. Comparison of blood-brain barrier disruption in intracarotid Iopamidol and methylglucamine iothalamate. *A.J.N.R.* 4:8938, 1983.

41. Savoiardo, M., Strada, L., and Passerini, A. Intracranial cavernous hemangiomas: Neuroradiologic review of 36 operated cases. *A.J.N.R.* 4:945, 1983.

42. Sclafani, S. Transcatheter control of arterial bleeding in the neck, mediastinum, and chest. *Semin. Intervent. Radiol.* 2(2):130, 1985.

43. Seeger, J., and Carmody, R. Digital subtraction angiography of the arteries of the head and neck. *Radiol. Clin. North Am.* 23(2):193, 1985.

44. Seeger, J., Carmody, R., and Goldstone, J. Intravenous digital subtraction angiography of the nearly occluded internal carotid artery. *A.J.N.R.* 5:35, 1984.

45. Sheldon, J., et al. Intravenous DSA of intracranial carotid lesions: Comparison with other techniques and specimens. *A.J.N.R.* 5:547, 1984.

46. Smith, D., Smith, L., and Hasso, A. Fibromuscular dysplasia of the internal carotid artery treated by operative transluminal angioplasty. *Radiology* 155:645, 1985.

47. Stanley, J., et al. Extracranial internal carotid and vertebral artery fibrodysplasia. *Arch. Surg.* 109:215, 1974.

48. Takahashi, M., Bussaka, H., and Nakagawa, N.

Evaluation of the cerebral vasculature by intra-arterial DSA. With emphasis on *in vivo* resolution. *Neuroradiol.* 26:253, 1984.

49. Taveras, J. M., and Wood, E. H. Diagnostic Neuroradiology. Section I in L. L. Robbins (ed.), *Golden's Diagnostic Radiology* (2nd ed.). Baltimore: Williams & Wilkins, 1976.

50. Teasdale, E., et al. Subselective preoperative embolization for meningiomas. A radiological and pathological assessment. *J. Neurosurg.* 60:506, 1984.

51. Toole, J., et al. Transient ischemic attacks due to atherosclerosis: A prospective study of 160 patients. *Arch. Neurol.* 32:5, 1972.

51A. Tsai, F. Y., et al. Percutaneous transluminal angioplasty of carotid artery. *A.J.N.R.* 7:349, 1986.

52. Vinuella, F., et al. Preembolization of superselective angiography. Role in the treatment of brain arteriovenous malformations with isobutyl-2 cyanoacrylate. *A.J.N.R.* 5:765, 1984.

53. Vitek, J., and Morawitz, R. Percutaneous transluminal angioplasty of the external carotid artery. *A.J.N.R.* 3:541, 1982.

54. Vitek, J., Ramon, B., and Oh, F. J. Innominate artery angioplasty. *A.J.N.R.* 5:113, 1984.

55. Weibel, J., and Fields, W. S. *Atlas of Arteriography in Occlusive Cerebral Vascular Disease.* Philadelphia: Saunders, 1969.

56. Weinstein, M., et al. Intraarterial digital subtraction angiography of the head and neck. *Radiology* 147:717, 1983.

57. Wendling, L. R., et al. Intracerebral venous angiomas. *Radiology* 119:141, 1976.

58. White, R., et al. Embolotherapy with detachable silicone balloons. Technique and clinical results. *Radiology* 131:619, 1979.

59. Wolfel, D., et al. Outpatient arteriography: Its safety and cost effectiveness. *Radiology* 153:363, 1984.

60. Wolpert, S., and Stein, B. Factors governing the course of emboli in the therapeutic embolization of cerebral arteriovenous malformation. *Radiology* 131:125, 1979.

61. Wood, G. W., et al. Digital subtraction angiography with intravenous injection: Assessment of 1000 carotid bifurcations. *A.J.N.R.* 4:125, 1983.

62. Zeitler, E., Berger, G., and Schmitt-Ruth, R. Percutaneous Transluminal Angioplasty of the Supra-aortic Arteries. In C. Dotter et al. (eds.), *Percutaneous Transluminal Angioplasty.* Berlin: Springer-Verlag, 1983. Pp. 254–261.

63. Zimmerman, R., et al. Aortic arch digital arteriography: An alternative technique to digital venous angiography and routine arteriography in the evaluation of cerebral vascular insufficiency. *A.J.N.R.* 4:266, 1983.

Parathyroid Angiography—Arterial and Venous

Indications

Parathyroid angiography is indicated for detection of parathyroid adenomas following unsuccessful surgical exploration. It should be performed only if the following studies are unsuccessful: high resolution ultrasonography of the neck; thallium 201– technetium 99m pertechnetate thyroid subtraction scans; computed tomography; or, magnetic resonance imaging (if available) of the neck and mediastinum.

Technique

APPROACHES

Arterial Studies

1. The percutaneous femoral artery approach allows bilateral selective superior and inferior thyroid and internal mammary arteriography with a single percutaneous puncture. A complete arteriographic study requires selective injection of these six vessels. The inferior thyroid arteries are usually the most productive in outlining parathyroid adenomas.
2. Alternatively, in elderly patients with tortuous ectatic vessels, each axillary artery may be used for ipsilateral inferior thyroid and internal mammary angiography.

Venous Studies

The percutaneous femoral vein permits catheterization of the inferior, superior, and middle thyroid veins, as well as the veins of the mediastinum, from a single approach.

CATHETERS

Arterial Studies

1. A 5 or 6 French polyethylene or polyurethane 100-cm catheter with a modified Hincks No. 1 curve may be used. It is modified by shortening the distal tip to 5 mm and increasing its angle to 80 degrees (Fig. 15-1A). All six vessels (the superior and inferior thyroid and internal mammary arteries) can often be selectively catheterized with this shape. An unmodified 5 or 6.5 French Hincks catheter tip shape is also useful (Fig. 15-1A).
2. Alternatively, the Muller USCI guided catheter system[1] may be used.

Venous Studies

The Muller guided catheter system may be used with a woven Dacron 6 French soft-tipped catheter without side holes. External manipulation permits curves of varying diameters on the distal catheter. The catheter can also be "paid out" over the fixed wire curve deep into the vein. Contrast medium can be injected through a side entry into the handle of the closed system, thereby allowing checks for catheter position.

CONTRAST AGENTS, PROJECTIONS, AND RADIOGRAPHIC PROGRAMMING

Details concerning contrast media, projections, and radiographic programs in parathyroid angiography are given in Table 15-1.

Anatomic Considerations

Normally there are four small (average $5 \times 3 \times 1$ mm [16]) parathyroid glands, which are too small to be seen by angiography. The superior parathyroid glands lie adjacent to the posteromedial surface of each thyroid lobe at the junction of the middle and superior thirds. The inferior parathyroid glands lie adjacent to the posterolateral aspect of each lower thyroid pole. In approximately 5 percent, the glands lie in ectopic positions, and even more rarely, there may be supernumerary glands (up to six). It is largely for these reasons that there is a 5 to 10 percent surgical failure rate in finding parathyroid adenomas; 70 percent of those missed at surgery are in ectopically located parathyroid glands [10]. When the superior para-

---

[1] USCI, a division of C. R. Bard, Inc., Box 566, Billerica, MA 01821.

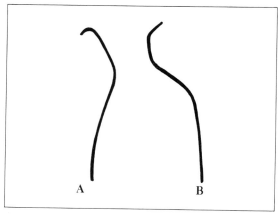

Fig. 15-1. Preformed catheter shapes for superior and inferior thyroid arteriography.
A. Modified Hincks No. 1 curve.
B. Hincks No. 1 curve.

thyroid glands are ectopically positioned, they usually lie more medially in a retropharyngeal or retroesophageal location, or they may descend into the posterior-superior mediastinum. When the inferior parathyroid glands are ectopically positioned, they may lie anywhere from the angle of the jaw (rare) (Figs. 15-2, 15-3) to the pericardium. More frequently, ectopic positions of inferior parathyroid glands are due to an extended descent during development into (1) the lower neck, (2) the anterior-superior mediastinum (with the thymus), or (3) the posterior-superior mediastinum. Supernumerary parathyroid glands are usually located in the mediastinum.

ARTERIAL STUDIES

The parathyroid glands are supplied by small arterial branches arising primarily from the inferior thyroid artery; this artery is therefore the most important vessel to inject [2, 3]. It arises from the thyrocervical trunk in conjunction with the ascending cervical branch and frequently with the transverse scapular branch. The thyrocervical trunk originates anterosuperiorly from the subclavian artery, most frequently in that short section lying between the vertebral artery and the costocervical trunk. Since it often arises in common with, or just superior to, the internal mammary artery, this artery is a good landmark during the procedure. If there is difficulty in selectively catheterizing the thyrocervical trunk, try entering the internal mammary artery first and then slowly

withdraw from it with the catheter tip directed anteriorly and superiorly.

Injection of the costocervical artery is dangerous because some of its branches may give off small feeding arteries that supply the spinal cord. Paraplegia has been encountered following overinjection of contrast medium into the costocervical trunk. Only very rarely is there a radicular branch to the anterior spinal artery arising from the thyrocervical trunk [2]. Familiarity with the anatomy of this area is essential.

The inferior thyroid artery is the most medial branch of the thyrocervical trunk and has two identifying loops, one cephalad and the other caudad (Fig. 15-3; see Fig. 15-8). The angiographer should make sure to identify these loops with small test injections prior to the arteriographic series. Since the loops are quite variable in location, displacement must not be considered diagnostic of a parathyroid mass. Small branches from the inferior thyroid artery descend downward to supply short segments of the esophagus. A poorly marginated muscular stain results, which must not be confused with the smooth margins of a parathyroid adenoma. Also, small inferior thyroid branches may arise proximally from the thyrocervical trunk to supply parathyroid ectopic adenomas, and a catheter advanced beyond this trunk may miss the lesion (see Fig. 15-7).

Less often, the superior thyroid artery may supply an adenoma. This usually occurs if the inferior thyroid artery has been surgically ligated, but it has also been described in patients with a lingual thyroid [8]. The superior thyroid artery arises anteriorly as the first branch of the external carotid artery and curves downward and medially to supply the superior pole of the thyroid gland (Fig. 15-4). It also supplies small branches to the neighboring muscles and portions of the pharynx.

The thyroid gland normally stains evenly throughout, following contrast injection, and the draining veins are well outlined on delayed films. A poorly marginated, nonhomogeneous stain results from opacification of small branches supplying adjacent muscles and portions of the larynx, and should not be mistaken for an adenoma.

Pay careful attention to anomalous vascular origins, particularly if an adenoma has not been uncovered following the routine six-vessel selective arteriograms. Sometimes a subclavian or innominate artery injection identifies these origins. The

Table 15-1. Technical specifications in parathyroid angiography

Angiographic procedure	Contrast agent[a]			Total films	Total time (sec)	Radiographic program[b] (films/sec)	Projections
	Density	Volume (ml/inj)	Rate (ml/sec)				
Arterial studies[c]							
Selective superior and inferior thyroid	L (NI)	7–10	2/sec (hand)	12	10	2/sec for 3 sec; 1/sec for 7 sec	AP (add oblique views if the tumor is seen)
Internal mammary	L (NI)	10–12	3/sec (hand)	12	10		
Venous studies[d]	L	10	4/sec (hand)	6	6	1/sec	AP

[a] Nonionic recommended.

[b] Start films 0.1 sec before start of injection to obtain film for subtraction mask. To ensure good subtraction films, do not permit breathing or swallowing during the injection. This is often difficult for the patient, who must be forewarned.

[c] Use the smallest possible focal spot for good detail. Center the films over the neck and upper half of the mediastinum for all selective thyroid artery injections. Repeat the study with oblique projections if a suspicious area is uncovered, since adenomas may lie retrotracheal (see Fig. 15-2) or behind the esophagus.

[d] A hand injection of 10 ml in one of the major draining veins will fill all the thyroid veins and will act as a "road map" for subsequent selective vein catheterization. A small test injection in the remaining veins with a single film will document the draining vein from which the sample is obtained.

L = low-density contrast agent; NI = nonionic (see Appendix 3).

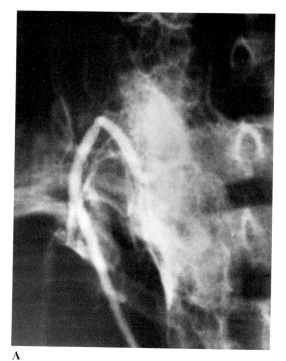

A

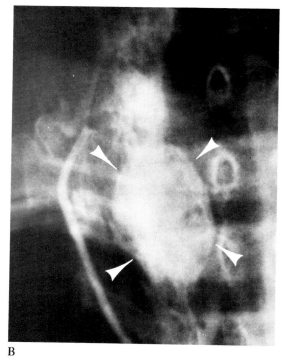

B

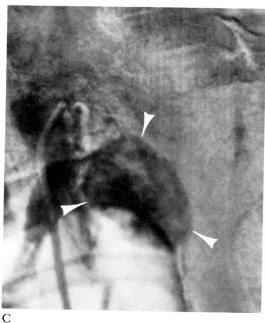

C

Fig. 15-2. Right-sided posteriorly located parathyroid adenoma arising from the right inferior thyroid artery.
A and B. Early and late phases of an inferior thyroid arteriogram, in AP projection. The adenoma is well marginated; it overlies but does not indent the tracheal air shadow.
C. RPO projection subtraction film determines the posterior position of the adenoma in the superior mediastinum.

thyroidea ima branch arises anomalously from the superior margin of the innominate artery. Occasionally the origin of the thyrocervical trunk is lateral to the costocervical trunk. Mediastinal parathyroid adenomas have an anomalous vascular supply either from the inferior thyroid artery, small branches arising from the thyrocervical trunk, or from the thymic trunk of the internal mammary artery. The thymic artery (the second branch to arise medially from the internal mammary artery) supplies the thymus and can enlarge to supply intrathymic parathyroid adenomas lying in the anterior-superior mediastinum. Previous surgery results in a distorted vascular pattern.

VENOUS STUDIES

The thyroid venous system is a diffuse anastomotic plexus of veins that surrounds the thyroid gland (Fig. 15-5). These veins drain via the superior and middle thyroid veins into the ipsilateral internal jugular vein. The paired inferior thyroid veins are most important to the angiographer. They usually join to form a single common inferior thyroid vein which enters into the superomedial border of the

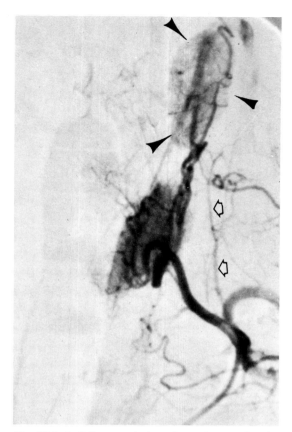

Fig. 15-3. Left thyrocervical trunk arteriogram showing a left parathyroid adenoma. The left inferior thyroid artery passes medially, opacifies a normal left thyroid lobe, and gives branches to an anomalously high and posteriorly positioned parathyroid adenoma (*arrowheads*). There is a normal ascending cervical branch (*open arrows*). The transverse scapular branch travels laterally. There is a high-lying parathyroid adenoma supplied by the inferior thyroid artery.

left innominate vein. The parathyroid glands drain into the lateral margins of these ipsilateral inferior thyroid veins, an important anatomic point during the catheterization for obtaining venous effluent. Samples from the medial aspect of the thyroid gland or of the isthmic segment are of little value [2].

Normal variants of draining thyroid veins are frequent and can be uncovered by a forceful hand injection (with three or four films exposed at one per second) into any thyroid vein first encountered. This serves as a helpful road map for subsequent catheter placement. An accessory left inferior thyroid vein may drain into the left innominate vein. The common inferior thyroid vein

may drain very medially into the superior border of the left innominate vein or at the junction of the left and right innominate veins. It may drain into the thymic vein, which enters the inferior aspect of the left innominate vein. Surgical ligation of the inferior thyroid vein distorts the anatomy, requiring catheterization of the middle or superior thyroid veins. Anterior mediastinal adenomas may drain into the inferior thymic vein. Since adenomas in the neck may also drain into this channel, the lesions in the low neck or in the anterior mediastinum may not be accurately localized by venous sampling alone. Adenomas in the neck and posterior mediastinum may also drain into the vertebral vein.

Approach to the Study

Studies should be performed in the following sequence prior to considering angiography for detecting operatively missed parathyroid adenomas.

1. High resolution ultrasonography of the neck [1, 14]. In the proper clinical setting, up to 80 percent of parathyroid adenomas *in the neck* can be located with high resolution ultrasonography using a 7.5- or 10-MHz transducer. Sonographic accuracy depends on both the size and the location of the lesion. It is most successful when adenomas lie within or adjacent to the thyroid glands (Fig. 15-6A). Those adenomas that lie in the retrotracheal and paraesophageal region are more difficult to see. Those in the superior mediastinum require other techniques such as CT or MRI. When lesions other than parathyroid tumors are suspected (thyroid adenomas, abnormal lymph nodes), direct puncture under ultrasonographic guidance for parathormone assay [5] or fine needle biopsy [13] may be performed.

2. Scintigraphic digital subtraction studies using technetium 99 pertechnetate and thallium 201 [6, 10, 12]. Thallium 201 localizes in abnormal parathyroid glands as well as in normal and abnormal thyroid tissue. A thyroid scan with ^{99m}Tc pertechnetate, performed to define the limits of thyroid tissue, is subtracted from the thallium image. The residual uptake image over the background represents an abnormal parathyroid lesion (Fig. 15-6B).

There is a high success rate with these sub-

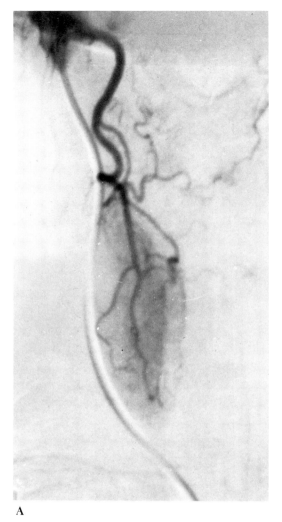
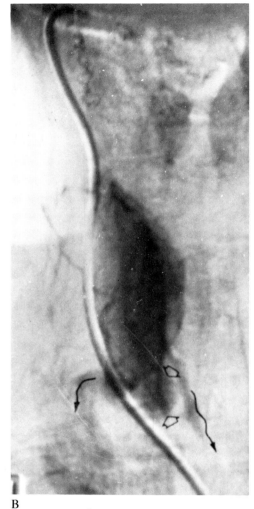

A   B

Fig. 15-4. Right parathyroid adenoma. This subtraction film of a right superior thyroid arteriogram clearly outlines the entire right lobe of the thyroid gland. Often only the uppermost portion is opacified.
A. Arterial phase.
B. Capillary and venous phases. The adenoma protrudes beyond the thyroid tissue (*open arrows*). The wavy arrows parallel the middle thyroid vein coursing laterally and the inferior thyroid vein draining medially. It is unusual for a superior thyroid artery to supply a parathyroid adenoma; if it does, usually the inferior thyroid artery has been surgically ligated.

traction techniques [6, 10]. False-negatives may be seen in lesions less than 5 mm in size. False-positive studies may occur with malignant thyroid lesions and metastasis to adjacent nodes. These studies are particularly helpful in lesions that are ectopic in position, such as in the superior mediastinum.
3. Computed tomography (CT) [14, 15] helps to uncover parathyroid adenomas in the superior mediastinum that cannot be observed by ultrasonography (Fig. 15-7). The diagnosis may be confirmed with direct CT-guided percutaneous puncture and aspiration for parathormone determination and/or biopsy. Magnetic resonance imaging is another screening method and has

shown an accuracy of 90 percent in detecting abnormalities of the parathyroid glands [13A].
4. Angiography is performed only if noninvasive methods are unsuccessful.

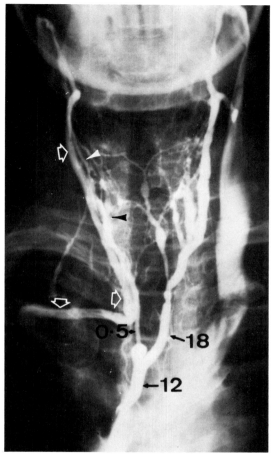

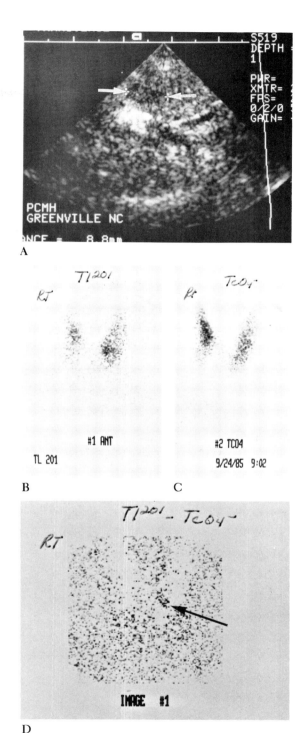

Fig. 15-5. Common inferior thyroid venogram. The left and right inferior thyroid veins drain into the common inferior thyroid vein; the left superior thyroid vein drains into the internal jugular vein. The right superior thyroid vein (*arrowheads*) and the anterior jugular vein (*open arrows*) are closely aligned. The numbers indicate the parathormone levels and show a parathormone gradient on the left which correctly identified a left-sided parathyroid adenoma.

Fig. 15-6.
A. Ultrasonography shows a parathyroid adenoma measuring 9 × 4 mm.
B. Thallium scan.
C. Technetium scan.
D. Thallium 201 minus technetium 99m pertechnetate digital subtraction scan demonstrates an area of increased uptake representing the parathyroid adenoma on the left (*arrow*).

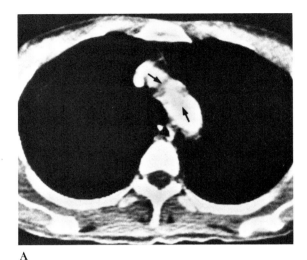

A

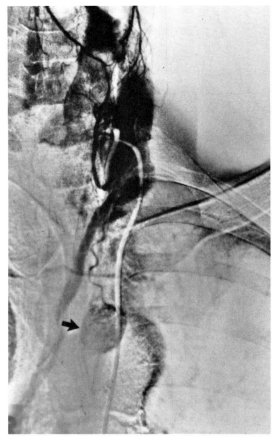

B

Selective six-vessel studies (bilateral inferior and superior thyroid arteries and internal mammary) are time consuming, require large doses of contrast medium and expertise, and have a potential for stroke or infarction of the spinal cord.

The dangers may be reduced by doing IA-DSA nonselective studies of the innominate artery, the left subclavian, and the left carotid arteries initially. These studies may detect up to half of the lesions [11], most of which are seen in the neck; they are less helpful in finding those located in the mediastinum [7]. The adenomas may be obscured by the blush of the normal thyroid gland or by overlying ectatic or tortuous vessels. IV-DSA has not been helpful in detecting parathyroid adenomas [9].

When all else fails, proceed with selective conventional magnification studies of the inferior thyroid, superior thyroid, and internal mammary arteries.

Fig. 15-7.
A. Computed tomography scan of superior mediastinum outlines a parathyroid vascular stain that was originally considered to be a mediastinal vessel (*arrows*).
B. Inferior thyroid arteriogram demonstrates the superior mediastinal tumor (*arrow*).

Selective Arterial and Venous Angiographic Studies

1. A linear dot thyroid scan should be obtained prior to angiography to determine the size and shape of the thyroid gland. The capillary parenchymal blush of the thyroid angiogram is then superimposed over the thyroid scan. Any vascular area not representative of functioning thyroid gland is considered to be tumor (Fig. 15-8).

2. Arterial and venous angiographic studies should be performed on different days, preferably with arteriography first. This procedure outlines the venous anatomy for subsequent venous studies. If considerable atherosclerosis is present, only venous studies should be performed because of the risks and the difficulties involved in arteriography. If a question still remains, it is easier and less risky to catheterize the inferior thyroid artery and internal mammary artery by bilateral axillary artery punctures. These are the most important vessels to determine the presence of ectopically positioned adenomas.

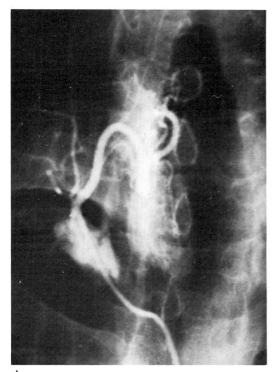

A

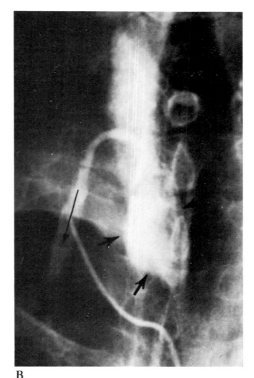

B

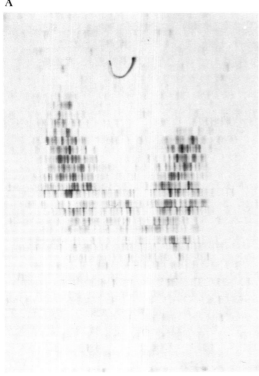

C

Fig. 15-8. Right parathyroid adenoma.
A and B. Arterial and venous phases of a right thyrocervical arteriogram. Short arrows point to the adenoma; the long arrow outlines the venous drainage.
C. The thyroid scan shows no radioisotope uptake over
  the corresponding area of angiographic stain of the
  parathyroid adenoma.

3. Arteriography localizes the adenoma as an abnormal but fairly well marginated vascular
   tumor blush, particularly if it extends beyond
   the normal thyroid gland as seen by thyroid
   scan [4]. It may be remote from the thyroid
   gland, lying in the upper neck or in the mediastinum. The inferior thyroid artery or a small
   proximal inferior thyroid branch usually supplies the adenoma, whether it is intrathyroid,
   juxtathyroid, or ectopic in location in the neck
   or in the posterior mediastinum. Rarely, these
   vessels supply ectopic adenomas seen in the anterior mediastinum, but anterior mediastinal
   adenomas usually are supplied by the thymic
   branch of the internal mammary artery.
4. The parathyroid adenoma may be flat and in
   one dimension and appear as a small pancake.
   It may be seen either on edge (Fig. 15-9) or en
   face. Small intrathyroid adenomas may or may

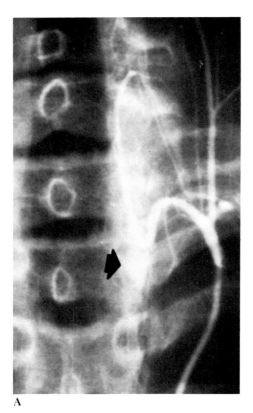

A

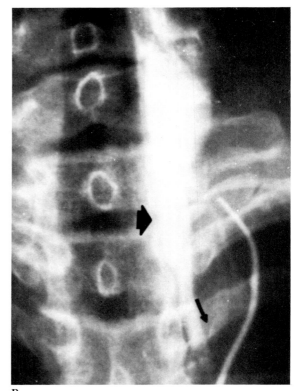

B

Fig. 15-9. Left inferior thyroid arteriogram. A parathyroid adenoma is seen on edge on the inferior part of the gland (*large arrows*). The inferior thyroid vein drains lateral to the adenoma (*small arrow*). At surgery, the tumor was flat and pancake-shaped, lying lateral to the trachea.
A. Arterial phase.
B. Capillary phase.

not be seen as delayed staining, late in the sequential films.

The later films of the thyroid arteriogram show the anatomy of the draining veins for subsequent selective collection of venous effluent. False-positive arteriograms will occur if thyroid adenomas are present.

5. Venous studies.

a. The primary function of venous studies is to localize veins for selective withdrawal of venous samples for subsequent parathormone assay [3, 17]. Since the vast majority of venous effluent from either the superior or inferior parathyroid gland flows into the ipsilateral inferior thyroid veins, these are the most important samples to obtain. Accessory laterally positioned inferior thyroid veins must be identified and sampled, because parathyroid glands generally drain into the lateral aspects of the thyroid lobe. A gradient of parathormone secretion tells the surgeon on which side the lesion is more likely to be present. Samples should be obtained from the superior and middle thyroid veins only if the inferior thyroid veins have been surgically ligated; otherwise they are not very rewarding. Samples should be obtained from those veins that drain into the mediastinum (such as the thymic and the azygous), if an anomalous position is suspected. Samples from both vertebral veins help to localize posteriorly placed adenomas. Adenomas both from posterior portions of the neck and the posterior aspect of the superior mediastinum may also drain into the vertebral veins. A peripheral venous sample is also studied for a background level of parathormone.

b. Occasionally venography will demonstrate a capsular circumscribed vein surrounding an adenoma.

c. The surgeon is helped most by seeing the adenoma, either by imaging methods or by angiography, rather than relying on the venous sampling alone. The latter should be used only as confirmatory evidence.

6. Pitfalls of parathyroid angiography.
   a. The arterial and venous anatomy may have been distorted by previous surgery.
   b. The vertebral and anterior jugular veins may be mistaken for veins draining the thyroid.
   c. The venous valves may be a barrier to catheter placement. They must be bypassed for successful study. Sometimes swallowing momentarily straightens out tortuous veins and allows the catheter tip to pass. Gentle suction, turning the patient's head to one side or the other, or using a Valsalva maneuver are other helpful techniques. The drip siphon technique of collection rather than that of active suction is often more successful. Hydrostatic pressure should be used with the catheter hub below the level of the patient. Heparinizing the patient at the start of the study (45 IU/kg) prevents clotting within the catheter. A small side hole at the very tip of the catheter may help, but the catheter tip and the side hole must be well within the draining vein.
   d. Atherosclerosis (tortuosity, aneurysms, plaques, stenosis) of the subclavian and carotid arteries makes the selective arterial procedures hazardous in the older age group.
   e. Even if adequately injected, small intrathyroid or retrotracheal parathyroid adenomas may be obscured by overlying normal structures. Oblique projections and subtraction studies will help to make these more visible. A thyroid adenoma may angiographically mimic an intrathyroid parathyroid adenoma; venous sampling or direct percutaneous puncture for parathormone helps differentiate these two tumors.

Interventional Procedures in Parathyroid Disease

Therapeutic ablation of solitary parathyroid adenomas has been reported as an acceptable alternative to surgery by some authors [2] provided the catheter can be selectively wedged into the feeding artery. Prior documentation that the tumor is indeed a parathyroid adenoma is obtained by needle aspiration for cytologic study and/or parathormone determination, or by selective venous sampling of the lesion. The procedure is performed by overinjecting undiluted contrast agent (15 to 20 ml of 76% high-density contrast agent) by hand injection. This results in sufficient cellular damage to cause infarction of the tumor with a subsequent decrease in serum calcium to normal levels. Ablation of abnormal glands in patients with secondary hyperparathyroidism by ultrasonographically guided percutaneous ethanol injection has also been reported [13]. Indications for this procedure are recurrence of parathyroid tumors after surgical resection, patients at high risk, or refusal of surgery. Absolute ethanol has been injected (1 ml per 2 or 2½ ml of gland tissue), reportedly with improved clinical and biochemical results.

References

1. Butch, R., Simeone, J., and Mueller, P. Thyroid and parathyroid ultrasonography. *Radiolog. Clin. North Am.* 23(1):57, 1985.
2. Doppman, J. Parathyroid localization: Arteriography. In H. Abrams (ed.), *Abrams' Angiography: Vascular and Interventional Angiography* (3rd ed.). Boston: Little, Brown, 1983. Pp. 977–999.
3. Doppman, J. Parathyroid localization: Arteriography and venous sampling. *Radiol. Clin. North Am.* 14:163, 1976.
4. Doppman, J., et al. Localization of abnormal mediastinal parathyroid glands. *Radiology* 115:31, 1975.
5. Doppman, J., et al. Aspiration of enlarged parathyroid glands for parathyroid hormone assay. *Radiology* 148:31, 1983.
6. Ferlin, G., et al. New perspectives in localizing enlarged parathyroids by technetium-thallium subtraction scan. *J. Nucl. Med.* 24:438, 1983.
7. Krudy, A., Doppman, J., and Miller, D. Detection of mediastinal parathyroid glands by non-selective digital arteriography. *A.J.R.* 142:693, 1984.
8. Krudy, A., et al. Arteriographic localization of parathyroid adenoma in the presence of a lingual thyroid. *A.J.R.* 136:127, 1981.
9. Krudy, A., et al. Work in progress: Abnormal parathyroid glands. Comparison on nonselective arterial digital arteriography, selective parathyroid arteriography, and venous digital arteriography as methods of detection. *Radiology* 138:23, 1983.
10. McFarlane, S., et al. Localization of abnormal parathyroid glands using thallium-201. *Am. J. Surg.* 148:7, 1984.
11. Obley, D., et al. Parathyroid adenomas studied by

digital subtraction angiography. *Radiology* 153:449, 1984.

12. Okerlund, M., et al. A new method with high sensitivity and specificity for localization of abnormal parathyroid glands. *Ann. Surg.* 200:381, 1984.

13. Solbiati, L., et al. Percutaneous ethanol injection of parathyroid tumors under ultrasound guidance. Treatment for secondary hyperparathyroidism. *Radiology* 155:607, 1985.

13A. Spritzer, C. E., et al. Abnormal parathyroid glands: High resolution MR imaging. *Radiology* 162:487, 1987.

14. Stark, D., et al. Parathyroid imaging: Comparison of high resolution CT and high resolution sonography. *A.J.R.* 141:633, 1983.

15. Stark, D., et al. Parathyroid scanning by computed tomography. *Radiology* 148:297, 1983.

16. Wang, C. The anatomic basis for parathyroid surgery. *Ann. Surg.* 183:271, 1976.

17. Wells, S., Jr., et al. The preoperative localization of hyperfunctioning parathyroid tissue utilizing parathyroid hormone radioimmunoassay of plasma from selectively catheterized thyroid veins. *NC Med. J.* 35:678, 1974.

Spinal Cord Angiography

Indications

1. Location of spinal cord arteriovenous malformations (AVMs), the site of origin of their feeding vessels, and the blood supply to the normal cord in candidates for surgical correction or embolization [1, 2, 3, 5, 11, 16].
2. Demonstration of certain hypervascular spinal tumors (hemangioblastomas, hypervascular gliomas, neurofibromas).
3. Preoperative localization of vessels feeding the anterior spinal artery (e.g., scoliosis repair, prolapsed disk, extramedullary tumors, aneurysm resections) [10].
4. Preoperative demonstration of relationship of radiculomedullary branches to a vascular lesion of the vertebral or perivertebral area.
5. Trauma to the spine [17].
6. Transcatheter embolic occlusion of feeding vessels to an AVM or of perivertebral branches of a hypervascular lesion [3, 6, 11, 15].

Technique

APPROACH

A percutaneous femoral artery approach is used in spinal angiography. The axillary artery may be necessary if aorto-iliac occlusion is present.

CATHETERS

1. For evaluation of the brachiocephalic components of an AVM, use a polyethylene or polyurethane catheter, as suggested in Fig. 14-5.
2. For catheterization of the lumbar and intercostal arteries, use an 80-cm 5, 6, or 6.5 French torque-controlled end-hold catheter with a thin 1-cm tapered tip (4 French), a 90-degree primary curve, and a secondary curve with a long, gentle obtuse angle. Alternate curves include a Mikaelsson curve and a modified Simmons No. 1 curve (Fig. 16-1). A "cobra head" curve (see Fig. 3-27) is also useful.

CONTRAST AGENTS, PROJECTIONS, AND RADIOGRAPHIC PROGRAMMING

Details concerning contrast agents, projections, and radiographic programs in both conventional and intraarterial digital subtraction angiography (IA-DSA) methods of spinal angiography are given in Table 16-1.

DIGITAL SUBTRACTION ANGIOGRAPHY

Intravenous digital subtraction angiography (IV-DSA) techniques have little or no role in angiographic evaluation of the spinal cord [7], for there is insufficient detail to make an accurate assessment regarding operability or other therapeutic approaches.

Intraarterial digital subtraction angiography (IA-DSA) provides a number of advantages [7, 8, 13, 18]. Since smaller volumes of dilute contrast medium are required, there is better patient tolerance (with less chance of motion artifact) and less neurotoxicity. The smaller volume makes the use of the expensive but less neurotoxic nonionic contrast agents more practical. IA-DSA considerably decreases the total time required for performing an often lengthy and arduous procedure. Midstream IA-DSA studies in the descending thoracic aorta (20 ml Conray 60 in 1 second) or subclavian arteries (10 ml Conray 60 in 1 second) may demonstrate major feeding arteries, but they often miss minor arterial feeders and other normal vascular anatomy (i.e., artery of Adamkiewicz) so vital for informed therapeutic decisions [7]. Selective studies (using 1 to 3 ml Conray 30 or nonionic contrast) can be rapidly performed [18], because the area investigated is centered at the time of fluoroscopy during the test injection, the imaging sequence follows this immediately, and the images can be viewed in "real time" and reviewed immediately without having to wait for lengthy film processing. The savings in time is considerable when 25 to 30 vessels must be individually studied. Both the mask and two images of each sequence must be recorded on the multiformat camera in order to promptly identify the location of the injected vessel.

The disadvantages of IA-DSA include motion artifact, smaller field size as compared with conventional angiographic methods, and somewhat poorer spatial resolution. Lateral projections with IA-DSA techniques are impractical because of

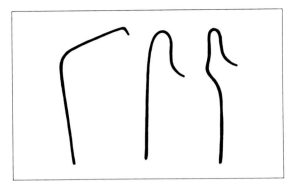

Fig. 16-1. Different catheter shapes useful for catheterizing the intercostal and lumbar arteries. From left to right: double-curved catheter with a tapered tip; modified Simmons No. 1 catheter shape; Mikaelsson curve.

artifacts by diaphragmatic motion and the sharp contrast between air-filled lung and abdominal density.

Since lateral projections are required to give precise detail of pathologic vessels, the examination should be supplemented with conventional angio-graphic studies once the abnormal blood vessels have been outlined. Optimal detail is provided by biplane selective magnification conventional seriographic cut-film angiography at these precise levels. Conventional filming provides the larger field size required for total coverage of a long lesion.

Anatomic Considerations [1, 2, 5, 12]

Just before the vertebral arteries join to form the basilar artery, each one gives off a branch; these branches join to form the anterior spinal artery (Figs. 16-2, 16-3). This lies in the ventral sulcus of the spinal cord and supplies (through small endartery sulcal branches) the anterior two-thirds of the spine. The posterior third of the spine is fed by posterior spinal arteries, which are very small discontinuous longitudinal vessels lying on the posterolateral portion of the spine. In normal circumstances they are not seen because of their small size. As the anterior spinal artery courses down the

Table 16-1. Technical specifications in spinal angiography[a]

Angiographic procedure	Contrast agent[b]			Total films	Time (sec)	Radiographic program[c]	
	Density	Volume (ml/inj)	Rate (ml/sec)			(films/sec)	Projections
Midstream injection							
Thoracic aortogram	M (NI)	50	30	15	18	2/sec for 3 sec; 1/sec for 3 sec; 1 every 2 sec for 12 sec	Biplane AP and lateral; AP or oblique with DSA
Abdominal aortogram	M (NI)	50	25	15	18		
Pelvic arteriogram	M (NI)	50	10	15	18		
Selective catheterization							
Vertebral artery	L (NI)	8	6	12	12	2/sec for 3 sec; 1/sec for 3 sec; 1 every 2 sec for 6 sec	AP and lateral; AP and obliques for DSA
Subclavian artery	L (NI)	18	8	12	12		
Costocervical trunk	L (NI)	2–4	Four films at 1/sec. Once an arteriovenous malformation has been detected, 10 films at 1/sec with unopacified first film for subtraction studies				AP; biplane AP and lateral if lesion detected
Intercostal or lumbar artery	L (NI)	2–4	Same as for costocervical trunk				

[a] For IA-DSA studies, use the same volume of contrast medium suggested for conventional studies but half-strength. Frame timing may approximate film timing.
[b] Nonionic recommended.
[c] Start films and frames before start of injection to obtain subtraction mask.
M = medium-density contrast agent; L = low-density contrast agent; NI = nonionic (see Appendix 3).

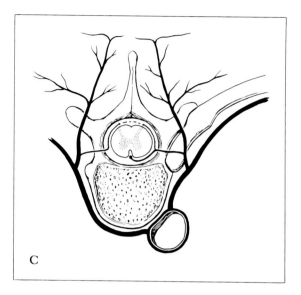

C

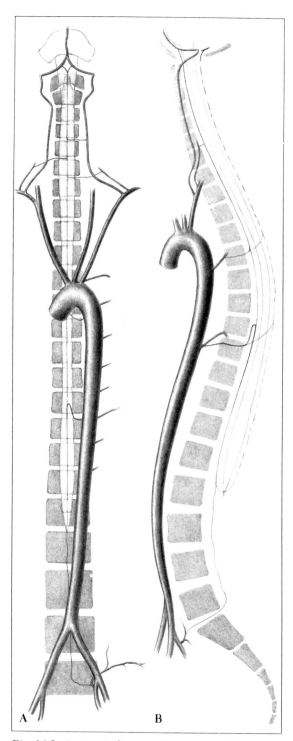

A   B

Fig. 16-2. Anatomic drawing of arteries supplying the spine.
A. AP projection.
B. Lateral projection.
C. Transverse projection (see text).

spine, it is nourished by a series of eight to twelve radiculomedullary feeding branches. In the *neck*, three or four of these branches arise from each side from the vertebral and the costocervical arteries (Figs. 16-2, 16-3, see Fig. 16-9C). Very rarely, small spinal feeding branches arise from the thyrocervical trunk. The costocervical trunk also gives off intercostal arteries in relation to the first four ribs (see Fig. 16-5).

There are only a few anterior spinal artery feeders in the upper thorax; they may arise from a high intercostal branch (T3 to T6). In this region also, the right bronchial artery often arises in common with the intercostal artery, which in turn may supply a radicular branch to the spine. The intercostal and bronchial arteries do not arise jointly on the left side. As a result of the sparse number of these feeding vessels to the spinal artery in the upper thorax, it is considered a watershed area; the anterior spinal artery is sometimes too small to be seen, and the spinal cord is particularly susceptible to ischemia in this region.

Intercostal and lumbar arteries branch into an anterior and posterior division soon after they arise from the dorsolateral aspect of the aorta. Any radicular branches that feed the anterior or posterior spinal arteries arise (together with muscular branches) from the posterior division (Fig. 16-2C).

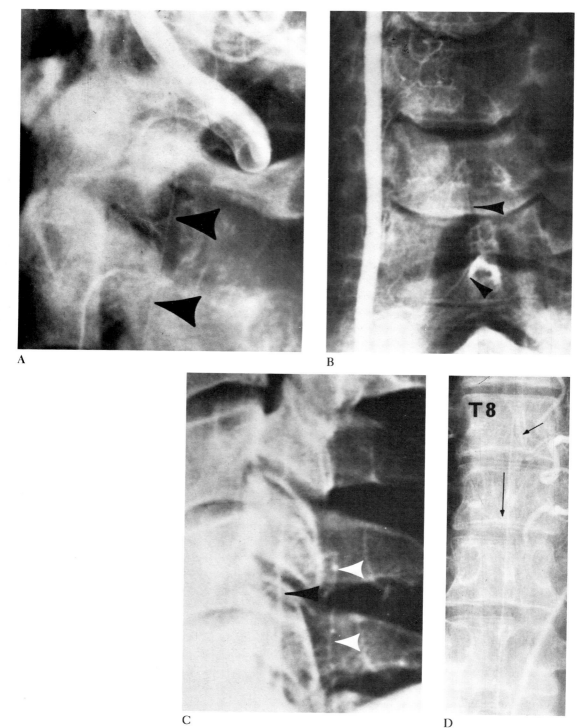

Fig. 16-3. Anatomy of the spinal arteries (see text for details).

A. Lateral projection. The anterior spinal artery (*arrowheads*) arising from the vertebral arteries runs the length of the cord in the anterior median fissure.

B. AP projection. The radiculomedullary feeding branch from the vertebral artery to the anterior spinal artery (*arrowheads*).

C. Lateral projection of the anterior spinal vein (*black arrowhead*) and posterior spinal veins (*white arrowheads*), which fill late in the study, following injection of the costocervical trunk.

D. AP projection. The artery of Adamkiewicz with its characteristic hairpin turn arising from the left eighth intercostal artery (*short arrow*) and feeding the anterior spinal artery (*long arrow*).

In the dorsal area, sometimes two intercostal arteries may arise from a common trunk. In this case, the posterior division of one of them (with its potential spinal feeder) may arise directly from the thoracic aorta and must be recognized or sought in order to complete the study. In the lumbar area, both right and left lumbar arteries may come off together, one of which may be missed angiographically if the catheter tip is advanced too far into the posteriorly located trunk.

In the thoracolumbar area, there is an important and prominent feeding vessel, the artery of Adamkiewicz, which arises from an intercostal or lumbar artery anywhere from the T6 to L2 level. It originates more frequently on the left side (Fig. 16-3D; see also Fig. 16-8C). It has a characteristic hairpin turn as it first ascends toward the midline and then descends down the ventral cord as the anterior spinal artery. The anterior spinal artery varies in diameter, being larger in the cervical cord and smaller in the upper dorsal cord, and then enlarging when it gets its major feeder from the radiculomedullary branch (artery of Adamkiewicz). At the conus, the anterior spinal artery divides and curves posteriorly to anastomose with the posterior spinal arteries. Angiographically the posterior spinal arteries do not quite meet the midline, an important feature to recognize and differentiate from the midline position of the anterior spinal artery. The posterior spinal arteries are supplied by a larger number (10 to 23) of the posterior radicular branches along the course of the cord.

The veins of the anterior portion of the cord drain toward its surface to join the anterior median spinal vein, which runs longitudinally just ventral to the median sulcus. The posterior and lateral portions of the cord drain in a radial manner to enter into the longitudinally draining coronal veins, located both posteriorly and anterolaterally along the surface of the cord. The anterior median spinal vein and coronal veins have laterally draining branches (anterior and posterior medullary veins), which also drain the dural perivertebral plexus into the azygous and caval systems [12]. The major spinal veins lie on the posterior aspect of the cord and usually drain cephalad. They may become elongated and tortuous in patients over 70 years of age and cause a serpiginous myelographic pattern that can be confused with a spinal AVM or hypervascular lesion.

Abnormalities of the Spinal Cord

ARTERIOVENOUS MALFORMATIONS OF THE SPINAL CORD

In spinal AVMs, the capillary bed fails to develop between the arteries and veins, with subsequent direct shunting between arteries and veins, resulting in venous hypertension, engorgement, and enlargement. The site of arteriovenous communication attracts a number of converging feeding arteries and emits a number of emerging enlarged veins; it may be a simple direct communication between a single artery and a single vein with the precise point of arteriovenous connection being difficult or impossible to determine. There may be associated aneurysms of arteries and/or veins in the complex vascular mass, which may bleed [3, 4, 12, 16].

AVMs can be classified as to their location in the longitudinal aspect of the cord (cervical, dorsal, dorsolumbar), whether or not they are extramedullary (dural or pial); and whether they are totally or partially intramedullary. Those AVMs fed entirely by the anterior spinal artery may be intramedullary or mixed intra- and extramedullary [15] but rarely are totally extramedullary.

AVMs can be further classified as to whether they are simple direct arteriovenous communications (type I), a glomus (type II) (Fig. 16-4), or juvenile (with a conglomerate of multiple arterial feeders and draining veins).

Fifteen percent of spinal angiomas have a segmental cutaneous angioma or a vertebral angioma at the same level (see Fig. 16-7).

The precise location of the AVM in relationship to the cord, the number and location of the feeding vessels of the AVM, and recognition of enlarging veins (as opposed to prominent feeding arteries) have important therapeutic implications.

Extramedullary Arteriovenous Malformations

In general, those AVMs in which the arterial feeders lie outside the cord, either on its posterior surface (supplied by the posterior spinal branches) or on the dura, are amenable to surgical resection. As a rule, these do not involve the anterior spinal artery. Rarely, some purely extramedullary AVMs are supplied by the anterior spinal artery with no intramedullary component and are in the form of a

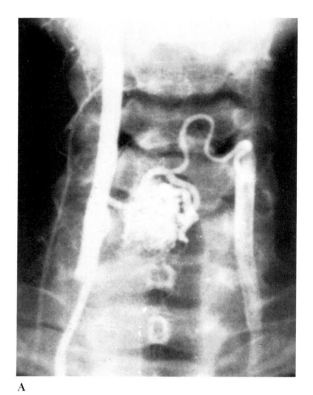

A

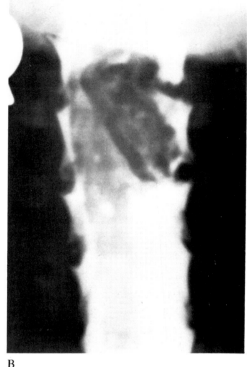

B

Fig. 16-4. Cervical glomus type spinal AVM.
A. Selective right vertebral arteriogram demonstrating multiple radicular feeding arteries arising from the vertebral arteries.
B. Cervical myelogram. (Courtesy of Dr. Ken Chow, University of Saskatchewan, Saskatoon).

direct fistulous communication between the spinal artery and spinal vein. They usually occur at the level of the conus [15].

The simplest and most satisfyingly treatable lesions are those AVMs *that involve only the dura*. These *extramedullary dural* AVMs have a single extradural tuft or nidus of fistulous vessels [16] and are usually seen in the lateral gutter of the intervertebral foramen immediately adjacent to a posterior nerve root sheath. They drain into dilated posterior or lateral coronal veins or into the anterior spinal vein, which courses longitudinally along the cord. In these dural AVMs the artery of Adamkiewicz is of normal size and generally arises from a different segment. Occasionally, however, this normal-size nonfeeding artery of Adamkiewicz can arise from the same intercostal lumbar segment, an important anatomic point for the surgeon to observe to avoid cord damage at the time of surgical resection [4] of these dural AVMs. Posterior spinal branches are usually not observed, and thus dural AVMs are differentiated from pial AVMs (Fig. 16-5). These dural AVMs are now thought to represent the majority of spinal vascular malformations.

Extramedullary pial AVMs that lie along the posterior aspect of the cord are supplied by large posterior spinal branches (Fig. 16-6). These can be recognized as one or more prominent feeders not quite meeting the midline of the spine on the AP projection. The artery of Adamkiewicz must be recognized as a normal branch arising at the same or a different level to ensure its lack of participation in the AVM. These lesions are more common in the dorsolumbar area.

Intramedullary Arteriovenous Malformations

Intramedullary AVMs (Fig. 16-7) have an intramedullary vascular component with feeding branches from the anterior spinal artery, posterior spinal arteries, or both. They drain into large anterior spinal, lateral, or posterior coronal draining veins.

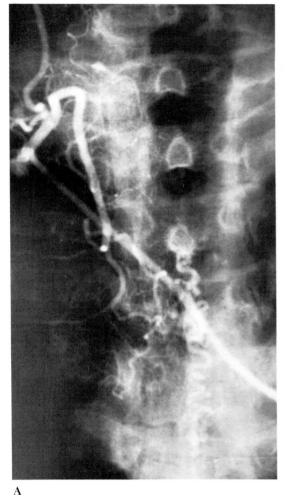

A

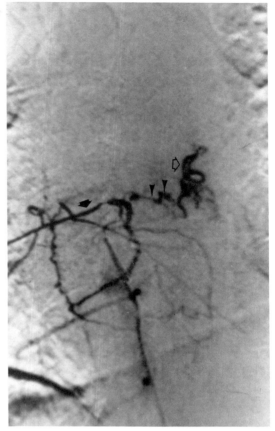

B

Fig. 16-5.

A. Thoracic dural spinal AVM supplied by the third and fourth intercostal branches of the right costocervical trunk. In this patient, the first four intercostal branches are supplied by this trunk. A small nidus of feeding dural branches enters into a longitudinal slowly draining central venous complex on the posterior aspect of the spine. The AVM was surgically removed.

B. Spinal dural AVM arising from T9 intercostal artery in another patient. Intraarterial digital subtraction arteriogram (AP projection, using 1.5 ml Renografin 60) shows the ninth intercostal artery (*closed arrow*) filling the dural AVM (*arrowheads*) and subsequent opacification of a pathologically dilated coiled spinal cord vein (*open arrow*) located in the center of the cord. The vein was surgically removed. (Courtesy Dr. Ralph Heinz, Duke University Medical Center, Durham, NC.)

With intramedullary AVMs in the *cervical region*, radicular branches may arise from the vertebral arteries or from the costocervical trunk, or both; often the anterior spinal artery is involved.

In the *dorsal region*, the intramedullary AVM may be focal and midline, supplied by sulcocommissural branches of the anterior spinal artery alone. The AVMs may be supplied by posterior spinal branches as well.

Intramedullary AVMs in the *dorsolumbar area* may be supplied by the anterior spinal artery as well as by hypertrophied abnormal posterior spinal branches. Sometimes normal posterior spinal branches may give important collateral branches around the base of the conus to the anterior spinal territory compromised by an AVM. These vessels

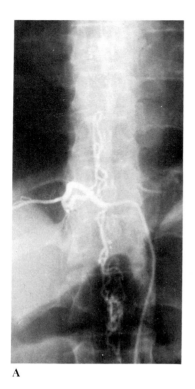

A

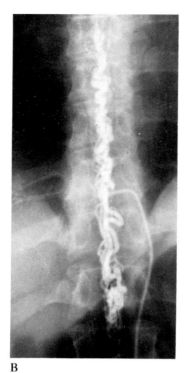

B

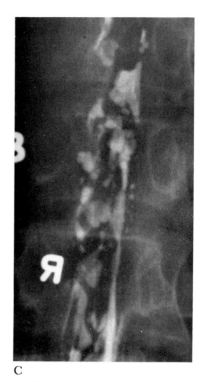

C

Fig. 16-6. An extramedullary spinal AVM extending the length of the thoracic spine and subsequently surgically removed from the dorsal aspect of the cord. There is a single feeding artery arising from the right tenth intercostal artery.

A. Early arteriogram showing the posterior arterial feeder extending just short of the midline.
B. Eight seconds following the start of the injection, long draining veins are seen extending up the midline of the cord. These vessels typically fill slowly, and the films should be programmed accordingly.
C. Serpiginous filling defect in a thoracic myelogram.

must be recognized as contributors to normal spinal function, and thus be spared, rather than as contributors to the AVM, and thus occluded. Although usually fed by branches from T6 to L2 on either side, AVMs in the dorsolumbar area may have feeding branches arising from the lower lumbar arteries or even the middle sacral artery or branches from the posterior division of the internal iliac artery.

OTHER LESIONS

Hemangioblastomas appear as a fine, fairly well marginated vascular network with a capillary blush that persists into the venous phase of the arteriogram. The lesion may be difficult to see, except by subtraction techniques, due to the overlying bones (Fig. 16-8). Usually there are a number of small feeding vessels from different segmental levels. There may be more than one lesion.

Other neural tumors are best defined by computed tomography or other studies. Occasionally, the relationship of these tumors to the normal major radiculomedullary spinal branches may require local spinal angiography.

Angiomas of vertebral bodies (Figs. 16-7, 16-9) may show marked hypervascularity, dense capil-

lary filling, and premature venous filling into large draining veins.

Prominent spinal vessels seen on a myelogram do not always reflect a tumor or vascular anomaly. They may hypertrophy (as with other surrounding collateral vessels) in response to occlusion of the adjacent aorta (e.g., coarctation).

Fig. 16-7. Glomus type intramedullary AVM and an accompanying vertebral angioma.

A and B. AP and lateral projections showing a large feeding radicular branch arising from T10 and a long dilated draining vein. Parallel line to the right of the cord in A is an artifact.
C and D. AP and lateral projections of angioma of T12 vertebral body.

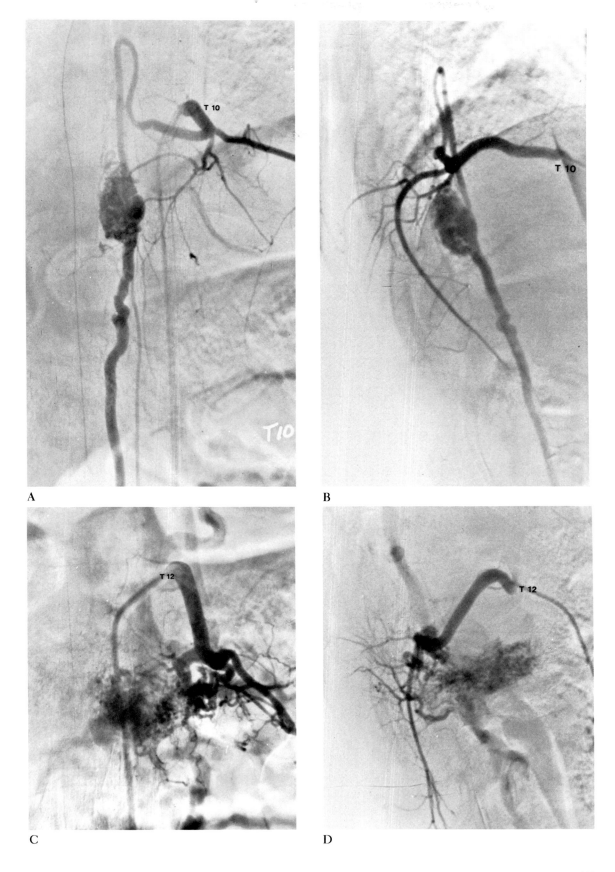

A

B

C

D

469

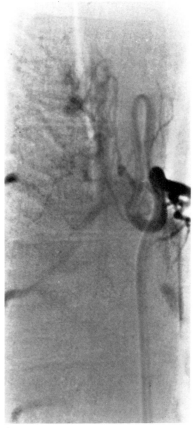

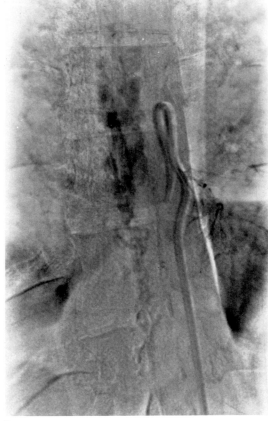

A

B

Fig. 16-8. Hemangioblastoma of the thoracic spinal cord supplied by multiple feeders.
A and B. Subtraction magnification arteriograms, early and late phases.
C. Artery of Adamkiewicz is normal and arises at a different level.

C

Comments and Techniques

An angiographic study is usually preceded by a myelogram, with the patient both prone and supine. Exceptions may be made in patients being studied preoperatively for a thoracic aortic aneurysm resection or a scoliosis repair. If the myelogram is negative, in our experience an AVM or cord lesion is probably not present. Serpentine myelographic defects can be found in lesions other than AVMs or vascular tumors (normally seen in elderly patients, they are collaterals in aortic obstruction).

An angiographic study must answer the following questions:

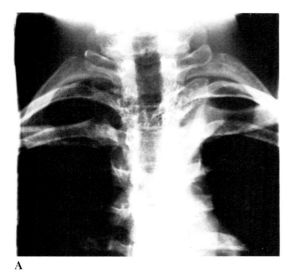

A

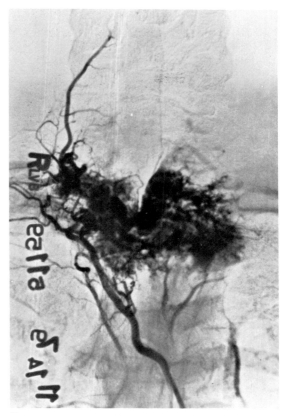

B

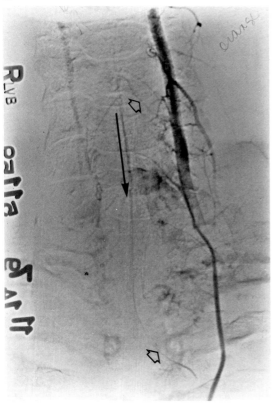

C

Fig. 16-9. Angioma of the second dorsal vertebra.
A. Coned view of upper dorsal spine.
B. Subtraction arteriogram of third intercostal artery showing angioma and communications with the costocervical trunk.
C. Subtraction left vertebral arteriogram shows a normal arterial supply to the cord (*open arrows*, radicular branches; *arrow*, anterior spinal artery).

1. The nature of the lesion (AVM, fistula, vascular tumor).
2. The number and location of all abnormal feeding vessels, the segments from which they arise, and whether they feed the anterior or posterior aspect of the cord. If the artery of Adamkiewicz is involved, treatment of the lesion is more hazardous and may result in cord damage.
3. The venous component of the lesion.
4. The position of the normal spinal arteries, particularly the artery of Adamkiewicz.

Spinal AVMs may extend the length of the spine, but usually much of the lesion represents longitudinal draining veins. Feeding vessels are often single, but may be multiple. The preceding myelogram may dictate the level of the initial examination and thus limit the extent of the arteriogram.

The angiographic procedure may be extensive. It is performed most expeditiously in the following manner:

1. IA-DSA midstream injection of each subclavian artery in AP projection, and of the descending thoracic aorta in AP or slightly LPO projection. These views may demonstrate major feeding vessels.

2. All subsequent selective studies should be performed in the AP projection with either well coned conventional filming or IA-DSA (see Fig. 16-5B). Only 2 to 3 ml of contrast agent is required for selective injections into the costocervical trunks and intercostal and lumbar arteries. The contrast medium is injected slowly by hand, and four arteriographic films are obtained at one per second (or one per second DSA frames) throughout the injection. When the feeding vessels to the abnormality are uncovered, additional injections are made into the feeding arteries with slightly more contrast agent (4 to 5 ml) using magnification and biplane studies and a larger number of films to cover a 15-second interval. An initial unopacified film must be available for subtraction purposes.

The location of lesions may be:

1. High thoracic and/or cervical region. Inject all vessels from T5 upward, including both vertebral arteries, the costocervical trunks, and occasionally the thyrocervical trunks. The costocervical trunks usually feed the upper three or four intercostal arteries.

2. Middle and lower dorsal regions. Study four segments above and four below the lesion bilaterally.

3. Below the eleventh dorsal vertebra. Study four segmental arteries above bilaterally and all of the lumbar arteries on each side, as well as the middle sacral artery and the posterior division of the internal iliac artery bilaterally.

4. In addition to the above, when any segmental vessel is seen feeding the lesion, include study of an additional three levels bilaterally above this vessel.

Try to see the anterior spinal artery in the region of the AVM, determine whether it is involved in the AVM, and demonstrate as well the radiculomedullary branch feeding the anterior spinal artery.

It is important to see if the lesion is either dural or posterior extramedullary in location, for these are the most suitable for surgical resection. Lateral projections are therefore important.

A complete evaluation outlines the vessels that can be safely resected. Some investigators [15] obtain additional angiotomographic and angiomyelotomographic sections at the level of the lesion to ensure a more accurate angiographic evaluation of the precise relationship of the lesion to the cord.

Preangiographic care is particularly important. The hazards of the study must be explained to the patient. Although the injections of the contrast agent into vessels supplying the spine are controlled, they may be painful and may bring on clonic muscle spasms of the legs. Adequate sedation and hypnotics are necessary. The spasms can be controlled with intravenous diazepam (Valium); if they are too frequent, the study may have to be terminated and continued on a subsequent day. Nonionic contrast agents, although expensive, are both less painful and less toxic; combined with IA-DSA, they can make the study less lengthy and much more tolerable.

In patients with progressive symptoms in whom the blood-cord barrier may have deteriorated, preangiographic steroids and steroid coverage during the procedure may be used to reduce cord edema. Despite these precautions, the symptoms may progress slightly following the procedure [12], but function usually returns fairly soon to preangiographic levels.

At the start of the study, mark the spine with a strip of lead numbers accurately positioned over the vertebrae. Record accurately each of the vessels studied. A negative angiographic study in the presence of an abnormal myelogram may indicate a missed dorsal intercostal or lumbar branch feeding the malformation. The film should be well coned and digital subtraction magnification studies made available. A lateral well-coned projection is an important part of the examination. One must be able to see whether the position of the lesion is posterior (usually resectable) or anterior (often not resectable) in relationship to the cord.

To avoid cord damage during the injection, do not wedge the catheter. The tip should be removed if there seems to be inadequate flow into the vessel.

Terminate the investigation if there are progressive neurologic symptoms. Injecting small doses of diazepam directly into the artery supplying the spine reportedly has helped to resolve the problem [9]. Although its efficacy has been questioned, some improvement has been reported if spinal fluid is replaced with Ringer's lactate. Slow replacement (10 ml every 4 or 5 minutes) of up to a total of 200 ml may help alleviate symptoms [14].

Catheter Treatment of Spinal Arteriovenous Malformations

It is obvious that a very thorough examination of the pathologic anatomy of an AVM, produced by an expertly performed angiogram, is necessary to decide the therapeutic approach. Complete surgical resection is the treatment of choice for all AVMs. This is often not possible. Embolization of all or portions of the lesion may be used either as a preoperative measure to facilitate surgery and prevent bleeding or for long-term palliation of unresectable lesions [3, 11, 15, 16]. Although spinal angiography is within the realm of an experienced angiographer, embolization is best left to those with active experience and adequate surgical backup.

References

1. DiChiro, G., and Wener, L. Angiography of the spinal cord: A review of contemporary techniques and applications. *J. Neurosurg.* 39:1, 1973.
2. Djindjian, R., et al. *Angiography of the Spinal Cord*. Baltimore: University Park Press, 1970.
3. Doppman, J. Spinal Angiography. In H. Abrams (ed.), *Abrams' Angiography: Vascular and Interventional Radiology* (3rd ed.). Boston: Little, Brown, 1983. Pp. 315–335.
4. Doppman, J., DiChiro, G., and Oldfield, E. Origin of spinal arteriovenous malformation and normal cord vasculature from a common segmental artery: Angiographic and therapeutic considerations. *Radiology* 154:687, 1985.
5. Doppman, J., DiChiro, G., and Ommaya, A. *Selective Arteriography of the Spinal Cord*. St. Louis: Green, 1969.
6. Doppman, J., DiChiro, G., and Ommaya, A. Percutaneous embolization of spinal cord arteriovenous malformations. *J. Neurosurg.* 38:48, 1971.
7. Doppman, J., et al. Intraarterial digital subtraction angiography of spinal arteriovenous malformation. *A.J.N.R.* 4:1081, 1981.
8. Enzman, D., et al. Intraarterial digital subtraction spinal angiography. *A.J.N.R.* 4:25, 1983.
9. Gordon, D., and Levin, D. Treatment of angiographically produced cord seizures by intra-arterial diazepam. *Cathet. Cardiovasc. Diagn.* 2:297, 1976.
10. Hillal, S., and Keim, H. Selective spinal angiography in adolescent scoliosis. *Radiology* 102:349, 1972.
11. Hillal, S., Sane, P., and Mowad, M. Therapeutic Interventional Radiologic Procedures in Neuroradiology. In H. Abrams (ed.), *Abrams' Angiography: Vascular and Interventional Radiology* (3rd. ed.). Boston: Little, Brown, 1983. Pp. 2252–2254.
12. Kendall, G. Spinal Angiography. In G. H. Dub Boulay (ed.), *Textbook of Radiological Diagnosis. Royal College of Radiologists. Vol. I. The Head and Central Nervous System.* Philadelphia: Saunders, 1984. Pp. 563–580.
13. Levey, J., et al. Digital subtraction arteriography for spinal arteriovenous malformation. *A.J.N.R.* 4:1217, 1983.
14. Miskin, M., Baum, S., and DiChiro, G. Emergency treatment of angiography-induced paraplegia and tetraplegia. *N. Engl. J. Med.* 288:1184, 1973.
15. Riche, M., Melki, J., and Merland, J. Embolization of spinal vasculature malformations via the anterior spinal artery. *A.J.N.R.* 4:378, 1983.
16. Symon, L., Kuyama, H., and Kendall, D. Dural arteriovenous malformations of the spine. Clinical features and surgical results of 55 cases. *J. Neurosurg.* 60:288, 1984.
17. Wener, L., DiChiro, G., and Gargour, G. Angiography of cervical cord injuries. *Radiology* 112:597, 1974.
18. Yeates, A., et al. Intraarterial digital subtraction angiography of the spinal cord. *Radiology* 155:387, 1985.

IV

Thoracic Vascular Procedures

Catheterization of the Right Side of the Heart and Pulmonary Angiography

Indications

1. Acquired pulmonary vascular diseases.
   a. Pulmonary thromboembolism.
   b. Pulmonary hypertension.
      (1) Pulmonary venous hypertension.
      (2) Obliterative parenchymal disease.
      (3) Pulmonary artery obstruction.
      (4) Hyperkinetic (left-to-right shunts).
   c. Arteritis.
   d. Aneurysm.
   e. Varix.
   f. Venous obstruction.
      (1) Tumor.
      (2) Mediastinitis.
      (3) Veno-occlusive disease.
   g. Primary tumor.
   h. Chronic inflammatory and obliterative conditions (e.g., emphysema, bullae).
   i. Trauma.
2. Congenital pulmonary vascular diseases.
   a. Unilateral congenital dysplasia of lung.
      (1) Hypoplasia.
      (2) Interruption of pulmonary artery.
      (3) Pulmonary agenesis.
   b. Anomalous origin of pulmonary arteries.
   c. Aneurysm.
   d. Peripheral pulmonary artery stenosis.
   e. Arteriovenous malformation.
   f. Pulmonary venous stenosis.
   g. Pulmonary varix.
   h. Anomalous venous return.
3. Miscellaneous conditions.
   a. Study of pulmonary emphysema to determine amount of functioning lung.
   b. Diseases of the atria (tricuspid valve insufficiency, clots, myxoma).
   c. Mediastinal mass assessment regarding operability.
   d. Sequestration.
   e. Pericardial disease.
   f. Study of congenital heart disease.

4. Endovascular therapy.
   a. Selective lysis or suction of pulmonary emboli.
   b. Angioplasty of pulmonary valve stenosis.
   c. Embolization of arteriovenous malformations.
   d. Removal of foreign bodies.

Technique

APPROACHES

The percutaneous venous approach is almost always possible and satisfactory. With some catheters (NIH, Gensini, Lehman, Eppendorf), approaches from the arm or neck permit easier intracardiac manipulation. The femoral venous approach is also feasible with these catheters, but other catheters (e.g., Grollman) are more suitable for the femoral venous approach since myocardial perforation is less likely to occur. Tightly coiled pigtail catheters, introduced from either approach, can be advanced through the cardiac chambers with the help of an external manipulator or preformed stiff guidewire. Balloon catheters can be advanced from either the femoral or the upper extremity venous approach through a catheter sheath. The following are the veins available for introduction of catheters.

1. Above the diaphragm (see Figs. 3-24, 3-25, 3-26):
   a. Antecubital fossa (basilic vein if possible, cephalic vein if necessary).
   b. Axillary vein (just posterior to the artery).
   c. External jugular vein (sometimes requires surgical exposure).
   d. Internal jugular vein (percutaneous approach for rapid emergency use; see Fig. 3-26).
   e. Subclavian vein.
2. Below the diaphragm: femoral vein. (The

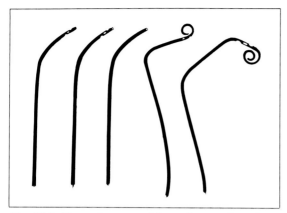

Fig. 17-1. The catheters used for evaluating the right heart and pulmonary arteries. From left to right: NIH catheter; Gensini catheter; Lehman catheter; Grollman catheter; double curve pigtail catheter.

reader should review the sections on methods of venous catheterization in Chapter 3.)
3. Surgical exposure of the superficial antecubital or brachial veins.

CATHETERS (Fig. 17-1)
1. NIH or Eppendorf catheters[1] are 100-cm Dacron catheters with a gentle single curve. They have a closed end with multiple side holes to minimize catheter recoil during high-volume rapid injections. An 8 French diameter is preferred in the adult. Shorter (80-cm) and smaller diameter catheters are available for children; these catheters require a special technique for percutaneous introduction, which includes previous insertion of a Mylar sheath into the veins (see Fig. 3-24).
2. The Gensini catheter is a single-curved 7 or 8 French 100-cm or 125-cm Dacron catheter with side holes and an end hole. No Mylar sheath is required for its introduction, but its blunt end requires adequate dilation of the vein with a vessel dilator prior to insertion. With this catheter and other end-hole catheters, high rates of injection of contrast medium into the main pulmonary artery (more than 20 ml per second) may cause the catheter to recoil back across the pulmonary valve, embedding its tip into the wall of the ventricle and causing serious myocardial damage, penetration, and peri-

cardial accumulation of blood and contrast medium. The catheter may recoil back into the right atrium or into the superior vena cava from its initial position in the pulmonary artery. This catheter should be used only in selective pulmonary artery positions, and injection rates should not exceed 15 ml per second.
3. The Lehman catheter is a 125-cm Dacron end-hole catheter used for recording pulmonary wedge pressures. A 7 or 8 French diameter is preferable. Alternatively, a Swan-Ganz balloon catheter[2] may be used for this purpose.
4. "Pigtail" catheters do not perforate the myocardium; they maintain a stable position during high-pressure injections. Subselective positioning is sometimes more difficult and often requires a curve on a guidewire or an external manipulator. The Grollman catheter has an end hole, side holes, and a reversed-shaped pigtail tip with the distal curve angled at approximately 100 degrees. Another useful catheter configuration has a double curve to its tip, with graduated side holes between the pigtail and its primary curve. These catheter shapes are useful for catheterization from the femoral vein.
5. A 7 or 8 French balloon tip catheter can be introduced through a sheath in a peripheral vein, and flow directed to the right or left pulmonary artery. It is deflated prior to a diagnostic angiography study. These catheters are prone to recoil if contrast agent is injected at high pressures.

Balloon occlusive angiography further improves the diagnostic quality of a study [4]. The balloon catheters are of much larger diameter than those routinely used to float up to the pulmonary arteries, for the balloons must be large enough to totally occlude the pulmonary artery during the injection. Optimal filling of a locally closed vascular system is possible by this method, without artifact caused by overlying partially filled and rapidly emptying vessels.

CONTRAST AGENTS, PROJECTIONS,
AND RADIOGRAPHIC PROGRAMMING
Details concerning contrast agents, projections, and radiographic programming in pulmonary angiography are given in Table 17-1.

---

[1] USCI, a division of C. R. Bard, Inc., Box 566, Billerica, MA 01821.

[2] Edwards Laboratories, 17221 Red Hill Ave., Santa Ana, CA 92705.

Table 17-1. Technical specifications in pulmonary angiography[a]

Angiographic procedure	Contrast agent[b]			Total films	Total time (sec)	Radiographic program[c]		Projections
	Density	Volume (ml/inj)	Rate (ml/sec)			Films/sec	Timing	
Adults								
Main pulmonary arteriogram	M	60	30	16	10	3/sec for 2 sec; 2/sec for 2 sec; 1/sec for 6 sec	Start films 0.4 sec after start of injection; use a biwedged filter (see Fig. 1-6)	(1) AP, alternately slight RPO; (2) in forward angiocardiogram, add a lateral view coned to heart
Alternate program (slow flow of increased resistance due to pulmonary hypertension, congestive heart failure)				16	18	2/sec for 4 sec; 1/sec for 2 sec; 1 every 2 sec for 12 sec		
Selective pulmonary artery study (for biplane studies with alternate film loading)	M	35–40	20[d]	15	9	3/sec for 2 sec; 2/sec for 2 sec; 1 every sec for 5 sec	Start films 0.4 sec after start of injection	Biplane[e] preferable; AP or appropriate oblique may be used (RPO for left, slight RPO for lower branches of right pulmonary artery)
Alternate program for large patients				15	10	2/sec for 4 sec; 1/sec for 2 sec; 1 every 2 sec for 4 sec	Start films 0.4 sec after start of injection	Biplane AP and lateral
Superselective studies[f]	M	5–30	5–15[d]			Same as for selective studies, coned to area of interest	Start films 0.4 sec after start of injection	Biplane AP and lateral
Children[g]								
Main pulmonary arteriogram								
Infants	L	1.5–2.0 ml/kg	Total within 1.0–1.5 sec	15	7	3/sec for 3 sec; 2/sec for 2 sec; 1/sec for 2 sec	Start films at onset of injection	Biplane AP and lateral
Others	M		Same					
Selective studies (infants, others)	Same	1.0–1.2 ml/kg	Same	15	7	Same	Same	Biplane AP and lateral

[a]For intraarterial digital subtraction angiography, use one-half to two-thirds the volume of contrast agent but half-strength.
[b]Nonionic contrast agents are recommended when right ventricular end-diastolic pressure is greater than 10 mm Hg (see text).
[c]Normal circulatory time in adults is 3 to 5 seconds; it is more rapid in children.
[d]Make a test injection with 5 ml at same injection rate with the catheter in final position, in full inspiration, and with arms above the head (for biplane) to preclude catheter recoil or wedge positions.
[e]Apply lateral changer to the side being studied for optimal object-film distance.
[f]Amount of contrast agent needed depends on size of vascular bed.
[g]Amount of contrast agent needed in children varies with body weight.
M = medium-density contrast agent; L = low-density contrast agent (see Appendix 3).

479

PHYSIOLOGIC MONITORING

Flow, pressure, and resistance within the cardiovascular system are closely interrelated. Flow is directly proportional to the pressure generated and inversely proportional to the resistance it meets. If intraluminal pressures and flow (cardiac output) can be measured, the resistance can be calculated. We can often assume an increased resistance to flow and show its morphologic cause, or demonstrate a high-flow system, by angiography. More meaningful functional data, however, are obtained by accurately measuring and calculating physiologic parameters [39]. Therefore, a physiologic monitoring unit should be included in all angiographic laboratories. It should be capable of recording or measuring the following factors: electrocardiogram (ECG), two simultaneous pressure recordings. Cardiac output and shunt measurements, although not essential, are helpful adjuncts. In this case, there should be easy access to oximetric evaluation of selectively obtained blood samples.

Pressure Measurements

TECHNIQUE. Continuous visual monitoring of pressures and ECG should be available on an oscilloscope during catheter manipulations through the chambers of the heart, the great vessels, or their branches. In addition, a permanent paper record allows data determinations. The following steps should be observed:

1. Set the transducer at the zero point (mid-chest level).
2. Fill the pressure transducer with sterile water at room temperature and keep it free of bubbles.
3. Accurately balance and calibrate the equipment immediately before the study, following the instructions of the manufacturer.
4. Fill the catheter within the vascular system with 5% dextrose, attach the rotating stopcock to its hub, and connect the catheter (via a three-way stopcock and connecting tube) to the transducer (Fig. 17-2) and to a flushing syringe. Beware of bubbles and blood leaking into the transducer.
5. Before each pressure reading, open the transducer to the air for final fine balancing of the recorder.
6. On the venous side (for right heart or pulmonary arteries), adjust the sensitivity to a low attenuation level in order to record the low-pres-

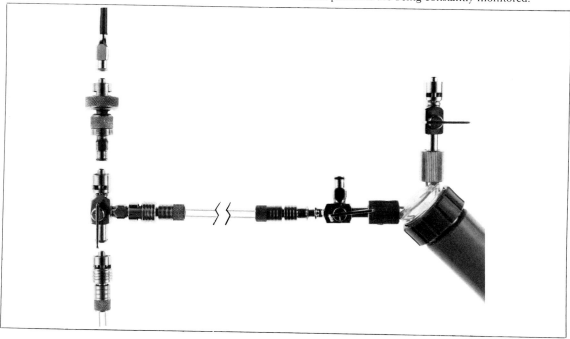

Fig. 17-2. Strain gauge and connecting tubes to catheter assembly. A rotating adapter intervenes between the stopcock and the catheter to allow more maneuverability of the catheter during intracardiac manipulations while pressures are being constantly monitored.

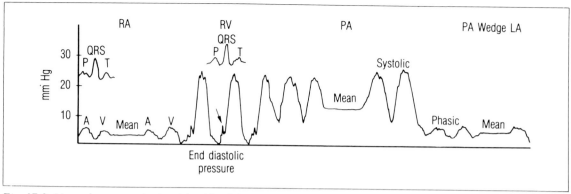

Fig. 17-3. Normal pressures in the right side of the heart: *Right atrium* (RA). The A wave (5 mm Hg) occurs after the ECG P wave and reflects atrial contraction. The V wave (5 mm Hg) is caused by right atrial filling and occurs during ventricular contraction when the atrioventricular valves are closed. It occurs roughly in conjunction with the T wave of the ECG. The normal mean right atrial pressure is approximately 3 mm Hg. *Right ventricle* (RV): The right ventricular end-diastolic pressure (RVEDP) is 6 to 7 mm Hg. This pressure corresponds to the first valley measured on the pressure recording after the QRS on the ECG (usually 0.06 second after Q) and reflects the immediate presystolic pressure. *Pulmonary artery* (PA): The pulse pressure is the difference between systole (23 mm Hg) and diastole (10 mm Hg). The mean pulmonary artery pressure measures 13 mm Hg. *Pulmonary artery* (PA) *wedge pressure* (mean 8 mm Hg): This reflects left atrial (LA) pressure and requires a catheter with an end hole but no side holes (Lehman). Advance the catheter out the pulmonary artery until it can be advanced no further. The wedge position is proved by a drop in pressure to the left atrial level, suction of red oxygenated blood, and a sharp jump to the pulmonary arterial pressure level on withdrawal.

sure signals. In the higher pressure arterial system, use a higher attenuation level. Be prepared to measure phasic pressure responses (systolic peaks and diastolic troughs) in the cardiac chambers and great vessels; to measure ventricular end-diastolic pressure; and to make mean (electronically averaged) pressure recordings in the atria and great vessels.

NORMAL PRESSURE MEASUREMENTS. Normal pressure measurements on the right side of the heart are given in Figure 17-3 and Table 17-2.

ABNORMAL PRESSURE MEASUREMENTS

1. Atrial pressures. Elevated *a* waves occur when there is difficulty in emptying the atrium (atrioventricular valve stenosis; ventricular outflow tract stenosis; pulmonary or systemic hypertension). The *a* waves are absent in atrial fibrillation. Elevated *v* waves occur with incompetence of atrioventricular valves. Elevated *a* and *v* waves with rapid down-slopes occur with pericardial constriction.

2. Elevated right ventricular end-diastolic pressures occur with right ventricular failure. In pericardial constriction these pressures tend to equalize with the right atrial and pulmonary wedge (left atrial) mean pressures and the diastolic pulmonary artery pressures.

3. Pulmonary hypertension (pulmonary artery pressures over 30 mm Hg).
   Mild: systolic pressure 30 to 40 mm Hg.
   Moderate: systolic pressure 40 to 70 mm Hg.
   Severe: systolic pressure over 70 mm Hg.

Table 17-2. Normal pressure values in the heart

Vessel	Systolic pressure (mm Hg)	Diastolic pressure (mm Hg)	Mean pressure (mm Hg)
Right atrium			0–5
Right ventricle	20–25	0–7	
Pulmonary artery	20–25	8–12	15
Left atrium (or wedge)			5–10
Left ventricle	110–130	5–12	
Aorta	110–130	75–85	100

4. Gradients. A gradient is a systolic or diastolic pressure difference across a valve or stenotic area. Its presence indicates an absolute or relative stenosis across the involved area. The most accurate means of recording a gradient is by simultaneously measuring pressures on either side of the involved area; this requires two catheters and two pressure manometers. Continuous monitoring of pressures as a single catheter is pulled back over a stenotic segment is also satisfactory. One should be wary of pressures measured on either side of a valve on temporally disparate occasions, since normal hemodynamic variations may give a false impression of a gradient. It is important to consider a gradient across a valve in relation to the cardiac output of the patient. Patients with a normal or high cardiac output may tolerate a given area of stenosis, whereas those with a low cardiac output may not. Gradients across atrioventricular valves are measured during diastole. Even a small gradient across the tricuspid valve (over 3 mm Hg) is poorly tolerated, whereas larger gradients across the mitral valve (over 10 mm Hg with normal or high cardiac output) are required to consider surgical correction. Gradients of up to 50 mm Hg are tolerated across the semilunar valves in patients with normal cardiac output, but surgery is usually considered if pressures rise much above this level.

Cardiac Output

Cardiac output can be measured using dye dilution techniques or by the Fick principle based on oximetric values. Commercially available computerized cardiac output units can perform the calculations with reasonable accuracy in the absence of shunts.

Shunts

Shunts within the cardiovascular system can be detected by a variety of means, the most common being green dye dilution techniques and measurement of a sudden change in the oxygen content at the site of the shunt. In right-to-left shunts using the dye dilution techniques, the major bolus of dye is diverted into the arterial circulation, and it obviously appears and peaks earlier at the sampling site. With oxygen saturation measurements, there is a sudden decrease in oxygen content on the systemic side of the circulation. In left-to-right shunts, since some of the dye is being diverted to the right side, the initial sample from the sampling site (usually the radial artery) is lower than normal concentration, but occurs at the proper time interval; there will be a step-up of oxygen saturation on the right side of the heart as oxygenated blood enters the system.

Pulmonary Vascular Resistance

The flow of blood through the lungs is normally accomplished at pressures that are one-sixth as great as those in the systemic circulation because of the low resistance in the pulmonary circulation. These low pressures are possible because the peripheral pulmonary vessels are thin-walled and respond less to neural, humoral, or pharmacologic agents. Because the pulmonary circulation is relatively passive and easily distensible, the flow through normal lungs can increase threefold before there is significant increase in pulmonary artery pressure. If pulmonary vascular or parenchymal disease supervenes, however, this reserve may markedly diminish.

The resistance to flow in the lungs can be calculated and its relationship to the resistance in the systemic circulation approximated. The *total* pulmonary resistance is that measured across the pulmonary vascular system *and* the left atrium. The pulmonary vascular resistance is that measured across the pulmonary arterial system, *excluding* that derived from the left atrium. The normal ratio of pulmonary artery resistance to systemic artery resistance is approximately one-sixth. A ratio lower than 0.25 is considered to be normal, but if it is 0.75 or higher, the pulmonary artery resistance is at a dangerous level.

TECHNICAL CONSIDERATIONS

1. The catheter should be filled with fluid prior to its insertion into the veins, because it may be difficult to replace the air column in the catheter with fluid by suctioning due to impaction of the venous wall against the catheter holes.
2. Problems may arise in advancing the catheter from the vein in the arm into the chambers of the right side of the heart.
   a. The catheter may not be within the lumen of the vein but rather in the periadventitial tissues. A small test injection shows a stain.

b. The catheter tip may lodge against a venous valve or enter into a small tributary. Careful withdrawal and readvancement obviates this problem.

c. The catheter may also become wedged into the lateral thoracic vein at the level of the axillary vein. It should be withdrawn and its tip rotated cephalad as the catheter is advanced.

d. The chosen vein, although prominent at the site of selection, may be hypoplastic or narrowed from previous phlebitis of the extremity. Small test injections of contrast medium define these problems.

e. Venous spasm may occur and may be difficult to overcome. It can be recognized when one has previously successfully advanced the catheter in the vein, but with subsequent prolonged catheterization further catheter advancement is unsuccessful. It can sometimes be overcome by slow (often painful) withdrawal of the catheter to the site of spasm and injection of 50 mg of lidocaine. Be judicious with the dose, since the drug acts directly on the myocardium. A thin film of sterile silicone ointment may be applied to the catheter surface. Only small amounts of silicone should be used, since this material embolizes to the lungs. A smaller catheter size may also prove helpful.

f. The cephalic vein should be avoided if possible for two reasons. First, it frequently becomes hypoplastic centrally, and second, it often has an acute angle at its juncture with the subclavian vein at the level of the shoulder. The latter difficulty may be overcome by very actively abducting and at the same time pulling on the patient's arm.

g. The left innominate vein, the right internal jugular vein, or the azygos vein may sometimes be entered inadvertently. Injections of contrast medium and appropriate manipulation, sometimes accompanied by moving the patient's arm and head in various directions, usually permit successful entry into the superior vena cava and the right atrium.

3. Catheter manipulation from the femoral vein is sometimes impeded when the catheter tip passes into the inferior epigastric veins or into the ascending lumbar veins. Again, contrast injection, various manipulations and rotations of the catheter, and, if possible, introduction of guidewires overcomes these problems.

4. The angiographer should be aware of the normal relationships of the cardiac chambers and valves (Fig. 17-4). When in the *right atrium*, form a loop on the catheter with the tip against the lateral atrial wall (Fig. 17-5); then rotate the tip anteriorly through the tricuspid valve into the right ventricle and on into the main pulmonary artery, advancing fairly rapidly. At this time pressures must be monitored; look for the normal elevation when in the right ventricle. If the ECG is sufficiently stable while the catheter tip is in the right ventricle, record the pressures for calculation of the systolic and end-diastolic pressures.

5. Difficulties manipulating the catheter through the chambers of the heart or into the pulmonary artery may be encountered.

a. The catheter sometimes appears fluoroscopically to be in the ventricle, but it may actually be in the coronary sinus or under a ventricular trabecula. The pressures are usually dampened at this point. A small hand injection of contrast medium demonstrates the curvilinear vein in the atrioventricular groove (Figs. 17-5 and 17-6) or the stain in the myocardium.

   If the soft myocardium has been penetrated, the stain may extend into the pericardium. The catheter tip may penetrate into the pericardium medial or lateral to the pulmonary valve. If the catheter tip position is too lateral in the cardiac silhouette, and if the catheter does not move freely with cardiac pulsations, penetration into the pericardium must be suspected. Inject 1 or 2 ml of contrast medium, and if the catheter tip position is verified, withdraw to the right atrium immediately. If penetration into the pericardium occurs, the patient must be monitored closely for signs of pericardial tamponade (see following section on complications).

b. Occasional premature ventricular contractions are to be expected when the catheter is passing through the tricuspid valve into the right ventricle. Quickly pull back into the right atrium if they become multiple or if ventricular tachycardia supervenes. Undue stress or dilation of the tricuspid valve may

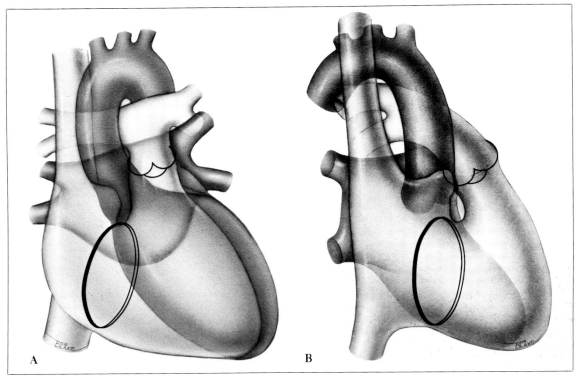

A   B

Fig. 17-4. Normal relationship of the cardiac chambers and the great vessels, showing the relationship of the tricuspid and pulmonary valves on both projections.
A. Anteroposterior projection.
B. Lateral projection.

initiate ventricular irritability; if this represents a problem, 50 to 100 mg of lidocaine may be given directly through the catheter. The recognition and treatment of myocardial arrhythmias are reviewed in Tables 17-3 and 18-2.

c. When approached from below, the tricuspid valve may be difficult to enter despite normal anatomy because of an insufficient curve or straightening of an NIH catheter tip. An increase in size of the right atrium or abnormalities of the tricuspid valve may also contribute toward difficulties in catheterization. If difficulties occur, form a loop in the catheter by catching the tip in a crevice in the wall of the atrium and rotate the U-shaped tip toward the anteriorly placed tricuspid valve, at the same time withdrawing to enter the valve. As soon as the tip flips through the tricuspid valve, rapidly rotate and simultaneously advance the catheter toward the posteriorly directed pulmonary valve (Fig. 17-5). If this maneuver is not accomplished rapidly, the natural tendency will be for the U loop to retain its shape and force the catheter tip into an un-

desirable location in the apex of the right ventricle. If this occurs, withdraw the catheter back into the right atrium and start again.

d. If great difficulty is encountered in advancing a closed-end NIH catheter from the right atrium to the main pulmonary artery, change to a catheter with an end hole (e.g., Gensini). A "floppy" curved-tip guidewire protruding through the catheter tip can often be manipulated through the right ventricular chamber to act as a leader over which the catheter can follow. Once the catheter has entered the main pulmonary artery it can usually be advanced to the right or left pulmonary artery. If difficulty is encountered, it may be overcome by using an externally manipulated catheter deflector.[3] Alternatively, a tight circular curve may be

[3]Cook Inc., P.O. Box 489, Bloomington, IN 47401.

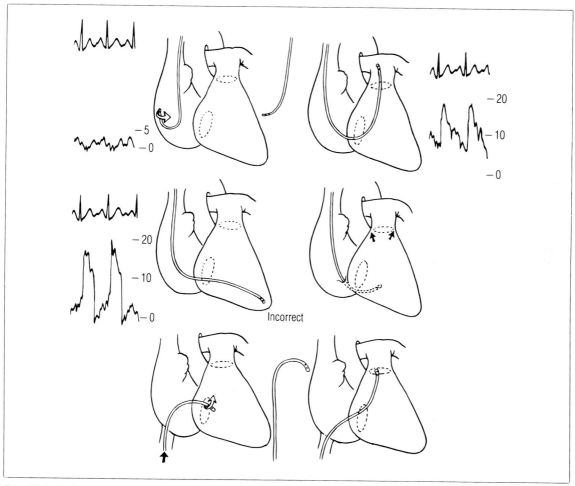

Fig. 17-5. Catheter manipulations for pulmonary artery catheterization. *Top row:* Normal ECG and pressure tracings in the right atrium and the pulmonary artery. Approach from above. *Middle row:* Normal ECG and right ventricular pressure tracings. The catheter is placed incorrectly into the apex of the right ventricle and into the coronary sinus. Withdraw the catheter to the right atrium and reform the curve as in the top illustration. The arrows point to possible sites of perforation on either side of the pulmonary valve. *Bottom row:* Approach from below, using an NIH catheter (see text for details).

formed on the stiff end of a guidewire and advanced to, but not beyond, the catheter tip. When pointed toward the appropriate vessel, the catheter may be "paid out" over the stiff wire to the desired level. All manipulations with guidewires must be performed rapidly to prevent fibrin accumulation.

e. The problem of perforating the myocar-dium with the catheter tip can be prevented by using a catheter with a pigtail tip config-uration. The Grollman catheter (Fig. 17-7) is ideally shaped for the femoral approach. Its pigtail tip prevents penetration of the myocardium, and its sharply angled 1-cm curve may be adapted for easy entrance through the tricuspid valve. This entrance may be facilitated by using an external catheter deflector, as previously described. Once the catheter tip has entered the right ventricle, it is rotated posteriorly to pass through the pulmonary valve.

Double-curved or straight catheters with a tight pigtail tip configuration can be ad-vanced from either the upper extremities or the femoral vein. Entry through the tricuspid valve with the straight catheter requires a U-

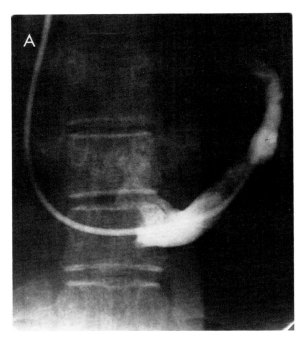

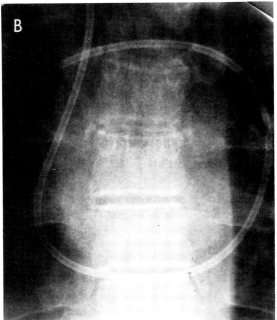

Fig. 17-6.
A. Catheter tip in coronary sinus.
B. Catheter was withdrawn and repositioned with its tip in the right pulmonary artery. (From I. S. Johnsrude, *Pulmonary Embolism. Current Problems in Diagnostic Radiology.* Chicago: Year Book Medical Publishers, 1982. Used by permission.)

shaped curve imposed on the distal 4 to 5 cm of the catheter by a guidewire with an external manipulator. This is directed anteromedially through the tricuspid valve and then paid out over the fixed guidewire curve to eventually advance through the main pulmonary artery. Selective right or left pulmonary artery placement is more easily obtained with the double-curved pigtail catheter.

f. No. 7 or 8 French balloon tip catheters are available for pulmonary angiography. By inflating the balloon with 1 cc of air, the catheter can be flow directed through the cardiac chambers to the main pulmonary artery. A curve on the distal tip, accompanied by transient inflations and deflations of the balloon, helps in manipulating the tip to the desired pulmonary artery under investigation. The tip should be deflated prior to the injection of contrast agent in order to prevent recoil. The large, rapid doses of contrast agent required for a conventional diagnostic major vessel arteriogram are sometimes not possible due to instability of the position of the catheter tip. These balloon tip catheters can be helpful for smaller injections (as with digital subtraction stud-

ies) in patients with difficult anatomy. They are expensive and are required only under unusual circumstances.

Injecting into a relatively closed vascular system through an occlusive balloon catheter (MediTech) may help reveal an underlying pathologic condition otherwise obscured by flow defects or overlying vessels. Be sure that the diameter of the inflated balloon is sufficiently large to occlude the vessel under investigation.

6. For selective placement of catheters in the left and right pulmonary arteries, recall that the left pulmonary artery lies more posterior in location, whereas the right pulmonary artery extends in a horizontal fashion. The catheter tip should always extend approximately 1 cm into the lower lobe branches prior to injection in order to accommodate the catheter recoil of high-pressure injection. Before the test injection, both of the patient's arms should be ele-

vated if biplane films are to be obtained, since this advances the catheter further into the artery if the approach is from the veins in the arms. In addition, there should be complete inspiration, since this tends to withdraw the catheter back toward the main pulmonary artery. The slight recoil during injection usually opacifies all the branches of the right or the left pulmonary vascular tree. Guard against wedge injections of large doses of contrast medium into small pulmonary artery branches; this is especially likely to occur with selective catheter placement in the left main pulmonary artery, when the catheter can wedge into the superior segment branch of the lower lobe. As little time as possible should elapse between the placement of the catheter and the final injection of contrast medium, since the catheter can advance itself with the thrust of each ventricular systole. For injections into the main pulmonary artery, be sure that the catheter tip is well inside the vessel but perfusing both sides equally. If the catheter tip slips into the ventricles, a poor angiogram results due to dilution, and there is increased danger of arrhythmias and perforation of the myocardium (this is particularly true if end-hole catheters are used).

The catheter may take an unusual course if there are intracardiac anomalies. These anomalies should be recorded on film or videotape, and appropriate injections of contrast medium and blood samples for determining oxygen saturation should be obtained prior to withdrawal (Fig. 17-8).

DIGITAL SUBTRACTION PULMONARY ANGIOGRAPHY

As in angiography in other parts of the body, digital subtraction angiography (DSA) should be used as one of the several methods available in any sophisticated modern angiographic facility to record angiographic information. DSA should be considered when the advantages of its high-density resolution (reduced contrast requirements) and "real time" capability (shorter examination time) outweigh its disadvantages of motion artifact, poorer spatial resolution, and often smaller available field size [20, 29].

The patient should not be too ill or aged to be cooperative, otherwise motion artifact presents a problem. A standard injection of contrast agent into the right atrium with the image intensifier centered over the suspicious area (predetermined by a previous perfusion lung scan or x-ray abnormality) may prove entirely satisfactory. This relatively noninvasive approach is not possible if the patient is severely ill, has renal problems (precluding large doses of contrast agent), or impending right heart failure. Under these circumstances the catheter should be selectively placed in the area of interest dictated by the previous perfusion scan. Using DSA with the catheter in this position requires less contrast medium and provides diagnostic information with greater safety and less chance of motion artifact. With either method, cardiac "gating" helps decrease artifacts due to cardiac motion, but the two frames per cycle provide fewer images per second for recording the information. Less time is required to perform the examination due to real time capabilities and shorter "darkroom time" for processing films. Under many circumstances, pulmonary DSA studies will demonstrate emboli as small as 2 to 3 mm in second- or even third-order branches.

Do not rely entirely on this method of recording information, for the overall consistency of the examination is dependent on many factors. The patient often cannot suppress respiration or may not have the cardiac output essential for a successful study. Other factors are the reliability of the radiographic equipment, the computer, and control of camera saturation. In addition, the field size is limited by the diameter of the image intensifier; when the field is small, multiple injections are necessary to cover the entire field of interest. Generally, both lungs can be seen when the image intensifier diameter is 14 in. or larger, most of one lung when it is 12 in., and only two-thirds of one lung when it is 9 in.

In the final analysis, all available modalities to make an accurate diagnosis as safely, efficiently, and cost-effectively as possible should be used. Despite being more invasive and time consuming, we prefer selective pulmonary arterial catheter placement and biplane serial filming as the initial diagnostic study in the typical patient. The diagnostic accuracy provided by the higher spatial and temporal resolution of this method makes patient cooperation less critical. Questionable areas may be further studied by additional examinations using

Table 17-3. Basic arrhythmia problems (seen on lead II of ECG)

Catheter location	Common problems		Comments	Treatment
Right atrium	Premature atrial contractions		Individual premature atrial contractions present no problem	No treatment is required. May have to pull back to the superior vena cava or inferior vena cava
Right atrium	Atrial tachycardia		Usually in runs with 1:1 conduction	Stop stimulating right atrium with catheter (i.e., pull back). If problem persists, (1) stimulate a PVC with catheter in right ventricle or left ventricle, or (2) perform carotid sinus massage
Right atrium	Atrial flutter or atrial fibrillation		These conditions have similar significance. They may decrease cardiac output (especially in mitral stenosis). There may be a rapid ventricular rate	(1) Rest and/or sedation (10 mg diazepam); usually converts spontaneously. (2) Synchronous shock may be applied (25–50 watt-sec)
Right atrium and/or right ventricle	RBBB		Occurs as a result of stimulation of the right atrium just above the septal leaflet of the tricuspid valve	No treatment; RBBB alone is not significant; it usually goes away within hours or days

Right atrium and/or right ventricle	Complete heart block	N.B.: Occurs if RBBB develops in patient with preexisting LBBB	(1) Hit patient's chest. (2) Stimulate a PVC by touching the walls of the right ventricle with the catheter. If a left heart catheter study is being simultaneously performed, it is preferable to stimulate the PVC in the left ventricle. (3) One can place, through a separate venous approach, a pacing catheter within the right ventricle and embed it under a trabecula. Alternatively, a noninvasive, temporary (external) pacer is available. * This should be performed before starting the study on all patients with a known LBBB. Test the pacing capabilities prior to angiography. If complete heart block persists, the pacing catheter must remain in the right ventricle, and a demand pulse generator must be attached.
Right ventricle	PVCs	Multiple repetitive PVCs in an irritable myocardium may progress to ventricular tachycardia	Find a "quiet spot"; usually advance the catheter tip across the pulmonary valve. May have to withdraw the catheter into the right atrium. May give a 50-mg bolus of lidocaine directly through the catheter (repeat in a few minutes if unsuccessful). May start lidocaine drip (2–4 mg/minute) if arrhythmia recurs.
Right ventricle	Ventricular tachycardia		Withdraw the catheter into the right atrium. Have patient cough, take deep breaths. Strike the precordium. Lidocaine push of 100 mg in 5 ml 5% dextrose or normal saline. Repeat with an 80-mg dose in a few minutes if tachycardia persists. Start a drip of 2–4 mg/minute. If blood pressure drops, and ventricular tachycardia persists, use synchronous cardioversion with ECG-controlled defibrillator: turn on the power, switch to synchronous mode (see highlight over QRS) and cardiovert with 50 watts-sec. Increase power if unsuccessful. If ventricular tachycardia progresses to ventricular fibrillation, switch off synchronous cardioversion, defibrillate, and institute full cardiopulmonary resuscitation.

*Manufactured by ZMI Corporation, 325 Vassar Street, Cambridge, MA 02139.

RBBB = right bundle branch block; LBBB = left bundle branch block; PVC = premature ventricular contractions. See also Table 18-2 (page 528).

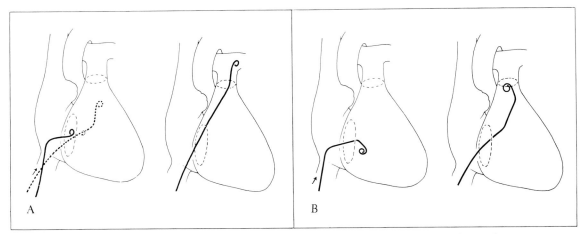

Fig. 17-7. The femoral approach to pulmonary arteriography.
A. The Grollman catheter.
B. A double-curved pigtail catheter.

either conventional films, photofluorographic spot films, or DSA studies. Some investigators prefer "panning" the pulmonary vascular bed using cineangiographic methods. The order of preference of these varied modalities will probably change as further advances in DSA technology occurs.

Complications and How to Handle Them

CARDIAC ARRHYTHMIAS

Basic arrhythmia problems are presented in Tables 17-3 and 18-2.

CARDIAC TAMPONADE

Although extremely rare, cardiac tamponade may be encountered during intracardiac catheterization. Be aware of this possibility, and try to avoid it with gentle catheter manipulations, and know how to recognize it. The patient becomes restless, dyspneic, and shocky, and the neck veins become prominent. As the cardiac output falls, the right-sided heart pressures (particularly the right atrial and the right ventricular end-diastolic pressures) increase rapidly, with an M- or W-shaped curve to the right atrial pressure tracing. The heart silhouette may increase in size, but not greatly so. Fluoroscopy is helpful, for intracardiac pulsations are evident by means of catheter movement, but the outer cardiac margin is virtually immobile.

Immediate action is required. Attach one end of a wire (with an alligator clamp on either side) to a

20-gauge spinal needle with attached syringe, and the other end of the wire to the unipolar lead of the ECG. Enter the pericardium with a shallow superior and dorsal subxiphoid approach, using continuous manual suction. An injury pattern (ST changes) signals when the needle has traversed the pericardium and has advanced too far into the myocardium. Prompt action and withdrawal of only small quantities of pericardial fluid may be lifesaving. If time permits, a cardiologic consultation should be urgently requested.

ACUTE COR PULMONALE

Normal pressure measurements are given in Table 17-2 and Figure 17-3. Pulmonary hypertension occurs if pulmonary artery systolic pressures are over 30 mm Hg. Since the vast majority of angiography of the pulmonary circulation is centered around pulmonary thromboembolism, the following discussion stresses hemodynamic abnormalities encountered in this condition. The same general principles pertain to other underlying causes of pulmonary hypertension.

Patients with a previously normal cardiopulmonary system suffering from acute pulmonary emboli demonstrate an elevation of pressures roughly linear in relation to the degree of angiographically demonstrated obstruction, up to a mean pulmonary artery pressure level of approximately 40 mm

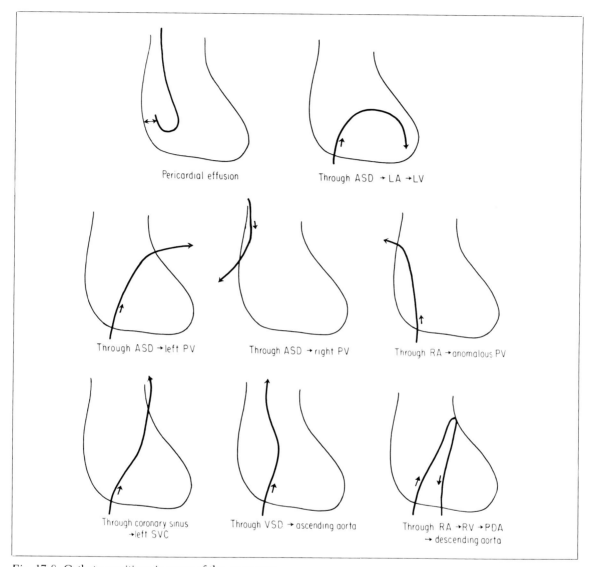

Pericardial effusion

Through ASD → LA → LV

Through ASD → left PV

Through ASD → right PV

Through RA → anomalous PV

Through coronary sinus → left SVC

Through VSD → ascending aorta

Through RA → RV → PDA → descending aorta

Fig. 17-8. Catheter positions in some of the more common cardiac abnormalities. Catheters may pass directly into anomalous veins draining into the right atrium. They may give a similar appearance on the anteroposterior projection when they pass through an atrial septal defect and then into a normally draining pulmonary vein. These positions should be recorded with injections of contrast medium.

Hg. Since those with a previously normal heart do not generate pressures much higher than this level, if higher mean pressures are recorded, there is usually some underlying cardiac or pulmonary cause for the hypertension; there may have been preexist-

ing recurrent pulmonary embolism. Right atrial mean pressure elevation is seen less frequently than high pulmonary artery pressures in patients with pulmonary embolism who had a previously normal cardiopulmonary status. When the pulmonary artery mean pressure exceeds 30 mm Hg, the right atrial pressure may be elevated. An important pressure measurement is the right ventricular end-diastolic pressure, for it is a measure of that chamber's ability to sustain the pressures in the pulmonary circulation. It rises when the right ventricle fails to keep up with the rising pulmonary resis-

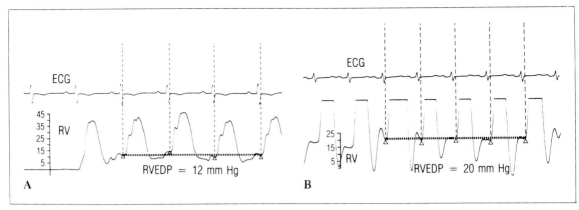

Fig. 17-9.
A. The right ventricular end-diastolic pressure
   (RVEDP) is higher than normal but not at a level
   dangerous for selective pulmonary arteriogram.
B. RVEDP measures 20 mm Hg in another patient
   with carcinoma of the lung and systemic pulmonary artery pressures. He developed cardiopulmonary arrest 30 minutes following the arteriogram. A
   segmental branch embolus to the right lower lobe
   was present. (From I. S. Johnsrude, *Pulmonary
   Embolism. Current Problems in Diagnostic Radiology.* Chicago: Year Book Medical Publishers, 1982.
   Used by permission.)

tance. The right ventricular end-diastolic pressure
is measured approximately 0.04 second after the
QRS on the accompanying ECG, or after the first
valley in the pressure curve after the QRS (Fig. 17-
3). Measurements under 7 mm Hg are normal.
Higher pressures often indicate an element of right
heart failure. When they reach 20 to 25 mm Hg or
higher, acute cardiac decompensation may follow
even small injections of ionic contrast medium
into the pulmonary arteries or chambers of the
right side of the heart (Fig. 17-9). This failure may
be due to the volume of contrast agent injected and
also to its hyperosmolarity. Under these circumstances the risk of not continuing the investigation
must be weighed with that of inducing an irreversible acute cor pulmonale.

If the study is continued, institute measures to
lessen the complications of angiography. Nonionic
contrast agents are known to induce less hemodynamic stress than ionic contrast media. Superselective injections of small volumes of contrast
agents in areas predetermined by perfusion scan
defects may more safely yield a diagnostic study.
Smaller doses of lower concentration contrast
media are required for selective intraarterial digital
studies. Oxygen should be administered during the
entire study. Inflow to the right side of the heart
can be decreased for several minutes during and
after the contrast injection by inflating blood pressure cuffs on the patient's thighs up to 80 mm Hg
(Fig. 17-10).

Precautions for dealing with acute cor pulmonale should be instituted. Under normal circumstances the pressures in the right side of the
heart increase slightly following contrast injections, but there is no decrease in the heart rate. If

bradycardia or rapidly increasing right-sided cardiac pressures occur, there should be immediate
withdrawal of 100 to 200 ml of blood through the
pulmonary artery catheter. Elevate the patient to a
sitting position. Morphine (up to ½ grain, or 15
mg) may also be administered intravenously. An
inotropic agent (sustaining left ventricular contractility) should be immediately available and administered through an existing intravenous line.
Dopamine is one agent that increases cardiac output without associated tachyarrhythmia. In seri-
ously ill patients, the initial recommended dose is
5 to 10 μg/kg/minute, rising by similar increments
up to 20 to 50 μg/kg/minute. One 5-ml (200-mg)
ampule mixed with 500 ml 5% dextrose or normal
saline gives a dilution of 400 μg per milliliter. In a
60 to 70-kg patient, the starting dose should be 1 to
2 ml per minute. Systemic blood pressure must be
monitored closely, and its rise is titrated with the
rate of intravenous administration. Be prepared to
institute cardiac and respiratory resuscitation.

Complications other than cardiac arrhythmias,
tamponade, and acute cor pulmonale can occur
[22]. Hematomas, extravasation in veins, reactions
to contrast media, and shaking chills have all been

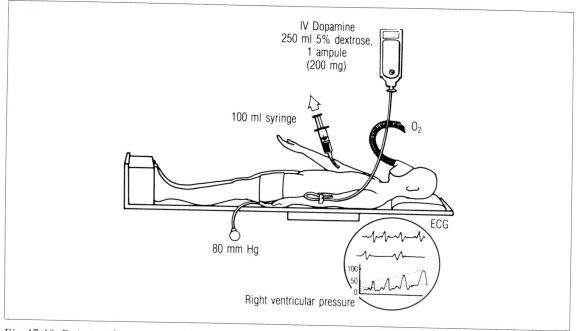

Fig. 17-10. Patient with acute cor pulmonale undergoing pulmonary angiography. Findings: bradycardia,
rapidly increasing right ventricular pressures, and decreasing left-sided pressures. Oxygen mask and restriction of venous inflow to the right side of the heart
(blood pressure cuffs on the legs) are prophylactic measures. Therapy consists of immediate withdrawal of 100
to 200 ml of blood from the pulmonary artery catheter
to reduce the load on the heart. Dopamine, a 1 to 2 ml
per minute drip, sustains cardiac output.

described. Of the deaths reported during pulmonary angiography (10 in a large composite series of
over 4000 studied), the vast majority were in those
with acute cor pulmonale [12]. Successfully converted cardiopulmonary arrest occurred in 9 patients, intimal injections in 6, perforations in 18,
and arrhythmias in 29.

Anatomic Considerations

As the left pulmonary artery arises from the main
pulmonary artery segment, it courses higher and
more posteriorly than the right. Since it is
foreshortened in its proximal portion on the anteroposterior projection, an additional lateral or
right posterior oblique projection is necessary for
complete evaluation. On both sides, the arteries
generally pass along the course of the bronchi.
There may be variations, for sometimes there is

not a separate branch for each segment. As the
contrast-laden vessels course out to the periphery
of the lungs, unopacified blood and crossing arteries may simulate filling defects of clot. In addition, bona fide filling defects may be obscured by
overlying vessels, a problem that is best resolved by
biplane studies. During the capillary phase (2 to 3
seconds into the injection), there is an even distribution of the capillary stain throughout both lung
fields. This is followed by a gradual but simultaneous centripetal filling of all of the pulmonary
veins, in both the upper and the lower lobes. In
the normal, supine patient there is no cephalo-
caudal differential in flow pattern. The pulmonary
veins lie more inferior to their corresponding arteries and pass in a more horizontal position as
they enter into the left atrium. In the upper lobes,
the veins lie a little more lateral than their corresponding arteries. Within 4 to 6 seconds, the left
atrium is densely stained and well marginated. If it
loses its sharply defined inferior margin, there may
be an atrial septal defect or other abnormal communication with the right atrium. In the absence
of a shunt there is sequential filling of the left
ventricle and thoracic aorta without further opacification of the right-sided cardiac structures. Figure 17-11 represents a normal selective right pulmonary arteriogram.

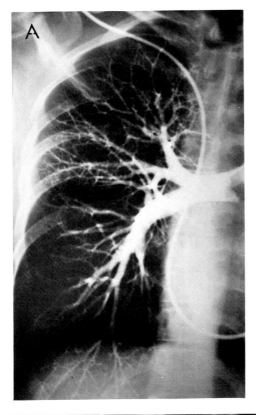

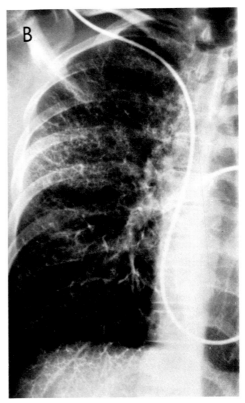

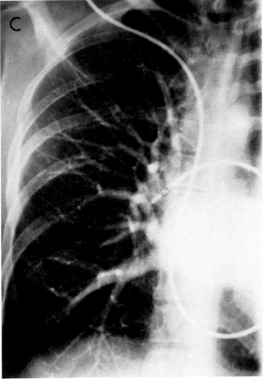

Fig. 17-11. Normal right pulmonary arteriogram in anteroposterior projections.
A. Arterial phase.
B. Late arterial phase.
C. Venous phase of the examination. (From I. S. Johnsrude, *Pulmonary Embolism. Current Problems in Diagnostic Radiology.* Chicago: Year Book Medical Publishers, 1982. Used by permission.)

Pulmonary Thromboembolism

Pulmonary thromboembolism is an often lethal, clinically confusing, and underdiagnosed condition [32]. Survival is considerably improved if the diagnosis is established and treatment instituted [2]. Insight into the factors predisposing to pulmonary embolism, the pathophysiology of the disease, the clinical manifestations, and the judicious combination of radiographic studies such as chest x rays, ventilation-perfusion lung scans, and pulmonary arteriograms help provide the answer to this often complex diagnostic puzzle.

FACTORS PREDISPOSING TO PULMONARY EMBOLISM

Those conditions resulting in venous stasis, a hypercoagulable state, or an abnormality of the veins predispose to venous thrombosis and pulmonary embolism [31]. Ninety percent or more of pulmonary emboli arise from thrombi in the deep venous system of the pelvis and lower extremities, from which they break off and flow to the lungs. There should be a high index of suspicion in patients with the following problems: heart disease (particularly myocardial infarction, myocardiopathies, and congestive heart failure), chronic obstructive pulmonary disease, prolonged immobilization due to trauma or surgery, malignancies, peripheral venous disease, obesity, pregnancy, or other medical conditions such as polycythemia vera, dysproteinemias, antithrombin III deficiencies, and sickle cell anemia. There is an increased incidence of pulmonary embolism in young patients on oral contraceptives.

PATHOPHYSIOLOGY

There are two major factors involved in the pathophysiology of pulmonary embolism. The first is the mechanical block to the pulmonary vascular bed and the second is the release of humoral substances by degranulation of platelets within the embolus. Both of these result in increased resistance to the occluded pulmonary artery and shunting of flow to uninvolved segments. Pulmonary arteriolar vasoconstriction is induced both by the accompanying hypoxia and by the humoral substances released by the platelets (serotonin, histamine, catecholamines, adenine nucleotides, prostaglandins, and others) [36]. The vasospasm is thought to account for the relatively larger perfusion defect seen on an accompanying perfusion scan than can be accounted for by the size of the occluded vessel. Peripheral airway constriction causes loss of lung volume, restricted ventilation, decreased lung compliance and an increase in total lung flow resistance.

The rise in pulmonary arterial pressure that occurs causes a strain on the right side of the heart, which, if severe, can progress on to acute cor pulmonale and rapid left heart failure with systemic hypotension and death. The result of continued ventilation in the nonperfused segments of the lung is an increase in dead air space, which leads to a decrease in gas exchange. There is resulting hypoxemia, which is relative to the extent of pulmonary vascular occlusion suffered and also to the amount of pulmonary reserve the patient enjoyed prior to the embolic event. Thus, a patient with chronic cardiopulmonary disease who develops pulmonary embolism suffers more severe hypoxemia than one who was previously healthy.

An accompanying loss of surfactant results in areas of subsegmental atelectasis.

All of these changes contribute to the dyspnea and tachypnea found in almost all patients with pulmonary embolism, and the elevated diaphragms seen on their chest roentgenograms.

Death of tissue distal to an occluded pulmonary artery (i.e., pulmonary infarction) occurs in only 10 percent of pulmonary emboli. This is because the systemic bronchial arteries and not the pulmonary arteries are responsible for maintaining pulmonary parenchymal viability. Pulmonary infarction is seen more often when the more peripheral pulmonary arteries are occluded, and when patients have underlying pulmonary disease.

CLINICAL MANIFESTATIONS

The most common symptoms are dyspnea, cough, pleuritic chest pain, and hemoptysis; the most striking of these is dyspnea. Frequent physical findings are tachypnea, tachycardia, rales, and fever (sometimes as high as 40°C). Pleural friction rub, wheezing, and a prominent second pulmonic heart sound may also be present. Acute left heart failure may supervene. Shock, severe dyspnea, a loud P_2 heart sound, and S_3 or S_4 gallop may signal onset of acute cor pulmonale. Symptoms and signs are for the most part nonspecific [23, 34].

LABORATORY TESTS

Laboratory tests are also often nonspecific. Oxygen tension is low in most patients with pulmonary embolism, but a low PO_2 is of limited value for precisely making the diagnosis of pulmonary embolus.

The $PaCO_2$ may be low because of the hyperventilation that usually accompanies pulmonary embolism [8]. Enzyme studies are equally nonspecific.

The white blood cell count may or may not be elevated. Suspicion of pulmonary embolism should be aroused if the white blood cell count is normal (or if the patient is afebrile) in a patient with pulmonary consolidation.

The ECG is rarely helpful, except to exclude myocardial infarction. It may show signs of right heart strain. Atrial flutter or atrial fibrillation may occur. Be cognizant of a left bundle branch block if catheterization of the right heart chambers is anticipated for fear of inducing a complete bundle branch block.

ROENTGENOGRAPHIC STUDIES

Roentgenographic studies include the following in suggested order of preference: chest x ray, perfusion and ventilation lung scans, pulmonary angiograms. Occasionally peripheral venography may be performed to look for a source of pulmonary emboli.

Chest X Ray

Chest film abnormalities may not be seen during the first 24 hours following thromboembolism. An elevated diaphragm and areas of subsegmental atelectasis may occur. Those patients who have emboli without pulmonary infarction show rapidly clearing areas of air space disease. Segmental or lobar oligemia due to occlusion of a major branch may occasionally be seen, together with increased flow to uninvolved segments due to shunting of blood. Stress on vascular structures and cardiac chambers proximal to the point of obstruction may be reflected by dilatation of the pulmonary artery, right ventricle, right atrium, superior vena cava, and azygos vein. There is a very high incidence of pleural effusion when pulmonary infarction develops. Here also, the areas of pulmonary consolidation take considerably longer (up to several weeks) to resolve.

Radioisotope Perfusion and Ventilation Lung Scans

Both perfusion and ventilation lung scans are necessary in the diagnostic work-up of almost all patients suspected of pulmonary embolism. For greatest accuracy, lung scans should be performed as soon after the embolic event as possible, before the body's inherent fibrinolytic activity modifies abnormal perfusion patterns. An accompanying recent chest x ray should be reviewed.

Pulmonary emboli usually occur at lobar or segmental levels, most frequently involve the lower lobes, are usually multiple, and are often bilateral. These, then, are the types of defects that are most

characteristically seen on perfusion lung scans in patients with embolic disease. A well performed normal perfusion lung scan showing a uniform distribution of tracer activity throughout both lung fields, is of great value for it virtually excludes pulmonary embolus.

Since any condition that alters pulmonary blood flow gives rise to a perfusion defect, the study is sensitive to these changes, but it is not specific. Careful analysis of the perfusion defect or defects, together with chest x rays and the addition of ventilation scans, improves specificity.

Ventilation scans help to identify airway parenchymal diseases that cause perfusion defects other than those caused by pulmonary emboli and are reported to improve the specificity of perfusion scans by as much as 30 percent. There are several inert gases available for these scans, but the most commonly used are xenon 133 and xenon 127. If [133]xenon is used, its low energy photons require that the ventilation scan precedes the perfusion scan. The higher photon energy provided by [127]Xe allows the xenon scans to be performed after the perfusion scan. Thus, the ventilation scan need not be performed at all if the perfusion scan is normal. Also, an optimal projection (reflected by the position in which defects are best observed on the perfusion scan) can be chosen during the ventilation scan. Normal ventilation lung scans show an even distribution of tracer throughout both lung fields on the initial image and at the termination of the equilibrium phase of the study, followed by gradual symmetric diminution of activity with complete washout in 2 to 3 minutes. Nonembolic parenchymal disease causing abnormal areas of ventilation result in a delay in uptake of the tracer, together with defects, in both the immediate and the equilibrium phases of the study. Air trapping is recognized as focal areas of retained activity on the delayed washout phase of the examination, in areas that earlier were normal or had abnormally decreased activity.

Ventilation-perfusion scans should be performed if the perfusion scan is not normal. If multiple large perfusion scans defects are recognized in the lung or portion of the lung with normal ventilation, this indicates a mismatching of ventilation and perfusion, which represents a high probability for pulmonary embolism. If the ventilation scan demonstrates a defect similar to that of the perfusion scan (matching ventilation and perfusion) and/or trapping of the xenon in the lungs, obstructive airway disease is most commonly present [21, 24, 28, 35].

The probability of ventilation-perfusion lung scans being diagnostic of pulmonary embolism can be classified as follows:

1. High probability (90 percent chance of embolus). Multiple large perfusion defects are seen at the lobar or segmental level with a normal ventilation lung scan. The accompanying chest x-ray should either be normal or, preferably, show areas of abnormality smaller than the corresponding areas seen on the perfusion lung scan.
2. Intermediate or indeterminate probability (40 percent chance of embolus). Single, segmental mismatching defects or multiple segmental defects, which may be either mismatching or matching. The perfusion defects match the size of the abnormality seen on the chest roentgenogram.
3. Low probability (approximately 10 percent or smaller chance of embolus). Ventilation defects match perfusion defects. There may also be subsegmental or diffuse mismatching defects. The defect may be smaller than the corresponding roentgenographic abnormality.

During the interpretation of the lung scan, the clinical probability of pulmonary thromboembolism should also be considered. A high clinical probability for thromboembolism, together with a high ventilation-perfusion scan probability, will have pulmonary emboli in well over 90 percent. It is those patients with an intermediate probability or indeterminate probability lung scans that generally require further investigation. In addition, patients with a high ventilation-perfusion scan probability but a low clinical probability and those with a low ventilation-perfusion scan probability but a high clinical probability should also be further studied.

In summary, all patients suspected of having pulmonary embolism should have ventilation-perfusion scans regardless of the appearance of the chest x ray. They provide excellent "road maps" for selective pulmonary angiography and act as baselines for future evaluation. Only patients who cannot physically undergo the procedure should be excluded. There should be an accompanying recent chest x ray. A normal ventilation-perfusion scan excludes pulmonary emboli. Matching defects should be analyzed closely; if the perfusion defect is larger than the ventilation defect, it increases the probability of emboli; if smaller, it decreases the likelihood. Only with high or low probability lung scans can the diagnosis be made with relative confidence, and then only if the clinical setting is correct.

One report found pulmonary embolism angiographically in 15 percent of patients with low probability scans and in only 66 percent of those with high probability scans. Intermediate probability or indeterminate scans were only 32 to 39 percent accurate in demonstrating emboli [3].

Pulmonary arteriography is recommended in all difficult decisions, for the cost and risk of long-term anticoagulation is far greater than that of pulmonary arteriography [30]. Approximately 10 percent of patients suspected of having pulmonary thromboembolism who have had ventilation-perfusion scans undergo pulmonary arteriography.

The examples in Figures 17-12, 17-13, and 17-14 illustrate the range of diagnostic presentation with ventilation-perfusion scans in patients suspected of pulmonary embolism.

Pulmonary Angiography
Pulmonary angiography is performed when the diagnosis is in reasonable doubt [18]. It acts as confirmatory evidence of pulmonary embolism in those patients suspected of pulmonary embolism who run a high risk of anticoagulant or thrombolytic therapy (e.g., those with recent surgery, cerebral hemorrhage, or bleeding ulcers) or in those in whom intervention (caval interruption, placement of an inferior vena cava filter, pulmonary embolectomy) is being considered. Approximately 30 to 40 percent of patients undergoing pulmonary angiography demonstrate pulmonary emboli.

Pulmonary angiography poses a greater risk in patients with suspected embolism who have severe right heart failure. Concurrent hemodynamic studies give additional information on the severity of the obstructive process (Fig. 17-9). Injections of contrast medium through a selectively placed catheter in each of the right and left pulmonary arteries provides greater safety than does a single large main pulmonary artery injection, because there is less volume load on an already overloaded right ventricle. Selective studies also permit biplane angiography (and therefore a more complete

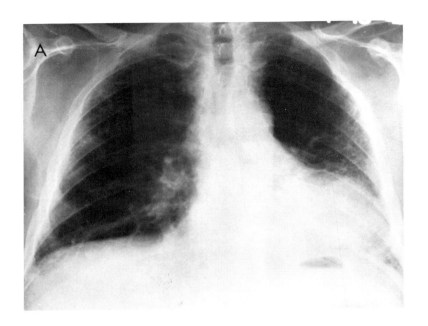

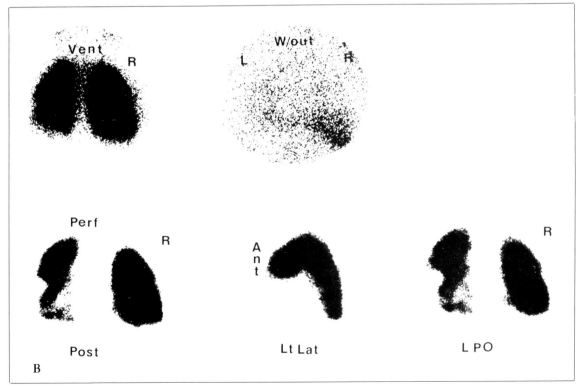

Fig. 17-12.

A. Left lower lobe consolidation on chest x ray.

B. Large mismatching perfusion defect in left lung. Ventilation scans show air trapping in the right base.

C. No emboli but slow flow seen on pulmonary arteriogram. Heparin therapy was withdrawn and final diagnosis of *Pneumocystis carinii* pursued. (From I. S. Johnsrude, *Pulmonary Embolism. Current Problems in Diagnostic Radiology*. Chicago: Year Book Medical Publishers, 1982. Used by permission.)

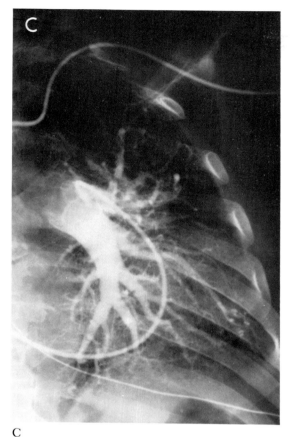

C

study) with a single bolus of contrast agent in each lung. A program of 15 films in each plane sequentially exposed over a period of 10 seconds captures not only morphologic pathology but also the dynamics of abnormal flow. Superselective studies, balloon occlusion, and occasionally magnification studies enhance the diagnostic capabilities in more difficult cases. Selective intraarterial DSA studies using nonionic contrast agent make the study safer in those with suspected right heart failure.

Because pulmonary arteriography is an invasive procedure, requiring skill and sophisticated angiographic equipment, it is wise to perform the procedure during the daytime hours when a full supporting staff is available. An emergency arteriogram is rarely required and is more prone to complications. If a patient has findings arousing suspicion of pulmonary embolism during the night and the scans are suggestive or equivocal, it is a good policy to treat the patient with heparin until the following morning, when anticoagulant therapy is discontinued during the angiographic proce-

dure. The only exception to this is if there is a contraindication to heparin or if the patient is critically ill and requires immediate angiographic confirmation, operative intervention, thrombolytic therapy, or an inferior vena cava filter.

ANGIOGRAPHIC FINDINGS. The primary angiographic signs of pulmonary embolism are an intravascular filling defect or a vessel cutoff. Overlying vessels must not be confused as filling defects, and defects should be seen on at least two consecutive films. Occasionally a small branch is occluded flush with the origin of the vessel; this makes detection difficult. When the sum of the diameters of branching vessels is less than that of the parent vessel, be suspicious of an embolus. Small fresh clots can lyse within 24 hours, but are usually seen angiographically up to 4 days after the embolic event, and sometimes even up to 16 days later. Figures 17-13 to 17-18 demonstrate a variety of presentations of acute pulmonary emboli.

There are secondary angiographic findings of pulmonary embolism, but these are also seen in other conditions. These include parenchymal staining, decreased perfusion (Fig. 17-16), crowded vessels, delayed venous return from the affected area, and shunting away from the involved lung. These associated findings, when seen by themselves, are nonspecific; they should lead to superselective and magnification arteriograms to help resolve the question. Microemboli may manifest themselves by tortuosity and pruning of peripheral vessels localized to segmental areas with accompanying slow filling and emptying (Fig. 17-19).

Subacute (see Fig. 17-24) and chronic changes (Figs. 17-20, 17-21) of pulmonary thromboemboli may sometimes be recognized.

Changes occur soon after pulmonary emboli are lodged within the pulmonary artery, and their fate depends on the type of thrombus from which they arise. If fresh, the emboli usually lyse and disappear. They can fragment, obstruct, organize, and recanalize to form intravascular webs and strands, mural thrombi, and plaques.

CHRONIC PULMONARY EMBOLISM. There is a small group of patients in whom pulmonary emboli fail to resolve, and who with repetitive bouts of pulmonary embolism so increase their pulmonary vascular resistance as to develop pulmonary hypertension. The embolic events may be large and involve whole segments, lobes, or lungs. The pa-

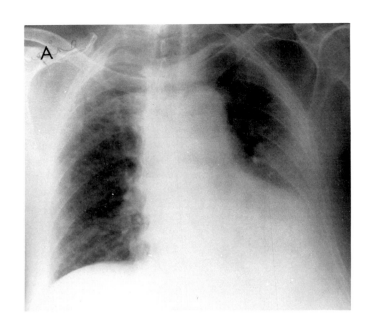

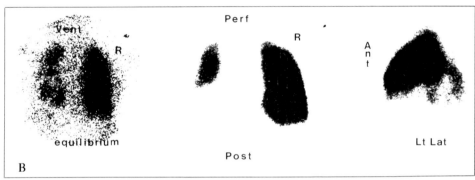

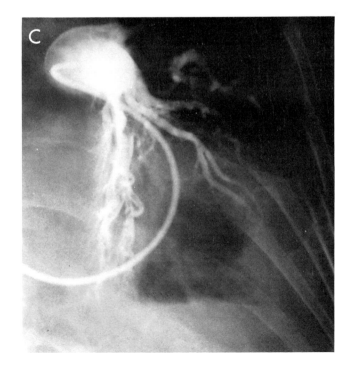

tients in this group are beyond conservative medical management, and surgical intervention to remove the organized fibrotic emboli has been advocated [6]. This procedure has been accomplished successfully when there are large areas of occluded vessels but the vessels peripheral to the obstruction are patent. In these patients, the heart (particularly the right-side chambers) and the main pulmonary artery are generally enlarged on the chest x ray (see Fig. 17-21). Pulmonary arteriography shows smooth convex-bordered occlusions (see Fig. 17-21), stenoses, intravascular webs, or strands (see Fig. 17-20A, B, and C).

An important addition to the angiographic evaluation of these patients (beyond pulmonary arteriography and right heart pressure determination) is bronchial arteriography. The lungs have a dual blood supply, provided by the pulmonary arteries and bronchial arteries. If pulmonary arteries are occluded, bronchial artery circulation hypertrophies, and the degree of hypertrophy depends on the extent and chronicity of the occlusion. The intercommunications between the peripheral pulmonary and bronchial arterial system are nicely demonstrated in Figure 17-21, in which the pulmonary artery branches distal to the chronically occluded pulmonary artery are filled during a bronchial arteriogram. This helps to predict healthy back-bleeding at the time of surgical removal of the fibrosed emboli and potential success of chronic embolectomy. One must always be aware of the dangers of pulmonary angiography in these patients with pulmonary hypertension. Be sure to measure pulmonary artery and right ventricular pressures, and in particular, the right ventricular end-diastolic pressure, during the procedure.

ACCURACY OF PULMONARY ANGIOGRAPHY. The accuracy depends on the compulsive, judicious search for emboli, selective catheter placement,

---

Fig. 17-13.
A. Chest x ray. Note air space disease and effusion in left base.
B. Intermediate to low probability for embolus. Left lower lobe perfusion defect larger than corresponding ventilation defect.
C. Large embolus seen on pulmonary angiogram. (From I. S. Johnsrude, *Pulmonary Embolism. Current Problems in Diagnostic Radiology.* Chicago: Year Book Medical Publishers, 1982. Used by permission.)

and the time lag between the embolic event and the angiographic procedure. If the interval between the embolic episode and the angiogram is long, there is a greater chance of the clot lysing and an angiographic false-negative result.

Once emboli are found, the presence and extent of other emboli may be inferred from the accompanying perfusion lung scan. With this approach in mind, it is doubtful that significant emboli will be missed. Those few patients with equivocal arteriograms should be anticoagulated if the lung scans and clinical findings show strong evidence for pulmonary embolism.

INTERVENTIONAL TECHNIQUES IN PULMONARY EMBOLISM

Once the diagnosis of pulmonary embolism has been firmly established, the majority of patients are successfully treated with standard anticoagulant therapy using heparin followed by dicumarol. This treatment inhibits further formation of clot while allowing the body's inherent thrombolytic capabilities to work on the obstructing clot. Some patients, however, may require more immediate treatment. These include: (1) Patients who have developed massive emboli (i.e., life-threatening events with emboli in two or more lobar arteries or their equivalent); (2) Pulmonary emboli of any size in patients who are hemodynamically unstable due to previous underlying cardiopulmonary problems; (3) Pulmonary emboli that do not respond to standard anticoagulation. In these patients, an attempt to actively dissolve, displace, or remove the clot by the following means may be life-saving (surgical embolectomy carries a high mortality):

1. Clots may be fragmented and dispersed manually with a catheter (Fig. 17-22), thus allowing perfusion of a larger number of otherwise obstructed vessels.
2. Special catheters with large suction cups at the tips can be surgically introduced into the femoral vein or the internal jugular vein [13].
3. Substituting anticoagulant therapy for thrombolytic therapy may bring about more rapid dissolution of the clot.

Systemic Thrombolytic Therapy
Systemic thrombolytic therapy results in significant improvement in pulmonary perfusion, a reduction in the mean pulmonary artery pressures,

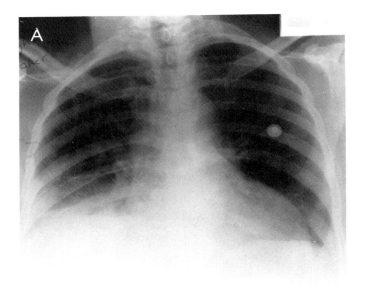

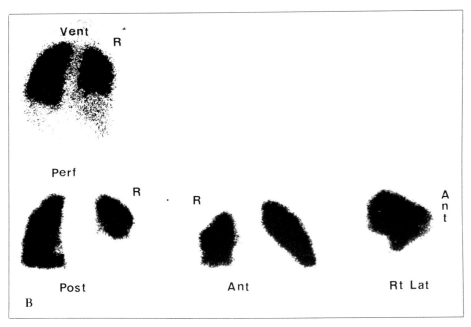

Fig. 17-14.
A. Chest x ray shows pleural effusion in right costophrenic angle.
B. Low probability ventilation-perfusion scans with
   segmental matching defects in the right lower lobe.
C and D. Anteroposterior (C) and lateral (D) projection
   pulmonary arteriograms. Pulmonary embolus demonstrated best on lateral projection. (From I. S.
   Johnsrude, *Pulmonary Embolism. Current Problems
   in Diagnostic Radiology.* Chicago: Year Book Medical Publishers, 1982. Used by permission.)

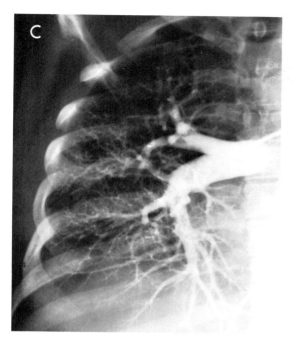

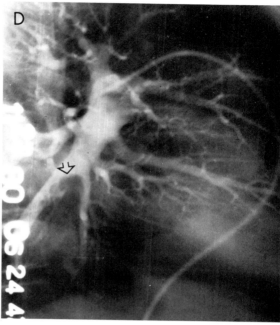

Fig. 17-15. Multiple small emboli to right lower lobe. A "racetrack" shape is formed as the contrast agent streams on either side of intraluminal clots in separate segmental arteries to the right lower lobe (*arrows*).

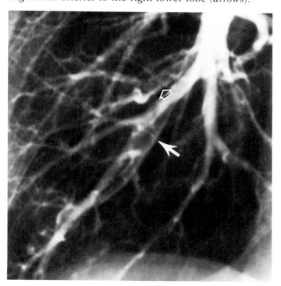

an increase in systemic oxygenation, and a slight improvement in cardiac output. It may have better long-term effect than heparin therapy alone, for it causes more complete resolution of pulmonary emboli than does heparin, and it provides better capillary perfusion [33]. The existing peripheral venous thrombi are also dissolved more thoroughly, thereby preventing recurrent pulmonary embolism.

The major risk associated with systemic doses of thrombolytic agents is bleeding, which occurs at surgical invasive, cut-down, and puncture sites. Thrombolytic agents are contraindicated in patients who have had surgery within the past 10 days (6 weeks for neurosurgical procedures), extensive trauma, or major invasive procedures. They are also contraindicated in patients with internal bleeding, recent strokes, cerebral metastases, aneurysm, or other similar diseases with a potential for bleeding. Intravenous punctures should be kept to a minimum; subclavian vein and intraarterial punctures should be avoided altogether. Thrombolytic agents should not be used for at least 12 hours after insertion of a vena cava filter. No anticoagulants or platelet altering drugs should be used during systemic thrombolytic therapy. In patients whose treatment started with heparin, bleeding parameters should be measured accurately and

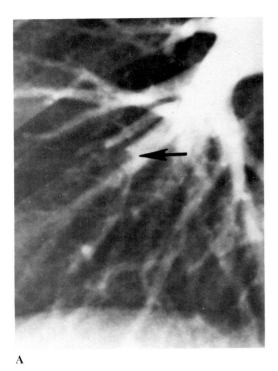

A

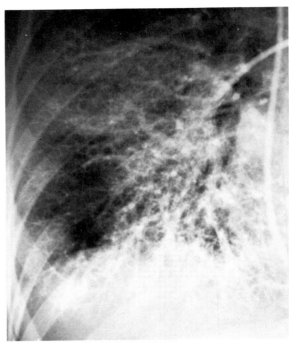

B

Fig. 17-16. Embolus to a segmental branch of the right lower lobe.
A. Arterial phase shows abrupt cutoff (*arrow*) of the segmental artery.
B. Capillary phase shows poor perfusion to the involved segment.

Fig. 17-17. Pulmonary emboli (selective biplane study).
A. Attenuated vessels extend out to peripheral infiltrate in the right costophrenic angle. Since no cutoff or filling defects are seen, the diagnosis cannot be made with confidence on the basis of this projection.
B. Lateral projection. Sharp cutoffs (*arrowheads*) confirm the diagnosis of pulmonary embolism.

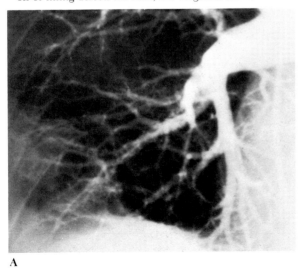

A

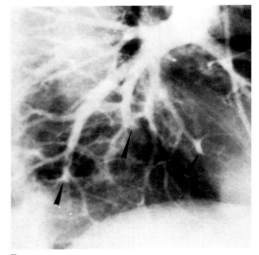

B

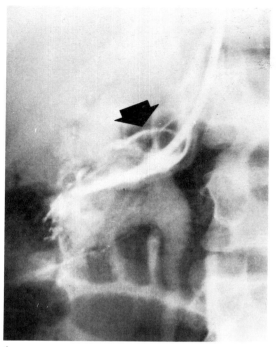

A

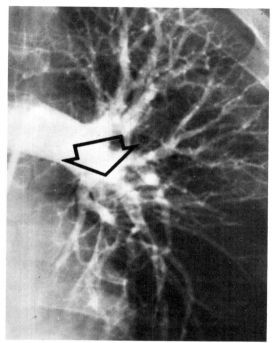

B

Fig. 17-18. Pulmonary embolism arising from a thrombus in the right renal vein.
A. Large filling defect (*arrow*) in the right renal vein.
B. Large pulmonary embolus (*arrow*) to the left lower lobe. The patient presented clinically with signs of pulmonary thromboembolism. Proteinuria was uncovered prior to the examination.

should be near normal before thrombolytic therapy is instituted.

Selective Low-dose Thrombolytic Therapy
The catheter tip is embedded within the clot and positive pressure infusion is instituted. An initial dose of streptokinase, 20,000 IU, followed by 5000 to 10,000 IU per hour for up to 24 hours may be used. (See Chap. 7 for details of administration.) Urokinase, although it is more expensive, appears to be a more efficient thrombolytic agent (Fig. 17-23; see Chap. 7).

Thrombolysis is less successful in subacute and

Fig. 17-19. Pulmonary hypertension, with prominent central pulmonary artery and tortuous peripheral vessels. Small peripheral vessels demonstrate peripheral emboli. Right ventricular pressure of 96 mm Hg with an end-diastolic pressure of 20 mm Hg.

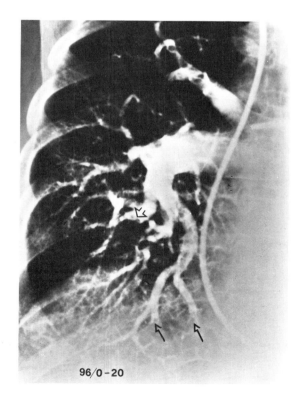

96/0-20

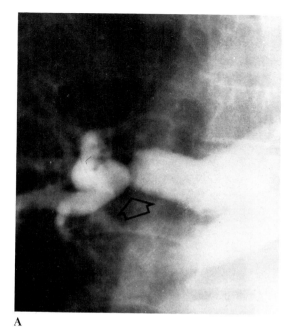

A

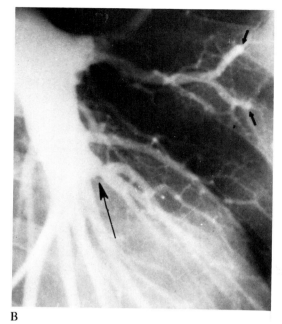

B

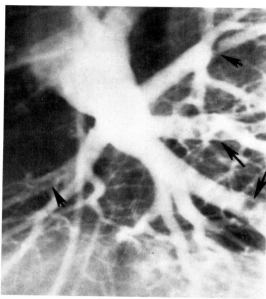

C

Fig. 17-20. Changes of chronic emboli in three separate patients.
A. Large web in artery to right upper lobe (*arrow*). The patient had pulmonary hypertension with multiple episodes of previous emboli.
B. Pulmonary web segmental branch to the left lower lobe (*long arrow*) and chronic rounded occlusions in arteries to the midlung (*short arrows*).
C. Changes of chronic and acute pulmonary emboli in the right lower lobe (lateral projection). There is a linear defect in the anterior segment of the lower lobe, and a web in the superior segment of the right lower lobe (*short arrows*). One can see filling defects of acute emboli in the posterior basilar segments (*long arrows*).

chronic emboli (Fig. 17-24). Newly discovered tissue plasminogen activators are clot selective thrombolytic agents that do not induce systemic thrombolytic action and hold promise for a safer, more effective form of therapy in the near future.

Inferior Vena Cava Filter
Another method of dealing with pulmonary embolism is interruption of the inferior vena cava.

This procedure may be used when anticoagulant and/or thrombolytic treatment fails or is contraindicated. Patients at high risk for bleeding, those who develop repetitive pulmonary embolism despite anticoagulation, or those who demonstrate large free-floating ileocaval thrombi may benefit from this approach. Filters being developed can be rapidly and safely introduced percutaneously through either the jugular or the femoral venous approach. (See Chap. 21 for the technical details of insertion.)

Pulmonary Hypertension

Pulmonary angiography and cardiac catheterization can sometimes help to differentiate the vari-

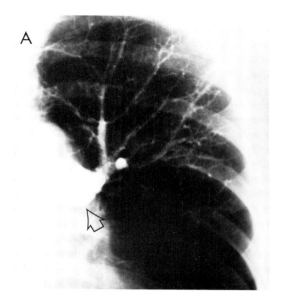

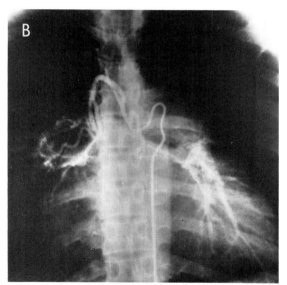

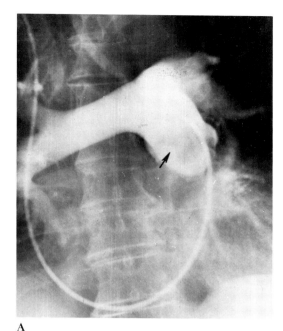

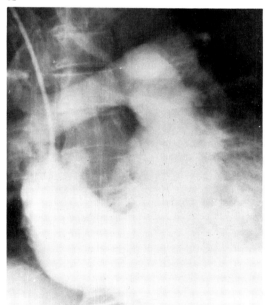

Fig. 17-21.
A. Chronic occlusion of all branches of pulmonary artery to left lower lobe (*arrow*).
B. Bronchial arteriogram demonstrates filling of these occluded pulmonary branches through bronchopulmonary arterial communications. (From I. S. Johnsrude, *Pulmonary Embolism. Current Problems in Diagnostic Radiology*. Chicago: Year Book Medical Publishers, 1982. Used by permission.)

Fig. 17-22.
A. A large central pulmonary artery embolus (*arrow*) 4 days postoperatively. The patient was hypotensive and unconscious at this time. The pressure measured at the catheter tip dampened during passage through the clot.
B. Repeat angiogram following purposeful fragmentation of the embolus was performed to rule out atrial clot prior to embolectomy. No central clot is now evident. The systemic pressures rose 20 mm Hg, and the patient improved without surgery.

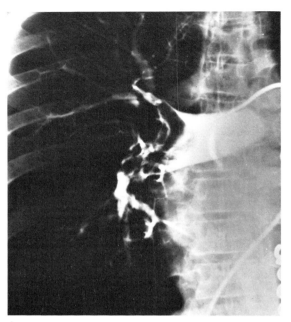

A

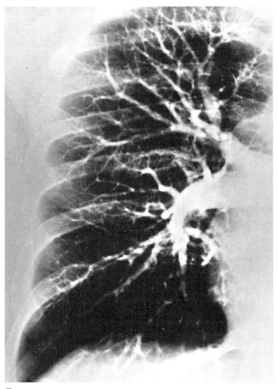

B

Fig. 17-23. Repeated pulmonary emboli despite Coumadin therapy, treated selectively with intraarterial urokinase followed by inferior vena cava filter.

A. Pulmonary angiogram (using 15 ml of nonionic contrast agent) 2 days following the acute episode demonstrates massive right pulmonary artery embolism. Pulmonary artery pressure measured 58/22 mm Hg (mean of 40 mm Hg). Urokinase, 500,000 IU mixed with 4 ml diluent, was injected directly into the clot, followed by 4000 IU per minute for 2 hours, then 2000 IU per minute for 20 hours. Heparin, 1000 IU per hour, was also administered. Fibrinogen level and partial thromboplastin time were followed closely.

B. Pulmonary angiogram 24 hours later shows almost normal perfusion of the right lung. Pulmonary artery pressure 30/12 mm Hg (mean 18 mm Hg).

ous causes of increased pulmonary pressures. Since pressure, flow, and resistance are interrelated, an increase in either flow or resistance may cause an elevation of pressure. Increased resistance may be at the postcapillary venous level (e.g., left heart obstruction or failure; obstruction to the mitral valve, left atrium, or pulmonary venous return). Resistance may also be increased as a result of obstructive pulmonary arterial disease

Fig. 17-24. Subacute (9-day-old) and chronic pulmonary embolus involving almost all of the right lower lobe. Selective intraarterial treatment with urokinase brought little change.

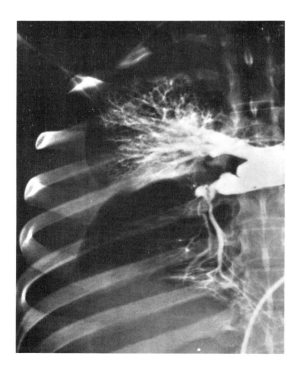

(pulmonary embolism, arteritis, primary pulmonary hypertension) or obliterative parenchymal disease (emphysema, pulmonary fibrosis). The angiogram in pulmonary hypertension due to increased resistance shows proximal arterial dilatation and tortuosity of vessels, disproportionate narrowing of small and medium-sized arteries, a patchy capillary density, and prolonged circulation time commensurate with reduction in blood flow. The venous phase of the pulmonary arteriogram may outline stenosed veins; it may also show delayed flow through attenuated lower lobe vessels if there is obstruction on the left side of the heart, such as in mitral valve disease. Sometimes chronic changes of pulmonary thromboembolism may provide a clue to the underlying etiology.

Increased flow resulting from left-to-right intracardiac shunts causes hyperkinetic pulmonary hypertension. On the venous phase of a pulmonary arteriogram, following opacification of the left cardiac chambers and aorta, there will be filling of the right heart chambers or refilling of the pulmonary artery, depending on the level of the shunt. Hemodynamically, higher than normal oxygen saturation makes its initial appearance at the site of the shunt, and increased pulmonary flow can be calculated.

Pulmonary Emphysema

In patients with pulmonary emphysema, angiography can help to determine the extent of functioning lung and can provide an anatomic road map for the surgeon wishing to excise segmental or lobar diseased portions. Angiographically, the vessels become attenuated and displaced around bullae, and there may be diminished peripheral pulmonary vascularity. There may be narrowing of small arteries, diminution in small arborizing vessels, and a decrease in capillary filling. Asymmetric pulmonary blood flow is often evident, and there may be indications of right heart enlargement.

Congenital Abnormalities

UNILATERAL CONGENITAL
DYSPLASIAS OF THE LUNG
In congenital dysplasia of the lung [10, 11, 17] there are developmental pulmonary anomalies that present as hypoplasia, interruption, agenesis,

or anomalous origin of the pulmonary vessels. Patients with these anomalies often present with a unilaterally contracted hemithorax, decreased or absent vascular markings, a small or absent hilus, a mediastinal shift to the affected side, and sometimes superimposed inflammatory changes.

The lung buds develop as a ventral outgrowth from the foregut and receive blood transiently from small systemic vessels arising from the paired dorsal aortae (Fig. 17-25). Pulmonary parenchymal vessels then develop, which eventually join on each side with the corresponding sixth arch. The ventral portions of each sixth arch are forerunners of the right and left major pulmonary arteries; the dorsal portions (connected on each side to dorsal fourth arch forerunners of the descending aorta) form each respective ductus.

The following developmental anomalies may occur:

1. Interruption of the right or left pulmonary artery (Fig. 17-26) occurs when the ventral portion of the sixth arch does not communicate with its corresponding pulmonary parenchymal plexus. There is usually a left-sided arch when the right pulmonary artery is interrupted; similarly, if the left pulmonary artery is interrupted, a right-sided aortic arch is present.

2. In agenesis of the lung, no pulmonary vessels or parenchymal tissue remain. As one would expect, if the left lung is agenetic, there is a right-sided aortic arch (Fig. 17-27). The left main stem bronchus ends here in a blind pouch.

3. In congenital hypoplasia, there is lobar or segmental absence of pulmonary tissue, bronchi, and vessels, with otherwise normal central connections. Occasionally there may be an anomalous systemic arterial supply, and sometimes a pulmonary vein drains the lung anomalously into the inferior vena cava or the right atrium (scimitar syndrome) (Fig. 17-28) [27].

4. The pulmonary artery can also arise anomalously from the aorta. This anomaly can be explained embryogenically by a persistence of the dorsal portion of the sixth arch (ductus) and agenesis of its ventral portion (Fig. 17-29).

Patients with certain acquired lesions can also present with a contracted thorax and increased radiolucency due to decreased vascularity. These

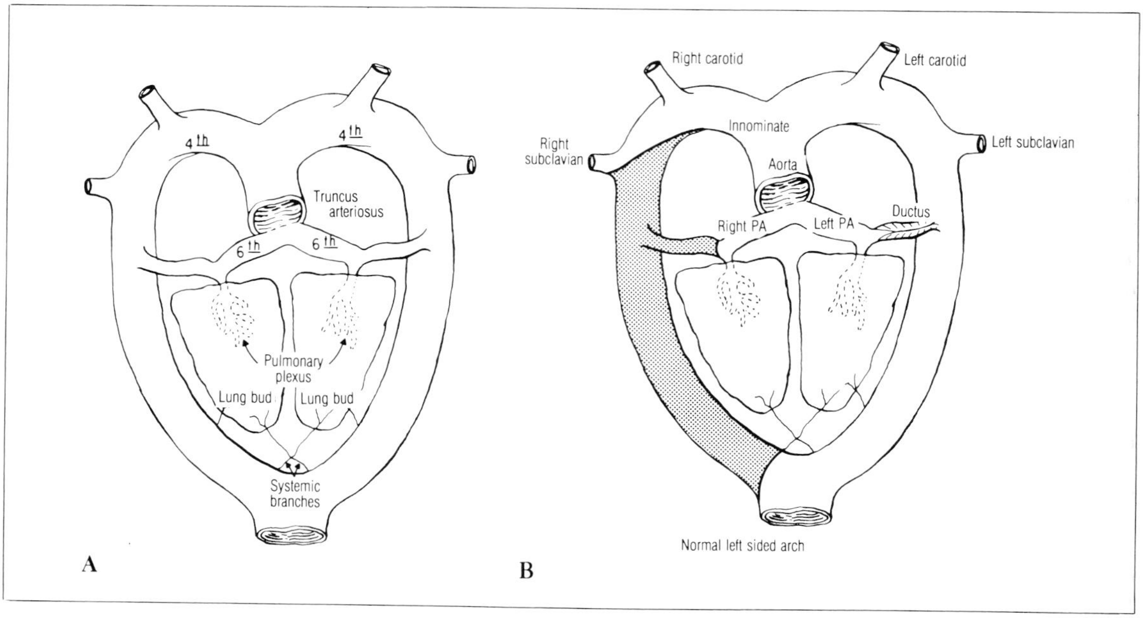
4th
4th
Truncus arteriosus
6th
6th
Pulmonary plexus
Lung bud
Lung bud
Systemic branches
A
Right carotid
Left carotid
Innominate
Right subclavian
Left subclavian
Aorta
Ductus
Right PA
Left PA
Aorta
Normal left sided arch
B

Fig. 17-25. Embryology of the lungs and pulmonary arteries (PA).
A. The aorta and main pulmonary artery arise from a common trunk, which eventually forms a septum that divides the main pulmonary artery from the ascending aorta. Ventral portions of the sixth arches bilaterally form the main left and right pulmonary arteries; dorsal portions form the ductus on the side that retains its fourth arch. A pulmonary plexus connects with the sixth arch on both sides. Systemic branches transiently supply the lung bud.
B. The right dorsal aorta and right ductus disappear (*gray area*), leaving a normal left-sided arch and ductus arteriosus.

patients include those with pulmonary artery occlusion resulting from a variety of causes, such as chronic emboli (see Fig. 17-19), primary or secondary pulmonary artery tumor [26], and bronchiolitis obliterans (Swyer-James syndrome; Fig. 17-30) [14].

PULMONARY SEQUESTRATION

In pulmonary sequestration [9, 15] there is an aberrant part of lung that is not connected with the pulmonary arterial system and sometimes not with the bronchial system. The arterial supply is from the low thoracic or upper abdominal aorta, and venous drainage is into either the systemic or, more commonly, the pulmonary venous system. The sequestration lies in or adjacent to the lower lobes on either side. Sequestrations may be explained embryologically as part of the spectrum of bronchopulmonary foregut malformations that result from the development of a supernumerary lung bud caudal to the normally located lung bud. They may be intralobar (that is, they share the same pleura of the surrounding lung), with pulmonary venous drainage to the left atrium. Conversely, they may have their own pleural covering and drain either into the pulmonary veins or the systemic venous circulation; these are termed *extralobar sequestrations*.

Sequestrations may be morphologically divided into the following types:

1. Bronchiectatic form. In this form there is bronchial communication between normal and abnormal lung.
2. Abscess form. A fluid-containing cavity is present, but there is no bronchial communication.
3. Pseudotumor. A pseudotumor is asymptomatic and has no communication with the bronchi (Fig. 17-31). The systemic vessels should be clearly defined prior to any anticipated surgery.

Patients with sequestrations must be differentiated from those with a systemic arterial supply that leads to acquired conditions involving the lung and the diaphragm (see Fig. 17-37).

ARTERIOVENOUS MALFORMATIONS

Arteriovenous malformations are congenital lesions that vary in size and number, are fed by

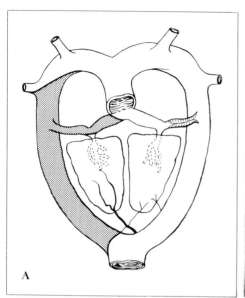

A

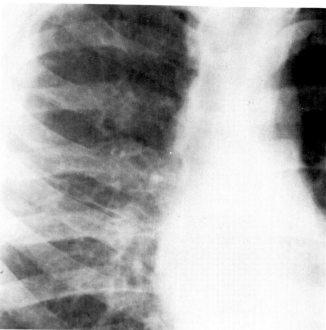

B

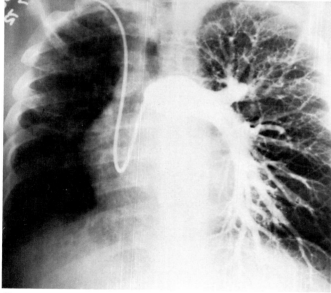

C

Fig. 17-26. Interruption of the right pulmonary artery.
A. Line drawing showing that the ventral portion of the sixth arch does not communicate with its corresponding pulmonary plexus. The systemic vessels hypertrophy to supply the lung. There must be a left-sided aortic arch.
B. Chest x ray of a patient with this condition. The hilus is absent.
C. Main pulmonary arteriogram, showing lack of communication to the pulmonary arteries on the right.
D. Thoracic aortogram. There is a left-sided aorta and prominent systemic vessels. The bronchial arteries develop later in fetal life and are therefore not prominent.
E. Delayed film of a thoracic aortogram shows filling of the pulmonary arteries by retrograde flow through these systemic collateral channels.

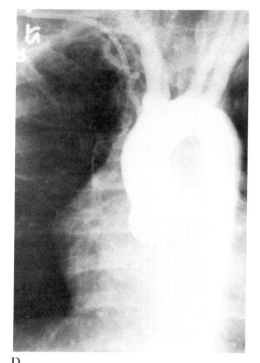

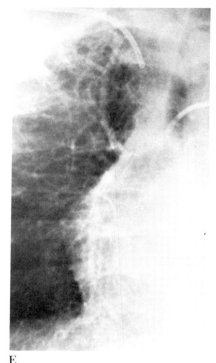

D   E

Fig. 17-26 (continued)

prominent pulmonary arteries, and are drained by large, prematurely filling veins (Fig. 17-32). They are often subplural in location. They may be solitary, multiple (in 50 percent), of varying size, diffuse, and telangiectatic, unilateral, or bilateral. They may be simple, with a simple pulmonary artery to pulmonary vein communication, which is usually aneurysmal and nonseptated. They may be more complex with multiple feeding arteries and aneurysmal septated draining veins. Up to 60 percent of patients with arteriovenous malformations have hereditary telangiectasia (Osler-Weber-Rendu disease). Pulmonary arteriovenous fistulas may result from trauma, schistosomiasis, mycotic aneurysms, long-standing hepatic cirrhosis, or vascular metastatic tumors (e.g., thyroid, choriocarcinoma; see Fig. 4-5). Pulmonary arteriovenous malformations may provide significant right-to-left shunts, with attendant complications of decreased PO_2, bacterial endocarditis, cerebral emboli and abscesses. If bleeding occurs, it can be severe. When the lesions are large or solitary, they may be removed surgically. When multiple, of varying size, involving many areas of one or both lungs, or when found in patients who are poor surgical can-

didates, intravascular embolization is another available therapeutic option. The occlusive device must be large enough to fit securely in the distal part of the feeding artery just proximal to the draining vein. This effectively occludes the arteriovenous malformation without infarcting normal areas of lung. Too small an embolus may migrate to the systemic circulation with potential for disaster. Both detachable balloons [41] and coils [5] have been used effectively.

PULMONARY ARTERY ANEURYSMS

Almost 90 percent of pulmonary artery aneurysms (Fig. 17-33) [23, 38] involve the main pulmonary artery and are asymptomatic. The remainder involve the peripheral vessels and are more likely to rupture. They may be congenital in origin, or they may be a result of Marfan's disease, syphilis, tuberculosis, Takayasu's disease, bacterial endocarditis, or trauma. Main pulmonary artery aneurysms must be differentiated from other conditions that can dilate this vessel, such as pulmonary hypertension, left-to-right shunts, pulmonary valve stenosis with poststenotic dilatation, and pulmonary valve insufficiency.

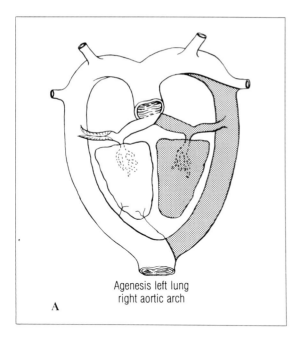

Agenesis left lung
right aortic arch

A

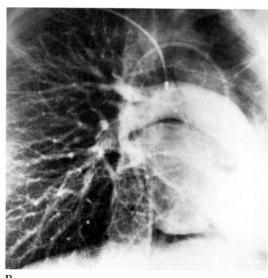

B

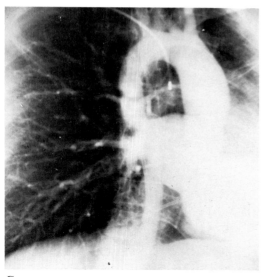

C

Fig. 17-27. Agenesis of the left lung (see text for details).

A. Line drawing. Neither the sixth arch nor the lung bud develops (*gray area*).

B. Forward angiocardiogram, showing absent pulmonary artery to the left lung. The heart is displaced to the left.

C. Levophase of the study, showing right-sided aortic arch.

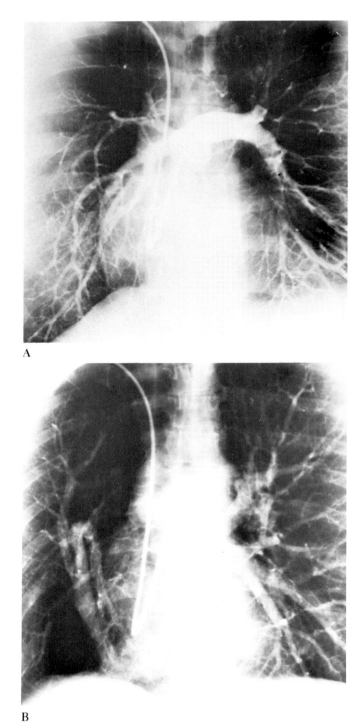

Fig. 17-28. Congenital hypoplasia of the right lung.
A. Arterial phase shows a segmental absence of pulmonary tissue.
B. On the venous phase there is an anomalously draining vein into the inferior vena cava (scimitar syndrome).

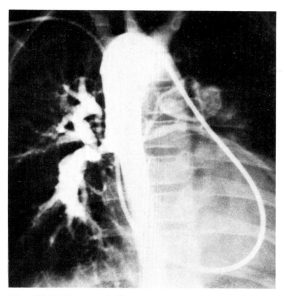

Fig. 17-29. Right-sided aortic arch with the right pulmonary artery arising from the descending thoracic aorta. The left pulmonary artery supply arises from the ascending aorta (which is not well seen due to catheter position) and in part from the descending thoracic aorta.

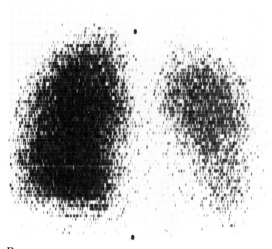

A

Fig. 17-31. Sequestration of the lung (left lower lobe).
A. Lateral projection chest x-ray shows unusual-appearing mass lying behind the heart.
B. The arterial supply to this sequestered segment of lung arises from the low thoracic aorta.
C. Venous drainage is into the pulmonary veins.

Fig. 17-30. Swyer-James syndrome (bronchiolitis obliterans).
A. Pulmonary arteriogram.
B. Perfusion lung scan. There is hypoperfusion by lung scan and hypoplastic arteries by arteriogram of the left lung. Poor filling of peripheral bronchi was seen on bronchography.

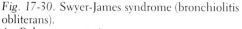

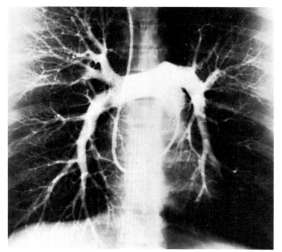

A

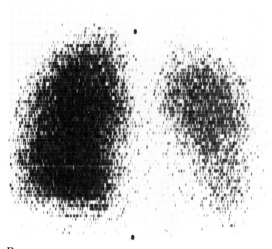

B

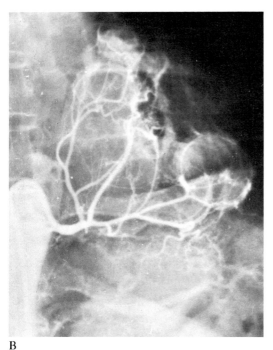

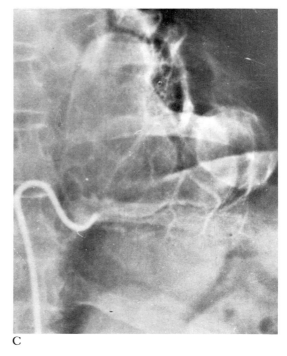

B

C

Fig. 17-31 (continued)

Fig. 17-32. Pulmonary arteriovenous malformation in the superior segment of the right lower lobe (right pulmonary arteriogram).

A. Anteroposterior projection, showing tangle of ves-

sels (*open arrow*) and prematurely draining pulmonary vein (*long arrow*).

B. Lateral projection, showing posterior subpleural location (*arrow*) of this lesion.

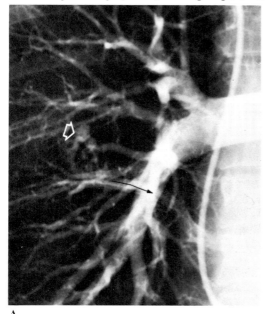

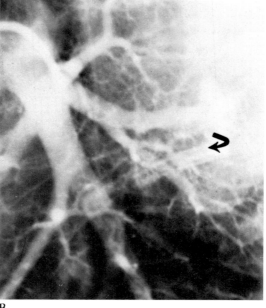

A

B

PULMONARY ARTERY STENOSIS

Pulmonary artery stenosis may occur centrally in the main pulmonary artery segment or in the major or peripheral branches (Fig. 17-34). Although the condition may be isolated in 40 percent of patients, it is usually accompanied by other lesions such as pulmonary valve stenosis, tetralogy, ventricular septal defect, patent ductus arteriosus, or supravalvular aortic stenosis. Congenital lesions are not hard to differentiate from acquired narrowing of pulmonary vessels, such as that occurring with organizing emboli (see Fig. 17-20), invasion by tumors (Fig. 17-35), extrinsic compression from aortic aneurysms, and obliteration or narrowing from arteritis, such as Takayasu's disease.

PULMONARY VARIX

On the chest x ray, pulmonary varices [1] are cylindric or oval-shaped densities, usually centrally located, and either unilateral or bilateral. They may be congenital or acquired; the latter type is most often associated with venous hypertension or mitral insufficiency. Although pulmonary varices have been known to bleed, they are usually asymptomatic, and their importance lies in correct recognition of the entity to prevent unwarranted surgery. Definitive diagnosis is provided by a contrast-enhanced computed tomography scan of the thorax.

ANOMALOUS PULMONARY VENOUS RETURN

Normally the pulmonary veins arise from a venous plexus around the foregut; in early embryonic life these veins anastomose freely with the systemic veins. An embryonic pulmonary vein forms from an outpouching of the primitive left atrium and joins the veins of the embryonic pulmonary venous plexus. If this main pulmonary vein develops improperly or not at all, the pulmonary veins retain their anastomosis with the systemic circulation (Fig. 17-36) [19].

The anomalous venous return may occur into the superior vena cava (Fig. 17-36A), the right atrium, the left innominate vein (Fig. 17-36B), the coronary sinus, the azygos vein, the inferior vena cava (see Fig. 17-28), the left subclavian vein, the portal vein, and the ductus venosus. There is frequently an associated patent foramen ovale or atrial septal defect. The right lung most often drains into the superior vena cava or the right atrium. The left lung usually drains into the left innominate vein, the coronary sinus, or a persistent left superior vena cava.

Totally anomalous pulmonary venous drainage occurs most often into the left superior vena cava, followed in order of frequency by drainage into the coronary sinus, the right atrium, the right superior vena cava, and least frequently below the diaphragm. These anomalies have associated atrial septal defects, which permit oxygenated blood to enter into the systemic circulation.

Anastomosis of Systemic Arteries with Pulmonary Arteries and Veins

The systemic arteries (bronchials, intercostals, phrenic, esophageal) can be stimulated to anastomose with pulmonary arteries and veins through pleural adhesions, mediastinal pleural reflections, pulmonary ligaments, and the diaphragm [37, 40]. This type of anastomosis occurs with a number of acquired conditions, which include the following:

1. Chronic inflammation of bronchiectasis or suppurative lung (Fig. 17-37).
2. Tumors of the lung.
3. Obstruction of the pulmonary arteries with a decrease in pulmonary artery pressure due to chronic embolization or primary vascular tumors (see Fig. 17-21).

The resulting systemic high pressure flow to the pulmonary artery can cause a hemodynamic block of this vessel.

Pericardial Effusion

Pericardial effusion can be diagnosed by fluoroscopy, radioisotope techniques, computed tomography, and magnetic resonance imaging, but is most easily and most often substantiated by ultrasonographic methods. Rarely, right atrial opacification with contrast agents may be used for this purpose. The right atrial "band" (right atrial wall, pericardium, and pleura) normally measures 2 to 3 mm, and when it is thicker than 5 mm, it is clearly abnormal (Fig. 17-38). Both radiopaque and radiolucent (carbon dioxide) contrast agents may be used. With carbon dioxide the patient is placed in a lateral decubitus position. One hundred milli-

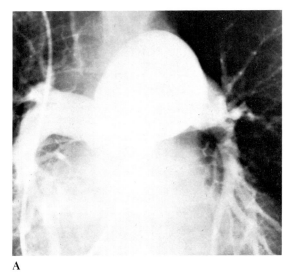

A

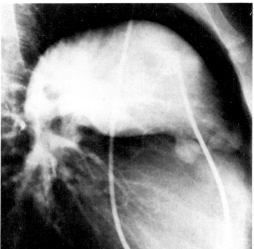

B

Fig. 17-33. Aneurysm of the main pulmonary artery in an asymptomatic patient.
A. Anteroposterior projection.
B. Lateral projection.

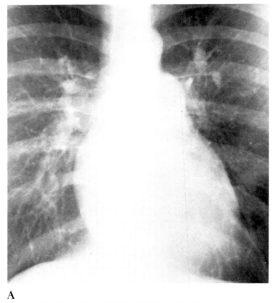

A

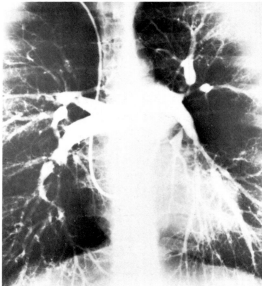

B

Fig. 17-34. Congenital peripheral pulmonary artery stenosis in a 23-year-old man with pulmonary hypertension. Right ventricular pressures 110/0 with a right ventricular end-diastolic pressure of 10 mm Hg. Main pulmonary artery pressure 95/40 mm Hg.
A. Chest x ray—the main pulmonary artery segment is prominent, and there is an irregular configuration to the segmental pulmonary branches.
B. Main pulmonary arteriogram shows multiple areas of constriction involving the pulmonary artery segmental branches bilaterally.

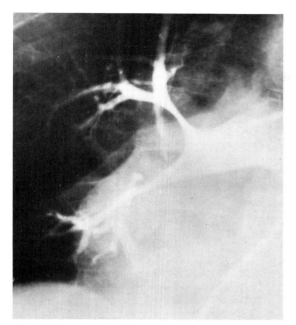

Fig. 17-35. Invasion of the right pulmonary artery by tumor. There is smooth constriction of the vessels by the tumor. This is a typical appearance of malignant invasion.

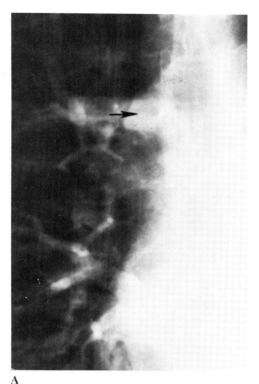

A

liters of pure carbon dioxide is injected through a large-bore needle in an antecubital vein with a 100-ml syringe that has been previously flushed with carbon dioxide. Four consecutive cross-table coned-down exposures at a rate of 1 per second are obtained, with the first exposure at the termination of the injection. The patient should remain in the same position for 10 minutes to allow total absorption. The pericardial disease may be confined entirely to the left side of the heart. A gated DSA or cine-radiographic forward angiocardiogram shows thickened pericardial space with a contracting left ventricular chamber and immobile external cardiac contour.

Fig. 17-36. Partial anomalous pulmonary venous return.
A. Vein draining the right upper lobe (*arrow*) enters into the superior vena cava (injection into the right pulmonary artery).
B. Vein draining the left upper lobe (*arrow*) enters into a left-sided superior vena cava, which connects with the left innominate vein (left pulmonary artery injection).

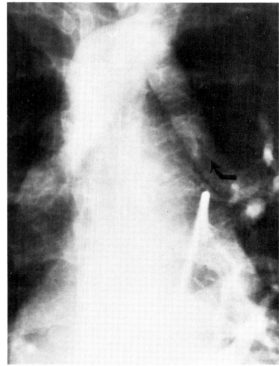

B

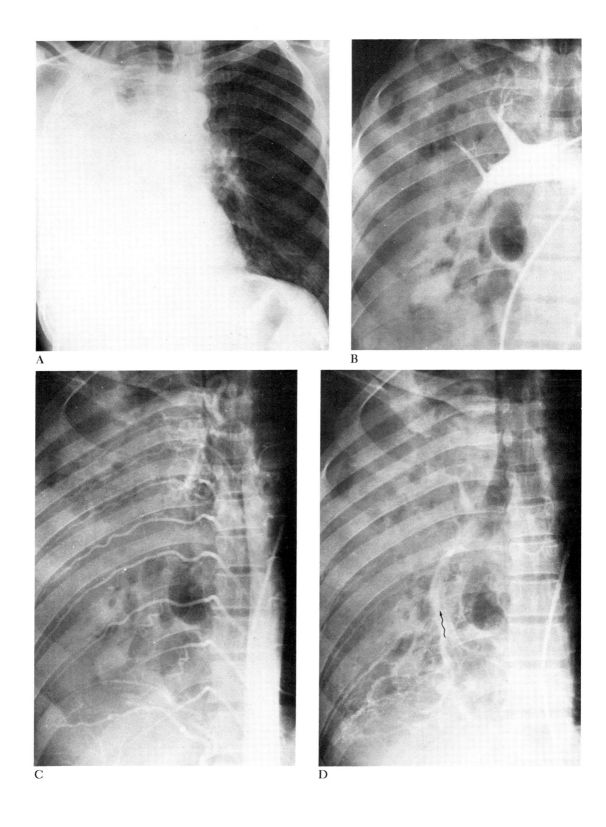

A

B

C

D

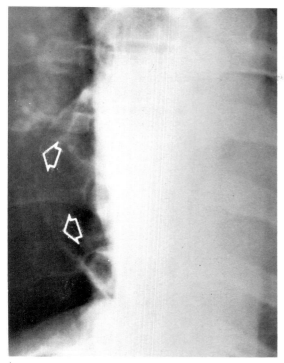

A

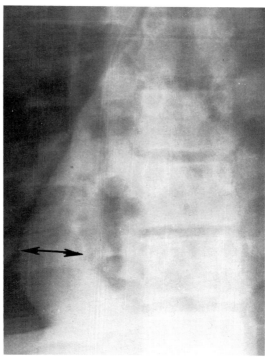

B

Fig. 17-38.
A. Right atrial injection with 100 ml of carbon dioxide (left lateral decubitus view). There is normal paper-thin thickness of the right atrial band (*arrows*). (See text for details.)
B. Marked thickening of the right atrial band, indicating a considerable degree of pericardial effusion (*arrows*).

Fig. 17-37. Chronic suppuration of the right lung.
A. Chest x ray.
B. Right pulmonary arteriogram, 4 seconds after the start of injection. There is very little flow through the pulmonary arteries of the right lung. There is a filling defect in the artery to the right lower lobe.
C. Thoracic aortogram shows prominent systemic arteries, which include bronchial arteries, inferior phrenic artery, and intercostal arteries.
D. Late phase of the aortogram shows retrograde flow through the pulmonary artery (*arrow*) due to numerous communications from the high-pressure systemic branches. This retrograde flow causes a hemodynamic block of the pulmonary artery to the right lower lobe, as seen in B.

References

1. Ben-menachen, Y., et al. The various forms of pulmonary varices: Report of three new cases and review of the literature. *Am. J. Roentgenol.* 125:881, 1975.
2. Benotti, J. R., and Dalen, J. E. The natural history of pulmonary embolism. *Clin. Chest Med.* 5(3): 403, 1984.
3. Braun, S., et al. Ventilation perfusion scanning and pulmonary angiography: Correlation in clinical high probability pulmonary embolism. *A.J.R.* 143:977, 1984.
4. Bynum, L. J., et al. Radiographic techniques for balloon occlusion pulmonary angiography. *Radiology* 133:518, 1979.
5. Castaneda-Zuniga, W., et al. Embolization of multiple pulmonary artery fistulas. *Radiology* 134: 309, 1980.
6. Chitwood, W. R., Sabiston, D. C., and Wechsler, A. S. Surgical treatment of chronic nonresolved pulmonary embolism. *Clin. Chest Med.* 5(3):507, 1984.
7. Chuly, R., et al. The role of noninvasive tests versus pulmonary angiography in the diagnosis of pulmonary embolism. *Am. J. Med.* 70:17, 1981.
8. Dantzher, D. R., and Bower, J. S. Alterations in gas exchange following pulmonary embolism. *Chest* 81:495, 1980.
9. Dux, A., and Felix, R. Diseases of the Lung: Disturbances of the Pulmonary Circulation. In H. R.

Schinz et al. (eds.), *Pleura, Mediastinum, and Lungs*. Vol. 4, part 2 in *Roentgen Diagnosis* (2nd American ed.). New York: Grune & Stratton, 1975.

10. Edwards, J., and McGoon, D. Absence of anatomic origin from heart of pulmonary artery supply: Clinical-pathologic correlations. *Circulation* 47:393, 1973.

11. Felson, B. Pulmonary agenesis and related anomalies. *Semin. Roentgenol.* 7:17, 1972.

12. Goodman, P. C. Pulmonary angiography. *Clin. Chest Med.* 5(3):465, 1984.

13. Greenfield, L. J., Bruce, T. A., and Nichols, N. B. Transverse pulmonary embolectomy by catheter device. *Ann. Surg.* 174:881, 1971.

14. Guzowski, J., and Duvall, A. Swyer James syndrome: A cause of hyperlucent lung. *Ann. Otol. Laryngol. Rhinol.* 84:657, 1975.

15. Heithoff, K., et al. Bronchopulmonary foregut malformations. *Am. J. Roentgenol.* 126:46, 1976.

16. Heitzman, R., Markarian, B., and Dailey, F. Pulmonary thromboembolic disease—A lobular concept. *Radiology* 103:529, 1972.

17. Hislop, A., Sanderson, M., and Reid, L. Unilateral congenital dysplasia of lung associated with vascular anomalies. *Thorax* 28:435, 1973.

18. Johnsrude, I. S. Pulmonary embolism. *Curr. Probl. Diagn. Radiol.* 11(1):4, 1982.

19. Lester, R., Mauck, H., and Grubb, W. Anomalous pulmonary venous return to the right side of the heart. *Semin. Roentgenol.* 1:102, 1966.

20. Ludurg, J. W., et al. Digital subtraction angiography of the pulmonary arteries for the diagnosis of pulmonary embolism. *Radiology* 147:639, 1983.

21. McNeil, B. J. Ventilation perfusion studies and the diagnosis of pulmonary embolism: Concise communication. *J. Nucl. Med.* 21:319, 1980.

22. Mills, S. R., et al. The incidence, etiologies, and evidence of complications of pulmonary angiography in a large series. *Radiology* 136:295, 1980.

23. Monchik, J., and Wilkins, E., Jr. Solitary aneurysm of the middle lobe artery: A case report and review of solitary peripheral pulmonary artery aneurysms. *Ann. Thorac. Surg.* 17:496, 1974.

24. Moser, K. M. Pulmonary embolism. *Am. Rev. Respir. Dis.* 115:829, 1977.

25. Novelline, R. A., et al. The clinical course of patients with suspected pulmonary embolism and a negative pulmonary arteriogram. *Radiology* 126:561, 1978.

26. Olson, H., Speitzer, R., and Erston, W. Primary and secondary pulmonary artery neoplasia mimicking acute pulmonary embolism. *Radiology* 118:49, 1976.

27. Osborne, A., and Silverman, J. Unusual venous drainage patterns in the scimitar syndrome. *Radiology* 113:601, 1974.

28. Pollock, J. F., and McNeil, B. J. Pulmonary scintigraphy and the diagnosis of pulmonary embolization. A perspective. *Clin. Chest Med.* 5(3):457, 1984.

29. Pond, G. D., Ovitt, T. W., and Capp, M. P. Comparison of conventional pulmonary angiography with intravenous digital subtraction angiography for pulmonary embolic disease. *Radiology* 147:345, 1983.

30. Robin, E. D. Overdiagnosis and overtreatment of pulmonary embolism: The emperor may have no clothes. *Ann. Intern. Med.* 87:775, 1977.

31. Rosenow, E. C., III, Osmundson, P. J., and Brown, M. L. Pulmonary embolism. *Mayo Clin. Proc.* 56:161, 1981.

32. Sasahara, A. A., Sonnenblick, E. H., and Leach, M. *Pulmonary Embolism*. New York: Grune & Stratton, 1975.

33. Sharma, G. V. R. K., et al. Effect of thrombolytic therapy on pulmonary capillary blood volume in patients with pulmonary embolism. *N. Engl. J. Med.* 303(15):842, 1980.

34. Sharma, G. V. R. K., et al. Clinical and hemodynamic correlates in pulmonary embolism. *Clin. Chest Med.* 5(3):421, 1984.

35. Sostman, H. D., et al. Problems in noninvasive imaging of pulmonary embolism. *Radiol. Clin. North Am.* 21:759, 1983.

36. Stein, M., and Levy, S. Reflex and humoral responses to pulmonary embolism. In A. A. Sasahara, E. H. Sonnenblick, and M. Leach (eds.), *Pulmonary Embolism*. New York: Grune & Stratton, 1975.

37. Tadavarthy, S. M., et al. Systemic to pulmonary collaterals in pathological states. *Radiology* 144:55, 1983.

38. Trell, E. Pulmonary arterial aneurysm. *Thorax* 28:644, 1973.

39. Verel, D., and Arainger, R. G. *Cardiac Catheterization and Angiocardiography* (3rd ed.). Edinburgh: Churchill Livingstone, 1978.

40. Viamonte, M. J., Jr. Intrathoracic extracardiac shunts. *Semin. Roentgenol.* 2:342, 1967.

41. White, R. I., Jr., et al. Angioarchitecture of pulmonary arteriovenous malformation. An important consideration before embolotherapy. *A.J.R.* 140:881, 1983.

Aortography and Left Ventriculography

Indications

THORACIC AORTOGRAPHY
[1, 3, 4, 5, 11–14, 21, 22, 23, 26, 28, 32, 35, 37, 41, 42, 46, 47, 50–54]

1. Acquired disease
    a. Aneurysms (atherosclerotic, syphilitic, cystic medial necrosis, traumatic, mycotic, and others)
    b. Aortic dissection
    c. Aortic trauma, blunt (aortic transections), penetrating injuries
    d. Aortic valve disease (aortic stenosis, aortic insufficiency, aortic prosthesis)
    e. Miscellaneous conditions (e.g., aortitis, neoplasm)
2. Congenital lesions
    a. Obstructing lesions (aortic valve stenosis, aortic valve atresia, supravalvular aortic stenosis, coarctation, tubular hypoplasia, aortic arch atresia)
    b. Left-to-right shunts or aortic runoff lesions (patent ductus arteriosus, aortopulmonary window, truncus arteriosus, coronary artery fistulas to the pulmonary artery or the cardiac chambers, aortic left ventricular tunnel)
    c. Aneurysms of the aortic sinuses, with or without rupture into the intracardiac chambers
    d. Anomalies of position (corrected or complete transposition of the aorta, double outlet right ventricle, right-sided aortic arch, double aortic arch, vascular rings, and other anomalies of development of the aortic arch and brachiocephalic vessels, such as pseudocoarctation and cervical thoracic aorta)

LEFT VENTRICULOGRAPHY
[1, 6, 7, 8, 10, 15, 16, 18, 19, 20, 24, 27, 36, 40, 48, 55]

Study of the left ventricle is sometimes a required progression in evaluation of the thoracic aorta. However, the hemodynamic and angiographic evaluation of the left side of the heart is beyond the scope of this book. Thus only a list of conditions in which such evaluation can be helpful is provided as well as some broad principles of technique and superficial comments on basic angiographic interpretation of some of the more common lesions encountered.

The following conditions can be studied by ventriculography:

1. The competence and appearance of mitral valves (rheumatic heart disease, myxomatous degeneration as in Marfan's syndrome, congenital incompetence, prolapsing mitral valve, and parachute mitral valve).
2. Ventricular configuration in acquired and congenital heart disease (aneurysms of the myocardium and membranous septum, idiopathic hypertrophic subaortic stenosis, fibrous subaortic stenosis, outflow tract deformity of endocardial cushion defects, and common ventricle).
3. Left ventricular function–left ventricular ejection fraction, and regional left ventricular wall motion (cardiomyopathies, idiopathic myocardial hypertrophy, coronary artery disease and myocardial infarcts, ventricular aneurysms).
4. Ventricular septal defects (membranous, muscular, and endocardial cushion defects).
5. Cardiac trauma (ruptured chordae, septal defects, and pericardial tamponade).

Techniques

APPROACHES
1. The percutaneous femoral artery approach is preferred.
2. The right (preferably) or left axillary artery approach may be used if the femoral approach is unavailable.
3. Occasionally, a brachial arteriotomy may be performed.
4. Transseptal (atrial) catheterization may be performed, using the femoral venous approach

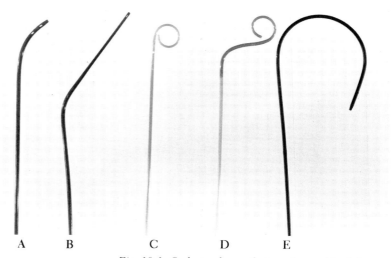

A B   C   D   E

Fig. 18-1. Catheter shapes that can be used for left ventriculography (right to left).
A. Gensini Dacron catheter with multiple side holes and an end hole.
B. Dacron catheter (Sones) for coronary arteriography (this catheter can also be used to study the left ventricle).
C. Pigtail polyethylene catheter with multiple side holes.
D. Grollman catheter with a second curve and multiple side holes.
E. Catheter used for the transseptal approach to the left side of the heart (see Fig. 18-3).

(see under Catheters, below). This technique is used in severe aortic stenosis when an approach from the extremities may be impossible.

5. Percutaneous cardiac (transapical) catheterization is performed when no other route is available. It is very rarely indicated.

CATHETERS

Midstream Aortic Root Injection
For the femoral artery approach, a 100- to 110-cm 7 French Teflon or polyethylene catheter with an end hole, multiple side holes, and a gentle curve over the distal 4 or 5 cm should be used. A "pigtail" catheter with multiple side holes proximal to the pigtail tip can also be used (Fig. 18-1C). In patients with elongation and tortuosity of the thoracic aorta, a longer catheter (125 cm) should be used. For use in children, 60- to 80-cm 5 or 6 French catheters are available.

For the axillary approach, a 60-cm 6 or 7 French catheter with similar tip configuration should be used.

Left Ventriculogram
The ideal catheter for left ventriculography should cross the aortic valve with ease, should remain in a stable position during the injection, should not perforate the myocardium, and should produce no disturbance of cardiac rhythm. The pigtail catheter fills most of the requirements, but a Grollman catheter may satisfy these requirements even better and may be the ideal catheter for left ventriculography (Fig. 18-1D) [34]. However, it is difficult to

cross a stenotic aortic valve with either of these catheters.

For the femoral artery approach, a 125-cm polyethylene or polyurethane pigtail or Grollman catheter should be used. Alternatively, a 125-cm woven Dacron Gensini catheter (with an end hole, multiple side holes, and a less rigid, softer tip) may be used (Fig. 18-1A).

For the axillary or the brachial artery approach, similar catheter configurations as in the femoral approach should be used, but with shorter lengths. Alternatively, an 80-cm 8 French diameter Sones woven Dacron or polyurethane catheter (Fig. 18-1B) may be used.

Transseptal Catheterization
A Brockenbrough 70-cm Teflon or polyethylene 8 or 9 French catheter should be used, with a tapered tip at the distal end shaped with a curvature to facilitate passage into the left ventricle (Fig. 18-1E). The radius of the curvature depends on the size of the left atrium; a selection of four loops

of different sizes is available (2.0, 2.5, 3.0, and 3.5 cm). Four spirally arranged side openings are located 0.5 to 1.5 cm from the distal tip. A flared proximal end accommodates a number of removable fittings, which include a detachable hub with stopcock and a 71-cm 18-gauge stainless steel tubing with a distal 1.5-cm tip of 21-gauge tubing and a sharp needle point. There is a gentle curve to the distal 4 cm of this needle. A large metallic arrow at the hub of the needle points in the same direction as this curve, in order to give the operator precise knowledge of the direction of the needle tip within the right atrium.

Contrast Agents, Projections, and Radiographic Programming

Details concerning contrast agents, projections, and radiographic programs in thoracic aortography and left ventriculography are given in Table 18-1 [31].

Cineradiography permits better appreciation of ventricular function (ejection fraction and regional wall motion) than does serial filming [6, 36]. Areas with akinesia or dyskinesia and small ventricular aneurysms are best studied by this technique [19, 55]. Cineradiography also detects smaller changes in contrast density than does seriographic filming. Whenever possible, it should be used to evaluate incompetent valves or small shunts. It may also be used in conjunction with a videotape or disk recorder, which allows instant replay capabilities. One disadvantage is the limited field size available; therefore, the larger ventricular chambers may be seen only by moving either the patient or the x-ray tube during the injection of contrast medium. The film rate should be 30 to 60 frames per second, with a pulse width as close to 4 milliseconds as possible. The filming should be started just prior to the start of the injection.

In left ventriculography, a steep right posterior oblique (left anterior oblique) projection of 45 degrees shows the ventricular septum in profile and better defines the location of septal defects. A 30-degree left posterior oblique (right anterior oblique) projection shows the mitral valve to advantage.

Digital subtraction angiography may ultimately play an important role in cardiac catheterization [34, 38, 39]. Digital subtraction angiography techniques not only permit a marked reduction in the concentration and volume of radiographic contrast material, but also allow objective quantitation of left ventricular function. Several reports have already emphasized the capability of this technology especially in the objective assessment of left ventricular ejection fraction and regional wall motion [38, 39].

Multiple limited serial injections of contrast agent (10 ml each) may be administered in left ventriculography to coincide with a predetermined phase of the cardiac cycle, particularly diastole [34, 43, 44]. This electrocardiogram (ECG)-gated technique of pulsed contrast material during diastole alone reportedly reduces arrhythmias and allows angiographic evaluation of multiple sequential cardiac cycles. Special ancillary attachments to the high-pressure injector are necessary to perform this technique. This phasic delivery of contrast in the ventricle during diastole is also useful with digital subtraction angiography.

In thoracic aortography, the heart should be included in the exposure field in order to record possible valvular insufficiency, patency of the proximal coronary arteries, or other runoff lesions. If only a single projection is available, a left anterior oblique projection "opens up" the aortic arch for better evaluation than the anteroposterior or lateral projection alone.

Technical Considerations

CARE OF THE PATIENT

Preangiographic care includes adequate sedation and the administration of atropine to prevent bradycardia. Drugs that may induce hypotension (e.g., meperidine) are usually avoided in evaluation of the heart and central vessels. Physiologic monitoring (of ECG and intravascular pressures) and cardiac resuscitative facilities should be available.

POSITIONING THE CATHETER

In thoracic aortography, the catheter tip should be approximately 2 cm above the aortic valve and lying free in the center of the aorta. The tip should not be directed toward a coronary artery. Proper positioning of the catheter for thoracic aortography should not only allow assessment of aortic valve abnormalities such as valvular insufficiency, but

Table 18-1. Technical specifications in thoracic aortography and left ventriculography

Disease	Contrast agent[a] Injection site	Volume (ml/inj)	Rate (ml/sec)	Total films[b]	Total time (sec)	Radiographic program[c] (films/sec)	Projections
Adults							
Aortic stenosis or insufficiency	AO root	50–60	30	Ciné 16	6–8 8	30 to 60 frames/sec[d] 3/sec for 3 sec; 2/sec for 2 sec; or 1/sec for 3 sec	Biplane AP and lateral; LAO
Disease of the thoracic aorta	LV AO root	40–50 60	20 30	12	8	2/sec for 4 sec;[e] 1/sec for 4 sec	Biplane AP and lateral; LAO
Mitral stenosis	LA PA	45 60	15 30	Ciné Ciné	6–8 8–10	30 to 60 frames/sec 30 to 60 frames/sec	Biplane AP and lateral; slight RAO or lateral
Mitral insufficiency	LV	50–60	20	Ciné	6–8	30 to 60 frames/sec	Biplane AP and lateral; slight RAO
Left atrial tumor	PA	60	30	Ciné	10–15	30 to 60 frames/sec	Biplane AP and lateral
LV abnormality	LV	45–50	15	Ciné 16	6–8 7	30 to 60 frames/sec 4/sec for 3 sec;[f] 1/sec for 4 sec	Biplane AP and lateral; biplane LAO and LPO
Ventricular septal defect	LV	45–50	15	Ciné 16	6 7	60 frames/sec 4/sec for 3 sec; 1/sec for 4 sec	Biplane AP and lateral; LAO or lateral
Children							
All of above diseases	Same as adults	Do not exceed 1.0–1.5 ml/kg	Total within 1.0–1.5 sec	Ciné 16	4–6	In shunts, film timing should be 4/sec or even 6/sec	As in adults

[a] Medium density. Use nonionic contrast agents in the left ventricle and other cardiac chambers; also in those with valvular and myocardial disease.
[b] Ciné or large films.
[c] Start films 0.4 sec after start of injection.
[d] With all ciné runs, start ciné just before the injection of contrast medium.
[e] For diseases with shunts (patent ductus arteriosus, aortopulmonary window) or patients with high cardiac output, use same program as for ventricular septal defect.
[f] For quantitative volume determinations, 6/sec for 4 seconds.
AO = aortic; LV = left ventricle; LA = left atrium; PA = pulmonary artery; ciné = cineradiography.

also evaluation of the proximal left and right coronary arteries, especially in patients suspected of aortic dissections.

In performing left ventriculography, it may sometimes be difficult to manipulate the catheter into the ventricular chamber. This difficulty may result from the presence of aortic stenosis, gross dilatation of the aortic root, or some other unfavorable anatomic consideration. A pigtail or Grollman catheter is occasionally more difficult to manipulate under these circumstances. With a somewhat straighter curved catheter, this problem can be overcome by extending the flexible portion of a straight-tipped guidewire beyond the catheter tip. With the catheter tip near the aortic root, the flexible wire tip is advanced over the opposite wall of the ascending aorta. As the wire is withdrawn, it flips across the valve into the ventricle, where it acts as a leader over which the catheter may be guided (Fig. 18-2). Catheters and guidewires too near the apex often elicit arrhythmias. Once the catheter is within the ventricle, the wire is removed. The catheter tip should be advanced in the long axis of the ventricle and should lie in midcavity, away from the walls. The catheter should be prevented from coiling too close to the mitral

Fig. 18-2. Helpful manipulative technique for placing the catheter in the left ventricle. The guidewire is withdrawn down the medial wall of the aorta until it drops into the left ventricle; it then acts as a leader for the catheter.

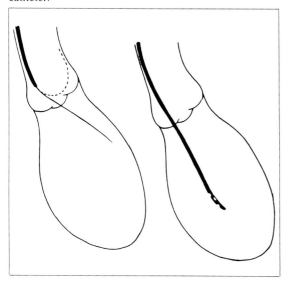

valve, because injection at this point may force contrast agent retrograde into the left atrium and give a spurious impression of mitral insufficiency. If the catheter tip is too close to the ventricular outflow tract, it may recoil into the aorta during the subsequent injection. If a pigtail-tipped catheter is used, frequent forceful flushings are essential to prevent clot formation in the distal "tail" of the tip. Heparin may be administered when not contraindicated by such conditions as aortic dissection. Pressure measurements must not be dampened; the catheter tip should be free and mobile within the chamber; if position is proved by a small test injection, the diagnostic injection of contrast medium will not enter the myocardium. Gradients across the ventricular chamber and outflow tracts should be accurately measured prior to catheter removal.

TRANSATRIAL SEPTAL APPROACH

A transatrial septal approach may be used to evaluate the left ventricle if the aortic valve cannot be transversed (Fig. 18-3) [20, 55]. It can also be used for thoracic aortography if the arteries of all four extremities are occluded and intravenous digital subtraction methods are not available. A Brockenbrough catheter (Fig. 18-1D) is introduced percutaneously into either femoral vein and is advanced to the right atrium over a guidewire with a flexible tip. This catheter has a 270-degree curve at its distal end; the diameter of the curve varies according to the size of the right atrium. The guidewire is removed and replaced by the transseptal needle; this procedure should be performed under fluoroscopy and, as in all other angiographic procedures, without excessive force. The long needle is advanced until its point lies just within the tip of the catheter. This maneuver straightens the curve of the catheter. The angiographer must take care not to perforate the wall of the catheter with the sharp point of the transseptal needle. The needle point must not protrude beyond the catheter tip at this time. A pointer on the hub of the transseptal needle shows the direction of the curved needle tip. With the tip of the catheter (not the needle point) facing posteromedially in the direction of the atrial septum, the angiographer should gently probe for the small depression representing the fossa ovalis. This residuum of the foramen ovale lies just above the openings of the inferior vena cava and the coronary sinus into the right atrium.

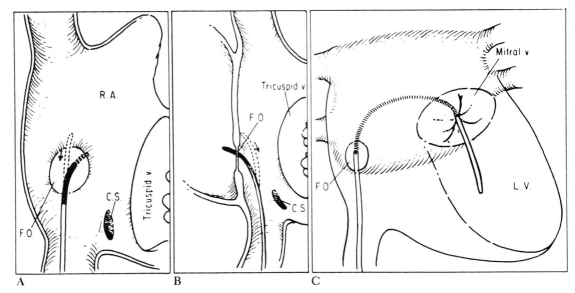

A   B   C

Fig. 18-3. Transseptal approach to catheterization of the left side of the heart (see text for details).
A. Anteroposterior projection. The curve of the catheter lies posteromedially and slips off the superior ridge of the fossa ovalis inferiorly into the fossa itself. A sharp, pointed internal needle then penetrates the septum, and the overlying catheter is advanced into the left atrium.
B. Lateral projection shows the catheter pointing posteriorly through the atrial septum into the left atrial cavity.
C. Anteroposterior projection. The catheter has now advanced through the mitral valve into the body of the left ventricular chamber. CS = coronary sinus; FO = fossa ovalis.

When the catheter tip is in this position, it cannot enter the anteriorly located tricuspid valve, and it cannot penetrate the septum into the anteriorly positioned thoracic aorta (this is not true, however, if there is a large aneurysm of the ascending aorta or the aortic cusps or if there is a malpositioned aorta). It can be fatal to force the catheter into the thoracic aorta.

As the catheter is withdrawn inferiorly from the superior vena cava, the catheter tip hesitates as it catches on the superior border of the fossa (limbus fossae ovalis). Sometimes the catheter will advance through the septum or through a small patent foramen ovale without further manipulation. As a rule, however, the transseptal needle must be advanced to the hub of the catheter, thus allowing the needle tip to protrude slightly beyond the catheter tip into the left atrium. During the septal puncture, elastic resistance of the septum is felt, a sudden decrease of which usually indicates that it has been perforated. At this point the patient usually experiences some transient sensations of fullness in the mediastinum or a sharp sensation of discomfort under the sternum. These sensations usually subside rapidly; if they persist, one should look for complications of inadvertent puncture of the atrial wall. Following perforation, the withdrawal of oxygenated blood confirms the left atrial position of the needle tip. The curved catheter should then be advanced over the needle into the

left atrium, the transseptal needle removed, and pressure measurements obtained. The most common cause of failure in puncturing the septum is right atrial enlargement. In addition, large mural thrombi within the left atrium will present difficulties. Once the catheter has entered the left atrium, the curve of the catheter allows it to be advanced gently through the mitral valve and into the left ventricle. Difficulties in traversing the mitral valve may be encountered in severe mitral stenosis or severe mitral insufficiency. Sometimes a curved guidewire with a flexible tip must be advanced into the left ventricle in order to act as a leader for the catheter. The catheter has several side holes at its distal tip, which allow an adequate injection of contrast medium into the left ventricle. The angiographer should make sure that the tip is not trapped under a trabecula and that it lies free within the ventricular chamber prior to injection.

Hazards of the transatrial septal approach include improper placement of the needle into the aorta and perforation of the heart into the pericardium and through the free atrial wall. Careful monitoring of pressures is necessary, through the advancing catheter as well as in a systemic artery. Pericardial tamponade due to blood accumulation is an infrequent but possible complication, and steps must be taken to perform pericardiocentesis if this should occur (see p. 490).

Measurements of Ventricular Dimensions and Volumes

Measurement of the left ventricular dimensions and volumes can be made from left ventriculograms, in order to provide additional information regarding myocardial function [7, 8, 18, 21, 24, 36, 40, 55]. Direct measurements of the longest axis of the ventricle, as well as determination of the minor axis of the chamber, are placed in the equation for the volume of an ellipsoid or a cone. This volumetric measurement is calculated with the ventricle in end systole as well as in end diastole. The stroke volume (end-diastolic volume minus end-systolic volume) and the ejection fraction (stroke volume/end-diastolic volume) can also be calculated. Ventricular volume can be calculated and the thickness of the ventricular mass can be measured directly from the radiograph, and the volume of the ventricular muscular mass can be estimated. Measurements of muscle thickness and calculations of ventricular volume and ejection fraction are particularly helpful to the cardiologist in evaluating patients with incompetent or stenotic valves, those with myocardiopathies, and those with coronary artery disease. These determinations require simultaneous recording of the electrocardiogram with the film exposures, either by cineangiography or very rapid biplane filming (six exposures per second) coned to the heart. Films obtained during extrasystoles are excluded from the calculations, and there must be correction for radiographic magnifications. Simultaneous ventricular pressure measurements give added information; the details of these measurements are beyond the scope of this book.

Complications

The following complications may occur in thoracic aortography and left ventriculography, in addition to those listed under general angiography [2, 20, 55]:

1. There may be inadvertent entry into and occlusion of the coronary artery (usually the left), which will be accompanied by complaints of angina. This can usually be detected by the catheter or guidewire position at fluoroscopy, as well as by dampened pressures measured at the catheter tip. It is often accompanied by QRS or T wave changes and by cardiac rhythm abnormalities, such as progressive bradycardia, pulsus alternans, or extrasystoles. This dangerous situation may lead to ventricular fibrillation if it is unrecognized and the catheter is not immediately withdrawn.

2. Perforation of the myocardium (atrium or ventricle) may occur. If this is recognized, the patient must be closely monitored for cardiac tamponade for at least 24 hours. A situation characterized by dampened ECG voltage, rising right and left atrial M-shaped pressure curves and rising ventricular end-diastolic pressures, pulsus paradoxus, decreased contractility of the cardiac silhouette by fluoroscopy, and increasing apprehension of the patient requires an immediate pericardial tap (see page 490). The angiographer should consult his cardiologic and surgical colleagues.

3. Intramural injections may occur when a catheter tip is trapped under trabeculae and/or is positioned too close to the endocardium. A freely moving catheter tip within the midventricle and a small high-pressure test injection reduce the chances of this complication. Often there are no symptoms, although angina, transient cardiac arrhythmias, and ST segment changes may occur.

4. Cardiac arrhythmias may occur (Table 18-2) [45].

5. Catheters and guidewires may become looped or kinked within the cardiac chambers. Usually careful, gentle manipulation under fluoroscopic guidance will resolve these problems. Often advancing instead of withdrawing the catheter will loosen the loop; advancing the guidewire through the looped catheter will also

Table 18-2. Basic arrhythmia problems (see on lead II of ECG)

Catheter location	Common problems	Treatment
Left ventricle	Premature ventricular contractions	Find a "quiet spot"; usually push the catheter in further toward the apex; may have to pull the catheter back into the aorta and then readvance it into the left ventricle. May give 50-mg intravenous bolus of lidocaine (10 mg/ml), to be repeated within a few minutes if unsuccessful. May start lidocaine drip of 50 mg/hour (1 gm in 1 liter of 5% dextrose) if arrhythmia recurs
Left Ventricle	Ventricular tachycardia	Withdraw the catheter into the aorta. Have patient cough, take deep breaths. Strike the precordium. Lidocaine push of 100 mg in 5 ml 5% dextrose or normal saline. Repeat with 80 mg-dose in a few minutes if tachycardia persists. Start a drip of 2 to 4 mg/minute. If blood pressure drops, and ventricular tachycardia persists, use synchronous cardioversion with ECG-controlled defibrillator, turn on the power, switch to synchronous mode (see highlight over QRS) and cardiovert with 50, 100, 150 watt-sec. Increase power if unsuccessful. If ventricular tachycardia progresses to ventricular fibrillation, switch off synchronous cardioversion, defibrillate, and institute full cardiopulmonary resuscitation
Left ventricle	Ventricular fibrillation	Immediate action is necessary. Defibrillate immediately. Apply 200, 300, 360 watts-sec in the adult. If immediate defibrillation is not possible, provide external massage, airway, and bag breathing until the defibrillator is ready
Coronary arteries	Progressive bradycardia to asystole*	Make patient *cough!!* Hit patient's chest. Insert pacer catheter; may pace from the right atrium (usually it is the sinoatrial node that is involved, and this usually occurs after right coronary artery injection). May pace during the coronary injections
Right	Transient depression of ST segment on lead II	
Left	Transient elevation of T segment on lead II	
Coronary arteries	Prolonged hyperacute T wave and ST changes signify ischemia	Check the pressure monitored at the coronary catheter tip to be sure it is not dampened; withdraw into the aorta if this is so. Wait for ST/T wave changes to get back to baseline level before further injections. Give nitroglycerine 0.4 mg sublingually

*More common with right coronary artery injection, but can occur on the left as well.

further uncoil it and permit safe withdrawal. Kinked guidewires should be immediately and carefully withdrawn, if necessary, together with the overlying catheter.

6. Hypotension and occasionally hypertension may follow cardiac and central vessel contrast injections. In patients with an unstable cardiovascular or cerebrovascular condition, complications such as myocardial infarction and stroke have occurred. Using nonionic contrast agents may help to reduce the complications.

7. Pulmonary edema may develop. It is usually caused by left heart failure in a severely compromised heart, which is further aggravated by hypervolemia of high doses of hyperosmolar contrast agent.

Anatomic Considerations (Figs. 18-4, 18-5, 18-6)

THE LEFT VENTRICLE

The left ventricle is a relatively smooth-walled, oval-shaped chamber with its apex pointing downward and to the left [19, 40]. The mitral valve and the aortic valve lie adjacent to each other, with the anterior leaflet of the mitral valve contiguous with the adjacent portions of the left and noncoronary (posterior) cusp of the aortic valve. On the anteroposterior projection ventriculogram, the smooth-walled outflow tract of the left ventricle is seen to be directed upward and to the right to meet the aortic valve; the three cusps of this valve are best seen in diastole. The posterior leaflet of the mitral valve is attached to the inferior portion of the mitral ring. On the anteroposterior projection, again in diastole, this ring is seen as a curvilinear structure defined by contrast agent trapped behind the mitral leaflet and unopacified blood entering the valve from the left atrium. Almost the entire right border of the left ventricle is formed by the intraventricular septum. The uppermost portion of the septum, the membranous portion, lies just inferior to the aortic cusps, whereas the rest of the septum is muscular. During systole, the aortic valves are no longer clearly identified, the mitral ring is obscured, and two unopacified structures (the papillary muscles) protrude into the ventricular lumen from each side of the ventricular chamber (see Fig. 18-16B) [29, 30, 33, 36, 40, 48, 55].

On the lateral projection, the anterior wall of the left ventricle is formed by the interventricular septum. The posteroinferior border of the left ventricle consists of the free ventricular wall, whereas its posterior boundary is the mitral valve. The close relationship of the anterior leaflet of the mitral valve with that of the aortic cusps is best appreciated on this projection and on the left posterior oblique projection. The right coronary cusp lies anteriorly. The left and noncoronary cusps lie posteriorly, with the noncoronary cusp lying lowermost. The relative levels of the aortic and pulmonary valves should be noted (Fig. 18-4).

Fig. 18-4. Normal anatomy of the cardiac chambers and the great vessels, showing relationship of valves on the left side of the heart.
A. Anteroposterior projection.
B. Lateral projection, as viewed from the right.

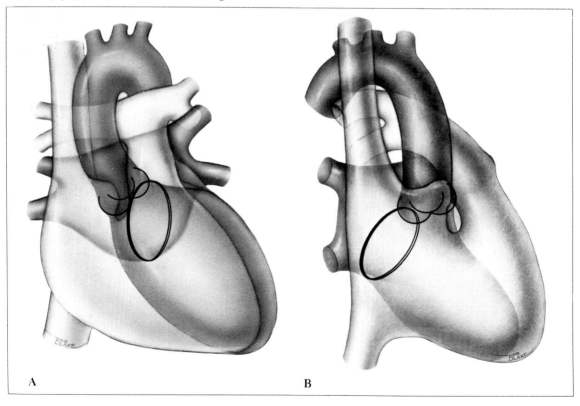

A   B

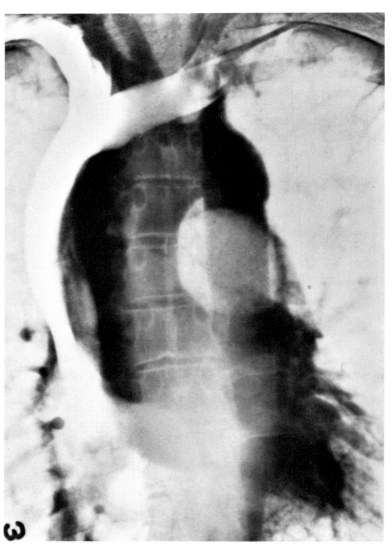

Fig. 18-5. Forward angiocardiogram. The chambers of the right side of the heart are seen as white areas; the left side of the heart and the aorta are black.

THE THORACIC AORTA

The aortic sinus meets the tubular portion of the aortic root at the sinotubular ridge. Above this ridge, the thoracic aorta ascends from the heart into the superior mediastinum to just below the manubrium sterni, where it passes posteriorly and obliquely to the left over the left mainstem bronchus. It continues inferiorly as the descending thoracic aorta, lying just anterior to and to the left of the vertebral column. The two coronary arteries are the first arterial branches from the aorta. These arteries originate just above the aortic valve cusps from the aortic sinuses. The left coronary artery arises from the left sinus and the right coronary artery arises from the anterior sinus. There is no artery originating from the right posterior sinus. The brachiocephalic vessels originate from the convexity of the arch. On the inferior aspect of the arch just distal to the left subclavian artery, there is often a small outpouching, a remnant of the fetal ductus arteriosus; in some patients this may be quite a prominent structure. Smaller branches arise from both sides of the descending thoracic aorta. These branches include the bronchial arteries, which arise anterolaterally at approximately the level of T5 to T6, and the fourth to the twelfth intercostal arteries. The relationship of the tho-

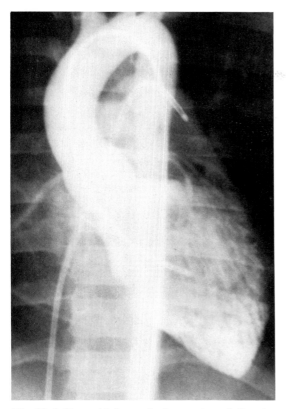

Fig. 18-6. Normal left ventriculogram in end diastole (anteroposterior projection).

racic aorta to the cardiac chambers, pulmonary arteries, and superior vena cava should be noted (Figs. 18-4 and 18-5).

Angiographic Findings

INCOMPETENCE OF THE LEFT HEART VALVES [20, 33, 55]

Incompetence of the valves of the left side of the heart is studied angiographically by contrast injections into the aorta (aortic insufficiency; Fig. 18-7) and the left ventricle (mitral insufficiency; Fig. 18-8). The position of the catheter during injection must be sufficiently distal to the valve (2 cm) to prevent reflux from purely mechanical artifacts. To be significant, the reflux should occur on more than one cardiac beat, and there should be persistent or progressive opacification of the chamber proximal to the involved valve. In the left ventricle, extrasystoles (induced by catheter recoil and the jet of contrast agent during injection) can cause artificial mitral insufficiency. Slight changes in

density encountered in a mildly insufficient valve are best observed by cineangiography.

STENOSIS OF SEMILUNAR VALVES [20, 48, 55]

Stenosis of the semilunar valves has some or all of the following characteristics: doming of the valve in systole; thickened valve; appearance of a jet of either unopacified blood (if the injection is distal to the valve) or opacified blood (if the injection is in the chamber proximal to the valve); poststenotic dilatation; slow emptying and hypertrophy of the proximal chamber (Fig. 18-9). Injections should be made in the left ventricular chamber in order to determine the ventricular configuration and the competence of the mitral valve, and to rule out subaortic stenosis or associated shunts. Injections should be made above the valve in order to rule out accompanying valvular insufficiency. Determinations of pullback pressures across the valve should be made in order to determine the extent of pressure gradients. Sometimes a markedly deformed valve may have a clinically insignificant gradient. It may be difficult to traverse the valve from the aortic root, in which case the transseptal approach should be used.

STENOSIS OF MITRAL VALVES [20, 55]

Mitral valve stenosis is best studied hemodynamically by catheterization of both the right and the left sides of the heart. Pressure measurements from the pulmonary artery wedge position back to the right atrium, pressure measurements and injections directly into the left atrium and the left ventricle, and determination of cardiac output are indicated. In addition to the pathologic anatomy, the abnormal hemodynamic effects of the stenotic valve, such as decreased cardiac output and increased pulmonary vascular resistance, should be assessed. It is important to demonstrate any associated shunts.

PREATRIAL AND ATRIAL SHUNTS [15, 20, 55]

Left-to-right shunts at the preatrial level (anomalous pulmonary venous return) and the atrial level are best studied angiographically by injection into the pulmonary artery and then following the contrast agent through to the levophase or venous phase of the study into the left atrium. Atrial septal defects may also be angiographically studied by

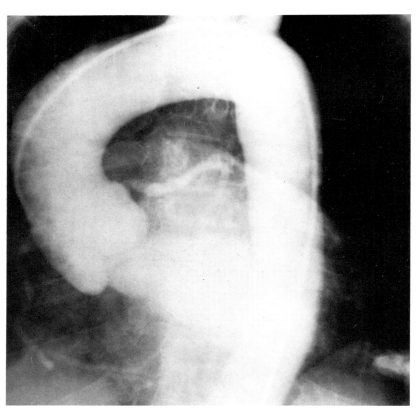

Fig. 18-7. Moderately severe aortic insufficiency resulting from rheumatic heart disease. The catheter is well above the aortic valve. The regurgitant flow into the left ventricle is well demonstrated.

direct injection into the left atrium. The right atrium fills following left atrial opacification, and the normally clear definition of the inferior wall of the left atrium is no longer apparent. There may also be reflux of contrast medium down the inferior vena cava. Opacification of the right ventricle and more delayed reopacification of the pulmonary artery occur. Ostium primum defects have a characteristic "gooseneck" deformity of the left ventricular outflow tract, an abnormal cleft of the anterior leaflet of the mitral valve, and often an incompetent mitral valve. There may be associated shunts at the ventricular septal level that make direct left ventriculography a useful procedure.

VENTRICULAR SEPTAL DEFECTS [20, 55]
Ventricular septal defects are best studied by left ventriculography, in which the location of the defect, the presence of multiple septal defects, or associated abnormalities of the left side of the heart and thoracic aorta may be demonstrated. Small shunts are best demonstrated by cineangiography, which provides better appreciation of minor density changes. With larger shunts, particularly when

they are associated with other complex cardiac abnormalities, a full view of the entire heart and associated vessels is often best appreciated by seriographic biplane anteroposterior and lateral large film angiography.

LEFT-TO-RIGHT SHUNTS ABOVE THE AORTIC VALVE
Left-to-right shunts above the aortic valve (e.g., aortopulmonary window, coronary artery fistula, patent ductus arteriosus, sinus of Valsalva fistula to cardiac chambers) are best seen with aortic root injections.

RIGHT-TO-LEFT SHUNTS
Right-to-left cardiac shunts are usually caused by obstruction to a right-sided chamber or to the outflow tract of the right ventricle or pulmonary arteries, and a more proximal communication between the right- and left-sided chambers. This type

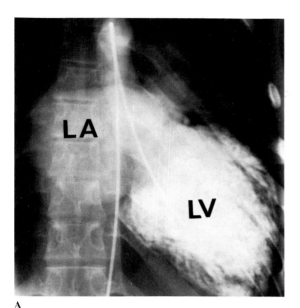

A

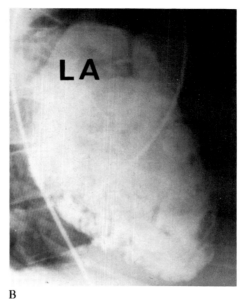

B

Fig. 18-8. Mitral insufficiency in a patient with idiopathic myocardial hypertrophy (injection into dilated left ventricle with regurgitation of contrast into the left atrium).
A. Anteroposterior projection.
B. Lateral projection. *LV* = left ventricle; *LA* = left atrium.

of shunt is studied by catheterization of the right side of the heart. Selective angiocardiography with right atrial and right ventricular injections coned to the cardiac structures, biplane projections (anteroposterior and lateral), and rapid film timing (four films per second for 2 seconds; two per second thereafter) will angiographically define the pathologic anatomy.

ENLARGEMENT OF THE AORTA

A large aorta may be caused by the following conditions [11, 15, 16, 26, 28, 37, 46]:

1. Aortic runoff lesions (aortic insufficiency, patent ductus arteriosus, aortic pulmonary window, aortic left ventricular tunnel, ruptured aortic sinus aneurysm).
2. Right-to-left shunts, with diversion of flow from the right side of the heart into the aorta (tetralogy of Fallot, pseudotruncus arteriosus, tricuspid atresia).
3. Poststenotic dilatation, as in aortic stenosis.

Fig. 18-9. Anteroposterior aortogram filmed during systole, showing aortic stenosis and mild coarctation of the thoracic aorta. There is doming of the aortic valve and poststenotic dilatation. A pressure gradient of 100 mm Hg was measured across the valve.

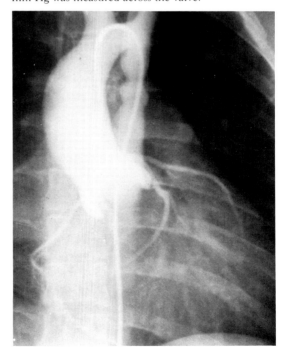

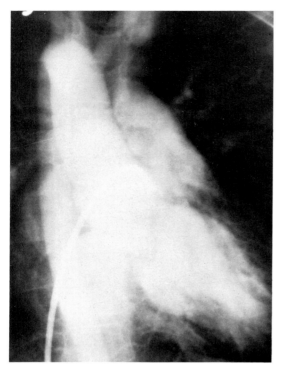

Fig. 18-10. Left atrial injection showing a mirror-image right-sided aortic arch in a patient with a tetralogy of Fallot and a left-sided Blalock shunt. This type of right aortic arch has an associated intracardiac anomaly in 98 percent of patients.

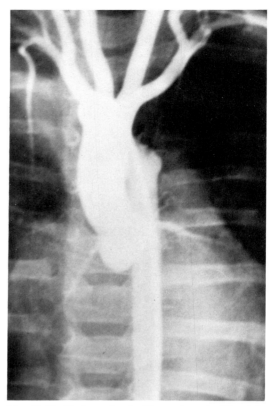

Fig. 18-11. Variant of a double aortic arch. The right arch is patent and rises high to the right of the trachea. The left brachiocephalic vessels are the first to arise from the aorta and represent the only remnant of the left arch. The remainder of the left arch was atretic at surgery and was replaced by a fibrous band. The aorta descends on the left. The patient had stridor and dyspnea together with recurrent pneumonia. There was an associated ventricular septal defect (not demonstrated here).

The ascending aorta may be enlarged in coarctation, in pseudocoarctation, and in interruption of the aortic arch. Acquired diseases such as atherosclerosis, hypertension, aortic stenosis, aortitis, and rheumatic aortic insufficiency may also cause an enlarged thoracic aorta.

SMALL THORACIC AORTA

A small thoracic aorta may occur as a result of a left-to-right intracardiac shunt (e.g., atrial septal defect) and in low-output conditions such as mitral stenosis or pulmonary venous stenosis [15, 29, 46]. Congenital lesions such as tubular hypoplasia, supravalvular aortic stenosis, and aortic valve atresia can also cause a small thoracic aorta.

POSITIONAL ABNORMALITIES
OF THE AORTA

Positional congenital abnormalities of the thoracic aorta include right-sided aortic arches (Fig. 18-10), a double aortic arch and its variants with symptomatic vascular rings (Fig. 18-11), and transposed ves-

sels (Fig. 18-12) [11, 15, 16, 26, 46]. These abnormalities are easily approached for angiography by the femoral route. Aberrant position of the great vessels and the cardiac chambers requires a combination of the injections into the right side of the heart, the left side of the heart, and the great vessels, as well as pressure measurements, since there are usually a variety of associated shunts and outflow tract obstructions to be evaluated [15, 16, 48].

OBSTRUCTIVE ABNORMALITIES
OF THE AORTA

Obstructive congenital abnormalities include coarctation (Figs. 18-13, 18-14), pseudocoarctation

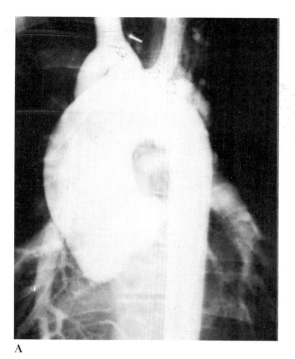

A

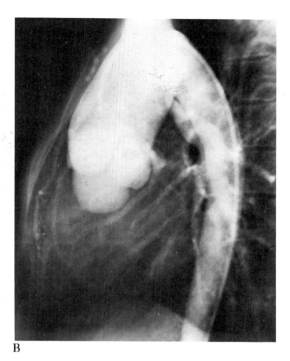

B

Fig. 18-12. Transposition of the great vessels. Thoracic aortogram shows an enlarged transposed aorta arising anteriorly from the right ventricle. Bilateral Blalock shunts (subclavian artery to the pulmonary artery) have been performed because of obstruction to the outflow tract to the pulmonary arteries.
A. Anteroposterior projection.
B. Lateral projection.

Fig. 18-13. Postductal coarctation of the thoracic aorta shown on a lateral projection. There are large collateral channels. There is a bicuspid aortic valve.

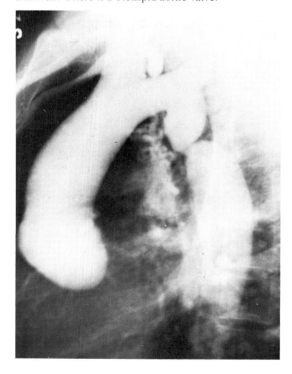

(Fig. 18-15) [9, 46], and interruption of the thoracic aorta. These abnormalities often require an axillary artery approach. Associated anomalies of origin of the subclavian arteries can occur where these arteries arise distal to the coarcted or atretic segment. The angiographer should be sure to check the blood pressures on both upper extremities prior to axillary artery catheterization. A localized posterior defect in the barium-filled esophagus may point to an anomalous origin of the right subclavian artery from the descending thoracic aorta, and this abnormality precludes a right axillary approach. Figure 18-14 shows this anomaly, together with an occluded left subclavian artery studied by levophase pulmonary angiography. It is important to identify angiographically the vessels that are both proximal and distal to the occluded segment.

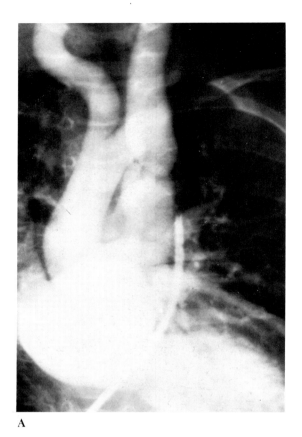

A

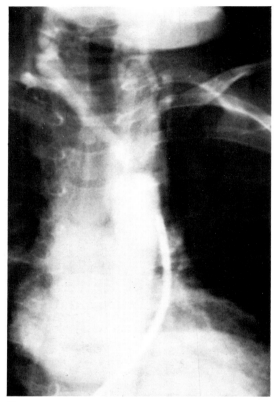

B

LEFT VENTRICULAR ANEURYSMS

Left ventricular aneurysms (Fig. 18-16) [10, 27, 40] generally occur as a complication of myocardial infarcts and most commonly are seen at the apex of the left ventricle. Rarely, they occur in the ventricular septum. These aneurysms can cause serious functional myocardial impairments; however, they can be surgically repaired. Calcium in the wall of the aneurysm, diminished or paradoxical pulsation, and an abnormal bulge on the anterior, posterior, or lateral aspects of the apex may be seen fluoroscopically and by standard roentgenographic methods. A full evaluation of the functional capabilities of the heart, a clear angiographic definition of the pathologic morphology of both the aneurysm and the rest of the left ventricle, together with the valves in multiple projections, and an angiographic demonstration of the underlying coronary artery abnormalities must be performed. Only then can a correct decision be made regarding surgery. A generally enlarged, poorly contracting heart, with a low ejection fraction and

Fig. 18-14. Coarctation of the thoracic aorta with interruption of the left subclavian artery and anomalous origin of the right subclavian artery demonstrated by the levophase of a pulmonary arteriogram.
A. The aorta arches to the left, and there is very severe stenosis of the descending thoracic aorta. Neither subclavian artery is filled.
B. Later in the study, one can see the right subclavian artery arising anomalously from the descending thoracic aorta distal to the coarctation. The left subclavian artery filled on subsequent films via large collaterals.

Fig. 18-15. Pseudocoarctation of the thoracic aorta in a 34-year-old female patient who underwent thoracotomy elsewhere for a mediastinal mass. The thoracic aorta is markedly elongated and kinked, and the left subclavian artery is grossly dilated. Patients with pseudocoarctation demonstrate no gradient across the kinked aorta. There may be associated congenital intracardiac defects.
A. Anteroposterior projection.
B. Lateral projection.

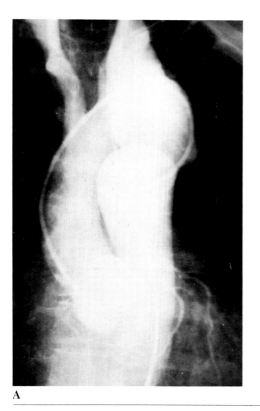
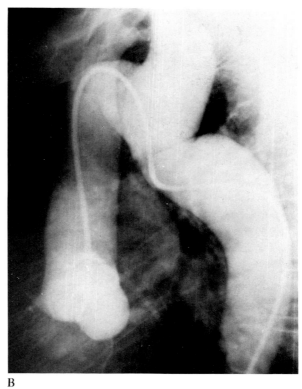

A   B

high left ventricular end-diastolic pressure, would mitigate against surgery.

Fig. 18-16. Aneurysm of the apex of the left ventricle, demonstrated by two frames of ciné left ventriculography.
A. Diastole.
B. Systole. Only the outflow tract and posterior free wall of the left ventricle contract. Note the papillary muscles protruding into the left ventricle above the aneurysm.

THORACIC AORTIC ANEURYSMS

An aneurysm is a dilatation—focal or diffuse—of an artery [1, 41]. Most aneurysms are *true aneurysms* and contain all three layers of the arterial wall. In contrast, a *false aneurysm* is one that is not bound by the three layers of the aorta and generally

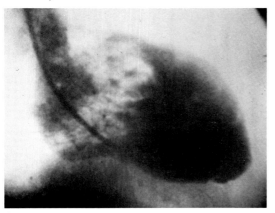
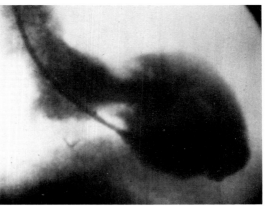

A   B

is contained only by the adventitia of the vessel. Other terms, such as *saccular* and *fusiform*, not only permit classification of aneurysms but also suggest an etiology. A saccular aneurysm usually arises from a distinct portion of the wall of the artery and possesses a mouth. The fusiform aneurysm represents a diffuse dilatation of the artery and involves the total circumference of the artery. Thus, a saccular aneurysm implies a traumatic or infectious (mycotic) etiology while a fusiform aneurysm generally represents a degenerative process, usually atherosclerosis, as an etiology. Moreover, most aneurysms are acquired rather than congenital in origin.

The following types of aneurysms are found in the thoracic aorta [2, 11, 41]:

1. Atherosclerotic aneurysms, which are the most frequent, are usually seen in the aortic arch or the descending thoracic aorta (Fig. 18-17). The calcification in their walls is usually thick and patchy, and there are associated findings of plaques, tortuosity, and elongation. The pathogenesis of these aneurysms is thought to be related to degenerative changes within the media that result in elastic fiber disruption with subsequent weakening and dilatation of the vessel wall.

2. Syphilitic aneurysms are caused by an obliterative endarteritis of the vasa vasorum, which frequently produces necrosis and fragmentation of the elastic fibers of the media. Saccular widening of the aortic lumen may develop. There is a characteristic fine, curvilinear line of calcium in the wall of the aneurysm, which most commonly involves the ascending aorta (Fig. 18-18). The descending aorta and, more rarely, the sinuses of Valsalva may also be involved. Accompanying aortic insufficiency due to distortion of the cusps and dilatation of the aortic ring is a common finding in syphilis.

3. Mycotic aneurysms are caused by bacterial infections within the wall of the aorta with resultant destruction of a vessel wall (Fig. 18-19) [2, 25, 41]. Moreover, since the aortic wall is resistant to infection, the development of a mycotic aneurysm usually requires both a source of infection and previous damage to or degeneration of the aortic wall. The damage could be from many causes, but the degeneration could be from atherosclerosis, cystic medial necrosis, or other causes. The infection arrives either through direct invasion from an adjacent suppurative process (e.g., tuberculosis) or by an infected embolus (e.g., bacterial endocarditis), or by way of vasa vasorum. The most common sites of mycotic aneurysms in the thoracic aorta are the sinuses of Valsalva (Fig. 18-20), the aortic root, the ascending aorta, and localized areas of narrowing such as coarctation or pseudocoarctation.

4. Aneurysms may be associated with arteritis, relapsing polychondritis, Reiter's syndrome, rheumatoid arthritis, and ankylosing spondylitis [28].

5. In cystic medial necrosis, there is dilatation of the aorta, particularly the aortic root, the ascending aorta, and the aortic ring, with an accompanying aortic insufficiency. These lesions are probably caused by a metabolic disturbance affecting the collagen and ground substance of the media resulting in reduced adherence of the media of the aorta, and they particularly predispose to aortic dissection (see Figs. 18-21 through 18-28).

Fig. 18-17. Large atherosclerotic aneurysm of the arch of the thoracic aorta. The lesion was gradually increasing in size, and the patient developed hoarseness.

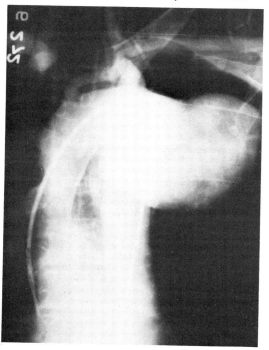

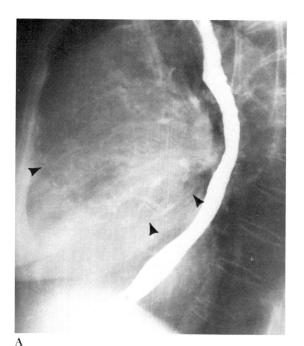

A

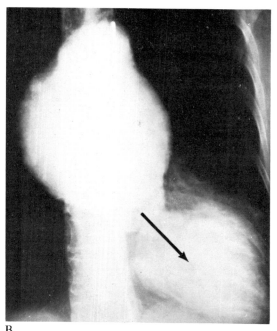

B

Fig. 18-18.
A. Syphilitic aneurysm. There is fine curvilinear calcium outlining the entire wall of the aneurysm of
the ascending aorta (*arrowheads*) and a large left
ventricle protruding behind the esophagus.
B. Thoracic aortogram outlines the aneurysm and
shows severe aortic insufficiency (*arrow*).

6. Aneurysms of the sinuses of Valsalva may be
either acquired or congenital (Figs. 18-20,
18-21) [2, 35, 41]. They can rupture and form
fistulas with various chambers of the heart.
These aneurysms are more frequent in the right
aortic sinus, and when they rupture, they do so
into the right ventricle or occasionally into the
right atrium. Aneurysms of the posterior noncoronary aortic sinuses, which are less frequent, usually rupture into the right atrium.
Aneurysms in the left aortic sinus are rare; if
they rupture, they do so into the left atrium or
into the pericardium (see Fig. 18-20).

The full extent of an aneurysm is often not angiographically demonstrated because of clots lying
within its wall. Thus, the angiogram represents
only the lumen of the aneurysm. Calcium in the
aneurysm wall, when present, helps to identify the
outside dimensions of the aneurysm. However,
the angiogram should always define the proximal
and distal extent of the aneurysms. Impending

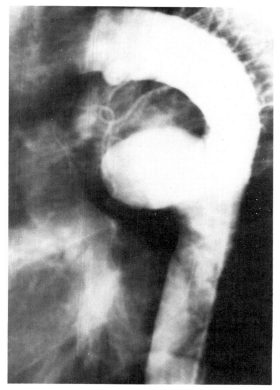

Fig. 18-19. Large infected (mycotic) aneurysm. A
fistula to the esophagus was found at surgery.

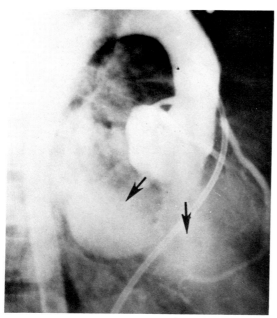

Fig. 18-20. A large (4-cm diameter) mycotic aneurysm arising from the left coronary cusp posteriorly, with a fistula to the left atrium. The patient is a 14-year-old boy with acute staphylococcal septicemia and bacterial endocarditis, myocarditis, and pericarditis. Lateral aortic root injection shows aortic insufficiency and direct communication between the aneurysm and the left atrium (*arrows*).

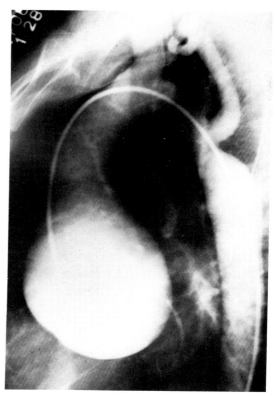

Fig. 18-21. Congenital aneurysm of the coronary cusps in a patient with Marfan's disease. There is mild coarctation of the thoracic aorta.

rupture of a thoracic aneurysm is suspected if there is associated chest pain, if there is an increase in the size of the aneurysm, or if there is pleural or pericardial fluid.

Guidewires and catheters can be safely passed through the lumen of an aneurysm from the femoral approach. A minimum of manipulation within the aneurysm is necessary to prevent embolization of friable clot. The catheter tip should be placed just above the aortic valve for the initial biplane (anteroposterior and lateral) thoracic aortogram, regardless of the position of the aneurysm. The heart should be included in the exposure area; this gives information regarding the integrity of the entire thoracic aorta, aortic valve, coronary arteries, and brachiocephalic vessels, and their relationship to the aneurysm. Often the contrast agent swirls and remains stagnant within the aneurysm, and the contrast column beyond the aneurysm is too dilute for adequate evaluation. A second injection (50 ml in 2 seconds) within the aneurysm is perfectly safe if the catheter tip lies free in the lumen and there is no stain on test injection. More than two projections may be required for complete evaluation. The optimal single projection for aneurysms of the aortic arch is the left anterior oblique; the relationship of the aneurysm to the brachiocephalic vessels is best defined in this projection.

AORTIC DISSECTION

Although a dissecting aneurysm of the aorta is not an aneurysm in the usual meaning of the word, it is considered with aortic aneurysms because of both diagnostic and therapeutic considerations. A dissecting aneurysm of the aorta, or, more appropriately, aortic dissection, represents an intramural hematoma of the aorta [3, 4, 5, 23]. As a result, these aneurysms have a true and a false lumen. The false lumen is the intramural hematoma of the aorta, and the true lumen is the anatomic lumen of the aorta. In 90 percent of patients there are intimal tears in more than one location, permitting free flow of blood through the false lumen that is thereby created within the dissected wall. The false lumen, representing the pulsating hematoma, may propagate blood in an antegrade or retrograde direction along the course of the artery. In the remaining 10 percent this does not occur and dissection is "incomplete," represented only by an intramural hematoma. In more than 90 percent of patients there is a predisposing weakness of the structures of the wall, cystic medial necrosis being the most common. The cystic medial necrosis may be either congenital or acquired in etiology. In both the basic underlying defect is a reduced adherence of the medial layer of the aortic wall with accompanying cystic changes and deterioration of the collagen and elastic tissues [3, 4]. When acquired, the underlying defect within the media is pathologically similar to that of congenital cystic medial necrosis but is less extensive. A certain amount of medial degeneration is associated with aging. Systemic hypertension is a usual accompaniment and may augment the changes in the media. With this background, once the intimal tear and intramural hematoma develop, the process is propagated by the shearing force of the systolic thrust induced by ventricular systole. Thus, a nontraumatic aortic dissection occurs when an intimal tear develops in the presence of degenerative or necrotic changes in the media with accompanying reduced intimal adherence.

Aortic dissection must be differentiated from traumatic aortic transection, which occurs when a deceleration injury results in differential rates of deceleration between the fixed and nonfixed segments of the aorta. An intimal tear occurs, and the shearing force of pulsating viscous blood as it pumps through the aorta allows an intramural hematoma to develop.

As an aortic dissection develops, it may progress in an antegrade or retrograde direction, or both, and may occlude arterial supply to adjacent structures (coronary artery, carotid artery, abdominal visceral arteries). The extent of the aortic dissection may be quite variable. DeBakey has developed a classification based on the location of the proximal intimal tear in the aorta. This classification includes three types of aortic dissection [13, 14]: type I involves the aortic root (often with aortic insufficiency) and extends to the descending thoracic aorta and sometimes to the abdominal aorta and beyond (Fig. 18-22); type II involves only the ascending aorta and possibly the brachiocephalic vessels (Figs. 18-23, 18-24, 18-25); type III arises distal to or at the level of the left subclavian artery and extends peripherally (Fig. 18-26). In addition, there is a type that commences at or near the diaphragm and has its major impact on the abdominal aorta.

Later, Daily and Anagnostopoulos reduced this classification from three to two types: those involving the ascending aorta, or type A (see Figs. 18-22, 18-23, 18-24, 18-25), and those involving the descending aorta, or type B (see Figs. 18-26, 18-28) [4, 12]. The newer classification reflects not only the different pathophysiologic mechanisms involved in these dissections but also helps dictate the therapeutic management of these patients. In addition, these aneurysms should be categorized as acute or chronic dissections whenever possible, predominantly for therapeutic considerations.

Computed tomography can be an important tool in studying patients suspected of a dissected aorta [49]. A normal, well-performed CT scan may obviate the need for an aortogram. CT can help to determine the presence and extent of a dissection and provides a baseline for follow-up evaluation. It may be used as the initial examination, particularly if chronic dissection is suspected or if the dissection is thought to involve only the descending aorta and there is no clinical suspicion of vascular compromise to essential organs. It is useful in studying those patients not considered operative candidates. CT may help determine if aortography is necessary and may guide the angiographer to the site of interest.

CT studies are performed with three bolus injections of 25 to 30 ml of contrast agent with rapid-sequence dynamic scans in each of three areas: the ascending aorta, the aortic arch, the low descending aorta. This is followed by 1-cm sections throughout the thorax with additional contrast infusion. Intimal flaps, double lumens (sometimes with differential contrast densities and flow rates), inwardly displaced media, and a distorted narrow true channel are some of the CT signs of aortic dissection (see Fig. 18-25).

Angiography helps to determine the diagnosis when it is in question and to define the full extent of disease. It should be performed in the acute phase as an emergency if the diagnosis is in doubt or if immediate surgical intervention is anticipated. Surgical intervention is considered in pa-

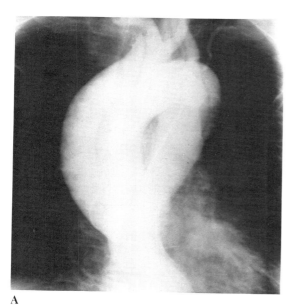

A

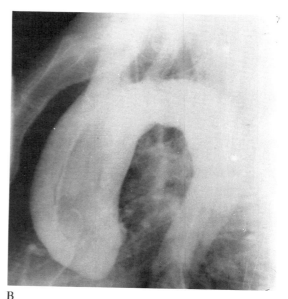

B

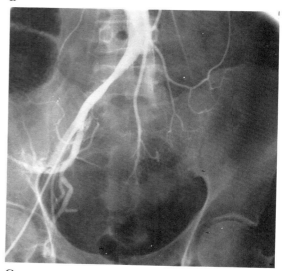

C

Fig. 18-22. Type A dissection.
A. Anteroposterior view.
B. Lateral view. There is aortic insufficiency present. Note intimal flaps involving the ascending and descending thoracic aorta, and entering the brachiocephalic vessels.
C. There is occlusion of the left iliac vessels by the dissection.

tients with severe aortic insufficiency (see Fig. 18-23), those who have leakage into pleural and pericardial spaces, those with impending rupture of a saccular component of the dissection (see Fig. 18-24), those with occlusion of vessels supplying vital structures, or those in whom there is uncontrollable hypertension. If the diagnosis is otherwise certain and surgery is not contemplated, angiography may be deferred until the condition of the patient stabilizes. In the interim, medical treatment with antihypertensive agents or beta-adrenergic blocking agents, or both, should be instituted [4, 12, 13, 14, 51, 52, 53, 54].

The study should be approached from the femoral arteries if one is patent, since dissections frequently involve the brachiocephalic vessels. Alternatively, an axillary artery approach may be used. If a direct arterial approach is not possible, an intravenous digital angiography study (or the levophase of a pulmonary angiogram, if digital equipment is unavailable) will often substantiate the diagnosis. However, aortic insufficiency cannot be assessed by these methods; in addition, poor detail of abdominal and peripheral vascular structures is obtained. The diagnosis may be subtle and requires at the very least biplane thoracic and abdominal aortography in all suspected cases.

The angiographic findings depend on the position of the catheter as it relates to the true and false lumina of the aorta and also on the proximity of the catheter tip to intimal tears (Figs. 18-22 to 18-28) [3, 21]. Absolute angiographic findings include the presence of an intimal flap, the filling (often delayed) of a false lumen, the shearing off of aortic branch vessels, and the finding of long,

In more than 100 patients with dissections who were studied angiographically at Duke University Medical Center, 50 percent had type III dissection, 41 percent had type I, and 9 percent had type II. Ten percent of the patients had no demonstrable intimal tears and presented with intramural hematomas; 90 percent had a false lumen and/or intimal flaps demonstrated. In our experience, 5 percent of patients with aortic dissection may not be diagnosed despite careful angiography; this occurs in patients with "incomplete" dissections, in whom the only abnormality is a thick aortic wall. A thick aortic wall can also be caused by an intramural clot in a thoracic aneurysm, periaortic fibrosis or fat, or tumor (Fig. 18-29).

TRAUMA

Trauma to the aorta may be caused by a penetrating injury such as a bullet or stab wound, by blunt trauma as in an automobile accident or, rarely, by iatrogenic factors [17, 22, 32, 42, 47, 54]. Penetrating injuries cause cardiac rupture with pericardial tamponade, as well as aortic, cardiac, and intracardiac shunts, vascular lacerations, and formation of false aneurysms and arteriovenous fistulas. Iatrogenic trauma can result from episodes of cardiac resuscitation and occasionally from mishaps occurring during diagnostic procedures (cardiac catheterization) or therapeutic procedures (surgical procedures) (Fig. 18-30). Penetration of the myocardium with or without resulting pericardial tamponade may occur.

Blunt trauma resulting from rapid deceleration injuries of automobile accidents, falls from high places, or crush injuries can cause trauma to the thoracic aorta and cardiac chambers and, more rarely, traumatic insufficiency of the aortic and mitral valves. The etiology of blunt thoracic aortic trauma usually is a deceleration injury to the chest. Sudden deceleration of the chest at the time of impact can be associated with differential rates of deceleration of the fixed and nonfixed anatomic structures within the chest and can therefore result in a traumatic injury to the aorta. Theoretically, these deceleration injuries may involve one, two, or three layers of the aorta. Involvement of the intima only is rare while involvement of the intima and media is most common. Moreover, since the adventitia provides approximately 60 percent of the tensile strength of the aorta, survival is dependent on this layer remaining intact. Involvement of all

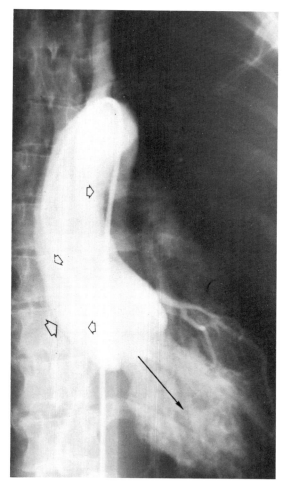

Fig. 18-23. Type A aortic dissection. The intramural hematoma extends from the aortic valve up the ascending aorta to involve the innominate artery. The true lumen is outlined by the small open arrows, and the outer margin of the false lumen by the large open arrow. The aortic valve is poorly defined, and there is considerable aortic insufficiency (*long arrow*).

smooth, extrinsic areas of aorta compromised by the intramural hematoma. Associated, but not entirely diagnostic findings include a thick aortic wall (more than 1 cm wide) on the left side of the thoracic aorta. The superior vena cava forms an unopacified column on the right side of the thoracic aorta (see Fig. 18-5) and can be of increased diameter in certain catastrophes other than dissection (e.g., pulmonary embolism, acute failure from myocardial infarct). Thus the diagnosis of a dissection of the ascending thoracic aorta should not be made solely on the basis of a thick aortic wall.

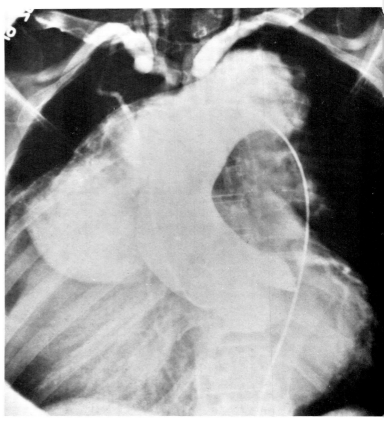

Fig. 18-24. Type A aortic dissection, with a large saccular component near the aortic root. The patient refused surgery and died 3 days later when the aneurysm ruptured into the pericardium.

Fig. 18-25. Chronic type A aortic dissection involving the ascending aorta anteriorly.
A. Lateral projection thoracic aortogram.
B. Computed tomography scan showing intimal flap (*arrows*).

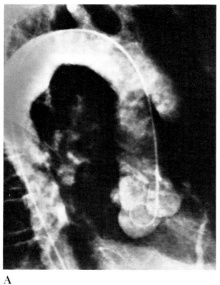

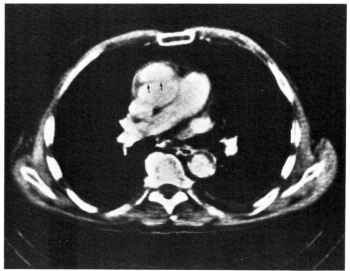

A

B

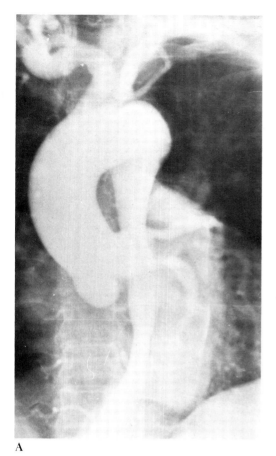

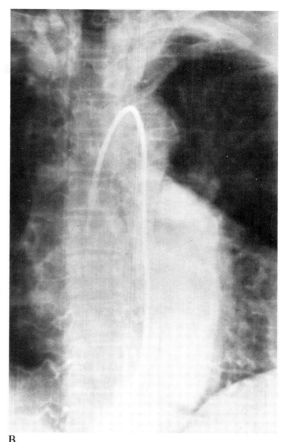

A   B

Fig. 18-26. Type B aortic dissection, arising distal to the left subclavian artery.
A. Narrowing of the true aortic lumen.
B. Filling of the false lumen late in the study.

three layers of the aorta—a complete transection—by the injury is usually fatal.

Since the aortic injury results from differential rates of deceleration of those anatomic structures within the chest, the anatomic locations of these traumatic aortic injuries can be predicted [4, 41, 52]. The most proximal anatomic point is in the ascending aorta at the level of the pericardial reflection; clinically, this injury location occurs second in frequency (Fig. 18-31). The most frequent location of injury is just distal to the origin of the left subclavian artery at the ligamentum arteriosum (Figs. 18-32, 18-33). The anatomically most distal but clinically least frequent location of injury is at the level of the diaphragm (see Fig. 10-28). If trauma to the aorta remains undetected,

exsanguination from secondary hemorrhage may occur, usually within 3 weeks.

Arteriography should be performed in any patient suspected of having aortic rupture, since additional trauma results from unnecessary surgical exploration in patients who are already severely injured [4, 32, 52]. Even when speed is important, aortography can be performed quickly while other life-saving measures are being carried out. Chest pain, increasing dyspnea, hypertension of the upper extremities, and a precordial systolic murmur may be clinically evident in less than half of these patients. A chest x-ray may show only minimal findings of irregularity of the aortic shadow. Mediastinal widening, deviation of the trachea and of the esophagus (outlined by a nasogastric tube), a downward displacement of the left mainstem bronchus, varying degrees of left hemothorax, and fractures of the first two or three ribs are suspicious findings and should be followed immediately by aortography. Bleeding from less significant vessels,

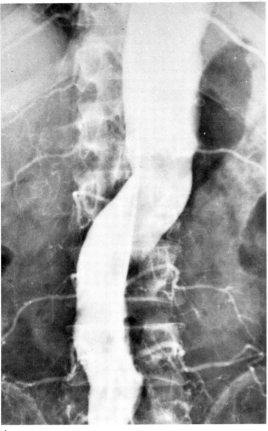

A

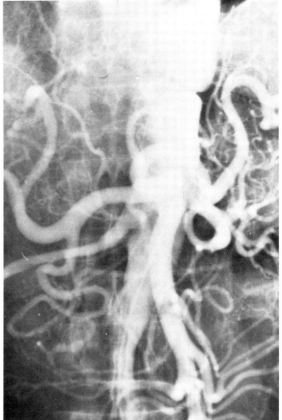

B

Fig. 18-27. Type A aortic dissection. The dissection started at the aortic root.

A. Abdominal aortogram with the catheter in the false lumen. There is no filling of the visceral vessels.

B. Injection into the true lumen fills the visceral vessels. A catheter was introduced through each femoral artery to produce this study.

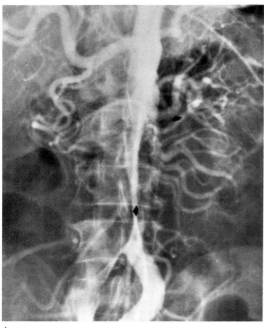

A

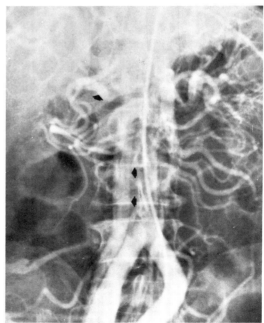

B

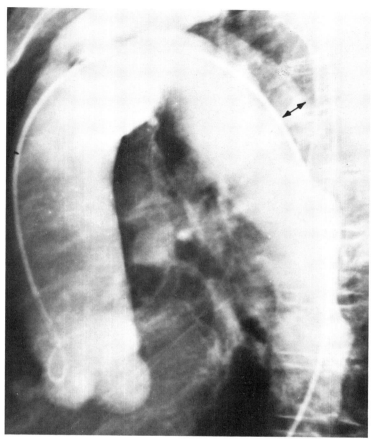

Fig. 18-29. Thick aortic wall (*arrows*) in a patient suspected of having a dissecting aneurysm. The thickness is caused by a clot lying in the wall of the diffusely ectatic thoracic aorta. There was an associated atherosclerotic aneurysm of the abdominal aorta.

Fig. 18-28.
A. Abdominal aortogram in a patient with type B dissection with the catheter in the true lumen. The true aortic lumen appears severely narrowed (*lower arrowhead*) and only the left renal artery fills (*upper arrowhead*).
B. Later phase of the same injection (during systole) shows the mobile aortic intimal flap (*lower paired arrowheads*) and delayed filling of the false lumen and the right renal artery (*upper arrowhead*).

such as small mediastinal arteries and veins, may be responsible for some of the suspicious chest x-ray findings.

Computed tomography scanning has a limited role in evaluating the thoracic aorta for blunt trauma. Periaortic bleeding does not necessarily implicate the aorta as its source. Associated injuries to the brachiocephalic vessels cannot be detected by CT. Although occasionally CT findings of false aneurysm, linear aortic lucencies, and intramural hematomas may be specific, CT scanning cannot consistently demonstrate reliable evidence of aortic rupture [17, 49]. Since each moment is valuable and may be life-saving, aortography should be undertaken directly.

The angiographic findings of a ruptured aorta may include that of a transverse radiolucent line caused by rolled-up edges of a lacerated intima and media (Fig. 18-32). There may be a localized, often irregular dilatation, which represents a false aneurysm with walls consisting of adventitia and

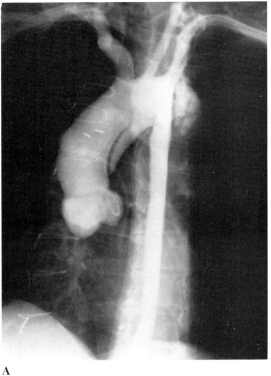

A

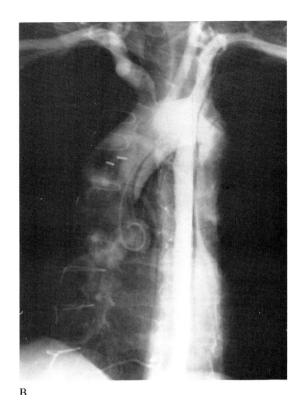

B

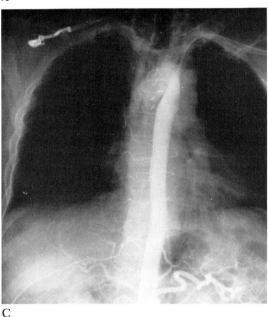

C

D

Fig. 18-30. Iatrogenic aortic dissection acquired during cardiopulmonary bypass for coronary artery bypass graft. The patient was perfused via the left femoral artery and had left leg claudication.

A. Note the intimal flap in the ascending aorta.
B. Note the delayed filling of the false channel in the descending aorta.
C. An injection in the true lumen of the descending

aorta demonstrates that the celiac axis is perfused from the true lumen.
D. Angiogram demonstrating the right and left renal arteries and right iliac artery system being perfused via the true lumen. The left iliac artery system is being perfused via the false lumen. The patient had a palpable left femoral artery pulse.

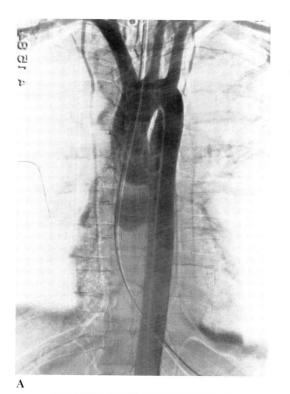

A

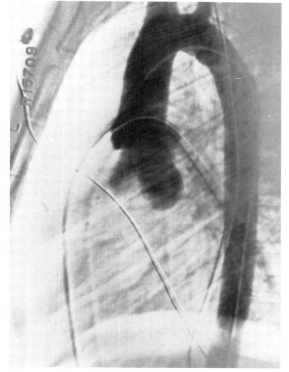

B

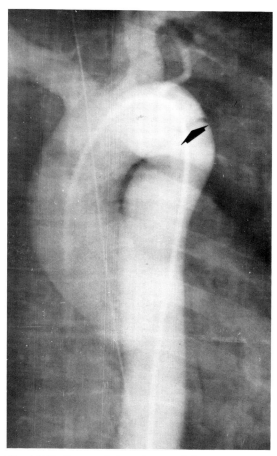

Fig. 18-32. Ruptured thoracic aorta following an automobile accident. A 270-degree circumferential tear was seen at surgery distal to the left subclavian artery. The radiolucent line is caused by rolled-up edges of lacerated intima and media (*arrow*).

Fig. 18-31. "Double" aortic valve sign demonstrated in ascending aortic transection at the level of the pericardial reflection. Note the position of the true aortic valve and coronary arteries in the anteroposterior (A) and lateral (B) projections.

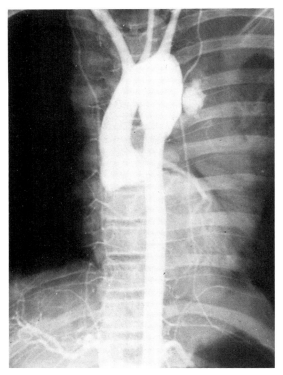

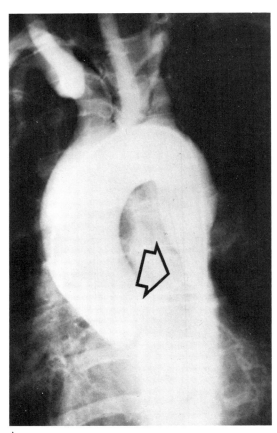

Fig. 18-33. Ruptured thoracic aorta following an automobile accident. There is severe left-sided hemothorax. There is a false aneurysm around the site of rupture, as well as free extravasation of contrast medium. There is considerable widening of the mediastinum.

A

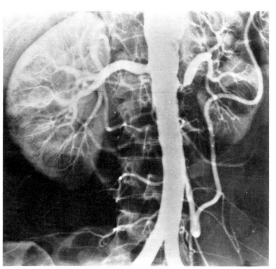

B

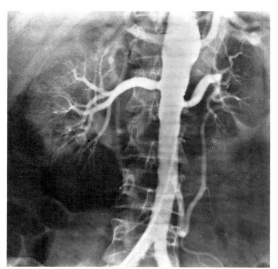

C

surrounding connective tissue; occasionally there may be extravasation of contrast agent at the site of rupture (Fig. 18-33). Sometimes there is disruption of one or more of the brachiocephalic vessels, without or in addition to a major traumatic aortic dissection.

In summary, an understanding of the pathophysiology of these blunt decelerating injuries to the chest and knowledge of the relative points of anatomic fixation of the aorta within the chest permits prediction of the anatomic location and angiographic findings of these injuries. The term *traumatic transection of the thoracic aorta* accurately reflects the underlying pathophysiology of this lesion.

TAKAYASU'S ARTERITIS

Takayasu's arteritis [28] is a panarteritis of unknown etiology; it is thought to be caused by an autoimmune process. It may involve the aorta and the proximal portions of its major branches, as well as the pulmonary artery. It can cause stenosis, which progresses to occlusion of the affected vessels. Often there are skip areas of noninvolvement. The disease is found worldwide, most commonly in females, and in any age group but with a peak incidence among persons aged 15 to 25. If a young patient demonstrates a long, constricting aortic lesion, particularly one involving the descending thoracic or abdominal aorta, the most likely diagnosis is Takayasu's arteritis. The brachiocephalic vessels have a high rate of involvement, as do the renal arteries (Fig. 18-34).

Fig. 18-34.
A. Takayasu's arteritis in a 28-year-old woman. There is a characteristic long area of stenosis involving the descending thoracic aorta (*arrow*); there is also occlusion of the left subclavian artery.
B and C. Takayasu's arteritis in another young hypertensive Chinese patient. There is an irregular abdominal aorta with occluded superior mesenteric artery and severe stenosis of the left renal artery (B). The left renal artery was dilated with a 6 mm and then a 7 mm diameter balloon (C). Arteries involved with acute arteritis should not be dilated for fear of rupturing the vessel. This chronic "burned out" lesion was dilated with difficulty, but blood pressure returned to normal. (Courtesy Drs. Chihan Yang and Jason Chen, West China University of Medical Sciences, Sichuan Province, People's Republic of China.)

References

1. Abrams, H. L. (ed.). *Abrams' Angiography* (3rd ed.). Boston: Little, Brown, 1983.
2. Abrams, H. L. Technique, Indications, and Hazards of Thoracic Aortography. In H. L. Abrams (ed.), *Abrams' Angiography* (3rd ed.). Boston: Little, Brown, 1983. Chapter 14.
3. Abrams, H. L. Dissecting Aortic Aneurysm. In H. L. Abrams (ed.), *Abrams' Angiography* (3rd ed.). Boston: Little, Brown, 1983. Chapter 20.
4. Anagnostopoulos, C. E. *Acute Aortic Dissections.* Baltimore: University Park Press, 1975.
5. Appelbaum, A., Karp, R. B., and Kirklin, J. W. Ascending Versus Descending Aortic Dissections. *Ann. Surg.* 183:286, 1976.
6. Behar, V. S. Contrast Ventriculography. In G. S. Wagner (ed.), *Myocardial Infarction: Measurement and Intervention.* The Hague: M. Nijhoff, 1982. P. 173.
7. Berenek, I., et al. Comparison of ejection fraction calculated by 9 different volume calculation methods: Description and evaluation of a new method. *Radiology* 120:553, 1976.
8. Carlsson, E. Functional evaluation of the heart by angiocardiography. *Radiol. Clin. North Am.* 14:209, 1976.
9. Cheng, T. Pseudocoarctation of the aorta: An important consideration in the differential diagnosis of superior mediastinal mass. *Am. J. Med.* 49:551, 1970.
10. Cheng, T. Incidence of ventricular aneurysm in coronary artery disease: Angiographic appraisal. *Am. J. Med.* 50:340, 1971.
11. Cornell, S. *The Roentgenographic Diagnosis of Diseases of the Thoracic Aorta.* Springfield, IL: Thomas, 1974.
12. Daily, P. O., et al. Management of acute aortic dissections. *Ann. Thorac. Surg.* 10:237, 1970.
13. Debakey, M., et al. Surgical management of dissecting aneurysm involving the ascending aorta. *J. Cardiovasc. Surg.* 5:200, 1964.
14. DeBakey, M. E., et al. Dissection and dissecting aneurysms of the aorta: Twenty-five year follow-up of 527 patients treated surgically. *Surgery* 42:1118, 1982.
15. Edwards, J., et al. *Congenital Heart Disease: Correlation of Pathologic Anatomy and Angiocardiography.* Philadelphia: Saunders, 1965. Vol. I.
16. Elliott, L., and Schiebler, G. *X-ray Diagnosis of Congenital Cardiac Disease.* Springfield, IL: Thomas, 1968.
17. Federle, M. P., and Brant-Zawadski, M. (eds.). *Computed Tomography and the Evaluation of Trauma* (2nd ed.). Baltimore: Williams & Wilkins, 1986. P. 180.
18. Gault, J. Angiographic estimation of left ventricular volume: Comprehensive review. *Cathet. Cardiovasc. Diagn.* 1:7, 1975.
19. Gensini, G. G. Left Ventriculography. In G. G.

Gensini (ed.), *Coronary Arteriography*. Mount Kisco, NY: Futura, 1975. Chapter 23.

20. Grossman, W. *Cardiac Catheterization and Angiography*. Philadelphia: Lea & Febiger, 1974.

21. Hayashi, K., et al. Aortographic analysis of aortic dissection. *Am. J. Roentgenol.* 122:769, 1974.

22. Hipona, F., and Paredes, S. The radiologic evaluation of patients with chest trauma: Cardiovascular system. *Med. Clin. North Am.* 59:65, 1975.

23. Itzchak, Y., et al. Dissecting aneurysm of thoracic aorta: Reappraisal of radiologic diagnosis. *Am. J. Roentgenol.* 125:559, 1975.

24. Jaffe, C. C., and Ellis, K. The angiocardiographic quantitation of ventricular volume, shape, and mass. *Curr. Probl. Radiol.* 4(1):1, 1974.

25. Jaffe, R., and Condon, V. Mycotic aneurysms of the pulmonary artery and aorta. *Radiology* 116:39, 1975.

26. Kerley, P., and Pattison, N. The Aorta and Great Vessels. In C. Shanks and P. Kerley (eds.), *A Textbook of Diagnosis*. Vol. II. *Cardiovascular System* (4th ed.). Philadelphia: Saunders, 1972. Chapter 13.

27. Kittredge, R., and Cameron, A. Abnormalities of left ventricular wall motion and aneurysm formation. *Am. J. Roentgenol.* 116:100, 1972.

28. Lande, A., and Berkmen, Y. Aortitis: Pathologic, clinical and arteriographic review. *Radiol. Clin. North Am.* 14:219, 1976.

29. McAlpine, W. *Heart and Coronary Arteries: An Anatomical Atlas for Clinical Diagnosis, Radiologic Investigation, and Surgical Treatment*. New York: Springer, 1975.

30. Meschan, I. *An Atlas of Anatomy Basic to Radiology*. Philadelphia: Saunders, 1975.

31. Meszaros, W. T. *Cardiac Roentgenology*. Springfield, IL: Thomas, 1969.

32. Moore, A. V., Putman, C. E., and Ravin, C. E. The radiology of thoracic trauma. *Bull. N.Y. Acad. Med.* 57:272, 1981.

33. Netter, F. *Heart* (The Ciba Collection of Medical Illustrations, Vol. 5). Summit, NJ: Ciba Corp., 1969.

34. Newman, G. E., et al. Digital Subtraction Left Ventriculography: A Technique with Gated Injections in Patients. Presented at 85th Assembly of American Roentgen Ray Society. April 1986, Washington, DC (abstract).

35. Ominski, S., and Kricum, M. Roentgenology of sinus of Valsalva aneurysms. *Am. J. Roentgenol.* 125:571, 1975.

36. Rackley, C. E. Quantitative evaluation of left ventricular function by radiographic techniques. *Circulation* 54:862, 1976.

37. Randall, P. A., and Jarmolowski, C. R. Aneurysms of the Thoracic Aorta. In H. L. Abrams (ed.), *Abrams' Angiography* (3rd ed.). Boston: Little, Brown, 1983. Chapter 19.

38. Rankin, J. S., et al. The effects of coronary revascularization on left ventricular function in ischemic heart disease. *J. Thorac. Cardiovasc. Surg.* 90:818, 1985.

39. Rankin, J. S., et al. Clinical and angiographic assessment of complex mammary artery bypass grafting. *J. Thorac. Cardiovasc. Surg.* (In press.)

40. Raphael, M. J., and Allwork, S. P. Angiographic anatomy of the left ventricle. *Clin. Radiol.* 25:95, 1974.

41. Sabiston, D. C., Jr. *Textbook of Surgery* (13th ed.). Philadelphia: Saunders, 1986.

42. Sanborn, J., Heitzman, E., and Markarian, B. Traumatic rupture of the thoracic aorta: Roentgenographic-pathologic correlations. *Radiology* 95:293, 1970.

43. Schad, N. Concentration of contrast material in angiocardiography during phased and continuous injection. *Am. J. Roentgen., Rad. Therapy, and Nuclear Med.* 104:25, 1970.

44. Schad, N., et al. The intermittent phased injection of contrast material into the heart. *Am. J. Roentgen., Rad. Therapy, and Nuclear Med.* 104:464, 1968.

45. Standards and guidelines for cardiopulmonary resuscitation (P4CPR) and emergency cardiac care (ECC). *J.A.M.A.* 255:2905, 1986.

46. Stewart, J., Kincaid, O., and Edwards, J. *An Atlas of Vascular Rings and Related Malformations of the Aortic Arch System*. Springfield, IL: Thomas, 1964.

47. Symbas, P. *Traumatic Injury of the Heart and Great Vessels*. Springfield, IL: Thomas, 1972.

48. Verel, D., and Grainger, R. *Cardiac Catheterization and Angiocardiography* (3rd ed.). Edinburgh: Churchill Livingstone, 1978.

49. Webb, W. R. CT of intrathoracic great vessels. In Siegelman (ed.), *Computed Tomography of the Chest*. New York: Churchill Livingstone, 1984.

50. Wheat, M. W., Jr. Acute dissecting aneurysms of the aorta: Diagnosis and treatment, 1979. *Am. Heart J.* 44:373, 1980.

51. Wheat, M., et al. Acute dissecting aneurysms of the aorta: Treatment and results in 64 patients. *J. Thorac. Cardiovasc. Surg.* 58:344, 1969.

52. Wolfe, W. G. Acute ascending aortic dissection. *Ann. Surg.* 192:658, 1980.

53. Wolfe, W. G., and Moran, J. F. The evolution of medical and surgical management of acute aortic dissection. *Circulation* 56:503, 1977.

54. Wolfe, W. G., et al. Surgical treatment of acute ascending aortic dissection. *Ann. Surg.* 197:738, 1983.

55. Zimmerman, H. *Intravascular Catheterization* (2nd ed.). Springfield, IL: Thomas, 1968.

Bronchial Artery Procedures

Indications for Arteriography

1. Location (and embolization) of feeding vessels in patients with life-threatening hemoptysis from bronchogenic carcinoma and from chronic inflammatory conditions such as tuberculosis, aspergilloma, bronchiectasis, suppurative lung conditions, cystic fibrosis, pneumoconiosis, hydatid disease, and certain rare mixed bronchial and pulmonary arteriovenous malformations (AVM)
2. Demonstration of hypervascular tumors and AVMs
3. Outlining bronchial pulmonary anastomoses in patients with chronic pulmonary embolism preparatory to surgical embolectomy

Technique

APPROACH
Approach is percutaneously by the femoral artery.

CATHETERS
An 80-cm 5 French thin-walled catheter with a Mikaelsson curve, a reversed curve, or a "cobra" curve. An alternative curve is one with a 1-cm tapered tip with a 90-degree primary curve and a secondary curve with a long, gentle obtuse angle (Fig. 19-1).

CONTRAST AGENTS, PROJECTIONS, AND RADIOGRAPHIC PROGRAMMING
Contrast agents with low neurotoxicity are required due to the occasional anastomosis of bronchial and intercostal branches with the anterior spinal artery. A preliminary thoracic aortogram is usually not helpful. Selective injections are necessary. Only small hand injections of 2 to 3 ml of low-density iothalamate (60% or less) or, preferably, nonionic contrast agent are used initially. Larger amounts, 5 to 10 ml, may be necessary if the vascular bed is considerably hypertrophied. Often 105-mm photofluorographic spot filming or intraarterial digital subtraction angiography (IA-DSA) is satisfactory for initial identification of bronchial arteries and for monitoring embolizations. Biplane seriographic films with magnification capabilities provide optimal detail as to extent of disease, important anastomotic channels, and final results of any therapeutic maneuver. Three films per second for 3 seconds, one film per second for 3 seconds, and one film every other second for 6 seconds suffices.

Anatomic Considerations [1, 6, 10]

There are a number of variations in the bronchial artery supply to the lungs (Figs. 19-2, 19-3). Most of them arise from the ventral surface of the descending thoracic aorta. Eighty percent or more arise just above the left mainstem bronchus, opposite the fifth and sixth thoracic vertebral bodies. As a rule (85 percent), the right bronchial artery arises in a ventrolateral position in a common trunk with the highest thoracic intercostal artery. The intercostal branches of this vessel may feed the upper four or five intercostal arteries. In approximately 5 percent of patients, these branches may supply small radicular vessels to the anterior spinal artery [6], an important consideration in avoiding overinjection of contrast agents and emboli. Less often, there are two bronchial arteries that supply the right lung. Occasionally a common trunk supplies both the right and the left bronchial vessels. Most commonly, there are two bronchial arteries on the left side, but there may be only one, or as many as three. There are a number of small, usually inconsequential accessory bronchial branches, which may enlarge when stimulated by pathology. These branches may arise from the aortic arch, subclavian arteries or their branches, and the descending thoracic and upper abdominal aorta. Thus, intercostal, phrenic, esophageal, thyrocervical, costocervical, lateral thoracic, internal mammary, and even coronary artery branches may hypertrophy in response to thoracic disease [9]. Many of these branches anastomose with pulmonary arteries and veins through pleural adhesions, me-

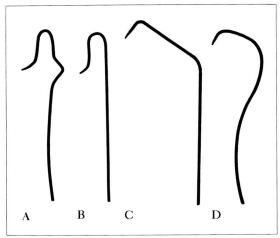

Fig. 19-1. Different catheter shapes used for catheterizing intercostal and bronchial arteries. From left to right: Mikaelsson curve; Simmons I, or Chuang reversed curve catheter shapes; double curved catheter with a tapered tip "cobra" curve.

diastinal pleural reflections, pulmonary ligaments, and the diaphragm.

Approach to Bronchial Bleeding
[5, 6, 8, 10]

Almost all bronchial bleeding is from erosion of systemic rather than pulmonary arteries. The two exceptions are patients bleeding from pulmonary

Fig. 19-2. Bronchial anatomy (see text).

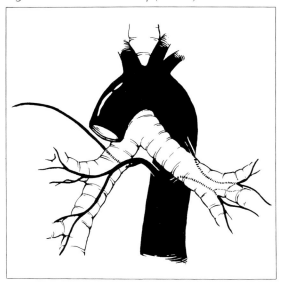

AVMs and those with pulmonary artery aneurysms. The latter are usually Rasmussen aneurysms, which are found in some patients with tuberculous cavities [7].

Patients are candidates for angiography and palliation by embolization only when hemorrhage is massive (over 600 ml per 24 hours, or less if repeated on successive days) and there are contraindications to surgery. Those with mild intermittent bleeding usually respond to supportive therapy with bed rest, sedation, and postural drainage. There is a high mortality in patients with massive hemorrhage who are left untreated, for they die not so much from shock due to blood loss as from asphyxiation. A chest x ray, followed by bronchoscopy to determine the site of bleeding, identifies the bleeding bronchus. At this time, a special two-lumen tube (one with an occluding balloon and the other for aeration) may be introduced by an anesthesiologist into the bronchus in an attempt to control the hemorrhage and prevent the escape of blood into other bronchi. With ventilatory support and replacement of blood volume, the patient should immediately undergo surgical resection.

Contraindications to surgery include inability to localize the side of bleeding; bleeding from both lungs; advanced pulmonary disease with poor pulmonary function studies; a nonresectable malignancy; recurrent postoperative bleeding; and refusal of surgery.

PROCEDURE

Approach the study anticipating an embolization procedure. Be aware from which side the bleeding is arising. Introduce and anchor a short 5 French sheath into the femoral artery. A hemostasis valve and sidearm allows constant infusion to prevent clot from forming around the catheter within the sheath. Rapid exchanges are possible through the sheath if the catheter becomes inadvertently occluded with embolic material. Advance the Mikaelsson, or reversed curved catheter to the aortic arch and manipulate its tip to face caudad (Fig. 19-4). A preliminary aortogram should be avoided for it is time consuming, adds unnecessary contrast medium to the study, and provides little helpful information. Concentrate on the T5 to T6 levels, with the catheter tip facing either directly anterior or slightly to the right. Make small, 1-ml test injections each time the catheter tip hesitates and becomes locked into a vessel orifice. When an

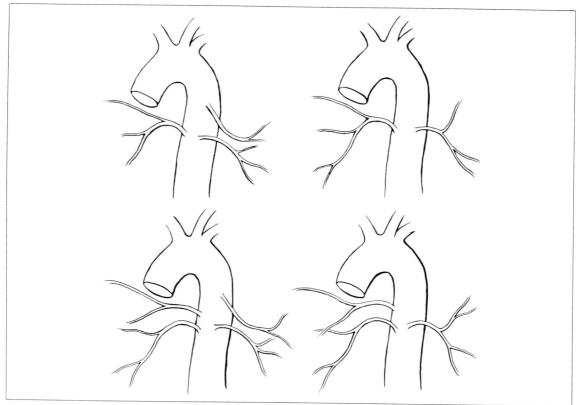

Fig. 19-3. The most frequent combinations of bronchial arteries as they arise from the ventral aspect of the thoracic aorta.

Fig. 19-4. Catheter manipulations for catheterizing bronchial and intercostal arteries using a Mikaelsson curve.

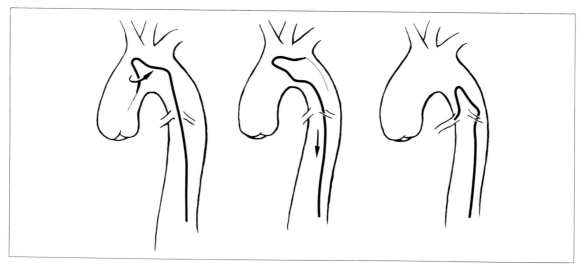

aortic branch is entered, determine whether it is a right or left bronchial artery, or a trunk common to both sides, or an intercostal artery. Document and record precisely the location of each vessel orifice for future entries. Determine the relative size of the vascular bed, for this dictates the amount of contrast required for the diagnostic study. For a normal intercostal artery, only 1 or 2 ml of contrast medium is necessary, with IA-DSA or 105-mm spot films used for documentation. If a large hypertrophied bronchial or intercostal feeder is entered, 5 to 10 ml is administered by hand injection, with serial films giving optimal detail. Check carefully for any anastomoses to the anterior spinal artery (Chap. 16) or other essential vessels; this may require digital subtraction views.

ANGIOGRAPHIC FINDINGS

Important angiographic findings suggesting a bleeding site include hyperplasia of vessels with hypervascularity, aneurysmal dilatation, a vascular hyperemic stain and focal areas of shunting into the bronchial and pulmonary veins, and some-

times even shunting into the pulmonary arteries (bronchopulmonary anastomoses) (Figs. 19-5, 19-6, 19-7) (see Fig. 17-21). Only rarely does one see extravasation of contrast medium into the bronchus. If these abnormal findings are present on the side predetermined by bronchoscopy and chest x ray, and feeders to the spinal artery are not seen, do not displace your catheter but instead prepare to embolize the vessel.

EMBOLIZATION

A number of particulate agents are available (see Chap. 5). We prefer microparticles of Ivalon (240

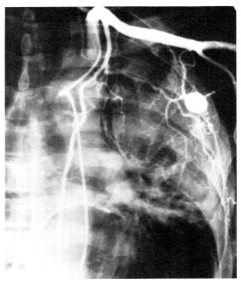

B

Fig. 19-5.
A. Left bronchial arteriogram demonstrates hypertrophied bronchial branches with vascular staining in the periphery of a large left upper lobe aspergilloma. A small branch supplies the right upper lobe.
B. Left subclavian arteriogram demonstrating hypertrophied systemic arteries supplying the lesion.
C. Postembolic arteriogram.

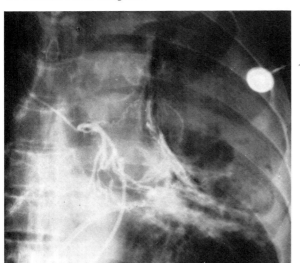

A

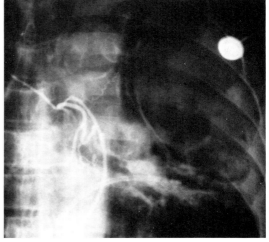

C

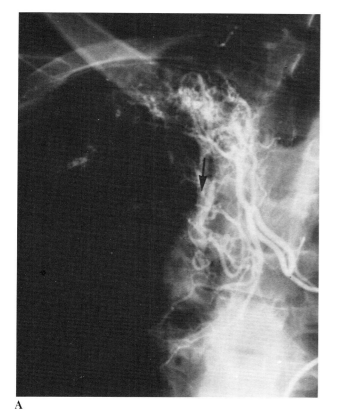

A

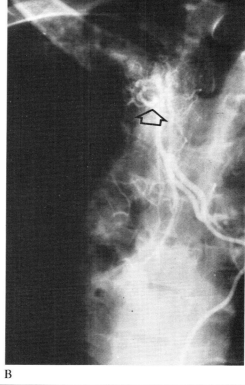

B

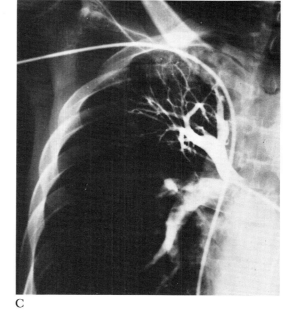

C

Fig. 19-6.
A. Right bronchial arteriogram demonstrating hypertrophied bronchial and highest intercostal branches with a vascular stain and arteriovenous shunting (*arrow*). There are no communications with the anterior spinal artery.
B. All hypertrophied branches on the right side are now occluded (*arrowhead*).
C. Normal pulmonary arteriogram.

to 500 μm). These are easily injected, inert, cause permanent occlusion, and are large enough that they do not penetrate into the capillary microcirculation. Isobutylcyanoacrylate may also be used as the embolic agent [3], but, unless care is taken, its low viscosity may penetrate to the capillary or precapillary level with possible danger of bronchial necrosis. Absolute alcohol should be avoided for fear of causing bronchial infarction [4]. Materials that penetrate vessels smaller than 150 μm should not be used.

Following embolization of the vessel, exchange the catheter for a new one and search for additional bleeding sites. All adjacent potential feeding vessels should be studied. In the lower thorax, this

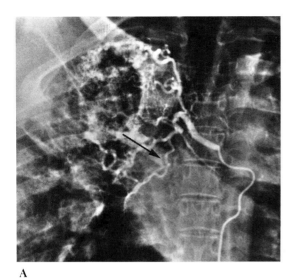

A

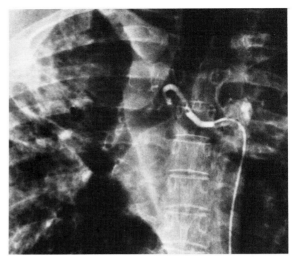

B

Fig. 19-7. Bronchiectasis and cavitation in right upper lobe.
A. Hypertrophied bronchial and intercostal arteries with arteriovenous shunting.
B. Postembolization.

includes the inferior phrenic artery; in the apex, it includes branches of the subclavian artery, particularly the costocervical trunk and lateral thoracic branch [8, 9]. Often multiple branches demonstrate hyperemia, staining, and shunting, and require vascular occlusion. In some conditions (e.g., cystic fibrosis), bilateral embolization must be performed [2].

COMMENTS AND PRECAUTIONS
1. IA-DSA considerably expedites the procedure.
2. Avoid injecting branches supplying the spinal artery.
3. Avoid vascular spasm or dissection by using gentle catheter manipulations.
4. Wedge the catheter tip well into the vessel to avoid reflux of emboli into the general circulation.
5. A 3 French coaxial catheter through a 6.5 French standard or 5 French thin-walled catheter allows passage of 250-µm size particles. Superselective catheter placement may be possible.
6. Start with small emboli to obstruct the more peripheral bronchial branches, then occlude the proximal larger vessels with larger emboli. Do not overinject with emboli; instead, occlude only 75 to 80 percent of the vascular bed. Proceed and follow each small bolus of emboli with half-strength contrast agent to check for

the earliest signs of reflux or opening of dangerous collaterals. When embolization appears complete, exchange the catheter for a fresh one before making a postangiographic diagnostic follow-up angiogram. This precaution prevents inadvertent release into the circulation of hidden emboli trapped in the catheter assembly.

COMPLICATIONS
Complications include:

1. Transverse myelitis. This results from occlusion of bronchial branches to the anterior spinal artery [9]. This complication occurs only rarely after injecting the right bronchial artery. The branch to the anterior spinal artery does not arise from the left bronchial artery.
2. Inadvertent reflux of emboli causes ischemia of vessels to other viscera or the extremities.
3. Changes in vascular resistance due to occluded vessels open up anastomoses and scatter emboli to branches of the subclavian artery.
4. Dysphagia, substernal pain, and fever due to ischemia of mediastinal structures may last for several days [3]. Rarely, there is necrosis of the bronchus or bronchoesophageal fistula.

RESULTS

Embolization is only a palliative procedure, and the underlying disease is not treated by this means. Good results have been described by a number of authors [2, 3, 6, 8] in tuberculosis, bronchiectasis, lung abscess, bronchogenic carcinoma, and cystic fibrosis. Hemorrhage can be controlled initially in 85 to 90 percent of patients. Hemoptysis recurs in some patients, usually due to initially insignificant collateral vessels revascularizing chronic bronchopulmonary lesions. Patients with aspergillosis do not fare well, probably due to the numerous systemic sites of vascular supply [8].

References

1. Botenga, A. S. J. Selective bronchial and intercostal angiography. Baltimore: Williams & Wilkins, 1970.
2. Fellows, K. E., et al. Bronchial artery embolization in cystic fibrosis. Technique and long-term results. *J. Pediatr.* 95:959, 1979.
3. Grenier, P., et al. Bronchial artery occlusion for severe hemoptysis: Use of isobutyl-2-cyanoacrylate. *A.J.R.* 140:467, 1983.
4. Ivanick, M. J., et al. Infarction of the left main stem bronchus: A complication of bronchial artery embolization. *A.J.R.* 141:535, 1983.
5. Pinet, F., and Froment, J. C. Angiography and Embolization of Thoracic Systemic Arteries. In H. Abrams (ed.), *Abrams' Angiography: Vascular and Interventional Radiology* (3rd ed.). Boston: Little, Brown, 1983. Pp. 845–867.
6. Remy, J., et al. Treatment of hemoptysis by embolization of bronchial arteries. *Radiology* 122:33, 1977.
7. Remy, J., et al. Treatment of massive hemoptysis by occlusion of a Rasmussen aneurysm. *A.J.R.* 135:605, 1980.
8. Uflacker, R., et al. Management of massive hemoptysis by bronchial artery embolization. *Radiology* 146:627, 1983.
9. Vujic, I., et al. Angiography and therapeutic blockade in the control of hemoptysis: The importance of control of nonbronchial arteries. *Radiology* 143:19, 1982.
10. Wholy, M. H., et al. Bronchial artery embolization for massive hemoptysis. *J.A.M.A.* 236:2501, 1976.

V

Venography and Lymphography

Venography of the Extremities

Indications

1. Evaluation of venous obstruction (due to thrombosis, phlebitis, invasion by tumor, trauma, or extrinsic compression)
2. Determination of the patency of deep veins in patients with superficial varices and venous insufficiency
3. Evaluation of congenital abnormalities (venous malformations, anomalous positions, hypoplasia)
4. Evaluation of venous components of arteriovenous shunts created for dialysis (see Chap. 8)

Technique

LOWER EXTREMITY VENOGRAPHY

Lower extremity venography is best performed on a radiographic tilt table with Bucky fluoroscopic and spot-film capabilities [5, 12, 17, 26]. The veins of the leg being studied must not be compromised by artifacts induced by extrinsic pressure or muscle contraction. The leg should hang freely, with the patient standing on a box on the opposite leg in a 60-degree upright position (Fig. 20-1). In this position, hydrostatic pressure retains contrast agent within the superficial and deep veins for longer periods. Obtain preliminary films of the leg. A 21- or 22 gauge butterfly needle (with attached connecting tube and syringe) is introduced into a peripheral vein, preferably laterally, on the dorsum of the foot. A total of 150 to 175 ml of 30 to 43% standard contrast medium is drawn up in three or four 50-ml syringes. The lower osmolarity of the diluted contrast agent and also that of the newer nonionic contrast agents, decreases the discomfort and complications sometimes associated with venography. The newer nonionic contrast agents are known to cause less endothelial toxicity and fewer other complications [24].

To evaluate the veins of the foot, the initial 40 to 50 ml of contrast is injected with a tourniquet applied above the ankle and the foot in a slightly oblique projection, and a film is obtained with the x-ray tube centered just over this area (Fig. 20-2A). The tourniquet is then removed, and the remainder of the contrast medium is injected. The contrast column is evaluated fluoroscopically and with appropriate spot films. If one is available, use a remote control room capable of taking 17 × 14-in. film cassettes with two or three in one spot films. If this is not possible, overhead films are obtained in a standard fluoroscopic room. When approximately 100 ml of the injection has been completed, expose the 14 × 17-in. overhead films (Fig. 20-2B, C). These are first coned to the extremity below the knee in the anteroposterior and lateral projections. Subsequently, the patient is lowered to a 45-degree upright angle while the contrast agent is continuously injected, and an anteroposterior view of the knee area is obtained (Fig. 20-2D). By the time 150 ml of contrast agent is injected, the patient is lowered to a 20-degree upright angle for an exposure of the thigh (Fig. 20-2E). At this point, trap the contrast medium in the leg by compressing the femoral vein. A final single film centered over the pelvis and lower abdomen is exposed to outline the iliac vein and inferior vena cava. This is best accomplished during the injection of the final amount of contrast agent, with the patient in a horizontal position. Just before exposure, the femoral vein compression is released and the extremity is quickly elevated in order to obtain maximum venous filling (Fig. 20-2F).

The large volume of low-density contrast agent injected into an upright non-weight-bearing extremity unencumbered with artifacts of tourniquets and muscle contractions provides sufficient hydrostatic pressure to fill both the superficial and deep and muscular branches of the leg under most circumstances. Direct puncture of the femoral vein may be required if the iliac venous system is not adequately opacified (Fig. 20-3).

UPPER EXTREMITY VENOGRAPHY

For upper extremity venography, the patient lies supine, either on a long film changer or on a radiographic table with Bucky capabilities. A 19- or

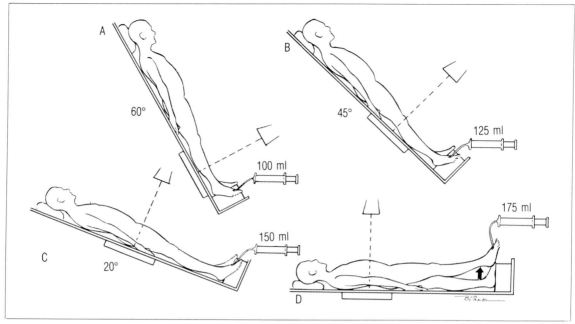

Fig. 20-1. Technique of lower extremity venography (see text for details).

21-gauge needle is placed in a peripheral vein on the dorsum of the hand, and 60 ml of low-density contrast agent is injected by hand. If the patient is supine, the radiographic filming is performed more rapidly than for lower extremity venograms, for here the slowing effect on the flow by the hydrostatic pressure of the upright position is not available. For better filling of the veins, the patient may be partially upright on a fluoroscopic x-ray table. Bucky films are obtained while the injection of contrast is continuing. Alternatively, if a long seriographic film changer is used, the films should be obtained every 5 or 6 seconds (see Fig. 8-4).

INTRAOSSEOUS VENOGRAPHY

Intraosseous venography is rarely needed and is seldom used. It is performed by injecting contrast agent through a trocar introduced directly through the cortex of the bone into the medullary space [20, 22]. The trocars are introduced into each of the greater trochanters in order to evaluate the pelvic veins, or into the lateral maleoli to evaluate the veins of the lower extremity. The procedure is painful, and general anesthesia is required. Aseptic techniques must be used, since the complication of osteomyelitis can occur. For examining the pelvic veins, 30 ml of low-density contrast agent is injected simultaneously into each of the two trocars at the rate of 6 to 10 ml per second, and

seriographic filming is performed, using 12 films exposed at a rate of 2 films per second for 3 seconds, then 1 film per second for 6 seconds.

Anatomic Considerations

LOWER EXTREMITY

The lower extremity is drained by superficial and deep venous systems (Fig. 20-2). These systems are connected by perforating branches, which flow from superficial to deep.

The veins of the foot consist of four venous systems which freely intercommunicate. There is a superficial venous system on the dorsum of the foot and one on its sole. There is a dorsal venous arch which receives drainage from the digital veins and, in turn, drains into the long and short saphenous veins of the leg. Finally there is a deep plantar venous arch which drains into the medial and lateral plantar veins which, in turn, enter into the deep veins (peroneal and tibial) of the leg.

The veins in the leg are smooth-walled vessels, often paired and with multiple valves, that follow the respective major arteries (the anterior and posterior tibial and peroneal arteries) to drain into the popliteal vein. The sural, or muscular, veins of the

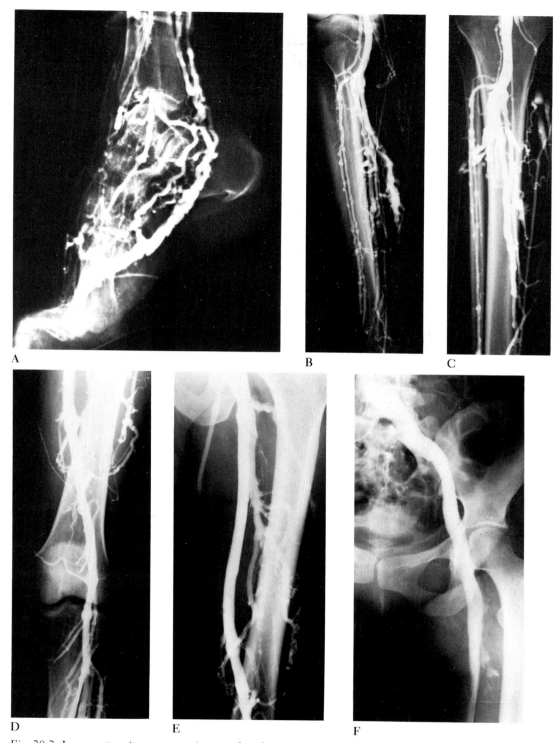

Fig. 20-2. Lower extremity venogram (a normal study). There are well-defined valves, and the walls of the veins are smooth. The soleal and gastrocnemius veins in the posterior calf muscles are well outlined. The profunda femorus vein is clearly seen in this study. Only the superior portion of the long saphenous vein is observed.

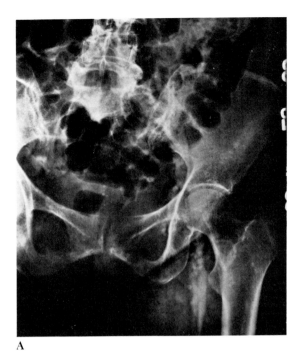

A

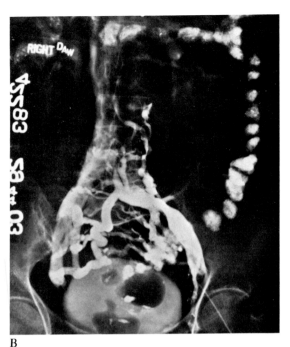

B

Fig. 20-3.
A. Inadequate opacification of the left iliac veins in a venogram performed in the routine fashion.
B. Direct left femoral venipuncture shows obstruction of left common iliac vein with large collaterals extending to the right side and subsequently to the inferior vena cava.

gastrocnemius and soleus muscles can be filled by angiographic techniques only if there is muscle relaxation during the contrast injection. They drain into the deep veins at the level of the popliteal vein. The popliteal vein also receives the posteriorly and superficially placed short saphenous vein and continues cephalad into the superficial femoral vein. The superficial femoral vein courses along beside the femoral artery to the inguinal ligament (where it lies just medial to the artery) to pass into the external iliac vein. Anomalously there may be two or more femoral veins, or the femoral vein may be replaced by a vein that accompanies the sciatic nerve. The deep femoral vein receives tributaries from the popliteal, inferior gluteal, and circumflex veins, and then joins the superficial femoral vein several centimeters below the inguinal ligament.

The superficial veins are comprised of a long and a short saphenous vein. The long saphenous vein lies along the medial foot, leg, and thigh. It begins in the foot, ascends in front of the medial malleolus, and eventually passes through the saphenous opening to join the superficial femoral vein below the groin. The short saphenous vein begins laterally in the foot, passes posteriorly in the leg, and eventually joins the popliteal vein at approximately the level of the knee joint.

Within the pelvis, in the absence of obstruction, only the external and common iliac veins are outlined by venography. The internal iliac veins, not being opacified, dilute the contrast column at their point of entry near the sacroiliac joint.

UPPER EXTREMITY
In the upper extremity (Fig. 20-4), veins from the dorsal venous network of the hand drain cephalad into two major superficial veins of the forearm: the basilic vein, lying medially, and the cephalic vein, lying laterally. An antecubital vein connects the two on the ventral surface of the elbow. The deep veins of the palm drain into the paired radial and ulnar veins (following the course of the radial and ulnar arteries), which join at the elbow. Here they form paired brachial veins, which follow the course of the brachial artery. The medially located basilic vein joins the brachial vein just before it becomes the axillary vein. The cephalic vein ascends laterally above and in front of the humerus

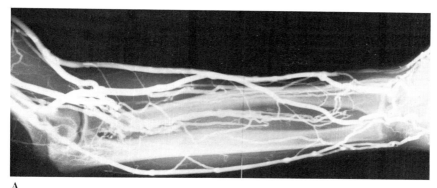

A

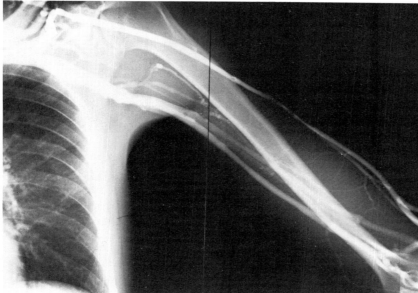

B

Fig. 20-4. Normal veins of the left upper extremity.
A. Forearm.
B. Upper arm.

Comments and Additional Technical Considerations

INTERPRETATION OF VENOGRAMS

Venous studies are difficult to interpret unless they are properly performed. Injection into a single vein causes a venous contrast column that can be diluted by blood from unopacified veins and produces artifacts due to flow defects (see Figs. 20-5,

to enter the axillary vein at a fairly acute angle. For purposes of catheterization of the right side of the heart, the basilic vein is the easiest to use because of its obtuse entry into the deep venous system.

20-6). Also, increased resistance in one system (or decreased resistance in the other) may divert flow with subsequent nonfilling of otherwise patent vessels. High-volume injections of diluted contrast agents, together with the hydrostatic pressure induced by the upright position, provide optimal filling of deep, superficial, and muscular veins of the leg with the least number of artifacts. If questions still arise, tourniquets may be applied at appropriate locations (above the ankle and/or above the knee) during repeat injections (Fig. 20-7).

TOURNIQUETS

Tourniquets may be applied at various levels of the leg to enhance the study. They should not be used routinely since their application may occlude deep

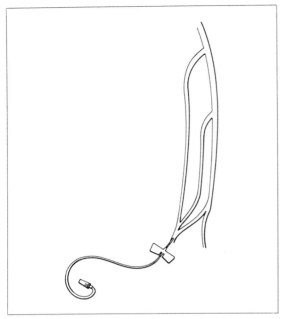

Fig. 20-5. Contrast injection into a peripheral vein provides room for artifacts. Unopacified veins drain into the contrast column causing dilution and flow defects. Increased resistance in one vein diverts flow into the other through communicating veins.

veins and thus introduce artifacts resulting from poor flow (see Fig. 20-6).

Tourniquets direct or force flow into the deep venous system and are used under the following conditions:

1. If the patient cannot be upright.
2. If the primary purpose of the study is to outline incompetent perforators and superficial varices. They are applied at the ankle, and the contrast medium is forced into the deep system. Any filling of superficial veins under these circumstances is accomplished by incompetent perforators (normally, perforating branches flow from superficial to deep), and their location can be recorded.
3. If resistance to the flow of contrast medium in a varicosed superficial system is lower than normal. In such cases, the preferential flow prevents adequate opacification of the deep system. A false impression of an occluded deep system can be prevented by forcing contrast agent into the deep system with the application of a tourniquet at the ankle. Sometimes it is necessary that the whole extremity be encased

in an ace bandage. It is only by seeing the deep veins that the cause for the diverted blood flow and increased resistance can be uncovered (see Fig. 20-10).
4. If there is incomplete filling of all the veins below the knee. Here a tourniquet may be applied above the ankle and/or below the knee in order to help retain the contrast medium and to direct its flow to the more deep and superficial veins.

LACK OF FILLING OF THE DEEP VEINS ABOVE THE KNEE

With the techniques described above, all the deep and superficial veins below the knee should fill if they are normal. If they do not, occlusive disease is assumed present (see Fig. 20-10). This is not true, however, of the deep veins above the knee. Approximately 50 percent of profunda femoris veins and the vast majority of internal iliac veins do not fill.

STUDY OF OCCLUSION

If venous occlusion is seen in the femoral vein on either side, try to determine if the disease extends to the iliac veins or to the inferior vena cava (see Fig. 20-3). If iliac venous occlusion and collaterals are seen on one side only, the inferior vena cava should be studied from the contralateral side. If iliac occlusion is seen bilaterally, the superior extension of the disease can be determined by one of two approaches:

1. Very gently pass a catheter retrograde starting from the antecubital vein and continuing through the superior vena cava and right atrium and down the inferior vena cava. This procedure is approached cautiously if a fresh thrombus is anticipated, for fear of embolization. The catheter tip should be placed near the iliac veins, and 10 to 20 ml of contrast agent injected per second, for a total of 40 to 50 ml (depending on the extent of occlusion). Digital subtraction studies require less contrast agent (see Chap. 21; Fig. 21-24).
2. Intraosseous venography, with trocars in each greater trochanter. This procedure is rarely performed, since it is painful and requires general anesthesia, and complicating osteomyelitis can occur.

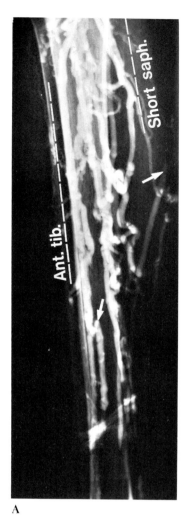
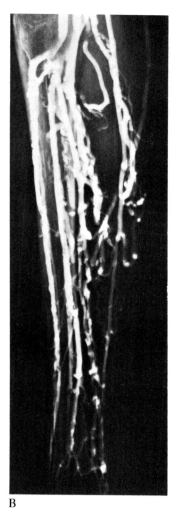

A   B

Fig. 20-6.
A. Venogram with tourniquet applied. There is nonfilling of portions of the short saphenous vein, and
   of the anterior tibial vein. Other deep veins fill by
   communicating channels.
B. Repeat study 10 minutes later without tourniquets
   shows all veins filling normally.

TECHNIQUES IN PATIENTS
WITH EDEMA

In patients with an edema of acute or subacute
nature, the superficial veins may be hidden and
may be difficult to locate for venipuncture. Generally, these veins are dilated and may be found if
the leg is placed in a dependent position and the
edematous subcutaneous fluid is digitally compressed away from the veins. The application of
warm compresses, tourniquets, nitroglycerine
patches, and the dependent position enhance ve-

nous filling. A modified retrograde study is sometimes successful under these circumstances [8]
(Fig. 20-8). With the legs dependent and the blood
pressure cuff applied above the knee, a dilated vein
in the calf of the leg may be cannulated and taped
in place. The cuff is removed and the patient is
positioned upright and non-weight-bearing, and
routine high-volume venography is performed.

CLOSED SYSTEM VENOGRAPHY IN
PATIENTS WITH ANGIODYSPLASIAS

Angiodysplasias are vascular abnormalities that
may occur at the arterial, capillary, or venous level
of the circulation (see Chap. 8). The larger arteriovenous malformations are best studied by direct
arteriography. Those lesions at the capillary and
venous levels (capillary, cavernous, and venous
hemangiomas) are often difficult to outline by

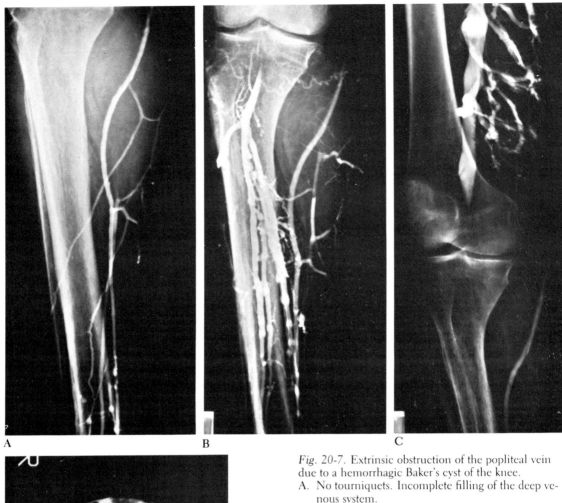

A   B   C

Fig. 20-7. Extrinsic obstruction of the popliteal vein due to a hemorrhagic Baker's cyst of the knee.
A. No tourniquets. Incomplete filling of the deep venous system.
B. Tourniquets applied. Deep veins of the calf are widely patent, but there is obstruction of the popliteal vein due to extrinsic compression at popliteal fossa.
C. Tapered reconstitution of popliteal vein above the knee.
D. Computed tomography scan shows large Baker's cyst, which was hemorrhagic at percutaneous puncture.

D

standard arteriography and venography. The full extent of the lesion can be demonstrated by "closed system" venography [4]. A peripheral vein is cannulated at the outset of the procedure. A blood pressure cuff, inflated well above systemic systolic pressures, is placed proximal to the lesion, and the entire limb is tightly wrapped with a rubberized Esmarch bandage. By keeping the blood pressure cuff inflated, but now removing the bandage, the

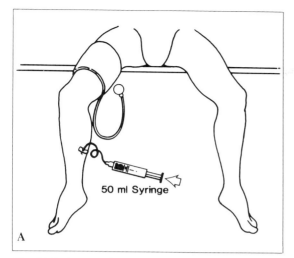

Fig. 20-8. Retrograde injection of contrast agent.
A. Apply blood pressure cuff above the knee, with patient's legs dependent. After cannulation of the calf vein, remove the cuff and inject contrast agent.
B. Extensive thrombosis in a patient with no superficial veins of the dorsum of the foot. Needle low and lateral in the midcalf.

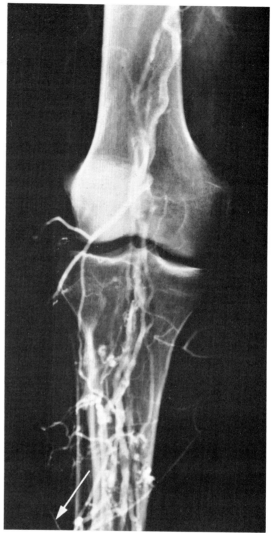

B

limb is converted to a "closed vascular system." By injecting 75 to 100 ml of dilute contrast medium into the previously cannulated vein, the full extent of the lesion can be clearly defined (Fig. 20-9).

RETROGRADE VENOGRAPHY
Venous insufficiency of the lower extremities is often due to incompetence of venous valves of the iliac region down to and below the popliteal area. The competence of these valves may be studied by retrograde venography. A catheter injection of 25 to 30 ml of contrast medium in the iliac vessels with the patient semiupright is evaluated fluoroscopically and with films. The catheter may have to be passed from the opposite femoral vein across the confluens of the common iliac veins. There is grade I incompetence if the contrast column passes retrograde and just below the inguinal ligament, grade II if to the midthigh, grade III if to a level at the knee, and grade IV if to a level below the knee.

PITFALLS
Pitfalls of venography of the extremities include the following:

1. Ankle tourniquets often occlude superficial and deep veins of the leg, particularly the anterior tibial vein (see Fig. 20-6).
2. Weight bearing prevents filling of muscular veins of the calf due to muscle contraction.
3. Needle placement too proximal in the foot sometimes causes the contrast medium to bypass the deep plantar veins (which eventually drain into the posterior tibial veins) and may produce artifacts simulating occlusion. Needle placement in the long saphenous circulation causes preferential flow to the superficial veins and prevents adequate deep venous filling.
4. Never assume a diagnosis on a suboptimally

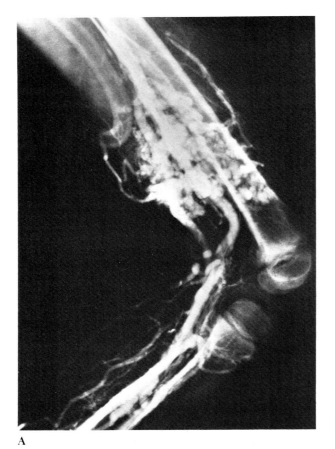

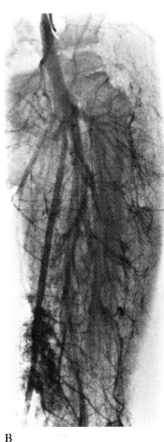

A   B

Fig. 20-9. Venous hemangioma in a 4-year-old boy.
A. Studied by "closed system" venography. Large venous and capillary hemangioma in distal thigh.
B. Late films on an intraarterial injection (following 15 mg tolazoline). Collection of abnormal venous structures observed in the thigh (better demonstrated by venography).

visualized vein. Try to see the site and nature of the occlusion (within limits of contrast tolerance) (Figs. 20-7, 20-10).

Complications of Venography

Various complications of venography of the extremities may occur. Mild discomfort to severe pain is sometimes felt during the injection, and this is usually worse if there are thrombosed veins present. The contrast medium is toxic to venous endothelium [1, 7, 13, 18] and can cause exacerbation of the symptoms in a patient with thrombophlebitis. In addition, phlebitis may occur at the puncture site or along the course of veins. This appears to be directly related to the osmolarity of the agent, and therefore the more dilute or nonionic agents should be employed. Also, the contrast agent should be thoroughly flushed from the

venous system as soon as the last x-ray film has been taken with at least 50 to 100 ml of 5% dextrose solution. The incidence of these problems may be reduced by adding 1000 to 2000 IU of heparin to the 100 ml of solution [2, 3]. Occasionally, an intense subcutaneous reflex arterial vasospasm occurs at the site of injection, accompanied by blanching of the skin and followed by a bullous discolored eruption. Eventually the skin will slough. This reaction is more likely to occur when contrast medium is extravasated, but it is also seen when the injection is entirely intravascular. Vasovagal and allergic reactions may occur.

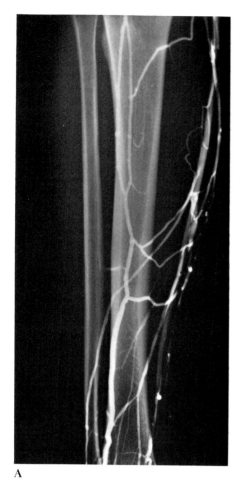
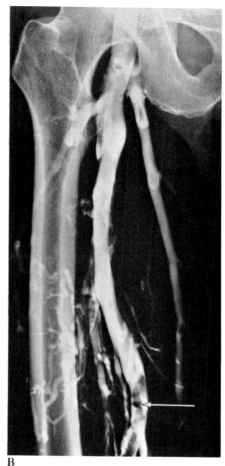

A   B

Fig. 20-10.
A. Nonfilling of deep veins below the knee. No tourniquets applied.
B. Fresh thrombus in proximal popliteal vein and distal superficial femoral vein (*arrow*). No tourniquets required.

Angiographic Findings

VENOUS THROMBOSIS

Phlebothrombosis usually starts by adherence of platelets to the venous endothelium, usually in the apex of venous valves [14, 17, 23, 25]. The addition of fibrin to these platelet aggregates forms the "white thrombus," and eventual entrapment of red cells produces the red thrombus. Recent thrombus appears as a radiolucent defect within an opacified vein outlined by a thin white line of contrast medium (Figs. 20-10, 20-11, 20-12), whereas with older thrombi the white line is thicker due to refraction. It may be obliterated by adherence of thrombus to the vein wall. The process may progress to complete occlusion. Filling defects due to clots must not be confused with the inconstant defects caused by inflow of unopacified blood. The thrombus may completely obstruct and organize, in which case the vein does not fill and drainage occurs through collaterals (Fig. 20-12A). The angiographer should try to demonstrate the actual point of obstruction in order to preclude misdiagnosis due to artifact. With healing, the thrombus retracts toward the wall of the vein, and the contrast column becomes narrow and irregular. Linear defects paralleling the vein wall or transverse webs may be seen; they represent fibrous, strand-like thrombus remnants. With recanalization, the appearance is one of irregular narrowed veins with no detectable valves (Fig. 20-13).

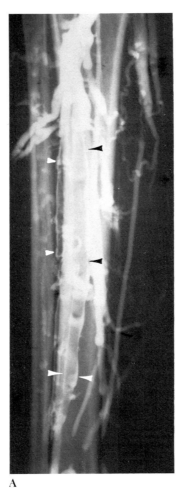

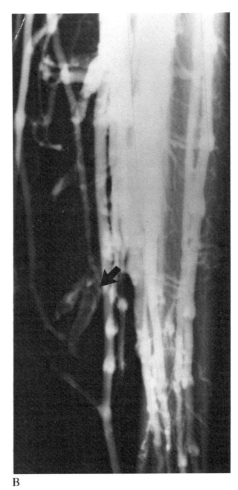

A   B

Fig. 20-11.
A. Fresh thrombus lying within the peroneal veins. A
   large filling defect bordered by thin white lines of
   contrast medium is evident (*arrowheads*).
B. Early acute thrombus in muscular veins.

VARICES

Varicosed veins are abnormally dilated, elongated,
and tortuous (Fig. 20-14). In the systemic circulation they are almost always confined to the lower
extremities. Exceptions occur in other parts of the
body when veins are obstructed (e.g., by tumor or
infection) or are involved in arteriovenous malformations or fistulas or in venous dysplasias of the
limbs (Figs. 20-15, 20-16; see also Fig. 20-9) [21].
Lower extremity varices that occur spontaneously
are caused by an inherent weakness in the venous
structural components. Venous dilatation and inadequate coadaptation of valves enhance venous
insufficiency and cause the veins to become more
dilated and tortuous. Incompetent perforating
veins allow retrograde flow from the deep to the
superficial veins, which in turn become overloaded, dilated, and tortuous. These changes are

easily demonstrated in venography by placing a
tourniquet above the ankle; normally the superficial system should not fill under these circumstances.

Superficial varices may occur secondary to deep
venous obstruction. They act as collaterals and enlarge to accommodate the increased flow. When
the deep vein obstruction is acute and extensive,
the venous collaterals are small and inadequate,
and this condition is accompanied by peripheral
edema. When the obstruction is chronic, venography shows varying degrees of deep vein recanalization and destruction of venous valves in addition

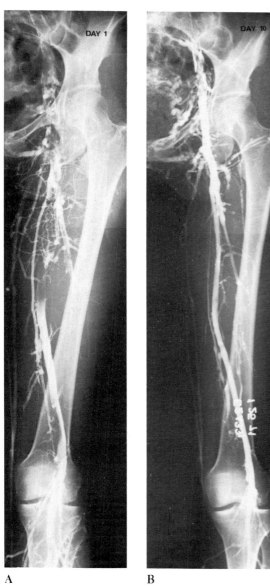

A **B**

Fig. 20-12. Extensive thrombosis of the left iliac, femoral, and popliteal veins, resolving partially with anticoagulant therapy.

A. Acute thrombosis.

B. Film taken after 10 days of therapy. Obstruction to the common iliac veins persists, and large collaterals have developed.

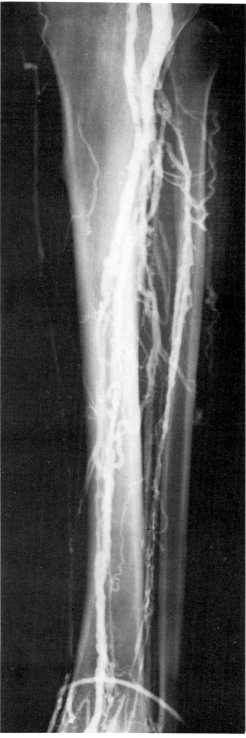

Fig. 20-13. Chronic changes of phlebitis. There are no valves present, and the walls of the veins are irregular. The linear filling defects represent strand-like thrombus remnants.

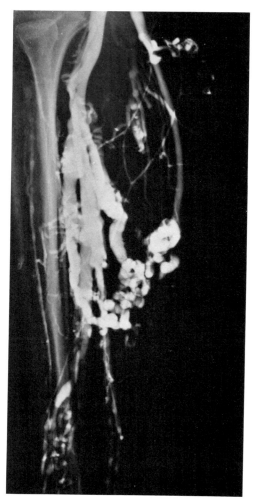

Fig. 20-14. Superficial and deep varicosed veins. Dilated deep veins with incompetent valves and perforators.

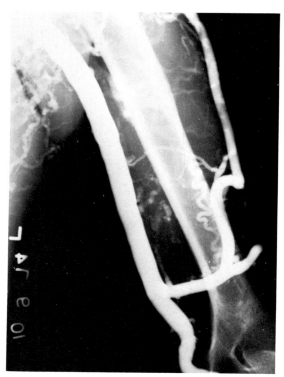

Fig. 20-15. Venous dysplasia of the left arm, showing grossly dilated, tortuous veins in a young patient with large systemic varices of the left upper extremity and thorax. No obstruction or arterial abnormality was present.

to the varices. It is important to show the surgeon the extent of deep vein involvement as well as the capacity of these veins to drain the lower extremity. The superficial varices that are demonstrated may be the only channels available for venous drainage; under these circumstances they should not be excised.

SWELLING OF THE EXTREMITIES
Swelling of the extremities may be caused by extrinsic compression of the veins by tumors (Fig.

Fig. 20-16. Multiple venous "aneurysms" of the hand in an asymptomatic child. (Courtesy of Dr. Phillip Howerton, Morganton, NC.)

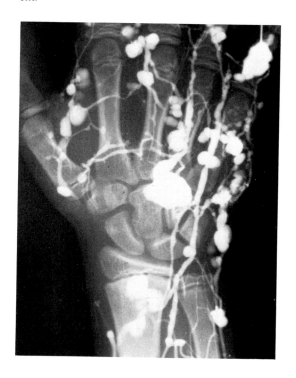

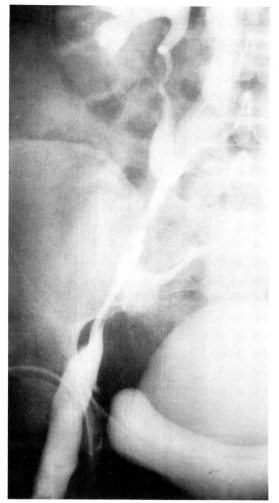

Fig. 20-17. Extrinsic compression of the right iliac veins by metastatic disease. There is also involvement of the distal right ureter.

20-17), cysts (see Fig. 20-7), aneurysms, or sometimes by adjacent muscles and bones (Fig. 20-18). It may be caused by acute or chronic changes subsequent to trauma [6]. Venous disruption or extrinsic compression often progresses to cause complete thrombosis of the involved segment of the vein.

Alternative Methods of Study

There are other methods of evaluating the venous system [9, 10, 15], which include Doppler ultrasonography [19], impedance phlebography [10,

15, 28], radioisotope techniques [7, 11, 27], and thermography [16].

IODINE 125 FIBRINOGEN VENOUS STUDIES

With this method, fibrinogen labelled with ^{125}I is injected into the bloodstream and is incorporated into the developing clot [1]. Increasing radioactivity due to the trapped fibrinogen is subsequently measured. To prevent uptake of the radioactive iodine by the thyroid, 100 mg of sodium iodide is introduced an hour before the study. Subsequently, 100 mCi of fibrinogen ^{125}I is injected, and counts are obtained at various levels along the extremities 4 hours following the injection and at 24-hour intervals for 3 days. These counts are compared with those of comparable areas on the opposite extremity and also with the background level counted over the precordium. Sustained areas of increased uptake signal the presence of phlebothrombosis. The advantages of this study are that it is a simple noninvasive test that is accurate below the knee and it allows serial studies to be performed. It is nonspecific, however, for increased levels of fibrinogen can be seen in conditions such as cellulitis or trauma. Also, the method is unable to detect clots above the thigh. Fully formed thrombus does not incorporate additional fibrinogen.

RADIONUCLIDE VENOGRAPHY

Radionuclide venography can be performed by injecting technetium 99m macroaggregates or technetium 99m pertechnetate [27]. With the patient supine and tourniquets placed above the ankles and below the knees, 2.5 mCi of the radionuclide is injected into a dorsal foot vein and is flushed with 20 to 30 ml of saline. Images are obtained of the calf, thighs, and pelvis, and repeat images are obtained after the tourniquet has been removed and also after exercise. Stagnation with increased radioactivity and collateral flow may be seen with occlusive disease. Similar techniques may be employed in the upper extremity (Fig. 20-19). Images of the lungs may also be obtained subsequently to determine the presence of pulmonary emboli. Although this study does not give fine anatomic detail, it is helpful in evaluating the venous system in patients who may be allergic to standard contrast agents.

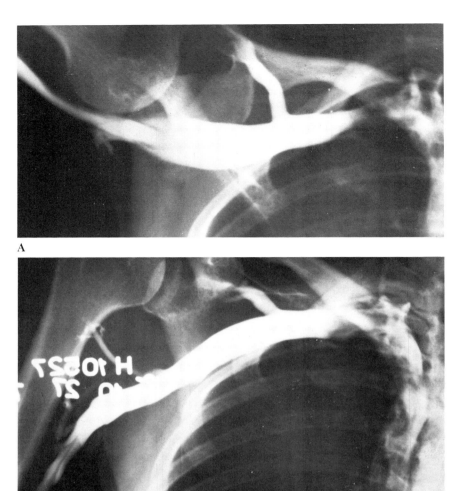

A

B

Fig. 20-18. Extrinsic compression of the right subclavian vein at the costoclavicular junction on stress maneuver in a symptomatic patient who was an active
swimmer. The patient's arm swelled following exertion.

A. Hyperabduction, showing narrowing of the subclavian vein.
B. Neutral position, showing normal caliber. There is
retrograde flow through the cephalic vein as it enters the axillary vein.

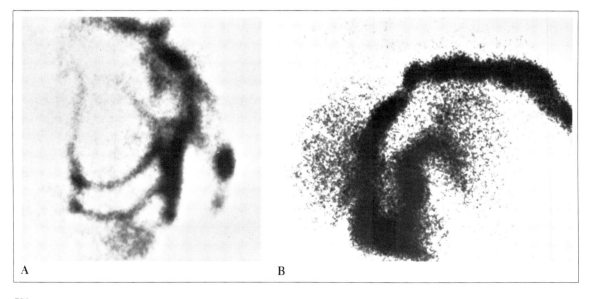

A   B

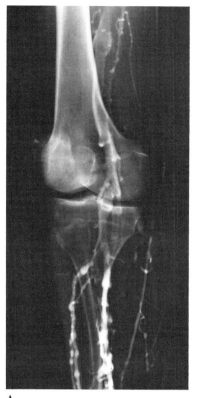
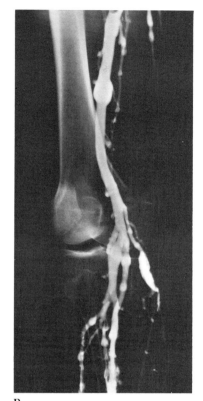

A   B

Fig. 20-20.
A. Acute thrombosis of popliteal vein.
B. Three days after systemic urokinase therapy. Venous system widely patent.

Fig. 20-19. Radionuclide venography using technetium 99m pertechnetate.
A. Thrombosis of left innominate and proximal subclavian vein with multiple collaterals.
B. Four days after streptokinase therapy. Venous system is now open with probable stenosis of left proximal innominate vein.

Interventional Techniques

THROMBOLYSIS

Selective low-dose thrombolytic treatment (using either streptokinase or urokinase) may be helpful when there are focal areas of involvement and the administered thrombolytic agent will not be drained away into uninvolved areas by collateral circulation. Standard methods of anticoagulation or systemic doses of thrombolytic therapy should be considered for more diffuse or extensive venous thrombosis, or thrombosis of the extremities (Fig. 20-20).

VASCULAR DILATION

Vascular dilation is sometimes successful in stenosed anastomotic sites of surgically created arteriovenous fistulas (see Chap. 8).

References

1. Albrechtsson, U., and Olsson, C. J. Thrombosis after phlebography: A comparison of two contrast media. *Cardiovasc. Radiol.* 2:9, 1979.

2. Arndt, R. D., et al. The heparin flush: An aid in preventing post venography thrombophlebitis. *Radiology* 130:249, 1979.

3. Bettmann, M. A., et al. Reduction of venous thrombosis complicating phlebography. *A.J.R.* 134:1169, 1980.

4. Braun, S., et al. Closed system venography in the evaluation of angiodysplastic lesions of the extremities. *A.J.R.* 141:1307, 1983.

5. Coel, M. N. Adequacy of lower limb venous opacification: Comparison of supine and upright phlebography. *A.J.R.* 134:163, 1980.

6. Gerlock, A., Jr., Thal, E., and Synder, W. Venography in penetrating injuries of the extremities. *Am. J. Roentgenol.* 126:1023, 1976.

7. Gomes, A. S., Webber, M. M., and Buffkin, D. Contrast venography versus radionuclide venography: A study of discrepancies and their possible significance. *Radiology* 142:719, 1982.

8. Gordon, D. H., et al. Descending varicose venography of the lower extremities. An alternate method to evaluate the deep venous system. *Radiology* 145:832, 1982.

9. Holden, R. W., et al. Efficacy of noninvasive modalities for diagnosis of thrombophlebitis. *Radiology* 141:63, 1981.

10. Hull, R., et al. Combined use of leg scanning and impedance plethysmography in suspected venous thrombosis. An alternative to venography. *N. Engl. J. Med.* 299:497, 1977.

11. Kakkar, V. Radioisotope techniques: The diagnosis of deep vein thrombosis using I125 fibrinogen tests. *Arch. Surg.* 104:152, 1972.

12. Kirschner, L., et al. Drip infusion venography. *Radiology* 96:413, 1970.

13. Laerum, F., and Holm, H. Postphlebographic thrombosis. A double blind study with methylglucamine metrizoate and metrizamide. *Radiology* 140:651, 1981.

14. Lipchick, E., DeWeese, J., and Rogoff, S. Serial long term phlebography after documented lower leg thrombosis. *Radiology* 120:563, 1976.

15. Moser, K. M., Brach, B., and Dolan, G. F. Clinically suspected deep venous thrombosis of the lower extremities. A comparison of venography, impedance plethysmography, and radiolabeled fibrinogen. *J.A.M.A.* 237:2195, 1977.

16. Pochakzevsky, R., Pillari, G., and Feldman, F. Liquid crystal contact thermography of deep venous thrombosis. *A.J.R.* 138:717, 1982.

17. Rabinov, K., and Pavlin, S. Roentgen diagnosis of venous thrombosis in the leg. *Arch. Surg.* 104:134, 1972.

18. Ritchie, W., Lynch, P., and Stewart, G. The effect of contrast media on normal and inflamed canine veins: A scanning and transmission electron microscopic study. *Invest. Radiol.* 9:44, 1974.

19. Sigel, B., et al. Diagnosis of lower limb venous thrombosis by Doppler ultrasound technique. *Arch. Surg.* 104:174, 1982.

20. Thomas, L. An improved intraosseous phlebography cannula. *Br. J. Radiol.* 42:395, 1969.

21. Thomas, L., and Andress, M. Angiography in venous dysplasias of the limbs. *Am. J. Roentgenol.* 113:722, 1971.

22. Thomas, L., and Fletcher, E. The techniques of pelvic phlebography. *Clin. Radiol.* 18:399, 1967.

23. Thomas, L., and MacAllister, V. The radiological progression of deep venous thrombus. *Radiology* 99:37, 1971.

24. Thomas, M. L., and Briggs, G. M. Comparison of triiodoisophthalidamide with meglumine iothalomate in phlebography of the leg. *A.J.R.* 138:725, 1982.

25. Thomas, M. L., and O'Dwyer, J. A. A phlebographic study of the incidence and significance of venous thrombosis in the foot. *A.J.R.* 130:751, 1978.

26. Tisnado, J., et al. An alternate technique for lower extremity venography. *Radiology* 133:787, 1979.

27. Webber, M., et al. Thrombosis detection by radionuclide particle (MAA) entrapment: Correlation with fibrinogen uptake and venography. *Radiology* 111:645, 1974.

28. Wheeler, H., Pearson, D., and O'Connel, D. Impedance phlebography: Technique, interpretation, and results. *Arch. Surg.* 104:164, 1972.

Inferior Venacavography, Abdominal Systemic Venography, and Interventional Procedures

Indications

1. Intrinsic obstruction due to thrombosis, phlebitis, webs, primary tumor (myxomas, leiomyomas, leiomyosarcomas, endotheliomas), or secondary tumor (e.g., hypernephromas, bowel carcinoma)
2. Extrinsic obstruction due to compression, deviation due to tumor, aortic aneurysm, retroperitoneal disease, herniated disk
3. Evaluation for obstruction of the venous outflow of abdominal viscera (renal vein thrombosis, hepatic vein thrombosis [Budd-Chiari syndrome], patency of portosystemic shunts)
4. Demonstration of congenital abnormalities
   a. Congenital variations in the inferior vena cava, with or without associated cardiac abnormalities (e.g., azygous continuation of the inferior vena cava)
   b. Evaluation for retrocaval ureter
   c. Congenital abnormalities of the renal veins
5. Biochemical analysis of selective venous effluent (adrenals, renal veins, gonadal veins, hepatic vein)
6. Intravenous interventional methods
   a. Inferior vena cava filter placement
   b. Testicular venous blockade for infertility due to varicocele
   c. Percutaneous transluminal angioplasty or thrombolysis for amenable venous stenoses and occlusions (portosystemic venous anastomosis, Budd-Chiari syndrome)

The images produced by ultrasonography, computed tomography, and nuclear magnetic resonance often provide sufficient detail regarding intrinsic and extrinsic abnormalities of the inferior vena cava, renal veins, the central hepatic veins, and the epidural venous plexus to obviate the need for direct vascular studies [17, 29].

Technique

APPROACHES

1. If the femoral and iliac veins are patent, the preferred approach is a percutaneous introduction of a needle sleeve into each femoral vein. If a unilateral approach is used, a catheter with multiple side holes is placed at the origin of the inferior vena cava.
2. If both femoral veins are occluded, the catheter should be passed gently retrograde from the antecubital vein, traversing the superior vena cava and right atrium, and down the inferior vena cava to the level of the iliac bifurcation. The angiographer should beware of dislodging fresh thrombus or tumor.
3. These same approaches, with the appropriate catheter shape, may be used to catheterize the hepatic and renal veins. In general, the hepatic vein is easier to catheterize from an approach above the diaphragm, and the renal veins are easier from the femoral vein approach (Fig. 21-1). The testicular veins can be approached from either femoral or jugular (internal or external) veins. The jugular venous approach [8] seems to provide greater ease in both entering the orifice and advancing the catheter down the length of both the left gonadal vein (as it enters the inferior aspect of the left renal) and the right gonadal vein, which enters the inferior vena cava at an acute angle anterolaterally just below the right renal vein (Fig. 21-2A). The left gonadal vein is easily catheterized from the femoral vein, but the right gonadal vein is more difficult to catheterize from this approach (Fig. 21-2B).

Catheterization of the adrenal veins is covered in Chapter 12. The epidural veins are approached from the femoral veins (Fig. 21-3).

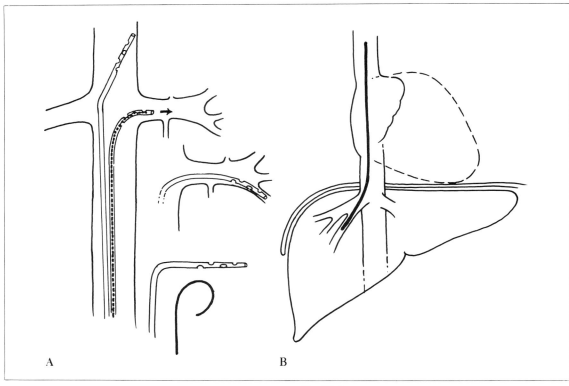

Fig. 21-1.
A. Catheter approach to renal venography.
B. Catheter approach to hepatic venography.

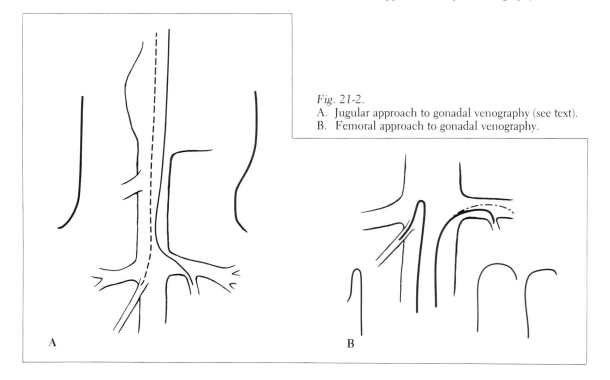

Fig. 21-2.
A. Jugular approach to gonadal venography (see text).
B. Femoral approach to gonadal venography.

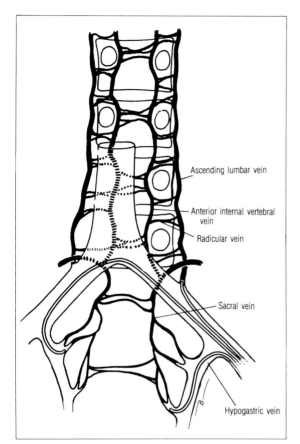

Fig. 21-3. Line drawing of the anatomy of the epidural veins. The catheter may be placed in the ascending lumbar vein or in a sacral vein on either side (see text).

CATHETERS

1. To catheterize the inferior vena cava, 4-in. long 5 French needle sleeves are used, one in each femoral vein. Alternately, advance a single 5 French 60-cm straight end-hole thin-walled catheter with multiple side holes or a "pigtail" catheter configuration to the origin of the inferior vena cava above the iliac venous confluens and approach the vein from below. If the vein is approached from above, a 90-cm 5 French pigtail catheter or an end-hole catheter with multiple side holes is used. A guidewire protruding just beyond the catheter tip presents a gentle curve at the catheter tip, which facilitates manipulation from the right atrium into the inferior vena cava. A selective catheter with a gentle curve of its tip and with two distal side holes can be passed into the hepatic vein, or into either renal vein.

2. To catheterize the renal vein (for purposes of renal venography) from the femoral approach, a 60-cm 5 or 6 French end-hole catheter with multiple side holes and a sharp right-angle curve approximately 6 cm proximal to the tip should be used (see Fig. 21-1). An external deflector or a sharp curve applied to the stiff end of a guidewire must be inserted to deform the catheter tip sufficiently so that it will enter the renal vein orifice. From this point, the catheter can be "paid out" deep into the renal vein. A "cobra" curve or simple right-angle curved catheter can be used when catheterizing for obtaining renal vein blood specimens. Side holes at the catheter tip assure prompt venous return on suctioning.

3. For catheterizing the gonadal veins from the jugular approach, a 5 or 6.5 French torque-controlled catheter with a Hincks I "head hunter" curve tip (Chap. 14) or one with a gentle curve to its distal tip engages the orifice of either the right or left gonadal vein (see Fig. 21-2A). It is advanced down the length of the gonadal vein over a guidewire once venography has been performed. For the femoral approach, differently shaped catheters are required. The left gonadal vein is entered with a modified "cobra" curve or a wide U-shaped curve (see Fig. 21-2B) to engage its orifice. The right renal vein requires a Simmons I or II curve (Chap. 14) to accommodate its sharp angulation from the inferior vena cava.

4. The hepatic veins can easily be catheterized from above with a catheter with a gentle curve to its tip. It may be catheterized from the femoral approach with a 60-cm 5 or 6 French end-hole catheter with a "cobra" curve. A flexible straight 6 French woven Dacron or polyethylene catheter may be advanced over a deflecting wire deep into the hepatic vein. If hepatic wedge pressures are being measured, the catheter should have no side holes. No. 7 or 8 French occlusive balloon catheters may be used in the hepatic veins. These are inflated to the diameter of the major draining hepatic vein immediately before the injection of contrast agent, allowing optimal opacification of the intrahepatic venous radicals. They are also useful for measuring intrahepatic venous wedge pressures.

5. For epidural venograms, a 5 French catheter

with a short "hockey stick" curve at its distal end can be used to pass easily into an ascending lumbar vein as it arises from the posterolateral surface of the common iliac vein. The catheter can be modified by the addition of a second, more proximal curve so that it can enter into the hypogastric vein on either side, and subsequently wedge into a lateral sacral vein (Fig. 21-3).

CONTRAST AGENTS, PROJECTIONS, AND RADIOGRAPHIC PROGRAMMING

Details concerning contrast agents, projections, and radiographic programs are given in Table 21-1.

INTRAVENOUS DIGITAL SUBTRACTION ANGIOGRAPHY

Intravenous digital subtraction angiography requires the bolus of contrast agent to be injected into the femoral or iliac vein, or into the low inferior vena cava. Its major advantage is that less contrast is required, which is useful in interventional procedures (see Fig. 21-24C).

Normal Anatomy

The inferior vena cava begins at the L5 vertebral body by the junction of the two common iliac veins [7]. It ascends vertically and to the right of the aorta until it reaches the liver, where it gently curves anteriorly in a groove on its dorsal aspect. The caudate lobe can cause a mild medial indentation on the inferior vena cava at this level. The anterior inclination of the vena cava continues as it pierces the diaphragm to join the right atrium at its posteroinferior margin. In the abdomen, the pancreas lies on the anterior wall of the inferior vena cava. At the L1 to L2 level the right renal artery passes behind the inferior vena cava and can cause an indentation on its posterior wall. During its central course it accepts lumbar veins on its posterior surface at appropriate vertebral levels, as well as the renal veins at approximately the L1 level. Three large hepatic veins drain into its ventral and lateral surfaces just below the diaphragm (see Chap. 13). Smaller hepatic veins may drain the caudate and right hepatic lobes somewhat lower in its course.

In the male, there is usually more than one venous branch that drains the pampiniform plexus

of each testicle. These veins pass upward through the inguinal ligament into the pelvis before they join to form the single left or right testicular vein. The right gonadal vein enters the inferior vena cava anterolaterally on the right below the renal vein, and the left gonadal vein enters the left renal vein inferiorly. Knowledge of the normal anatomy of these veins and their variance from normal is important when trying to perform an adequate intravascular therapeutic blockade in patients with varicoceles [12]. There may be two left testicular veins. There are frequent cross-communications with adjacent ascending lumbar veins, with renal capsular veins, and occasionally with the left colic vein. The optimal point of occlusion of the veins in treatment of varicoceles is just above the inguinal ring. The pampiniform plexus is a collection of tortuous veins surrounding the testicle, which acts as a marker for their location when searching for undescended testicles not detected by computed tomography scanning (Fig. 21-4).

The right suprarenal vein enters the inferior vena cava posterolaterally above the renal vein (at the T11 to T12 level); the left suprarenal vein enters the left renal vein from above (see Chap. 12).

The veins draining into the inferior vena cava are not normally seen during cavography; their location may be marked by transient, changing filling defects due to unopacified blood.

Figures 21-3 and 21-5A, B show a line drawing and a venogram demonstrating normal epidural venous anatomy. The catheters are inserted into either a lateral sacral vein or an ascending lumbar vein. These veins communicate freely with each other, have horizontal communicating veins that drain into the inferior vena cava, and eventually course up to the thorax as the azygous and hemiazygous venous systems. In addition to this external paravertebral plexus of veins, there is a freely communicating internal epidural plexus that lies between the dura and the vertebrae. These epidural veins form two main vertebral chains on the posterior aspect and two on the anterior aspect of the vertebral canal. It is these anterior internal epidural veins that lie on the posterior vertebral bodies and disk spaces and that can be disrupted or displaced by protruding disks or tumors (Fig. 21-5C) [5, 9, 14].

Sacral and lumbar veins may be seen as an artifact during inferior venacavography if Valsalva maneuver is performed or if the catheter is inad-

Table 21-1. Technical specifications in inferior venacavography and renal and hepatic venography

Location of angiographic procedure	Contrast agent			Total films	Total time (sec)	Radiographic program		
	Density	Volume (ml/inj)	Rate (ml/sec)			Films/sec	Timing	Projections
Adults								
Inferior vena cava								
Single catheter	M	50	20	10	7	2/sec for 3 sec; 1/sec for 4 sec (delay if obstruction is anticipated)	Start films 0.4 sec after start of injection	Biplane AP and lateral. Cone, with central beam just to right of spine
Needle sleeve in each femoral vein	M	25[a]	10[b]	10	7	Same as above	Same as above	Same as above
Selective renal vein	L	30[c]	15[d]	10	6	3/sec for 2 sec; 1/sec for 4 sec	Same as above	AP
Selective hepatic vein (not in wedge position)	L	30	10	10	7	2/sec for 3 sec; 1/sec for 4 sec	Same as above	AP or biplane AP and lateral
Children								
Inferior vena cava	L or NI	1.0–1.5 ml/kg	Total within 1–2 sec	10	7	Same as adult	Same as adult	Same as adult

[a]Injected simultaneously in each vein.

[b]This requires two injectors. A single injector and a Y connector joining both needles can be used if there is no obstruction to one side. Unilateral obstruction causes preferential flow through the unobstructed side.

[c]Use less if there is obvious obstruction on fluoroscopy.

[d]Immediately following epinephrine in same renal artery (see text, page 590).

M = medium-density contrast agent; L = low-density contrast agent; NI = nonionic 300 mg (see Appendix 3).

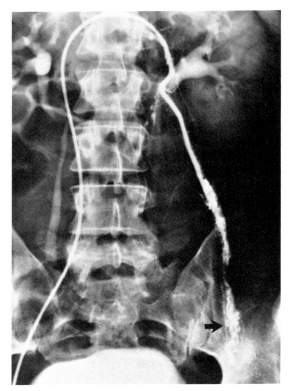

Fig. 21-4. Venogram of left testicular vein. Undescended testicle. Pampiniform plexus (*arrow*).

vertently advanced into the ascending lumbar vein as it arises from the iliac vein. Valsalva maneuver promotes filling of both the testicular and epidural venous plexuses during venography. It should be avoided during cavography, however, because it causes incomplete filling of some of the cranial portions of the inferior vena cava. Sacral and lumbar veins also fill if there is stenosis or obstruction of the iliac veins or the inferior vena cava.

VARIATIONS FROM NORMAL

The following variations from normal anatomy may occur [2, 17]:

1. A left-sided vena cava may exist to the level of the left renal vein, where it crosses to the right. When this occurs, usually there are two venae cavae to this level (caval duplication), but more rarely, there is a left-sided vena cava alone.
2. The inferior vena cava may continue superiorly as a persistent azygos vein that drains directly into the superior vena cava. The large roent-

genographic shadow cast by this dilated vessel may be mistaken for a mediastinal mass.
3. There may be a left-sided inferior vena cava, as in situs inversus.
4. Two left-sided renal veins may arise, one ventral and one dorsal to the aorta, to act as a sling [18].

VENOUS COLLATERAL CHANNELS

Occlusion of the inferior vena cava results in multiple alternate routes of drainage [7]. These alternate routes include the following:

1. Drainage may occur primarily through the ascending lumbar veins and the vertebral plexus into the azygous and hemiazygous venous systems to the superior vena cava (Fig. 21-6). Anastomoses with the intercostal and supreme intercostal veins drain directly into the innominate veins and thence into the superior vena cava.
2. Ureteral and gonadal venous channels bypass low caval obstructions by draining directly into the inferior vena cava on the right and into the left renal vein and thence into the inferior vena cava on the left.
3. Another bypass is through the hemorrhoidal plexus, through the inferior mesenteric vein, and thence into the portal venous system. Engorged abdominal wall veins drain into the paraumbilical veins and thence into the portal system; the reverse occurs in some patients with portal hypertension.
4. Abdominal veins can also drain into the mammary and the lateral thoracic veins and thence into the innominate veins.
5. When obstruction is below the renal veins, all of these channels are available. When obstruction is above the renal veins or possibly above the hepatic veins, the renal venous drainage is not available, but the remaining collateral routes are used.

Additional Technical Points

1. The femoral vein can be distended by Valsalva maneuver, which facilitates puncture under difficult circumstances.
2. Retroperitoneal disease causing anterior displacement of the inferior vena cava can be missed if biplane studies are not performed (Fig. 21-7). The angiographer should be sure to

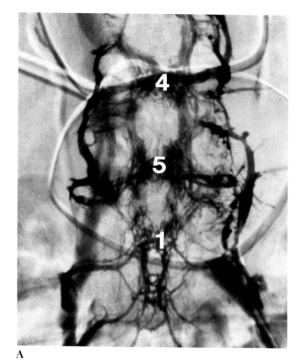

A

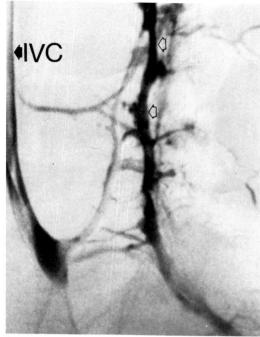

B

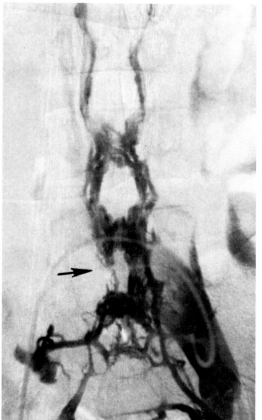

C

Fig. 21-5.

A. Normal epidural venogram (anteroposterior digital subtraction film following injection into the left ascending lumbar vein). The numbers are placed directly over the vertebral bodies of the corresponding lumbar and sacral vertebrae. The radicular veins on each side pass both above and below the vertebral pedicles. (See text for anatomic details.)

B. Lateral projection shows densely stained anterior internal vertebral veins lying on the posterior wall of the vertebral bodies (*open arrows*). Communicating veins join the ascending lumbar veins to the anteriorly located inferior vena cava (IVC).

C. Epidural venogram (left ascending lumbar vein injection). The anterior intervertebral veins on the right at L5–S1 are compressed and do not fill well despite adequate filling above and below this level (*arrow*). Similar findings were present on the right ascending lumbar venogram. The findings indicate disk herniation at this site.

include the diaphragm, since obstruction may be high in the course of the cava (Fig. 21-8).

3. Renal vein thrombosis may be difficult to substantiate. Selective catheter placement in a clot- or tumor-filled vein is dangerous and should be performed with caution. Moreover, retrograde injection into a venous system with adequate anterograde flow may present a false impression of filling defects, which may in fact be due to unopacified blood. The techniques

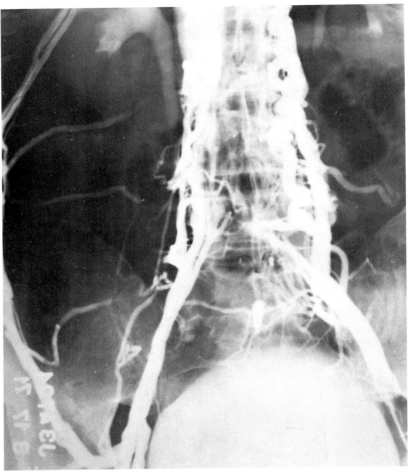

Fig. 21-6. Complete segmental occlusion of the lower inferior vena cava and both common iliac veins, with chronic changes of recanalization of the iliac veins. Collateral flow occurs primarily through large ascending lumbar veins and anterior abdominal wall collaterals.

that are available to the angiographer to make the diagnosis of renal vein thrombosis include the following:

a. Inferior venacavogram. Watch carefully for the normal radiolucent washout of unopacified blood (see Fig. 21-13). Occlusion or very sluggish renal flow should be suspected if this washout is not present. This washout is not an entirely reliable indicator, however, since it may be present despite renal vein thrombosis, particularly if the vein is not completely occluded (Fig. 21-9). Occasionally a constant, sharp filling defect will protrude into the cava from the renal vein, outlining a clot or tumor (Fig. 21-10).

b. If the cavogram is normal, selectively place a catheter with multiple side holes deep within the renal vein and inject 30 ml of contrast medium at a rate of 15 ml per sec-

ond. Retrograde flow of contrast medium into the vein may be enhanced by decreasing the renal arterial flow; this can be accomplished by Valsalva maneuver, using an occlusion balloon catheter, or by selective renal intraarterial injection of 5 to 20 μg of epinephrine immediately before the venous injection. The effect of the epinephrine is to decrease renal arterial flow momentarily and thus to allow retrograde renal venous injection of contrast medium (Fig. 21-11). The effect of epinephrine is very short-lived, and the drug is not hazardous except in a patient with severely compromised renal

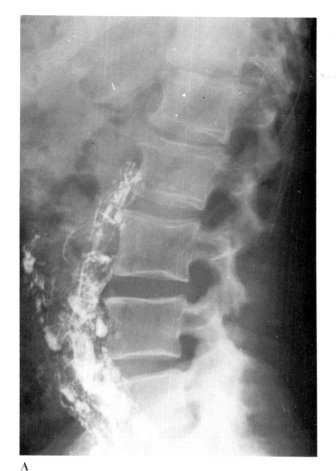

A

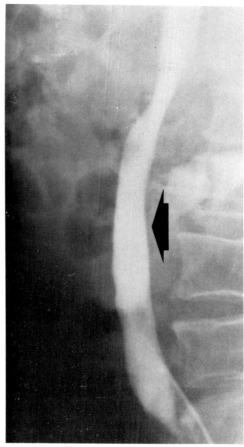

B

Fig. 21-7. Anterior displacement of the inferior vena cava by large lymphomatous lymph nodes [4].
A. Lateral projection lymphogram, showing abnormal lymph nodes.
B. Lateral projection inferior vena cavogram, showing anterior displacement (*arrow*).

function. In patients with poor renal function, the renal blood flow is usually so compromised that epinephrine is not required to give an adequate venous study.

4. Similar problems of diagnosis are present when evaluation of hepatic vein occlusion and selective venous studies are required (see Chap. 13) [4]. In addition, there are multiple veins entering the inferior vena cava, and some of these veins form a confluens before entering the cava. Multiple injections are required with a side- and end-hole catheter or sometimes with a balloon occlusion catheter to evaluate this structure completely. Approach from above often facilitates the study.

5. Adrenal venous studies are described in Chapter 12.

6. The gonadal veins may be selectively entered to obtain venous effluent for hormone determinations, to detect anomalous location of the testicle (see Fig. 21-4), or to treat varicoceles by venous occlusion with embolic materials (see Fig. 21-16). With a femoral vein approach, a catheter with a sharp angle approximately 2 cm proximal to the tip can search the right gonadal vein orifice as it enters into the inferior vena cava anterolaterally on the right, just below the right renal vein. For the left gonadal vein, a double-curved catheter must first enter the left renal vein and then seek out the left gonadal vein as it enters the inferior border of the left renal vein. Venospasm can be induced when catheters or guidewires are manipulated deep into the testicular veins, which in turn prevents

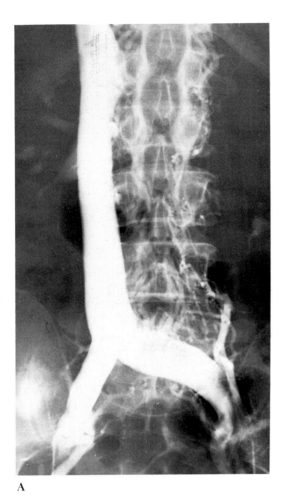

A

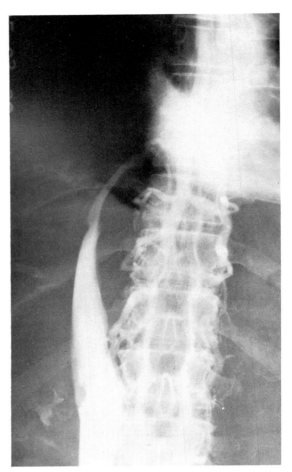

B

Fig. 21-8.

A. An inferior vena cavogram centered low. The only abnormality is hemodynamic, showing collateral flow into the vertebral veins. There is a sclerotic metastasis from the prostate in the ileum.

B. A repeat study centered at the level of the diaphragm shows extrinsic compression and displacement by intrahepatic metastatic disease found at surgery.

an adequate study. Therefore, venograms should be performed with the catheter tip in the orifice of the vein. Occasionally competent venous valves prevent retrograde flow; the catheter tip or guidewire must be passed beyond the valve before the study can be completed. Selective venography may be facilitated if the patient is in a semiupright position and a Valsalva maneuver is employed. If the patient is supine (and a film changer is available), four films are obtained at one film per second with filming commencing half-way through an injection of 10 to 20 ml of low-density contrast medium by hand (given in 2 to 3 seconds). In the semiupright position, only a single film is available for exposure, and this is performed near the termination of the injection.

When the venous anatomy is outlined, the catheter is advanced further down the vein over

a flexible-tipped guidewire if intravascular therapeutic procedures are to be performed. Occasionally, on the left side, with a femoral approach, a heavy-duty guidewire is necessary for optimal catheter tip placement. Impose a curve on the firm portion of the shaft of this guidewire in order to accommodate the 180-degree curve that the testicular vein makes in relation to the inferior vena cava.

7. Epidural venography can be used to study both primary metastatic tumors of the spine and the

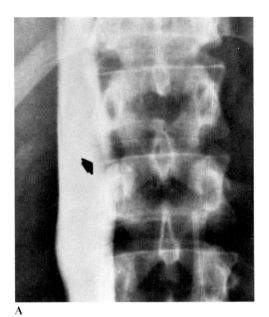

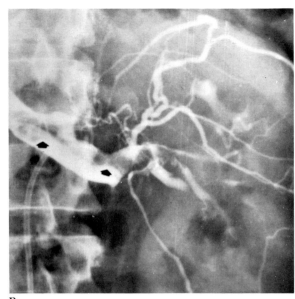

A   B

Fig. 21-9. Thrombosis of the left renal vein.
A. The inferior vena cava shows a faint defect of un-opacified blood (*arrow*) due to an incompletely occluded left renal vein.
B. Obvious thrombus lying within the left renal vein (*arrows*).

presence of herniated disks. Its usefulness has largely been supplanted by imaging with computed tomography and nuclear magnetic resonance.

An ascending lumbar vein or, alternatively, a small sacral branch ipsilateral to the suspected lesion is selectively catheterized (see Fig. 21-3). A long slow injection (3 to 4 ml per second for a total of 30 ml) of contrast medium is made into this vein during the Valsalva maneuver, with external midline abdominal compression. This ensures that the contrast medium enters the epidural venous plexus through the freely communicating valveless venous system rather than into the inferior vena cava. The initial film of the angiographic series should have no contrast medium; it is used as a mask for subsequent subtraction studies (see Fig. 21-5).

Angiographic Abnormalities

Angiographic abnormalities in a number of conditions involving the inferior vena cava and its branches are shown in Figures 21-4 to 21-10 and 21-12 to 21-16.

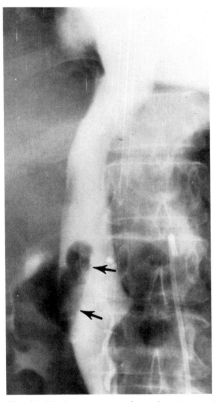

Fig. 21-10. Large tumor thrombus (*arrows*) extending from the right renal vein into the inferior vena cava detected during a total angiographic work-up on a patient with a right-sided hypernephroma. Overlying bowel gas blends in with the filling defect of the thrombus.

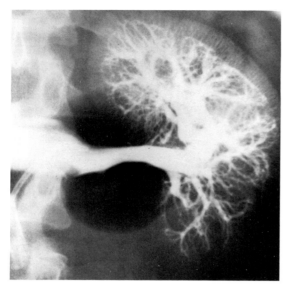

Fig. 21-11. Normal left renal venogram. Thirty ml of contrast medium was injected in 2 seconds immediately following the injection of 20 µg of epinephrine into the left renal artery.

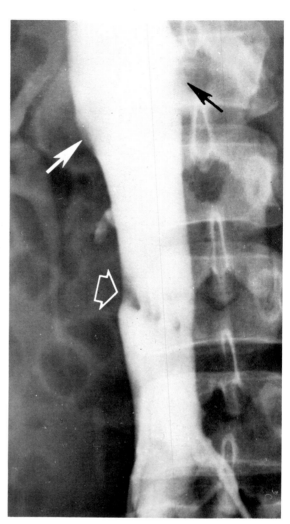

Fig. 21-13. Inferior vena cava showing plication (*open arrow*) well below the renal veins in a patient with past recurrent pulmonary thromboembolism. There are faint filling defects at the level of the renal veins, representing unopacified blood (*arrows*).

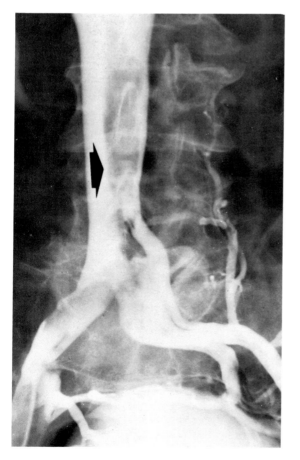

Fig. 21-12. A large filling defect representing clot (*arrow*) lying within the right iliac vein and the inferior vena cava. There is filling of the lumbar vein and retrograde flow into the hypogastric and sacral veins. These latter veins represent collaterals that developed as a result of obstruction [24].

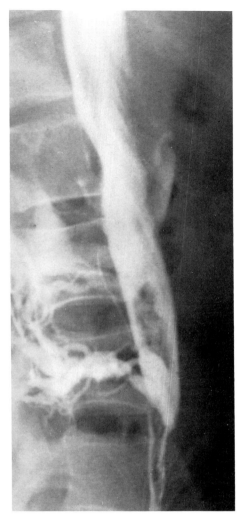

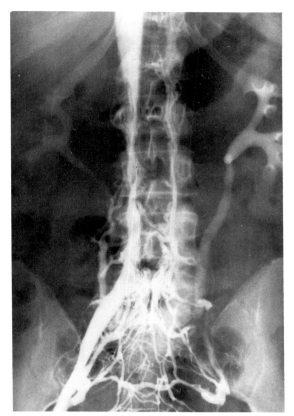

Fig. 21-15. Extrinsic compression of the inferior vena cava in a patient with retroperitoneal fibrosis. Collateral channels are developing through the ascending lumbar and sacral veins. There is a medial displacement of both ureters and slight dilatation of the left ureter [13].

Fig. 21-14. Ligated inferior vena cava resulting from recurrent pulmonary thromboembolism. This lateral projection cavogram shows clot lying above the point of ligation. Large collaterals extend posteriorly in the ascending lumbar region. The catheter was passed retrograde down the inferior vena cava to approximately the L2 level.

Intravenous Interventional Procedures

EMBOLIZATION OF VARICOCELES

Varicoceles may develop due to obstruction of the testicular vein, but much more frequently due to incompetence of its venous valves [11, 12]. Although usually left-sided, they may be bilateral. They are often associated with infertility, thought due to inhibition of spermatogenesis by the warmer testicular temperatures induced by the surrounding collection of abnormally prominent blood-filled veins. The condition may be corrected by either surgical or nonsurgical interruption of the spermatic vein [1, 8, 11, 12, 21, 22]. If performed at the correct level, distal to any associated communicating incompetent veins, the varicoceles regress and testicular drainage is induced through alternate internal iliac and epigastric collateral veins. The optimal site for occlusion is just above the inguinal ring; one must be sure to occlude any possible communicating vein that may enlarge and contribute to recurrence of the condition. Therapeutic blockade should therefore follow careful venographic examination unobscured by incomplete filling due to improper catheter placement or induced venospasm.

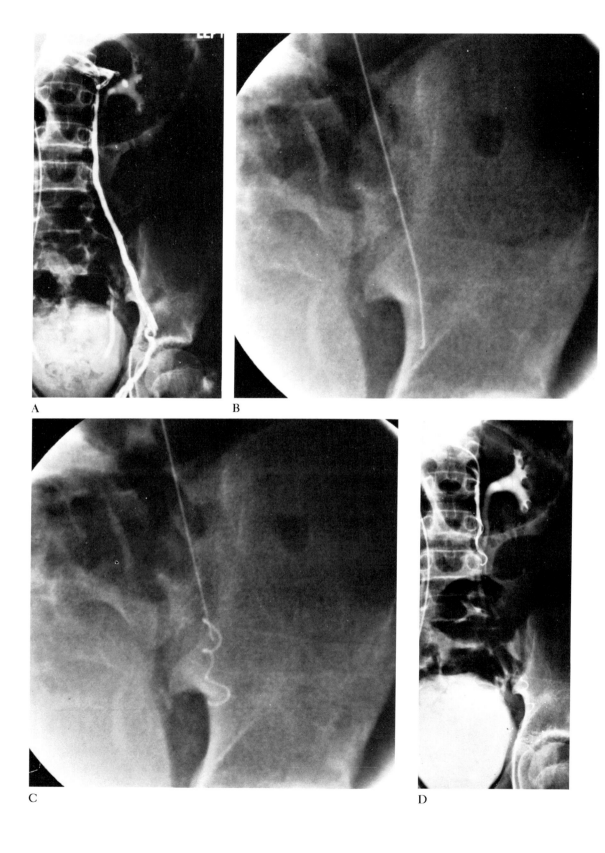

A

B

C

D

Once venography has been performed, a floppy-tipped guidewire can be gently advanced down the length of the spermatic vein, followed by the 5 or 6.5 French catheter into the upper portion of the testicular vein. Occasionally, a heavy-duty guidewire, a Lunderquist guidewire with a preformed curve, or one with a variable stiffness is required for this maneuver. Since the therapeutic occlusion of the spermatic veins is accomplished by injecting a variety of substances, the delivery systems of these embolic agents are also varied. See Chapter 5 for details. Gianturco coils (see Fig. 5-6, 5-7, 5-8) require the catheter tip to be advanced well down into the testicular vein, a provision best accomplished by the jugular approach. A modification of the delivery system allows advancement of the coil beyond the catheter to a peripheral location [16]. This technique allows a femoral vein approach (Fig. 21-16 A and B). Tissue adhesives and other liquid sclerosing agents such as hot contrast agent [21] may be administered through a coaxial system with a 3 French inner catheter or an injectable (open-ended) guidewire. Detachable balloons [11, 12, 22] require a 9 French (for 8-mm diameter balloon) or a 7 French (4-mm balloon) catheter tip in the orifice of the testicular vein. These large diameter outer delivery catheters may be advanced into the testicular veins over a guidewire that has been previously advanced into suitable position by standard renal vein catheterization techniques. Once in position at the orifice of the testicular vein, the inner 2 French Silastic catheter bearing the balloon can be easily injected to the appropriate level and inflated with isosmolar contrast agent, and its position and occlusive properties checked by injecting contrast agent through the delivery catheter. It can be deflated and repositioned if its position is unsatisfactory.

Complications are few, but they include migration of embolic material to nontarget areas, perforation of the testicular vein, and testicular

phlebitis. Recurrence can occur (in 10 percent [11]) and approximately 20 percent of patients undergoing embolization can father children.

INFERIOR VENA CAVA INTERRUPTION

Inferior vena cava filters are indicated in certain patients who have proven pulmonary emboli and occasionally in some patients with no documented pulmonary emboli but are at high risk for their development. They may be used when anticoagulant and/or thrombolytic treatment fails or is contraindicated. Patients at high risk for bleeding, those who develop repetitive pulmonary emboli despite anticoagulation, those who may be survivors of major pulmonary emboli or who have cor pulmonale, and those who demonstrate large free-floating iliocaval clots may benefit from this procedure. Also, patients with septic emboli or those with emboli in the first trimester of pregnancy may be candidates for a filter. Rarely, a filter has been used prophylactically in elderly, high-risk patients with orthopedic procedures.

Surgery (see Figs. 21-13, 21-14), intracaval balloons, and other devices have been used in the inferior vena cava in order to prevent the central flow of emboli [19, 25].

The most widely used filters, the Mobin-Uddin "umbrella" and the Kimray-Greenfield (K-G) filter, were devised for placement (lodged within a delivery capsule measuring 7 mm or 8 mm in diameter, respectively) following surgical venotomy of either the internal jugular vein or the femoral vein. Techniques have been modified to deliver these filters percutaneously through large-bore catheter sheaths (earlier models up to 30-mm diameter, but soon down to 12-mm diameter) [26]. The K-G filter is more simply introduced percutaneously than the Mobin-Uddin.

Percutaneous Technique for Placing K-G Filter (Figs. 21-17, 21-18, 21-19)

An inferior vena cavogram is performed first. This identifies and evaluates the location, patency, and direction, and anomalies of the renal veins and the inferior vena cava as well as the width of the inferior vena cava.

There are two approaches for percutaneously introducing a K-G filter, one from the femoral and the other from the jugular vein, and the delivery systems are different. The K-G filter is carefully

Fig. 21-16.
A. Surgical failure of left-sided varicocele. A 5 French "cobra" catheter in left proximal gonadal vein.
B. Modified coil attached to inner core of 0.025-in. guidewire advanced beyond the catheter tip low into the left pelvis (see Chap. 5).
C. Coil released.
D. Second coil placed higher in testicular vein.

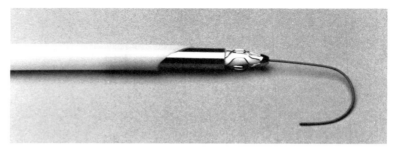

A

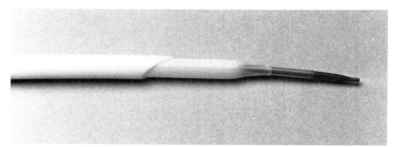

B

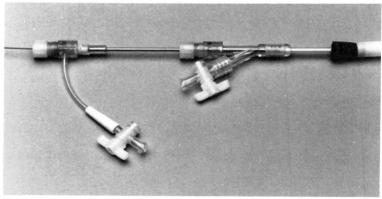

C

Fig. 21-17. Kimray-Greenfield (K-G) filter.
A. Filter encased in delivery capsule. The delivery system lies within a 24 French sheath.
B. Telescoping catheter with overlying 24 French sheath.
C. Hub of delivery catheter in overlying sheath (see text).

loaded onto the capsule, making sure that its tines do not cross or project beyond the capsule walls.

If the *femoral vein* approach is chosen, a large 40- to 50-cm long (24 French) catheter sheath system is required. The vein is entered and gradually dilated to a 24 French diameter using seven or eight dilators of gradually increasing size introduced over a rigid guidewire. Generous quantities of local anesthetic are required to counteract pain. Next a telescoping large-bore catheter system with an overlying 24 French sheath (Fig. 21-17B) is advanced over the guidewire to a point previously selected as the optimal site for filter placement. Expeditious meticulous care must be exercised to avoid air embolism and clot formation.

The 24 French catheter sheath is left open the brief instant when the inner telescoping catheters are exchanged for the capsule delivery system; this is rapidly closed from air by placing a hemostasis valve (an enclosing rubber stopper) on the hub of the sheath surrounding the large-bore introducing catheter (Fig. 21-17C). The K-G filter-capsule delivery system can be advanced over a previously placed guidewire, facilitating its passage through the iliac veins and into the inferior vena cava (Fig. 21-17A). If the inferior vena cava shows no clots and is of normal caliber (up to 25 or 28 mm), the capsule is advanced within the protective 24 French sheath to a point just below the renal veins (Fig. 21-18A). Accomplish the following maneuvers in rapid succession (Fig. 21-18): Keep the capsule with encased filter stationary, and withdraw the 24 French sheath to fully uncover the capsule (Fig. 21-18B). If it is not totally uncovered, the filter will be ejected partially into the sheath with subsequent malposition [Fig. 21-19]. The sheath should remain in the low inferior vena cava, to act as a conduit for an atraumatic withdrawal of the capsule following completion of the study. Next, keeping the inner wire fixated and the filter stationary, withdraw the capsule-bearing catheter. This disengages the filter at the precise planned location, with little chance of its tilting (Fig. 21-18C). If the filter is actively ejected by keeping the capsule stationary and pushing the inner wire, the filter springs forward into the cava, and there is less control of its final position and angle (Fig. 21-20). The longitudinal axis of the filter should remain in the vertical axis of the inferior vena cava (Fig. 21-18D). Once the filter has been ejected, withdraw the capsule-bearing catheter into the sheath (Fig. 21-18E). A digital subtraction study of the inferior vena cava through this same catheter documents the correct orientation and position of the filter.

Problems can occur during the femoral approach that are related primarily to the occasionally small caliber of the femoral vein or the iliac vein, since tortuosity of the iliac veins makes manipulation of large-bore catheters difficult; the presence of clots must be recognized. When clots occur, an alternate approach must be used.

The *jugular approach* is preferred by some angiographers; it is necessary if clots are seen in the inferior vena cava. If this *jugular* approach is selected, a shorter 24 French catheter sheath system (the one used for percutaneous renal stone extraction) is advanced into the proximal superior vena cava over a heavy-duty guidewire, previously advanced beyond the right atrium and into the inferior vena cava [26]. With this approach, it is absolutely critical to have a closed system in order to avoid air embolism. This is best accomplished by introducing the delivery capsule catheter with the patient in inspiration, and immediately withdrawing the sheath (within seconds) from the venous system as soon as the capsule enters into the superior vena cava. The subsequent techniques and precautions used in delivering the filter are similar to those in the femoral approach. Subsequent manipulations into the right atrium and the inferior vena cava are made *after* the sheath has been removed. The delivery capsule is simply withdrawn through the jugular vein when the procedure is completed. Compression of the puncture site for 10 to 15 minutes is all that is required.

The configuration of the K-G filter and its high record of patency allows it to be positioned above the renal veins when clot extends above this site. If the diameter of the inferior vena cava is 30 mm or greater, a K-G filter should be introduced into each iliac vein in order to avoid central migration of the 28-mm diameter filter [20].

Technical problems may occur during introduction of the filter through the internal jugular vein. These include spasticity and small diameter of the jugular vein, and a tortuous bend in the internal jugular vein as it enters into the thorax. Dilating the vein with a Foley balloon catheter and maneuvering the right shoulder might aid in passing the catheter and capsule. A prominent eustachian valve in the right atrium, guarding the inflow of the inferior vena cava, can be bypassed by a guidewire that has been previously positioned across the area. The right renal vein may lie almost parallel to the inferior vena cava, and the delivery system may be mistakenly positioned either in this vein or in the hepatic vein. Test injections through the delivery catheter during the act of positioning, and placing the patient's left side down to work with gravity prevent this malposition from occurring. One must take full precautions to avoid an air embolism.

Complications of filter placements include misplacement into a renal or hepatic vein. The filter may migrate higher up the inferior vena cava or even into the right atrium or the pulmonary artery if not properly seated. Improper alignment of the filter with the axis of the inferior vena cava (Fig. 21-20) results in inadequate filtration and may cause one or more prongs to penetrate the walls of the cava. Usually this is of no consequence, but there is a potential for retroperitoneal bleeding and perforations into adjacent structures such as bowel, ureter, and aorta. Delayed complications of filter placement are recurrent pulmonary embolism, oc-

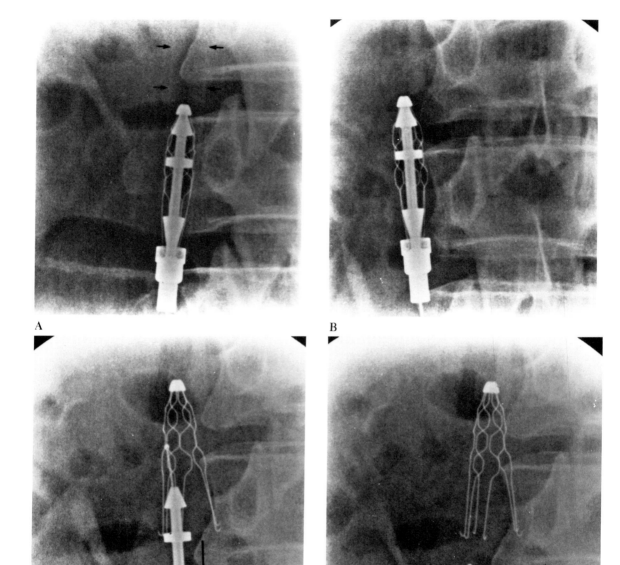

A

B

C

D

Fig. 21-18. Steps in delivering K-G filter percutaneously.

A. Protective sheath (*arrows*) lies just below renal
   veins. K-G filter advancing to this point.
B. The sheath is now withdrawn into low inferior vena
   cava, just beyond the common iliac vein.

C. Filter is disengaged by keeping the inner wire
   fixated and the filter stationary, and withdrawing
   the capsule-bearing catheter.
D. Filter in stable position well aligned with inferior
   vena cava.
E. Capsule withdrawn into low-lying sheath.

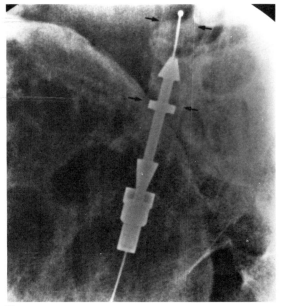

E

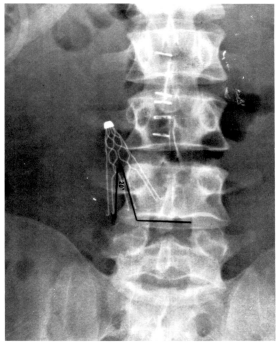
A

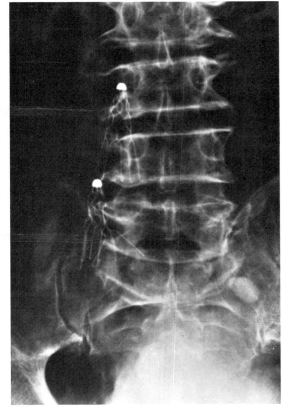

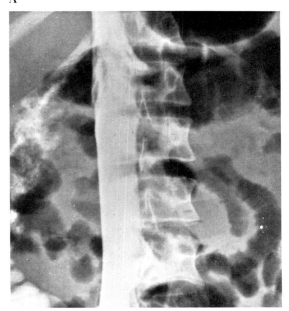
B

Fig. 21-19. Malposition of low-lying K-G filter into right common iliac vein. One of the filter tines has penetrated the vein wall. Second filter subsequently positioned from a jugular approach.

Fig. 21-20.
A. Misaligned filter, tilted in the inferior vena cava, due to actively ejecting the filter from the capsule rather than withdrawing the capsule from the filter.
B. Inferior vena cava prior to placing the filter. Note its vertical position.

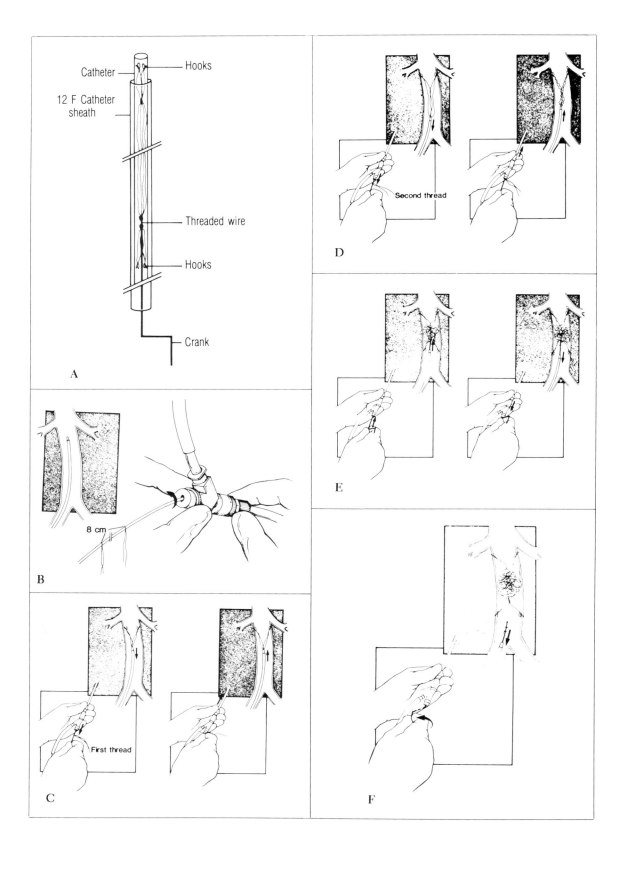

Catheter

Hooks

12 F Catheter sheath

Threaded wire

Hooks

Crank

A

8 cm

B

First thread

C

Second thread

D

E

F

Fig. 21-21.

A. Twenty-five cm long 0.016-in. wires with proximal and distal paired prongs encased in a 10 F catheter is introduced through a 12 F sheath.

B. Catheter sheath introduced percutaneously to a level below renal veins over a 10 F catheter. The 10 F catheter is replaced with the catheter assembly containing the filter. The O-ring adapter is loosened to allow easy withdrawal to the thread markers.

C. Hold the wire immobile and now withdraw the catheter and sheath 6 cms (to the first thread marker). This bares the emerging leading prongs, which spring out to engage the IVC wall. Gently advance the system 1 to 2 ml to secure the tynes into the wall.

D. Hold the wire immobile and withdraw the catheter sheath assembly another 6 cm (to the second thread marker) which uncovers the juncture of the uppermost prongs. One can now advance the whole assembly upwards approximately 1 cm.

E. Now fixate the catheter assembly and advance the wire up to the crank shaft; this pushes both the 0.016-in. wires out of the catheter (which coil in the IVC as the filter) as well as the distal fixating prongs which spring out to meet the IVC walls. The juncture of the proximal prongs lie slightly above that of the leading prongs. Gentle traction on the assembly secures their position.

F. Turn the crank counterclockwise a number of turns to disengage the filter and remove it from the sheath. Perform an angiogram through the sheath to outline the filter's position.

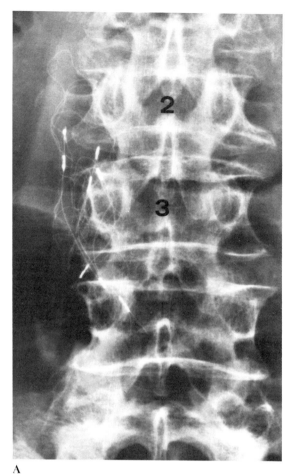

A

Fig. 21-22.

A and B. Satisfactory position of bird's nest filter in the inferior vena cava below the renal veins.

C. Autopsy specimen of bird's nest filter. Many clots were trapped within the wire mesh.

clusion of the inferior vena cava, migration of the filter, and infection. Fortunately, these complications are rare.

Other Filters

Although the inferior vena cava filters currently available are generally effective in reducing the incidence of pulmonary emboli, the large size of their delivery system makes percutaneous introduction cumbersome. There has been experimental and clinical research into newer inferior vena cava filters delivered more easily through small diameter catheters [3, 6, 15, 23, 25]. These have not as yet been approved for use by the FDA and are still considered experimental devices. One of these entails a filter that not only can be delivered from either the jugular or femoral vein approach but also can be retrieved [15]. Another uses

nitinol [3, 25] (an alloy of tin and titanium), which retains a memory for shape at certain temperatures. The material can be preformed to the shape of an effective filter at the temperature of the patient's blood, but can be straightened at room temperature into an easily delivered system.

BIRD'S NEST FILTER. Another concept [23] is that of introducing several elongated narrow-gauge wires, hooking their distal and proximal tips into the caval wall at a preselected site, and then coiling the wires into a tight mesh or network in a controlled confined area within the cava (Figs. 21-21, 21-22). This system is nonretrievable. It is easy to

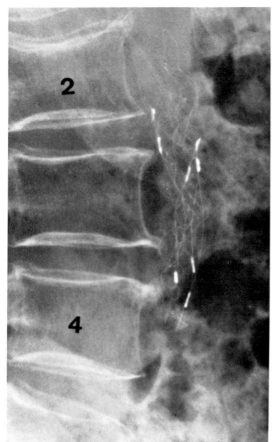

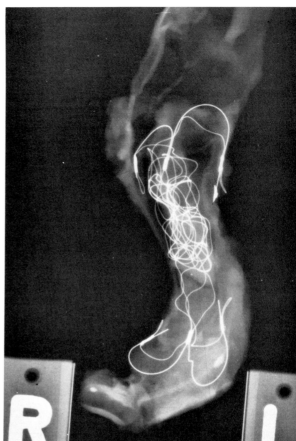

B

Fig. 21-22 (continued)

C

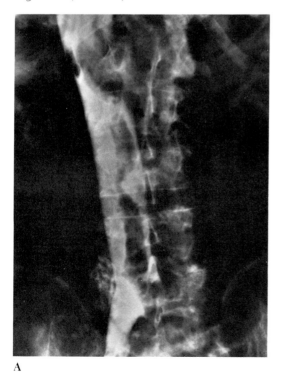

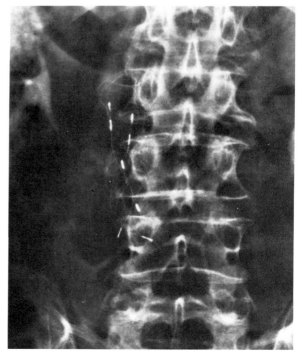

A

B

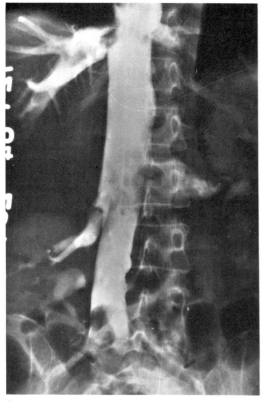

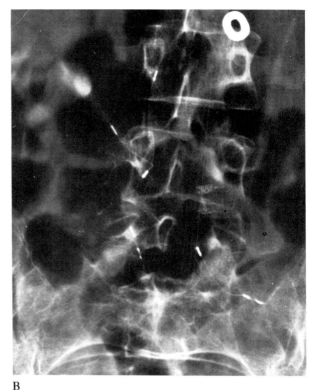

A   B

Fig. 21-24.
A. Occlusion of distal inferior vena cava by clot requiring jugular approach. Note low level of right
   renal vein.
B. Filter pushed into low inferior vena cava, trapping
   clot.
C. Intravenous digital subtraction study following filter
   placement.

introduce from either the femoral or the jugular
approach for it uses conventional size delivery systems, which can be passed up beside inferior vena
cava clots (Fig. 21-23A) or even into clots (Fig. 21-
24). The thin wire of the mesh of this system permits it to be placed across renal veins or above the
renal veins.

PERCUTANEOUS TRANSLUMINAL
ANGIOPLASTY

Percutaneous transluminal angioplasty is performed when there are focal areas of stenosis in-

Fig. 21-23. Large clot in the low inferior vena cava.
Catheter easily passed from a right femoral approach
beyond the clot, and a bird's nest filter was subsequently positioned across the renal veins.

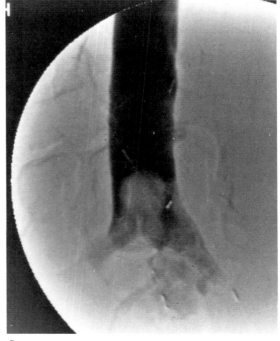

C

volving the systemic venous system. Thus patients with Budd-Chiari syndrome due to focal stenosis of the large hepatic veins [27] or the upper inferior vena cava [28] may be successfully treated. Stenosis of surgical portosystemic venous shunts may also be dilated (Fig. 7-5).

References

1. Berman, W., et al. Varicoceles. Coaxial coil occlusion system. *Radiology* 151:73, 1984.
2. Brener, B., et al. Major venous anomalies complicating abdominal aortic surgery. *Arch. Surg.* 108:159, 1974.
3. Cragg, A., et al. A new percutaneous vena cava filter. *A.J.R.* 141:601, 1984.
4. Deutsch, V., Rosenthal, T., and Adar, R. Budd-Chiari syndrome: Study of angiography findings and remarks on etiology. *A.J.R.* 116:430, 1972.
5. Draisin, G., et al. Epidural venography: Diagnosis of herniated lumbar intervertebral disc and other disease of the epidural space. *A.J.R.* 126:1010, 1976.
6. Dunne, M., and Goldstein, W. Computed tomographic and ultrasound appearance of Kimray-Greenfield vena caval filters and potential for non-invasive localization. *C.T.* 7:375, 1983.
7. Ferris, E., et al. *Venography of the Inferior Vena Cava and Its Branches.* Baltimore: Williams & Wilkins, 1969.
8. Formanek, A., et al. Embolization of the spermatic vein for treatment of infertility. A new approach. *Radiology* 139:315, 1981.
9. Gershater, R., and Holgate, R. Lumbar epidural venography in the diagnosis of disc herniation. *A.J.R.* 126:992, 1976.
10. Huberman, R., and Gomes, A. Membranous obstruction of the inferior vena cava. *A.J.R.* 139:1215, 1982.
11. Kadir, S., et al. Mechanism of recurrent varicocele after balloon occlusion or surgical ligation of the internal spermatic vein. *Radiology* 147:435, 1983.
12. Kadir, S., *Selected Techniques in Interventional Radiology.* Philadelphia: Saunders, 1982.
13. Kittredge, R., and Nash, A. The many facets of sclerosing fibrosis. *A.J.R.* 122:288, 1974.
14. LePage, J. Transfemoral ascending lumbar catheterization of the epidural veins: Exposition and techniques. *Radiology* 111:337, 1974.
15. Lund, G., et al. New vena cava filter for percutaneous placement and retrieval. Experimental study. *Radiology* 152:369, 1984.
16. Lund, G., et al. Detachable spring steel coils for vessel occlusion. *Radiology* 155:530, 1985.
17. Mayo, J., et al. Review. Anomalies of the inferior vena cava. *A.J.R.* 140:339, 1983.
18. Mitty, H. Circumaortic renal collar: A potentially hazardous anomaly of the left renal vein. *Am. J. Roentgenol.* 125:307, 1975.
19. Novelline, R. Practical points on transvenous insertion of inferior vena cava filters. *Cardiovasc. Intervent. Radiol.* 3:319, 1980.
20. Prince, M., et al. Diameter of the inferior vena cava and its implications for the use of vena caval filters. *Radiology* 149:687, 1983.
21. Rholl, K., et al. Spermatic vein obliteration using hot contrast medium in dogs. *Radiology* 148:85, 1983.
22. Ridel, P., Lungimayer, G., and Staki, W. A new method of transfemoral venous obliteration for varicocele using a balloon catheter. *Radiology* 113:323, 1981.
23. Roehm, J., Jr., et al. Percutaneous transcatheter filter for the inferior vena cava. A new device for the treatment of patients with pulmonary embolism. *Radiology* 150:255, 1984.
24. Rudikoff, J., Clapp, P., and Ferris, E. Ileocaval thrombi in pulmonary thromboembolic disease. *A.J.R.* 126:1019, 1976.
25. Simon, M., and Palestrant, A. Transvenous devices for the management of pulmonary embolism. *Cardiovasc. Intervent. Radiol.* 3:308, 1980.
26. Tadavarthy, S., et al. Kimray-Greenfield filter. Percutaneous introduction. *Radiology* 151:525, 1984.
27. Uflacker, R., et al. Percutaneous transluminal angioplasty of the hepatic veins for treatment of Budd-Chiari syndrome. *Radiology* 153:641, 1984.
28. Yamadea, R., et al. Segmental obstruction of the hepatic inferior vena cava treated by transluminal angioplasty. *Radiology* 149:91, 1983.
29. Young, R., Friedman, A. C., and Harman, D. Computed tomography of leiomyosarcoma of the inferior vena cava. *Radiology* 147:99, 1982.

Superior Venacavography and Azygos Venography

Many conditions involving the superior vena cava and major systemic veins of the thorax may be evaluated by dynamic computed tomography imaging [5, 7, 11, 12], ultrasonography, nuclear magnetic resonance [6, 8], and radionuclide flow studies. Cavography is reserved for those occasions when specific anatomic or pathologic detail is not provided by these techniques.

Indications

1. Evaluation of mediastinal diseases.
   a. Mediastinal masses. These may be benign or malignant neoplasms, thoracic aortic aneurysms, or abnormal mediastinal venous dilatations (e.g., continuation of azygos vein). Some of these conditions may cause extrinsic compression, deviation, obstruction, and narrowing of the superior vena cava and the azygos system. Venous occlusion by malignant neoplasm in the mediastinum is considered to be a sign of inoperability.
   b. Superior vena cava syndrome. Obstruction of this structure may occur by malignant or benign neoplasm (80 percent); fibrosing mediastinitis; tuberculosis; histoplasmosis; pyogenic mediastinitis [3, 4, 9].
   c. Thrombosis of the superior vena cava or innominate veins due to long-term placement of catheters, shunts, tubes, and pacing wires.
2. Forward angiocardiogram in the evaluation of cardiovascular abnormalities.
   a. Anomalies of pulmonary and systemic venous drainage (e.g., bilateral superior venae cavae).
   b. Surgical intervention, e.g., mustard procedure.
   c. Congenital and acquired cardiopulmonary disease.
3. Selective venous sampling of the azygos and vertebral venous plexus in search of extraadrenal paravertebral functioning tumors (pheo-

chromocytomas); thyroid and thymic venous sampling in search of parathyroid adenomas (see Chap. 15).
4. Planning therapy for obstructive lesions.
   a. Radiotherapy of obstructing tumor.
   b. Surgical bypass of superior vena cava.
5. Interventional procedures.
   a. Removal of foreign bodies (see Fig. 7-11) [10].
   b. Thrombolysis of thrombosed veins [2].
   c. Percutaneous transluminal angioplasty [2].

Technique

APPROACHES

1. Superior vena cava.
   a. A large-bore needle may be inserted in a vein in each antecubital fossa.
   b. Preferably, for a more rapid injection, one should introduce percutaneously a small-diameter catheter on each side and advance it as close to the subclavian veins as the obstruction permits. Only a single catheter is required if it can be advanced to the superior vena cava.
2. Azygos vein. The percutaneous femoral vein approach is used.

CATHETERS

1. Superior vena cava. A 16- or 17-gauge needle or a 60-cm 5 or 6 French "pigtail" catheter with side holes is used.
2. Azygos vein. A preformed polyethylene or polyurethane 5 or 6 French 100-cm catheter with a 270-degree circumferential curve of 2.5-cm radius is used (Fig. 22-1). This catheter is advanced well into the azygos vein.

CONTRAST AGENTS

1. Superior venacavogram. Forty to fifty milliliters of medium-density contrast agent is required. This may be hand injected if significant obstruction is anticipated; if not, and if the catheters are in place, simultaneous injection

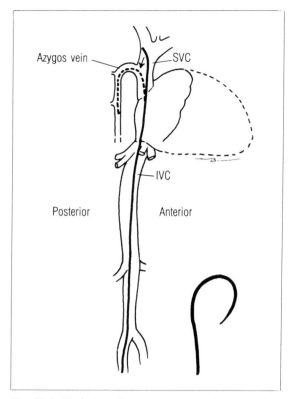

Fig. 22-1. Technique for azygos venography. Lateral projection of inferior and superior vena cava. IVC = inferior vena cava; SVC = superior vena cava.

of 10 ml per second for 2 to 2½ in each upper extremity is used. Separate injectors should be used if possible; otherwise, both catheters should be connected to a Y adapter. If injected through a single catheter in the superior vena cava, 50 ml at 15 to 20 ml per second is sufficient.

2. Azygos venogram. Forty milliliters of medium-density contrast agent is injected at a rate of 5 ml per second.

PROJECTIONS

1. Superior vena cava. Anteroposterior and lateral biplane projections are used; they should be coned to the superior vena cava and the cardiac chambers. Both hilar regions should be included. The superior vena cava lies just anterior to the center of the thorax on the lateral projection (Fig. 22-2).

2. Azygos venogram. Anteroposterior and lateral projections are used.

FILMS

1. Superior vena cava. Fifteen films should be taken. The filming should be started near the beginning of the injection. The film rate will vary, depending on the disease process under investigation.

    a. If complete obstruction is anticipated, 1 film per second will show the point of obstruction, the collateral flow, and the point of reconstitution, if any.

    b. For mediastinal deviation or compression, one should take 2 films per second for 4 seconds, and then 1 film per second for the remainder, for a total of 20 films over 16 seconds. This film program demonstrates the superior vena cava, the pulmonary arteries and veins, the structures of the left side of the heart, and the thoracic aorta.

    c. If the possibility of anomalous pulmonary venous drainage is being considered, film timing must be protracted to include not only the systemic venous system but also the pulmonary arterial system and then the pulmonary venous drainage. Under these circumstances, up to 100 ml of contrast medium may be used in an adult. Film timing here would be on the order of 1 per second for 5 seconds (to outline the superior vena cava and right-sided heart chambers), 2 per second for 5 seconds (to outline the faster flowing pulmonary circulation), and then 1 per second for the remainder, for a total of 20 films in 15 seconds.

2. Azygos vein. Eight films should be taken at a rate of 1 per second.

Other Techniques

INTRAVENOUS DIGITAL
SUBTRACTION ANGIOGRAPHY

Intravenous digital subtraction angiography requires smaller quantities and more dilute contrast agent as compared with conventional angiography. A smaller field size, limited by the size of the image intensifier, may require more than one injection. Cooperation from the patient is necessary to avoid motion artifacts.

RADIONUCLIDE STUDIES

Dynamic radionuclide angiography, using a frame rate of 0.5 to 0.9 per second, with the patient

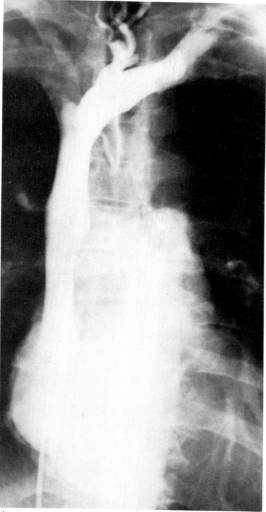

A

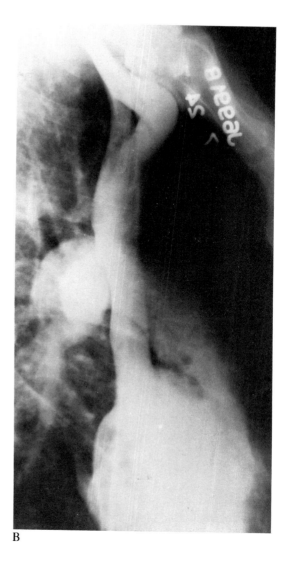

B

Fig. 22-2. Normal superior venacavogram (catheter was introduced from the femoral vein).
A. Anteroposterior projection. There is fortuitous retrograde filling of the inferior thyroid veins from the superior aspect of the left innominate vein, and filling of the thymic veins from the inferior aspect.
B. Lateral projection.

supine over the gamma camera, often provides adequate information. Either one or both antecubital veins are injected, using a total of 5 to 8 mCi of technetium 99m pertechnetate as a bolus and are flushed with isotonic saline through large-bore needles. The point of obstruction and the collateral vessels are easily identified in the patient with subclavian vein thrombus in Fig. 20-19B. Follow-up study after systemic thrombolytic therapy with streptokinase shows normal flow.

ELECTRONIC DIGITAL IMAGING AND COMPUTED TOMOGRAPHY SCANNING

A superior venacavogram may be recorded during the preliminary electronic image acquired for a thoracic computed tomography scan. Hand injections of 50 ml of medium-density contrast agent are rapidly introduced through 16-gauge needles in each antecubital vein during the 3 to 5 seconds required for the image [7].

Bilateral injections preclude the confusion in interpretation that may arise due to flow defects of unopacified blood. Subsequent axial computed tomography images can be obtained using bolus injections of contrast agent centered over the area of interest. By this means, the site and extent of an obstructing thrombus, extrinsic compression or invasion from a mediastinal mass, and the nature of the mass may be determined. Major collateral circulation can be identified, and the feasibility of surgery or radiotherapy planned. An added advantage is the guidance provided for percutaneous biopsy of the lesion.

Anatomic Considerations [1, 3]

The superior vena cava (Fig. 22-2) is formed by the junction of the two innominate veins in the

Fig. 22-3. Normal azygos venogram (see text).

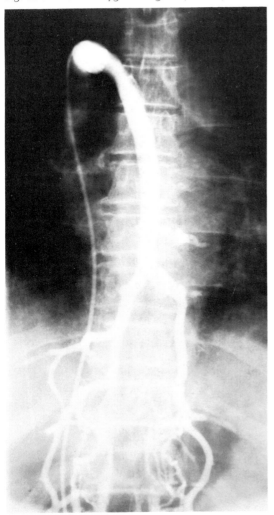

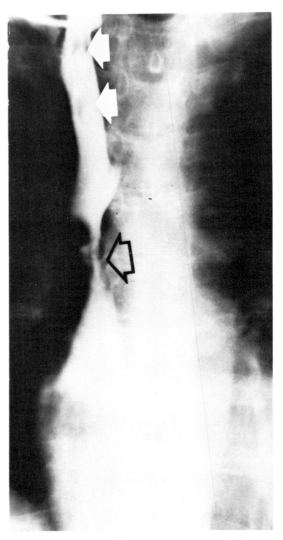

Fig. 22-4. Invasion of the superior vena cava by bronchogenic carcinoma (*open arrow*). Developing thrombi are within the partially obstructed superior vena cava (*solid arrows*).

superior mediastinum behind the sternum on the right side. It lies just in front of the root of the right lung and empties into the right atrium at the level of the third right costal cartilage.

The azygos vein arises as a direct continuation of the right ascending lumbar vein (Fig. 22-3). It ascends in the posterior mediastinum anterior to the twelfth to fourth thoracic vertebral bodies (receiving right-sided intercostal veins) and arches anteriorly to join the superior vena cava just as it is about to enter the pericardium. The hemiazygos vein (its counterpart on the left of the thoracic spine) crosses behind the aorta to join the azygos at the T8 or T9 level. The accessory hemiazygos vein arises high within the thorax and descends on the left to the T8 level, where it either joins the hemiazygos before it crosses to the right or joins the azygos directly. Veins from the esophagus, mediastinum, and pericardium drain into the azygos system. The uppermost intercostal veins drain into a common trunk and thence into the innominate veins on each side.

When there is obstruction of the superior vena cava or innominate veins, a number of collaterals develop in order to attempt to return blood to the right atrium. These collaterals occur through the azygos, internal mammary, lateral thoracic, and vertebral venous systems. Often a combination of systems is used. Various manifestations of obstruction are seen in Figures 22-4, 22-5, 22-6, 22-7. If

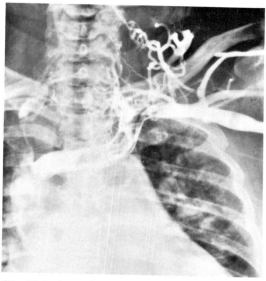

Fig. 22-6. Acute thrombus formation in the left innominate vein due to placement of an intravenous catheter for monitoring central venous pressures.

Fig. 22-5. Total occlusion of the superior vena cava and the innominate and subclavian veins. There are numerous collaterals: (1) azygos vein; (2) intercostal vein draining into the accessory hemiazygos vein; (3) lateral thoracic and thoracoepigastric veins; (4) vertebral plexus; (5) musculophrenic veins.

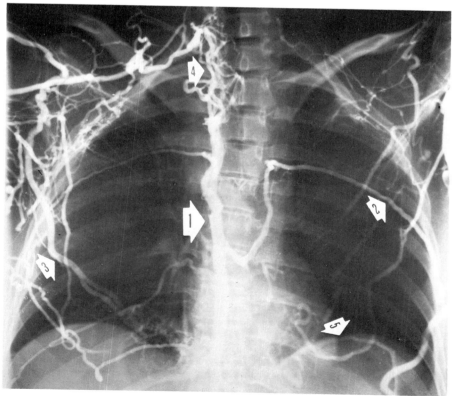

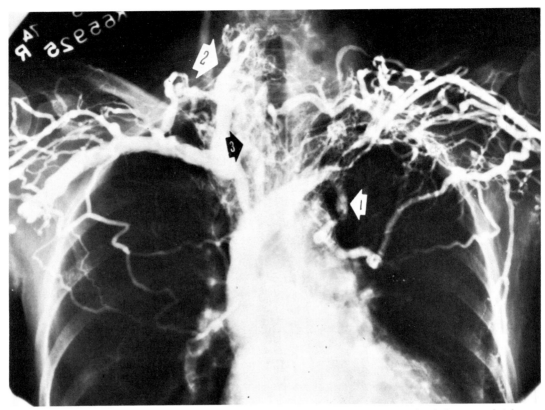

Fig. 22-7. Occlusion of the left subclavian and right innominate veins by sclerosing mediastinitis. Extensive collaterals bypass the areas of obstruction: (1) left superior intercostal vein; (2) right vertebral plexus; (3) thyroid venous plexus.

the obstruction is below the azygos vein, the azygos and hemiazygos veins drain caudad to the ascending lumbar veins and thence to the inferior vena cava and right atrium. If obstruction is above or involves the azygos septum, the other venous systems play a major role. These routes include the following: the internal mammary vein to the superior and inferior epigastric; musculophrenic, and superficial veins of the thorax to the iliac veins and thence to the inferior vena cava; the lateral thoracic, thoracoepigastric, superficial circumflex, and femoral veins and thence to the inferior vena cava; and the vertebral plexus, intercostal, lumbar, and sacral veins to the inferior vena cava. Another route has been reported [5], which drains through pleural adhesions directly into pulmonary veins.

References

1. Abrams, H. Vertebral and Azygos Veins. In H. Abrams (ed.), *Abrams' Angiography: Vascular and Interventional Angiography* (3rd ed.). Boston: Little, Brown, 1983.

2. Becker, G., et al. Local thrombolytic therapy for subclavian and axillary vein thrombosis: Treatment of the thoracic inlet syndrome. *Radiology* 149:419, 1983.

3. Bettman, M., and Steinberg, I. The Superior Vena Cava. In H. Abrams (ed.), *Abrams' Angiography: Vascular and Interventional Angiography* (3rd ed.). Boston: Little, Brown, 1983.

4. Brown, R., Nelson, M., and Lerona, P. Angiographic demonstration of collateral circulation in a patient with a superior vena caval syndrome. *A.J.R.* 119:543, 1973.

5. Engel, I., et al. CT diagnosis of mediastinal and thoracic inlet venous obstruction. *A.J.R.* 14:521, 1983.

6. Farmer, D., et al. Calcific fibrosing mediastinitis: Demonstration of pulmonary vascular obstruction by magnetic resonance imaging. *A.J.R.* 143:1189, 1984.

7. Moncada, R., et al. Evaluation of superior vena cava syndrome by axial CT and CT phlebography. *A.J.R.* 143:731, 1984.

8. O'Donovan, P., et al. Pictorial essay. Magnetic resonance imaging of the thorax: The advantages of coronal and sagittal planes. *A.J.R.* 143:1183, 1984.

9. Okay, N., and Byrk, D. Collateral pathways in occlusion of the superior vena cava and its tributaries. *Radiology* 92:1493, 1969.

10. Rossi, P. Percutaneous Removal of Intravascular Foreign Bodies. In R. Wilkins and M. Viamonte, Jr. (eds.), *Interventional Radiology*. St. Louis: Blackwell Scientific, 1982.

11. Smathers, R., et al. Pictorial essay. The azygos arch: Normal and pathologic CT appearance. *A.J.R.* 139:477, 1982.

12. Webb, W., et al. Pictorial essay. Computed tomographic demonstration of mediastinal venous anomalies. *A.J.R.* 139:157, 1982.

Direct Portal Venography

Direct portal venography is performed if indirect techniques (see Chap. 13) are inadequate. There are six methods available:

1. Percutaneous splenic puncture [1, 9]
2. Percutaneous transhepatic puncture and catheterization of the portal vein [7, 11, 19]
3. Percutaneous transjugular vein approach [5, 16]
4. Direct catheterization of a surgical systemic portal shunt
5. Surgical exposure of the umbilical vein and catheterization of the portal system [6, 8]
6. Cannulation of a portal tributary at laparotomy

Indications

1. Portal hypertension and varices.
   a. Diagnostic.
      (1) Defining pathologic anatomy and measuring pressures.
      (2) Localizing bleeding varices.
      (3) Determining patency of portosystemic shunts.
   b. Therapeutic.
      (1) Embolic occlusion of bleeding varices (transjugular and transhepatic).
      (2) Transluminal dilatation of stenosed portosystemic shunts.
      (3) Transluminal formation of portal-hepatic venous shunt [3].
2. Localizing functioning pancreatic tumors (hormonal assays of venous effluent) [2, 4, 10].

Contraindications

1. Blood dyscrasia (splenic puncture and transhepatic catheterization). Platelet count less than 50,000, prothrombin time more than 5 seconds, and partial thromboplastin time more than 15 seconds greater than control.
2. Severe ascites (splenic puncture and transhepatic catheterization). This is a relative contraindication. Ascites causes ballottement of the spleen and liver making the puncture more

challenging and hemostasis more difficult after the needle has been removed.

3. Avoid splenic puncture if a Warren procedure is contemplated. Here portal decompression is achieved by bisecting the splenic vein and anastomosing its distal segment with the renal vein. The spleen must not be jeopardized.

Technique

APPROACHES

Percutaneous Splenic Puncture
Prior to splenic puncture (Fig. 23-1), palpate the spleen and evaluate its position and size roentgenographically. The needle puncture site is in the midaxillary line at the tenth intercostal space; the site is located more posteriorly and higher if the spleen is small, more anteriorly and lower if it is large. The 20-gauge needle used for the puncture is approximately 10 cm long and has an inner sharp stylet and an outer flexible Teflon sleeve. Add two or three side holes to the sleeve for more even dispersion of the contrast agent. With a measured, even thrust, aim the needle superomedially 3 to 5 cm into the central portion of the spleen. Introduce 0.5 to 1.0 ml of saline solution to loosen the pulp. Correct insertion is indicated by the nonpulsatile return of venous blood. Remove the inner metal needle, leaving the flexible Teflon sleeve in place. Check the puncture with a few milliliters of 60% contrast agent, which pools and rapidly clears through the splenic and short gastric veins. If the contrast medium stains densely in the subcapsular area or the extrasplenic area due to needle misplacement, remove the needle completely and repuncture. Simple withdrawal of the needle into the body of the spleen is not enough because the needle track remains, and contrast medium injections follow this track. Measure splenic pulp pressure after the clearance of all contrast medium. Tape the Teflon sleeve to the skin and prepare for injection and filming. The needle sleeve is not held securely by the splenic pulp and can be displaced by exaggerated respiratory movements. Admonish the patient to breathe lightly, and perform the study as expeditiously as possible. The sleeve

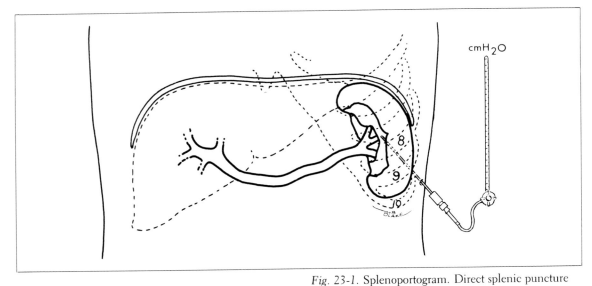

Fig. 23-1. Splenoportogram. Direct splenic puncture (see text for details).

should be removed as soon as the injection is completed. One may plug the needle track with small quantities of Gelfoam to reduce the likelihood of hemorrhage. Mechanical compression of the spleen can be obtained if the patient lies on the left side for 2 or 3 hours. Extrasplenic collections of contrast medium are associated with slowly subsiding pain but are otherwise usually of little consequence.

An alternative method of study is digital splenic portography (see Fig. 13-52) [1]. A thin needle, lesser quantities of contrast agent, and "real time" capabilities expedite the procedure and make it safer. Occasionally, two or three separate injections are required to cover the entire field (see Chap. 13 for details).

Percutaneous Transhepatic Catheterization

Percutaneous transhepatic catheterization (Figs. 23-2, 23-3) is generally not performed for purely diagnostic studies unless other maneuvers have proven unsuccessful. Patients with a bleeding diathesis or large amounts of ascites present a greater risk. The portal venous phase of a preliminary celiac and superior mesenteric arteriogram outlines both the patency and the location of the portal vein.

TECHNIQUE OF TRANSHEPATIC PORTOGRAPHY. Transhepatic portography requires transhepatic cannulation of the intrahepatic portal vein radicles and a subsequent catheter exchange. For the puncture, a needle is introduced percutaneously at the right midaxillary line during midrespiration. It

is performed at a level that is variable, depending on the depth of the costophrenic angle. It generally passes almost horizontally but slightly anteriorly to a point 2 to 3 cm lateral to and approximately one vertebral body width anterior to the vertebral body (usually T11). The initial puncture may be facilitated by ultrasonographic guidance with a special needle-guiding transducer [13].

There are a variety of needle and guidewire combinations available from which to choose:

1. A 25-cm 19-gauge needle with an overlying sleeve, or a Teflon sleeve overlying a metal stylet, is the standard needle [11]. It is introduced percutaneously at the chosen level, and the stylet removed and withdrawn until venous blood is suctioned. If an injection of contrast medium is seen fluoroscopically flowing rapidly toward the periphery of the liver, the needle is in the portal vein; if the contrast flows toward the high inferior vena cava, the needle is in the hepatic vein. Sometimes multiple punctures are necessary for successful cannulation. When the needle is in the portal vein, replace the metal shaft with a flexible-tipped guidewire with a 15-mm curve and advance both guidewire and sleeve deep into the portal vein and on into the splenic vein. A 30-cm 5 French sleeve-needle combination, with a preformed curve at the tip of the sleeve, precludes the need for subsequent catheter exchanges. The sleeve itself can be

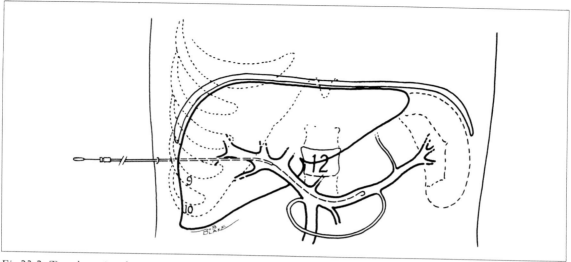

Fig 23.2. Transhepatic splenoportogram (see text for details).

used directly for selective placement once the metal needle shaft has been removed.

2. A thin (21-gauge) needle is less traumatic to the liver and allows more punctures with greater safety. Once it is placed in the portal vein, however, special measures are necessary to gradually increase the puncture diameter to a workable size. A variety of methods are available.

   a. Manipulate a small 0.018-in. flexible-tipped guidewire (with a firm steel shaft)

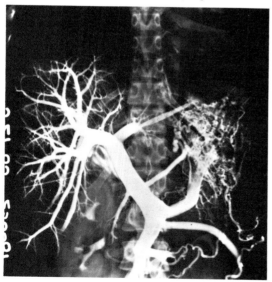

Fig. 23-3. Direct transhepatic portal venogram. Note gastric varices extending to distal esophagus.

through the thin needle deeper into the portal vein. Replace the thin needle with a long thin 3 French catheter with a shorter overlying 5 French coaxial Schwartz catheter system.[1] The 3 French catheter is sufficiently supple to follow the 0.018-in. guidewire into the portal vein, and it provides added body for passing the overlying 5 French catheter. With the 5 French catheter in the portal vein, the 3 French catheter and the 0.018-in. guidewire are replaced with the standard 0.035- or 0.038-in. guidewire for further manipulations or catheter exchanges.

   b. A similar approach uses the COPE[1] introducer system. After the 0.018-in. guidewire is advanced into the portal vein, the thin needle is replaced with a polyethylene introducer specially designed with a distal tip that snugly fits and follows the 0.018-in. guidewire but with a side hole that allows passage of a 0.035-in. guidewire. The introducer follows the 0.018-in. guidewire into the portal vein and the 0.018-in. guidewire is replaced with the 0.035-in. guidewire, which can only leave the introducer through the side hole to enter the portal vein. The introducer is then replaced with standard catheters.

   c. Another approach uses a long (45-cm) thin

[1]Cook Inc., P.O. Box 489, Bloomington, IN 47401.

needle with a removable hub [7].[2] This is introduced into the portal vein from the midaxillary line and, once the vein is entered, a 0.018-in. guidewire is introduced 5 to 10 mm beyond the needlepoint into the vein. With the flexible distal tip of the guidewire leading, both needle and guidewire are advanced together into the vein. The hub of the needle is removed, and the needle-guidewire combination provides sufficient length and rigidity for passing a 5 French catheter over it into the portal vein [7].

Once the 5 French catheter is in the portal vein, catheter exchanges can be performed over heavy-duty guidewires (Rosen, Amplatz, or Lunderquist exchange guidewires). The firm steel shaft of the Lunderquist and Amplatz exchange guidewires, with attached floppy tip, is particularly useful when a hard and fibrotic liver causes resistance to passing the catheter, which can buckle between the liver edge and abdominal wall. Under these circumstances, an additional helpful maneuver is to introduce an overlying thin-walled sheath together with the catheter over the guidewire. This helps when an existing fluid-filled space must be bridged as with ascites or when there is a particularly firm cirrhotic liver. Catheter manipulations and exchanges are considerably easier with this approach [19].

SELECTIVE CATHETERIZATION OF PORTAL VEIN RADICALS. This requires a catheter with a simple multipurpose "hockey stick" distal curve or a "cobra" curve. A 5 French diameter often is satisfactory if advanced over a leading guidewire with an easily reshapable flexible tip (Ring, USCI).[3] This guidewire-catheter combination can be very effective. Larger 6.5 French torque-controlled catheters may be more manageable if cirrhosis or ascites prevents use of these smaller catheters.

At this point, pressure measurements should be made. Contrast injections outline portal venous pathology (Fig. 23-4). At the completion of the study, a clot or a small plug of Gelfoam is injected into the liver parenchyma as the catheter is being removed to prevent intraperitoneal bleeding from the puncture site.

TRANSJUGULAR VEIN APPROACH. The right inter-nal jugular vein is entered percutaneously (see Chap. 3), and an 8 French catheter with a gentle distal curve is introduced and passed beyond the superior vena cava, right atrium, and inferior vena cava to enter the right hepatic vein (Fig. 23-5). A long needle of matching curvature but 2 cm longer (cardiac transseptal needle) is introduced with its tip still sheathed within the distal catheter. The direction that the curved needle tip is pointing is marked externally by a directing arrow. With the catheter and needle securely in the right hepatic vein, the tip is directed posteromedially toward the portahepatis. The needle is advanced 2 to 3 cm beyond the catheter tip into the liver parenchyma, and the catheter advanced to the needle tip. The needle is then withdrawn, and test injections with slow withdrawal show either contrast medium accumulation within the parenchyma, flow of contrast medium peripherally into the portal veins, slow filling of biliary ducts, or central flow into the hepatic veins. Occasionally, small vascular structures representing hepatic lymphatics are opacified. When the portal vein is recognized, advance a guidewire through the catheter deep into the vein and follow this with the catheter. An angiogram is performed following pressure measurements. If the 8 French catheter cannot be manipulated beyond the portal vein and into the target vein, a 5 French polyethylene catheter may be advanced coaxially and positioned through the 8 French catheter. Angiographic procedures or embolic therapy can then be performed.

INTRAOPERATIVE STUDY. An intraoperative technique as the primary method of evaluating the portal system causes increased operation time. Since seriographic film changers are often not available in the operating room, complete angiographic evaluation by this method is rarely available. A small surgical "minilaparotomy" may be performed in the angiography room. A jejunal portal radicle is isolated and catheterized. Diagnostic angiographic and intravascular therapeutic embolic procedures may be done under fluoroscopic guidance and recorded with standard or digital subtraction techniques [1].

CONTRAST AGENTS, PROJECTIONS, AND RADIOGRAPHIC PROGRAMMING

Details concerning contrast agents, projections, and radiographic programming in direct portal venography are given in Table 23-1.

---

[2]Cook, Inc.
[3]USCI, a division of C. R. Bard, Inc., Box 566, Billerica, MA 08121.

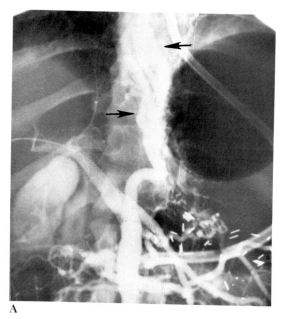

A

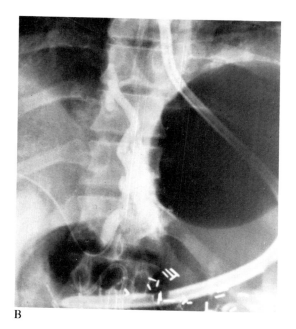

B

Fig. 23-4. Esophageal varices in a young cirrhotic man with occluded Warren shunt. Variceal bleeding (identified by endoscopy) could not be controlled by vasopressin infusion or other methods.

A. Transhepatic portal venogram shows large coronary vein feeding esophageal varices (*arrows*).

B. Bleeding stopped after the varices were occluded by Gelfoam emboli introduced through a catheter selectively placed (with the help of an external deflector) into the coronary vein.

Comments

PRECAUTIONS

1. Prior to direct portal venography, check for blood dyscrasias, noting particularly the prothrombin time and platelet count. Ascitic fluid should be removed if a direct splenic or transhepatic approach is being considered.

2. Inform the surgeons of the projected time of study. Emergency surgery may be required on rare occasions in case the spleen or liver is lacerated or bleeding occurs.

3. Both measured speed and minimal manipulation are essential in splenic punctures; the total

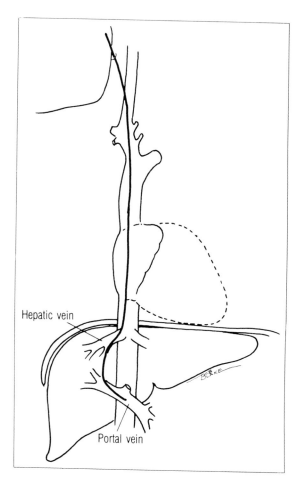

Fig. 23-5. Transjugular approach to direct portal venography. The same approach may be used for cholangiography and for liver biopsy.

Table 23-1. Technical specifications in direct portal venography[a]

Angiographic procedure	Contrast agent			Total films	Total time (sec)	Radiographic program (films/sec)[b]	Projection
	Density	Volume	Rate (ml/sec)				
Adults	M	40 to 50	8	20	16	2/sec for 4 sec; 1/sec for 12 sec	AP[c] (include lower thorax and upper abdomen with patient in mid-respiration)
Children	L	1.5–2.0 ml/kg	5–8	20	16	Same as for adults	Same as for adults

[a] See Chapter 13 for direct-puncture DSA technique using a thin needle and smaller doses (15–25 ml) of low-density (30 to 40%) contrast agent.
[b] Start filming at the start of the injection.
[c] May be performed in the prone position in order to obtain more complete filling of the intrahepatic venous radicles.
M = medium-density contrast agent; L = low-density contrast agent (see Appendix 3).

time from puncture to injection of contrast medium should be less than 5 minutes. A more leisurely approach is permissible with the other techniques.

4. While removing the needle in a transhepatic or direct splenic approach, close the needle track as a potential source of hemorrhage by injecting small quantities of clot or Gelfoam. Do not inject these emboli into the hepatic or portal veins.

NORMAL FINDINGS

1. The normal pressure of the splenic pulp and splenic vein is 10 to 15 cm H_2O (1.32 cm H_2O equals 1 mm Hg).
2. The diameter of the splenic vein is normally 1.0 to 1.5 cm, and that of the portal vein 2 cm. Both veins have a relatively straight course. The intrahepatic portal radicles are straight and extend out to the periphery of the liver. The normal transit time from spleen to liver is 2.5 seconds. The hepatogram lasts for 10 to 20 seconds. See Chapter 13 for a description of the normal portal venous anatomy.

Localizing Functioning Pancreatic Tumors by Portal Venous Sampling

Since venous sampling helps to localize functioning pancreatic tumors [2, 10], it is important to stress the *pancreatic venous anatomy* [15]. The distribution of the pancreatic veins corresponds roughly to that of the pancreatic arteries. Blood from the head of the pancreas drains into the superior mesenteric vein (SMV) and directly into the portal vein. Both the anterior superior pancreaticoduodenal vein (ASPDV) and the common trunk of the inferior pancreaticoduodenal vein (IPDV) drain into the SMV; the former (ASPDV) by way of a gastrocolic trunk on the right and the latter (IPDV) into a proximal jejunal branch on the left side of the SMV. The posterior superior pancreaticoduodenal vein (PSPDV) enters the portal vein directly, on its posteroinferior border approximately 2 cm distal to its origin. The dorsal pancreatic vein receives blood from the proximal body and head of the pancreas and enters the junction of the SMV and splenic vein. Many small veins drain from the body and tail of the pancreas into the adjacent splenic vein. Much of the pancreatic body is also drained by the transverse pancreatic vein, which enters into the inferior mesenteric vein, the upper part of the SMV, or the distal portion of the splenic vein.

ISLET CELL TUMORS

Islet cell tumors may be nonfunctioning or may secrete insulin, gastrin, glucagon, somatostatin, or vasoactive intestinal or pancreatic polypeptides. They may be solitary or multiple, diffuse or malignant (particularly gastrinomas). Instead of tumors, there may be islet cell hyperplasia or proliferation of endocrine cells in the pancreatic duct (nesidioblastosis). The precise location of a functioning tumor is sometimes difficult to determine. If imaging methods fail, selective pancreatic arteriography may be necessary and is sometimes successful.

Surgery may be difficult because of the variety of presentations of these tumors, their soft consistency, and their sometimes small size. Selective pancreatic venous sampling may help direct the surgeon to the area of concern.

Selective pancreatic venous sampling may present a precise localizing hormonal gradient (Fig. 23-6) at the site of the tumor. If multiple areas show high readings, a more diffuse process is suspected and the surgeon is forewarned. Falsely high readings may be seen as a result of collateral draining veins. Instead of selective pancreatic venous sampling of the pancreatic veins, multiple samples obtained 1.5 to 2 cm apart along the course of the entire splenic vein, upper SMV, and extrahepatic portal vein may also be useful [2].

Fig. 23-6. Functioning gastrin-secreting islet cell tumor.
A and B. Pancreatic arteriogram. Tumor blush seen on capillary phase of examination (B, *arrows*).
C and D. Collection of venous samples from pancreatic veins. Catheter tip in right gastrocolic trunk (C) (the anterior superior pancreaticoduodenal vein drains into this). Catheter tip in dorsal pancreatic vein (D). Marked elevation of gastrin levels from the dorsal pancreatic vein. (See text; see also Chap. 13.)

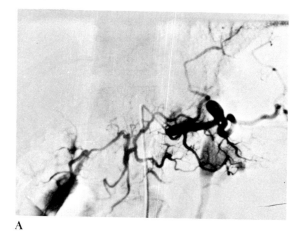

A

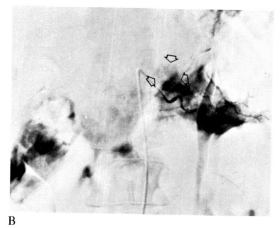

B

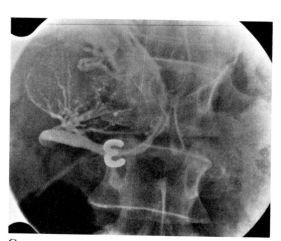

C

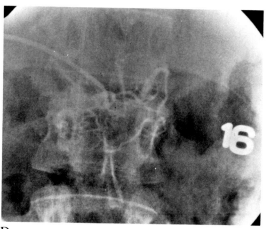

D

Angiographic Abnormalities

1. Demonstration of collateral portal veins indicates *portal hypertension* (see Chap. 13). Other findings include increased angulation of the junction between splenic vein and portal vein, and increased diameter and tortuosity of the splenic vein. As increasing hepatic resistance decreases portal venous flow, the diameter of the portal vein decreases. In severe cirrhosis this diameter progressively decreases until there is complete occlusion due to thrombosis. Since percutaneous transhepatic entry is difficult or impossible under these circumstances, prior indirect portal venography is justified. In portal hypertension with severe liver disease, intrahepatic portal branches show gnarling, tortuosity, and poor filling out to the periphery of the liver. Large collateral channels may replace the portal vein in the region of the portahepatis in patients with cavernous transformation due to old portal vein thrombosis. Primary or secondary tumors may invade, displace, stenose, or occlude the portal vein.
2. The splenic vein may be occluded by surgery or trauma or by diseases in nearby organs (e.g., chronic pancreatitis, carcinoma of the pancreas). Both the portal and splenic veins can occlude spontaneously subsequent to hypercoagulable states.

Pitfalls of Direct Portal Venography

A patent portal vein may not fill by direct splenic pulp injection, erroneously suggesting thrombosis. This nonfilling is due to preferential flow to a low-resistance variceal collection that diverts the contrast medium from the high-resistance portal venous bed. To confirm the diagnosis of thrombosis, one must demonstrate the collateral channels surrounding the portal vein by other techniques, such as indirect portography or hepatic venous wedge injections.

Direct Versus Indirect Portal Venography

DIRECT PORTAL VENOGRAPHY
The advantages of direct portal venography are as follows:

1. There is better opacification due to direct injection of contrast medium into the venous system.
2. Direct pressure measurements of the splenic pulp or portal system can be obtained.

The disadvantages are that

1. It cannot be performed if there is not a spleen present, and it is dangerous if the spleen is very friable.
2. A severe bleeding diathesis precludes direct organ puncture.
3. Complications related to splenic or hepatic trauma and hemorrhage are possible.

INDIRECT PORTAL VENOGRAPHY
The advantages of indirect portal venography are

1. It does not injure the spleen or liver.
2. It can usually be accomplished in the presence of a bleeding diathesis.
3. One can evaluate the portal system if the spleen is absent.
4. One can evaluate any underlying pathologic condition by studying the arterial pattern of liver, pancreas, gut, and spleen.

The disadvantages are as follows:

1. The venous opacification may not be adequate, particularly in severe portal hypertension. It is improved by using vasodilating drugs. These drugs are contraindicated in patients who are actively bleeding at the time of the study.
2. Splenic pulp and direct portal venous pressure measurements are not possible.

These different approaches are not mutually exclusive; if one approach does not give the required information, another should be tried.

Transcatheter Therapy in the Portal System

EMBOLIC OCCLUSION OF PORTAL VARICES
Indications
Transhepatic embolic occlusion of acutely bleeding varices is a stopgap measure to arrest hemorrhage and provides an opportunity for elective

rather than emergency portosystemic shunt procedures [11, 12, 20]. It is occasionally indicated in patients who have recently stopped bleeding but who refuse surgery or who are poor operative risks. It can be used when previous surgery did not include ligation of the gastric veins or in patients with failed surgical shunts. It should be performed after endoscopy confirms the varices as the source of the bleeding and after failure of other less invasive methods of therapy (e.g., intravenous vasopressin infusion [see Chap. 13], fresh frozen plasma, inflated Sengstaken-Blakemore tube, endoscopic sclerotherapy).

Comments
Conditions are rarely optimal for therapeutic embolization of gastroesophageal bleeding. Embolizations are usually performed as an emergency procedure in a patient with poor liver function, often with an encephalopathy and suboptimal bleeding parameters (Childs class C). Ascites and a fibrotic liver distort the anatomy, and a small or occluded portal vein may further frustrate both entering it and passing a catheter. Venous collaterals from multiple areas often drain into the gastroesophageal veins, requiring a prolonged procedure if the embolization is to be complete. Radiation exposure both to the operator and to the patient is high. Possible complications of the procedure include intraabdominal bleeding, bleeding or effusion into the pleural space, laceration of the liver, and infected ascites. Emboli reflux into the intrahepatic portal venous radicles with resulting portal vein thrombosis. They can pass through portosystemic collaterals into the lungs or through portopulmonary venous anastomoses [12, 17].

The natural history of the disease is progressive and rebleeding often occurs, if not through recanalized venous channels, then through other newly opened collateral channels.

Despite these often desperate conditions, the success rate for occluding veins and helping patients in the acute state is reported variably from 40 percent [13] to 95 percent [20]. Absence of recurrent bleeding for 1 year (in those successfully occluded) has been reported in up to 70 percent, and after 2 years in approximately 60 percent [20]. In general, the outcome for most of these patients is dismal, and the majority of those who survive are those who were initially in better clinical condition (Childs class B).

Preliminary indirect portography determines the patency and location of the portal vein, the location of portosystemic venous collaterals, and the extent of hepatofugal (partial or complete) versus hepatopetal flow. Those with complete hepatofugal flow are poor candidates for percutaneous transhepatic embolization of varices [12].

Technique
Review earlier sections in this chapter regarding technique of percutaneous transhepatic catheter placement, and Chapter 5 for details on the methods and materials for embolization. Consider the following additional points:

1. After successfully advancing the catheter, perform an angiogram with the catheter tip close to the splenic hilum, sometimes with the catheter in the superior mesenteric vein, and subsequently selectively in the veins feeding the varices. Deflate the Sengstaken-Blakemore tube before the angiogram to encourage filling of all veins and possible portosystemic anastomoses.

   All veins feeding the bleeding varices must be uncovered to ensure a complete embolization procedure. Try to uncover all spontaneous portosystemic shunts and portohepatic anastomoses and anomalies prior to embolization to preclude emboli entering into nontarget areas. Be particularly aware of potential anastomoses or communications between the gastric and renal veins (more often on the left) (Fig. 23-7); mesenteric and retroperitoneal veins; gastric and pericardial veins; paramediastinal and paraesophageal veins and the pulmonary veins [17]. Emboli deposited here may go directly to the lungs. The left branch of the portal vein may arise anomalously from the left gastric vein. The left gastric vein has an anterior branch, which typically feeds the esophageal varices; it should be embolized. The left gastric vein also has a posterior branch that enters the azygos and hemiazygos system; it must be avoided [18]. If there has previously been a Warren shunt that has occluded, or the splenic vein pressures in the venous system feeding the varices are much higher than in the portal vein, emboli may migrate to the portal vein.

2. The catheter tip must be well within the target vein feeding the varices prior to embolization.

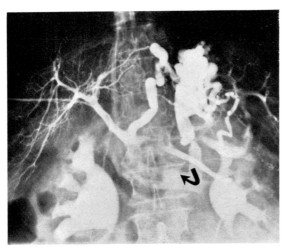

Fig. 23-7. Transhepatic portogram demonstrating a large gastrorenal anastomosis and narrowed anastomotic site.

A variety of embolic agents may be used. These include liquid (absolute alcohol, tissue adhesives [bucrylate]); particulate materials (Gelfoam mixed with Sotradecol; coils [with added thrombin]; Ivalon; Ivalon and Gelfoam mixture). If esophageal azygos communications are open, inflate the Sengstaken-Blakemore tube before embolizing esophageal varices to prevent embolization into communicating systemic and pulmonary veins.

LIQUID EMBOLIC AGENTS

1. Bucrylate [11]: Advance a small 3 French coaxial catheter 1 cm beyond the tip of the overlying 5 French thin-walled catheter. Infuse isotonic glucose solution through both catheters. Mix 1 ml bucrylate with 1 ml of Pantopaque or Lipiodol and attach to a three-way stopcock on the inner catheter.

   While continuously infusing the outer catheter with glucose solution, inject 0.5 to 1.0 ml of the bucrylate mixture (in a tuberculin syringe) into the inner catheter and follow immediately with a flush of nonionic 5% glucose solution attached to the other port of the three-way stopcock. Immediately withdraw both catheters slightly to prevent fixation of the catheter tip to the wall of the vein. Repeat the angiogram, and follow with additional injections either into the same vein or into additional veins as required.

2. Absolute alcohol: Absolute alcohol can be injected through a similar coaxial system described for tissue adhesives or through open-ended injectable guidewires fed well up into the target vein. Five or six milliliters of absolute alcohol is injected at one time; this dose may be repeated. A slow injection prevents reflux into the portal vein. A 6 French occlusive balloon catheter may be advanced through an overlying 7 French sheath into the orifice of the gastric vein feeding the varices and inflated before administering the alcohol. Since emboli may enter the systemic arterial circulation through portal pulmonary venous anastomoses, absolute alcohol may be the embolic agent of choice for occluding esophageal varices; the alcohol is too dilute to cause damage once it enters the pulmonary vein.

PARTICULATE MATERIALS

1. Gelfoam dipped in 3% Sotradecol (sodium tetradecyl sulfate, a sclerosing agent). Cut pieces of Gelfoam, soak in Sotradecol, and place in a tuberculin syringe. Inject slowly, forcing the embolus along the course of the catheter into the varix. When resistance to the injection is decreased, the embolus has extruded into the vein, and the force of the injection should be eased. Repeat the procedure until the varices are occluded (Fig. 23-8). Reflux of the emboli into the portal vein may be prevented if contrast agent or saline is injected as the catheter is removed from the occluded vein. A steel coil of appropriate helix diameter may also be used for this purpose.

2. Ivalon particles (250 to 500 μm), either alone or mixed with Gelfoam particles, may also be introduced, but large quantities would be required to fill the vascular bed.

TREATMENT OF OCCLUDED SURGICAL PORTOSYSTEMIC SHUNTS (See Chap. 7)

Surgical portosystemic decompression shunts may become stenosed or totally occluded. They may be catheterized through the systemic side of the shunt, and the clot suctioned through a large sheath or lysed with local urokinase infusion. The dangers of bleeding from the underlying varices due to focal thrombolytic therapy must be care-

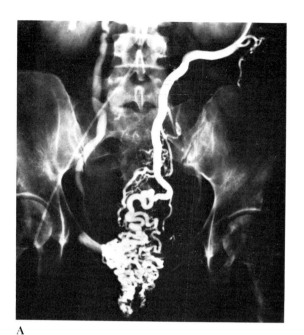

A

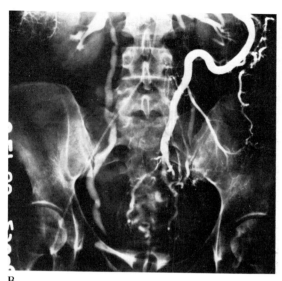

B

Fig. 23-8.
A. Massive hemorrhoids in patient with severe rectal bleeding and portal hypertension. Inferior mesenteric portal venogram.
B. Postembolization. Bleeding stopped, but recurred 6 months later.

fully weighed against those of an occluding shunt. Any stenosis present may be dilated with appropriate diameter dilation balloon catheters.

TRANSCATHETER FORMATION
OF PORTOSYSTEMIC SHUNTS

If there is severe portal hypertension and the patient is not a good surgical candidate, a portosystemic shunt may be attempted using intravascular catheter techniques. A catheter is introduced through a standard transjugular approach, advanced into the posteromedial right hepatic vein, and the portal vein entered as described earlier. Once the 8 French catheter lies within the portal vein, a long heavy-duty guidewire is passed well into the superior mesenteric vein or splenic vein. The catheter is replaced with an 8 or 9 French diameter catheter with a 10-mm 4-cm inflatable balloon. Following inflation, the portosystemic shunt is formed and tends to remain open. Expandable shunt stents between the portal vein and the hepatic vein are still in the experimental phase [14].

References

1. Braun, S., Newman, G., and Dunnick, N. Digital splenal portography. A.J.R. 144:1003, 1985.
2. Cho, K., et al. Localization of the source of hyperinsulinism. Percutaneous transhepatic portal and pancreatic vein catheterization with hormone assay. A.J.R. 139:237, 1982.
3. Colapinto, R., et al. Formation of intrahepatic portosystemic shunts using a balloon dilatation catheter: Preliminary clinical experience. A.J.R. 140:709, 1983.
4. Doppman, J., et al. The role of pancreatic venous sampling in the localization of occult insulinomas. Radiology 138:557, 1981.
5. Goldman, M., Fajmen, W., and Galambos, J. Transjugular obliteration of the gastric coronary vein. Radiology 118:452, 1976.
6. Gothlin, J., et al. Technique and complications of transumbilical catheterization of the portal vein and its tributaries. Am. J. Roentgenol. 125:431, 1975.
7. Hawkins, I., Jr. New fine needle for cholangiography with optimal sheath for decompression. Radiology 131:252, 1979.
8. Kessler, R., and Zimmon, D. Umbilical vein angiography. Radiology 87:841, 1966.
9. Leger, L. Splenoportography: Diagnostic Phlebography of the Portal Vein System. Springfield, IL: Thomas, 1966.
10. Lunderquist, A., Erikisson, M., and Ingenmansson, S. Selective pancreatic vein catheterization for hormone assay in endocrine tumors of the pancreas. Cardiovasc. Radiol. 1:117, 1978.

11. Lunderquist, A., Hoevels, J., and Owman, T. Transhepatic Portal Venography. In H. Abrams (ed.), *Abrams' Angiography: Vascular and Interventional Radiology* (3rd ed.). Boston: Little, Brown, 1983. Pp. 1505–1529.

12. Mendez, G., and Russel, E. Gastrointestinal varices: Percutaneous transhepatic therapeutic embolization in 54 patients. *A.J.R.* 135:1042, 1980.

13. Ohto, M., et al. Ultrasonically guided percutaneous contrast medium injection and aspiration biopsy using a real-time puncture transducer. *Radiology* 136:171, 1980.

14. Palmay, J., et al. Expandable intrahepatic portocaval shunt stents: Early experience in the dog. *A.J.R.* 145:821, 1985.

15. Reichardt, W., and Cameron, R. Anatomy of the pancreatic veins. A post mortem and clinical phlebographic investigation. *Acta Radiol. [Diagn.] (Stockh.)* 21:33, 1980.

16. Rosch, J., and Dotter, C. Retrograde pancreatic venography: An experimental study. *Radiology* 114:275, 1975.

17. Sano, R., et al. Portopulmonary venous anastomosis in portal hypertension demonstrated by percutaneous transhepatic cineportography. *Radiology* 144:479, 1982.

18. Takahasi, M., et al. Esophageal varices: Correlation of left gastric venography and endoscopy in patients with portal hypertension. *Radiology* 155:327, 1985.

19. Viamonte, M., Jr., et al. Pitfalls in transhepatic portography. *Radiology* 124:324, 1977.

20. Widrich, W., Robbins, A., and Nabseth, D. Transhepatic embolization of varices. *Cardiovasc. Intervent. Radiol.* 3:298, 1980.

21. Yune, H., et al. Absolute ethanol in thrombotherapy of bleeding esophageal varices. *A.J.R.* 138:1137, 1982.

Lymphography

The lymphatic system includes several hundred grams of highly organized lymph tissue connected centrally and peripherally by a network of lymph vessels. These vessels originate peripherally in perivascular spaces and form a fine, freely anastomosing capillary system into which fluid collects from the body tissues by osmosis, diffusion, and filtration. The system is involved in the defense of the body against invading organisms and in immunologic reactions, which include the production of antibodies and lymphocytes. It is also involved in the return of excess tissue fluid, especially proteins, to the circulation.

A variety of diseases, both benign and malignant, affect the lymph nodes and vessels. A number of radiologic methods have been used to evaluate the lymph system, particularly the portion, difficult to evaluate clinically, in the abdomen and thorax. Lymphography is the radiographic study of contrast-filled nodes and vessels. In this procedure, oily contrast medium is injected into a surgically exposed peripheral lymphatic vessel, and its course is followed radiographically to the more centrally located nodes; opacification remains for several months. There are other methods that may be used to study the lymphatic system. Imaging modalities, which include ultrasonography and computed tomography (CT), also provide useful information.

Because CT and lymphography are complementary, many authors suggest using both in the staging of carcinoma and lymphoma. Computed tomography provides excellent delineation of enlarged lymph nodes and also contributes information about tumor spread beyond the lymphatic system. Lymphography can detect tumor in normal size lymph nodes by demonstrating an abnormal internal nodal architecture. In some cases lymphography can differentiate benign from malignant causes of lymphadenopathy.

Indications for Lymphography

1. Malignant adenopathy
   a. Lymphoma: Determining stage of disease, response to therapy, radiotherapy portals
   b. Metastatic disease: Particularly from primary disease of the cervix, ovary, uterus, testicle, and prostate; occasionally other tumors, such as melanoma
2. Pathologic conditions of lymph vessels
   a. Lymphedema
      (1) Secondary: Obstruction of lymph vessels by tumor, radiotherapy, surgery, trauma, inflammation, parasitic infestation
      (2) Primary: Congenital abnormality of lymph vessels: hypoplastic (Milroy's disease, lymphedema praecox, lymphedema tarda); aplastic; hyperplastic
   b. Lymph vessel tumors
3. Study of chyluria, chylous ascites, chylothorax, and protein-losing enteropathy
4. Aid in adenectomy
5. Aid in localizing abnormal nodes for percutaneous biopsy

Anatomic Considerations [31, 41]

In the lower extremities, superficial and deep lymphatic vessels follow the saphenous and deep veins of the leg to drain into inguinal nodes (Figs. 24-1, 24-2). As in nodes elsewhere, afferent lymphatic vessels enter the capsule of each node on its convex side. They drain through a collection of sinusoids, which radiate to the hilus of the node and leave the node through efferent vessels. From the inguinal chain, the lymphatics drain into external and common iliac chains. There are usually three of these chains, coursing in close relationship to the iliac arteries and veins to join the paraaortic chains (Fig. 24-3). The hypogastric nodes receive drainage from the pelvic viscera, perineum, and gluteal area. Not being primarily injected with contrast medium, these nodes are rarely opacified during pedal lymphography. The paraaortic chains are comprised of four general groups of glands, which are named according to their relationship to the aorta: left and right lateral, retroaortic, and preaortic glands. Generally these nodes lie within 2 cm lateral and 3 cm anterior to the vertebral bodies (Fig. 24-4). Afferent vessels that drain structures such as the kidneys, adrenals, gonads, gut, and

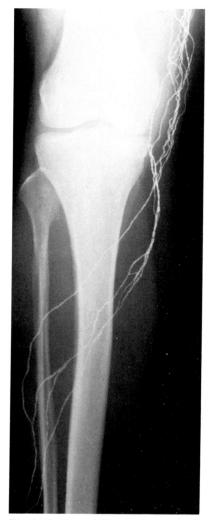

Fig. 24-1. Normal lymphatic vessels of the lower extremity.

retroperitoneal area also drain into these paraaortic chains. Under normal circumstances, nodes in the right paraaortic chain often do not fill above the third lumbar vertebra. In addition, one may see retrograde flow of contrast medium into lymphatics surrounding the celiac axis farther than the

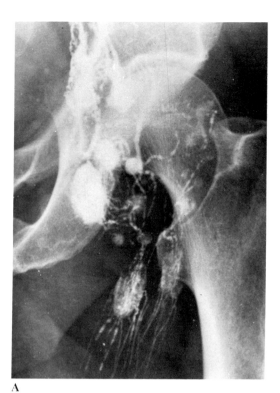

A

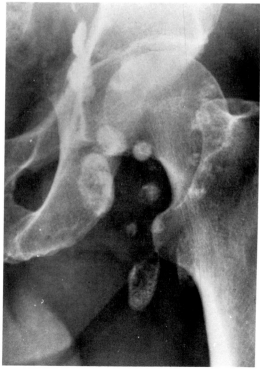

B

Fig. 24-2. Superficial inguinal nodes (inferior chain) filled by pedal lymphography.
A. Vascular phase. The afferent vessels enter the periphery of the node, and efferent vessels leave through the hilus of the node.
B. Well-marginated lymph nodes. The most inferior node is partially replaced with involutional changes of fibrosis and fatty replacement (fibrolipomatosis).

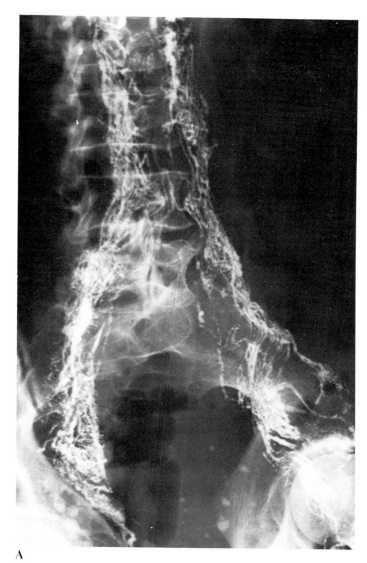
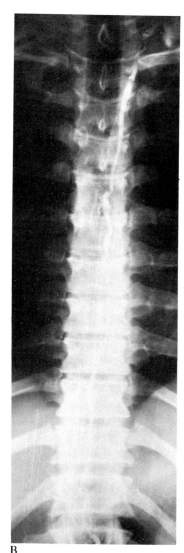

A

B

Fig. 24-3.
A. Normal lymphogram (LPO projection). Vascular phase.
B. Normal thoracic duct.

usual 3 cm from the anterior boundary of the vertebral bodies. In the abdomen, lymph collects into a localized dilatation that lies just anterior to the first two lumbar vertebrae, a structure called the *cisterna chyli*. From here lymph flow continues cephalad through the thoracic duct to enter the systemic circulation at the junction of the left subclavian and internal jugular veins.

Roentgenograms taken during or immediately after the injection outline lymphatic vessels as slightly beaded channels following fairly straight lines that communicate between the various nodal chains. The lymph vessels are usually emptied of contrast agent 4 hours after completion of the injection, and the contrast agent remains sequestered within the network of the nodes for periods of 6 to 18 months.

Normal lymph nodes have the following characteristics:

1. They are variable in size (less than 3 cm), oval or kidney-shaped, and usually flat in one dimension. They are largest in the inguinal chains and smallest in the paraaortic chains.

630

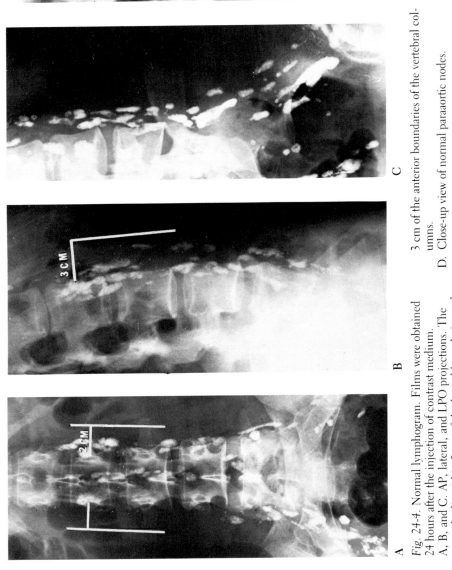

Fig. 24-4. Normal lymphogram. Films were obtained 24 hours after the injection of contrast medium. A, B, and C. AP, lateral, and LPO projections. The nodes lie within 2 cm of the lateral boundaries and 3 cm of the anterior boundaries of the vertebral columns.
D. Close-up view of normal paraaortic nodes.

2. They have a regular contour.
3. They have a smooth margin except in the paraaortic nodes, where they have a slightly feathery appearance.
4. There may be a central filling defect corresponding to the hilus; this can be recognized by referring to the vascular phase of the study and identifying the site of efferent vessels.
5. They have a homogeneous, reticular, somewhat granular pattern.
6. They have a close relationship to larger vessels, with little displacement from adjacent bony structures (within 2 cm lateral to the vertebral body and 3 cm anterior to it).

Technique

When radiopaque contrast medium is introduced into the lymphatic channels, not only the lymphatic vascular system but also the nodal component of the lymphatic apparatus may be studied. The slow rate of flow and the small size of the vessels requiring cannulation require special considerations in techniques of opacification of the lymphatic system.

SURGICAL TECHNIQUE (Fig. 24-5A, B, C)
Equipment
The equipment required for performing a lymphographic procedure is listed below:

1. FD&C blue dye No. 1.[1] This dye is specially prepared and sterilized.[2]
2. Sterile tray, containing:
   Lidocaine 1% (do not use a mixture with epinephrine).
   Commercially available 27- or 30-gauge needle with attached polyethylene tubing[3] or Tegtmeyer lymph duct cannulator.[4]
   Thumb forceps.[5]
   Mosquito forceps.[6]
   4-0 silk.

[1] Allied Chemical, Industrial Chemical Division, Morristown, NJ 07960.
[2] See Appendix 14.
[3] Becton-Dickinson, Rutherford, NJ 07070.
[4] North American Instrument Corp. (Hospital Supply Division), Hudson Falls, NY 12839.
[5] Iris forceps 3-154, Weck Eye Instruments, Long Island City, NY 11101.
[6] Jacobson mosquito forceps CVD CH8610, American Hospital Supply Corp., Chicago, IL 60648.

5-ml syringe with 25-gauge needle (for local anesthetic).
   10-ml syringe (for injecting sterile saline).
   Sterile saline solution.
   Sterile drapes.
   Sterile sponges.
3. Contrast medium and injector:
   Ethiodol,[7] two 10-ml vials.
   Simple 10-ml syringes powered by gravity and weights, *or* automatic injector.[8]
4. Binocular magnification glasses.
5. Adequate lighting.
6. Radiographic facilities for monitoring contrast medium injection.

Procedure
Blue aniline dye (FD&C No. 1), 0.25 ml, is injected intracutaneously into the two webs between the first three toes of each foot. The dye is absorbed by the lymphatic vessels and becomes visible on the skin of the dorsum of the foot within 20 minutes. (Warn the patient that he will excrete the dye in his urine.) Once experience in identifying these lymphatic channels has been gained, lymphography may be performed without the use of blue dye [27]. This eliminates one of the more painful steps in the study and precludes the possibility of an allergic response. Prepare the feet with antiseptic solution, and make a short, very superficial incision over the largest visible lymphatic channel. Choose the more medial lymphatic vessels lying over the upper third of the dorsum of the foot, since these vessels are generally larger. The incision can be transverse or longitudinal. Dissect the vessel free from surrounding tissues, and place a loosely knotted suture just distal to the intended site of entry. Loosely drape the attached saline-filled polyethylene tube over the toes so that when released, the needle will not recoil due to unwanted torque. Securing one of the ties in the forefingers of the hand holding the lymphatic-draped forceps, lightly elevate the lymphatic vessel and (with the bevel of the needle facing upward) pierce its anterior wall. The needle should be almost parallel to the vessel at this point in order to prevent piercing the posterior wall. Magnifying glasses are particularly helpful at this point in the procedure. Now advance the needle until the

[7] Savage Laboratories, Missouri City, TX 77459.
[8] Cordis Corporation, Miami, FL 33137.

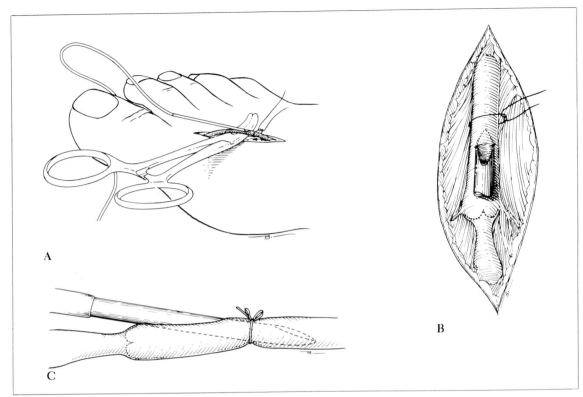

Fig. 24-5. Surgical technique of lymphography (drawing is not to scale; actual size of the vessel is considerably smaller). See text for details.

A. A longitudinal incision is made over the mid- to upper third of the dorsum of the foot medially, directly over a lymphatic vessel that has been made visible by blue dye. Clean off the surrounding perivascular tissues. Drape the needle and attached polyethylene tubing through the toes of the foot. Apply a loosely knotted tie.

B. With the fingers of the hand holding the forceps, secure one end of the tie. Advance the needle parallel to the lymphatic vessel, bevel up, through the anterior wall of the vessel. Dilate the vessel with saline as soon as the bevel is covered.

C. Advance the needle into the dilated lymphatic vessel and secure the knot.

bevel is completely covered. A slow injection of saline solution through the needle by an assistant will dilate the vessel and protect the lymphatic walls from inadvertent puncture as the needle is advanced another 2 or 3 mm. Release the needle and tighten the knot. Fixate the polyethylene tubing with tape and attach the injector for the slow injection of oily contrast medium.

An alternate method of entering the lymphatics by using a lymphatic duct cannulator has been described by Tegtmeyer [44] (Fig. 24-6). The greatest advantage of this method is that it is a guided system for the less experienced lymphographer. It is also a more stable method and prevents the displacement of the needle in the restless patient. This technique also has disadvantages, however. If the vessel is punctured with unsuccessful entry, it can no longer be distended. In addition, there are limitations as to the size of the vessel that can be cannulated; this is particularly true in patients with sclerosed small lymphatics as seen in chronic lymphedema.

Technical pitfalls to be avoided are as follows:

1. Stripping off small lymphatic tributaries that will subsequently leak.
2. Penetrating the posterior wall of the lymphatic. To avoid this, keep the needle parallel with the bevel up, dilate the vessel with saline, use magnifying glasses.
3. Placing the needle in perivascular tissues rather

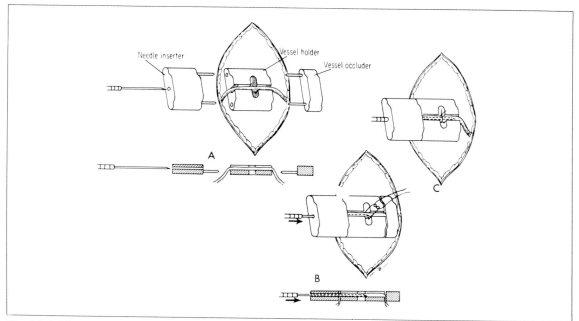

Fig. 24-6. The Tegtmeyer technique. The lymph duct cannulator has three separate components made of plastic: a lymph duct holder, a lymph duct occluder, and a needle inserter.

A. The lymphatic vessel is surgically isolated using a transverse incision and is placed in the groove of the lymph duct holder. The proximal duct is occluded by a lymph duct occluder, which distends the lymphatic vessel preparatory to puncture.

B. A needle inserter with a precut hole is moved into place, and the needle is guided into the distended lymphatic. The inserter anchors the needle in place, but for added safety a 4-0 silk suture is tied around the lymphatic.

C. The lymphatic occluder is removed prior to the injection of contrast medium.

than within the lumen. Milk the blue dye cephalad into the lymphatic just prior to insertion by massaging the webs of the toes. Clean the vessel adequately.

4. Inserting the needle at the level of the lymphatic valves. These valves narrow the lymphatic diameter considerably. Introduce the needle cephalad to their location.

5. Injecting contrast medium into a venule rather than a lymphatic (even experienced lymphographers may do this occasionally). Radiographs of the legs should be obtained before 1 ml of contrast has been injected. Look for multiple oily globules (the "caviar" sign) within the vein (Fig. 24-7) as compared with the normal ap-

Fig. 24-7. Oily globules of contrast medium in the vein (*arrowhead*) detected after the injection of 0.5 ml of contrast medium. Compare with the normal lymphatic, which was subsequently cannulated.

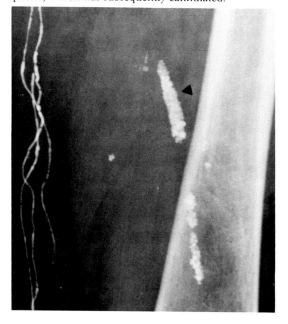

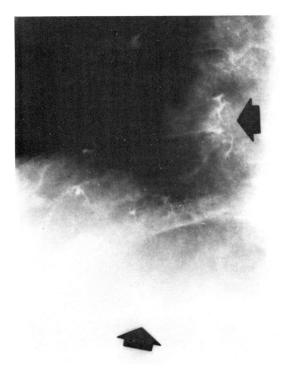

Fig. 24-8. Oily emboli (*arrows*) to the pulmonary microvasculature.

pearance of lymphatics (see Fig. 24-1). This contrast medium will flood the lungs with oily emboli.

6. Injecting large doses of contrast medium in the presence of severe lymphatic obstruction. In such cases there may be a direct communication with a vein as an alternate pathway of central flow, and the lungs may receive an unusually large dose (Fig. 24-8).

7. Extravasation of contrast medium may occur through ruptured lymph vessels. This occurs if too great a pressure is applied to the pump. The patient often complains of pain in the extremity, and the contrast medium does not advance to the pelvic nodes (Fig. 24-9).

CONTRAST AGENT

The contrast medium used in lymphography is a viscid, nondiffusible, radiopaque iodinated ester of poppy seed oil (Ethiodol), which does not diffuse from the lymph vessels and nodes as does aqueous material. The adult dose varies from 5 to 7 ml in each foot, administered slowly over a period of 45 to 60 minutes. In children, the dose is appropri-

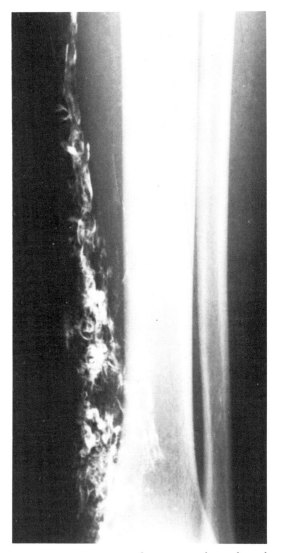

Fig. 24-9. Extravasation of contrast medium along the course of the lymphatic vessel. Another lymphatic must be cannulated for successful completion of the study.

ately lower. There is usually a sufficient amount injected when the contrast column is seen in the lower paraaortic chain.

RADIOGRAPHIC TECHNIQUE

Films of the extremities and of the pelvis are taken early and then again later in the course of the injection for monitoring purposes. The set of films taken immediately postinjection shows the vascular filling phase and allows evaluation of the dynamics of lymph flow. Another set, taken 24 hours later, shows the lymph nodes alone after the channels have emptied. High-contrast, well-coned films, usually with a maximum of 75 kV on the lateral projection and 60 to 65 kV on the anteroposterior and oblique projections, with high milliamperage and short exposure times, are obtained in multiple projections. The usual films taken are as follows:

1. Anteroposterior (AP) pelvic (17 × 14 in.). For the patient with pelvic metastatic disease, two additional views may be obtained, one with the tube tilted 25 degrees cephalad, the other 25 degrees caudad.
2. AP lumbar.
3. AP thoracic coned to the mediastinum.
4. 45-degree oblique views (right and left) of the abdomen. These films should be centered sufficiently low to capture the pelvic nodes.

All films must be coned to the area of interest. Tomographic studies and magnification films of the opacified lymph nodes occasionally give added information.

LYMPHOGRAPHIC BLIND SPOTS

Even with maximal doses of contrast medium, there are certain areas in which the nodes often do not become opacified and thus remain as "blind spots." These areas include both the deep and the superior group of the superficial inguinal nodes, the hypogastric nodes draining the pelvic viscera, those paraaortic nodes that drain the gonads and gut, and the nodes in the epigastric paraaortic region. Since drainage from the testicles lies centrally in the paraaortic region at the L2 to L3 level, only some of these nodes are seen with bilateral lower extremity injections. Additional nodes may be opacified by cannulating lymphatics within the spermatic cord (Fig. 24-10). Although it is not the rule, occasionally mediastinal and supraclavicular nodes may be filled by the injection of contrast medium into the lymphatics of the legs.

Lymphographic studies of the arms are performed much the same as those of the lower extremities. The vessels on the dorsum of the hand are slightly smaller than those on the feet. Not all of the lymph nodes in the axilla are filled by this technique, particularly those in the first line of

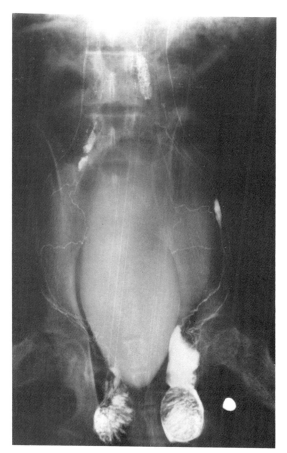

Fig. 24-10. Direct injection of the testis of a dog demonstrates the primary lymphatic pathway to lymph nodes in the paraaortic chain near the renal hilus.

involvement of breast lesions, such as the pectoral, subscapular, and central groups.

Lymphograms of the neck are not generally satisfactory, because all of the cervical nodes on one side cannot be opacified by cannulating a single proximal lymphatic channel.

If lymphedema is of prime concern, films of the extremity obtained during the injection will outline the abnormal vascular patterns accompanying this disease.

Fate of Contrast Medium [20, 21, 45]

That amount of oily contrast medium that is not trapped within the node eventually reaches the pulmonary circulation, since the thoracic duct empties into the junction of the left subclavian vein and the jugular vein. Within the lungs the contrast medium causes a transient blockage of the pulmonary capillaries, causing abnormalities of pulmonary function. These abnormalities include a decrease in pulmonary diffusion capacity, a decrease in capillary blood volume, a decrease in arterial oxygen tension, and an increase in the arterial pH. The contrast medium leaves the lung by (1) entering into the alveoli, (2) passing through the capillaries, (3) passing through shunts into the venous system, and (4) being broken down by enzymatic activity.

Complications

Complications of lymphography [11, 13, 14, 21, 23] may occur, such as chemical pneumonitis and pulmonary infarcts. Other very rare complications include hypotensive reactions, hypertensive reactions, collapse and loss of consciousness, and acute cardiac failure and death. These complications occur only when an overdose of contrast medium enters the lungs or the general arterial circulation (no more than 7 ml of contrast agent is required in each lower extremity in the adult). The elderly patient's lymphatic system undergoes a certain degree of atrophy and may not be able to tolerate a full adult dose. Therefore, a smaller dose should be given to the elderly patient or anyone with atrophy of the lymphatic system. Allergic reactions may occur. Fever with general malaise is a frequently associated finding. Since most of the complications are pulmonary and are related to oily emboli, the dose administered must be related to the tolerance of the lungs. A chest x ray must always be obtained prior to the study. Local complications may also occur in lymphography; these include wound infections, dermatitis, and lymphangitis.

Treatment of complications is symptomatic. Allergic and anaphylactic reactions are treated with steroids, oxygen, antihistamines, and other supportive measures. Rarely, tracheotomy may be necessary if edema of the glottis occurs. If acute cor pulmonale occurs, the patient should be treated for shock with oxygen, digitalis if necessary, and vasopressor drugs. The rate of hydrolysis of the fat may be delayed, with subsequent decrease in chemical toxicity; this is done by administering a lipase inhibitor such as ethyl alcohol either intravenously (2000 ml of 5% ethyl alcohol in 5% dextrose) or orally (30 ml of 50% alcohol every 3 hours).

Contraindications

Contraindications to lymphography include the following:

1. Severe respiratory insufficiency.
2. Right-to-left intracardiac or intrapulmonary shunts.
3. Concurrent radiotherapy to the lungs. Abnormal amounts of contrast medium may pass through the pulmonary circulation and produce cerebral symptoms from oily emboli [13].
4. The presence of marked obstruction, which may open lymphatic venous communications and thereby flood the lungs with contrast medium (see Fig. 24-12).

In the vast majority of patients, lymphography is a minor procedure with no complications.

Angiographic Findings

Lymphography is a rather gross radiographic study. Microscopic pathologic changes may not be detected, and the many areas that are "blind" to evaluation detract from a negative study. Lymphography is helpful when interpreted in the light of a known disease, and when insight into the extent of disease is required. When obvious lymphographic abnormalities are present, the cause of the pathologic process may still be in question. Biopsy or other clinical information is usually required to make a definitive diagnosis.

As in other vascular systems, both morphologic and dynamic abnormalities may be encountered. The dynamic concepts can be studied by evaluating the vascular channels with their portrayal of lymph flow. The static picture of the morphologic anatomy of nodes can be best observed on the 24-hour films.

LYMPHATIC OBSTRUCTION
AND LYMPHEDEMA
Since the lymphatic system is dynamic, it responds to stress as do other vascular systems [47, 50]. If the system is overloaded or obstructed, the vessels become dilated; there may be stasis and collateral flow (Fig. 24-11). Fistulas into the venous system (Fig. 24-12), the peritoneal and pleural spaces, the lumen of the bowel, or the urinary system may occur. The paralymphatic pathways may be filled

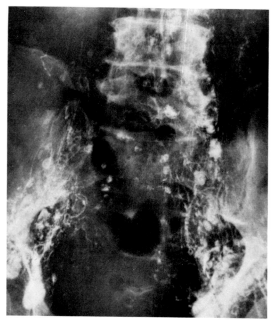

Fig. 24-11. Numerous pelvic and paraaortic collateral channels filling as a result of obstruction in a patient with advanced stages of malignant lymphoma.

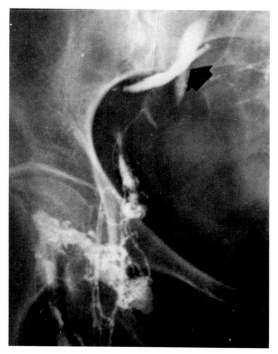

Fig. 24-12. Lymphogram in a patient with metastatic carcinoma of the cervix, causing obstruction of the iliac lymph channels and a lymphatic venous communication in the pelvis. The arrow points to large venous channels.

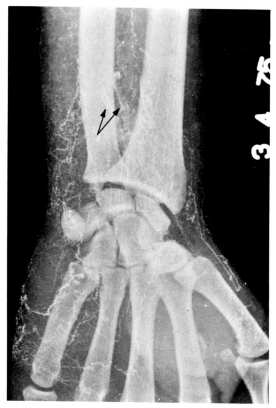

Fig. 24-13. Primary hypoplastic lymphedema of the right arm of a young woman. This film shows "dermal backflow," a fine network of dermal lymphatics that ordinarily do not fill. The arrows point to non-endothelium-lined pathways in the perivascular spaces.

in situations of stress; these are nonendothelium-lined pathways used for the transport of large molecular particles and include potential spaces in the interstitium, pleura, pericardium, peritoneal cavity, submucosal and subadventitial spaces, and perineural and perivascular spaces. *Dermal backflow* is the retrograde filling of dermal lymphatic vessels in the face of obstruction; it has a characteristic appearance (Fig. 24-13). Occasionally, dermal backflow may extend further into small, lymph-filled dermal vesicles.

Acquired Lymphedema

Acquired lymphedema may be secondary to tumor, infection, trauma, surgery, radiotherapy or chemotherapy, and parasitic infestations. In this condition, lymphography can show the abnormal morphology and the site of obstruction. Together with venography, it can show the underlying cause of a swollen limb.

Primary Lymphedema

In primary lymphedema [29, 31] there is no recognized cause for swelling. This condition can be classified on a clinical basis as to the time of appearance, other associated abnormalities, and hereditary characteristics. It can also be classified according to the lymphographically demonstrated morphologic pattern of the lymph structures.

CLINICAL CLASSIFICATION

1. Disease present at birth: Milroy's disease (hereditary autosomal dominant, more frequent in males and in lower limbs).
2. Disease occurring after age 5: Lymphedema praecox (gonadal dysgenesis, pes cavus, other vascular anomalies).
3. Disease occurring after age 35: Lymphedema tarda (more frequent in females).

LYMPHOGRAPHIC CLASSIFICATION (AFTER KIN-MONTH [29])

1. Hypoplastic lymphedema: Occurs in 87 percent of cases; lymph vessels are underdeveloped; includes Milroy's disease, lymphedema praecox, lymphedema tarda (Fig. 24-13).
2. Aplastic lymphedema: Occurs in 5 percent of cases.
3. Hyperplastic lymphedema: Numerous varicosed lymphatics; associated capillary angiomata; is usually unilateral; is more frequent in males (Fig. 24-14).
4. Proximal hypoplasia, distal hyperplasia.

Hyperplastic lymphedema is thought to be caused by incompetence of those structures (vessel walls, valves, and sphincters) that normally prevent retrograde flow of lymph. This incompetence may be sufficiently severe to allow retrograde flow of intestinal lymph (chyle) into the pelvic and lower extremity lymphatics, a condition called *congenital chylous reflux.*

Other abnormalities of development may occur. The embryologic primary lymph sacs can persist to form large, multilocular, cystic, lymph-filled structures called *cystic hygromas.* Termed *lymphangiomas,* they can occur in a simple or a cavernous form. An example of this abnormality is seen in Figure 24-15 in a patient with tuberous sclerosis, a condition with multisystem hamartomatous

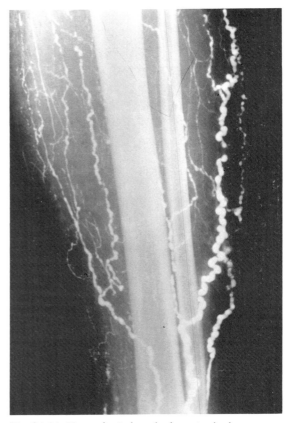

Fig. 24-14. Hyperplastic lymphedema in the lower extremity of a 10-year-old girl with many enlarged lymph vessels.

proliferation. Similar structural abnormalities are seen in *lymphangiomyomatosis,* which is characterized by multiple scattered lymphangiomas and varying amounts of proliferating smooth muscle, connective tissue, and endothelium (Fig. 24-16) [35]. Following trauma, lymph may escape into surrounding tissue, where it is encapsulated by nonendothelialized walls; these formations are called *lymphoceles* or *pseudocysts* (Fig. 24-17).

PATHOLOGIC CHANGES IN NODES
[3, 25, 31, 41, 46, 48]

The following pathologic changes may occur in lymph nodes:

1. Alteration in shape (round, cylindrical, irregular)
2. Variation in size
   a. Enlarged (tumor, inflammatory processes, lymphoid hyperplasia, lymphoma)

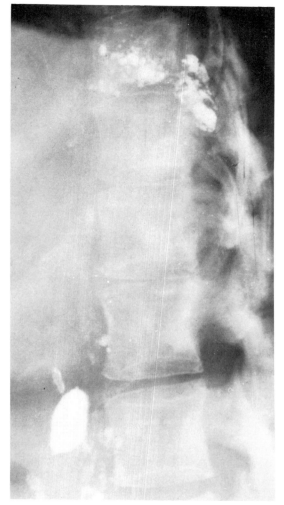

Fig. 24-15. Lymphangiomata in a patient with tuberous sclerosis. A cavernous form is seen overlying the T11–T12 vertebrae and a cystic form anterior to L2–L3. Note the mottled densities in the bone.

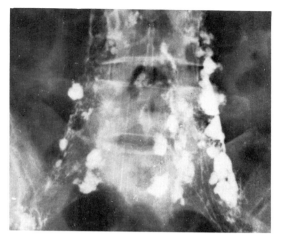

Fig. 24-16. Lymphangiomyomatosis. There is widespread replacement of pelvic and retroperitoneal nodes with cystic spaces.

Benign Processes that Cause Changes in Nodes [2, 12, 15, 38]

Many benign processes may cause large, abnormal nodes:

1. Acute infection
2. Chronic infection
   Tuberculosis
   Fungus
   Brucellosis
   Syphilis
   Tularemia
   Toxoplasmosis
   Infectious mononucleosis

Fig. 24-17. Lymphatic pseudocyst on the right (the patient had a biopsy at this site prior to lymphography). Compare the pseudocyst with the density of the lymphomatous lymph nodes on the left.

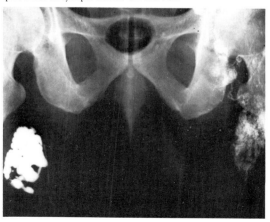

   b. Smaller than normal size (congenital hypoplasia, irradiation, chemotherapy and steroid therapy, replacement by tumor)
3. Variation in number
   a. Increased number (lymphomas)
   b. Decreased number to absent (congenital conditions; surgery; radiotherapy, chemotherapy, and steroid therapy; replacement by tumor)
4. Alteration in architecture (defects, foamy, finely lacy, granular, ghost-like, confluence, disintegration, density changes)

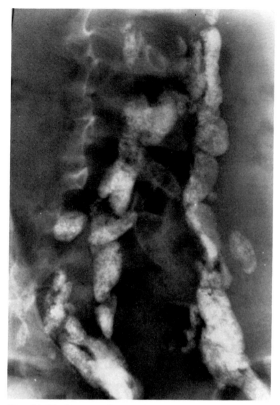

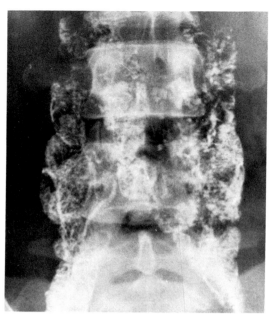

Fig. 24-19. Sarcoidosis. There are generally enlarged paraaortic nodes that are indistinguishable from those in lymphoma.

Fig. 24-18. Reactive hyperplasia. The reticular pattern is evenly distributed throughout the individual node as well as throughout the entire chain of nodes. This appearance contrasts with that of lymphoma, which has a more lacy appearance.

3. Reactive hyperplasia secondary to tumor and surgery (Fig. 24-18)
4. Sinus histiocytosis
5. Miscellaneous conditions
   Collagen disorders, especially rheumatoid arthritis
   Sarcoidosis (Fig. 24-19)
   Whipple's disease
   Dermatopathic lymphadenopathy, e.g., psoriasis
   Immunoglobulin abnormalities
   Hypersensitivity reaction to contrast media (rare)

Involutional changes may occur in lymph nodes, a condition known as *fibrolipomatosis*. Portions of nodes are replaced with fat and connective tissue. These changes are most frequently seen in

areas draining the extremities (the axilla, inguinal areas, external iliac chains), in which repeated infections may cause these nonmalignant architectural changes (see Fig. 24-2). The nodes are flat in one dimension, which is a good reason for evaluating all nodes in more than one projection. Afferent lymph vessels traverse these areas freely, in contrast to the findings of obstruction seen in nodes that are partially replaced with malignant disease.

Nonspecific reactive hyperplasia of nodal tissue can occur anywhere in the body; it is manifested by a loose reticular pattern with small, evenly distributed filling defects in normal size or enlarged nodes (see Fig. 24-18). This appearance is sometimes indistinguishable from that of lymphoma or metastases.

Effect of Metastases on Lymph Nodes and Vessels [16, 24, 26, 33, 36, 39, 40, 42, 43, 49]
Metastases (Figs. 24-20, 24-21, 24-22) are formed by tumor emboli that have become trapped, usually in the marginal sinus of the node in one or more places. These emboli enlarge, infiltrating, compressing, and displacing surrounding lymphatic tissue. They destroy the capsule and ob-

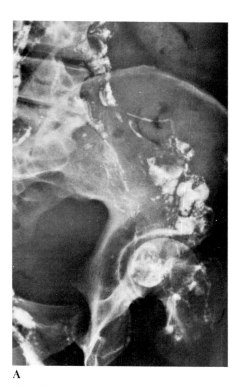 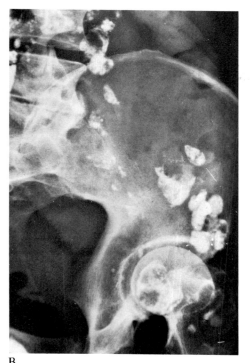

A   B

Fig. 24-20. Carcinoma of the prostate, with metastases
to the left inguinal, pelvic, and low paraaortic nodes.
A. Vascular phase of lymphogram.
B. Nodal phase showing multiple filling defects, primarily in the margin of the nodes.

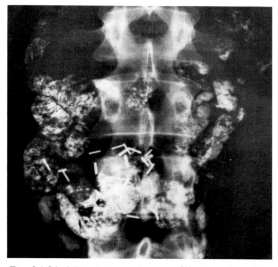

Fig. 24-21. Metastatic seminoma of the testicle, with
massive enlargement of paraaortic nodes. There is a
similarity in this condition to the foamy enlargement
seen in Hodgkin's disease. The metal clips are in position for radiotherapy localization.

struct lymphatic vessels, forcing open alternate
pathways and spreading tumor cells to these channels. Since malignant tissue is impervious to oily
contrast material, filling defects are seen. The disease may completely obstruct the lymphatics, preventing a central flow of contrast medium and
causing nonopacification of more central, although possibly normal, nodes. The regional
nodes may be enlarged and foamy due to a reactive
hyperplasia secondary to the toxic debris of the
tumor. The two abnormalities that are required for
a confident diagnosis of metastatic involvement of
a node are a filling defect in the node and an
obstructed lymphatic vessel. With the addition of
enlargement of the node, these abnormalities con-
stitute the *malignant triad*.

The node may be enlarged or normal in size,
globular or round, cylindric or irregular, depending on the size and number of defects. Defects are
usually marginal but may be central. They should
be larger than 3 mm or more than 25 percent of
the size of the node to be considered pathologic.
However, many of these defects are still due to
benign changes. If filling defects are 10 mm or
greater in diameter, the diagnosis of tumor can be
made with a high degree of confidence.

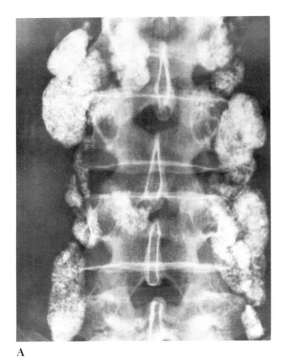

A

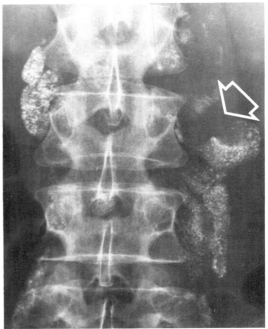

B

Fig. 24-22. The value of follow-up lymphogram, showing metastases developing in previously uninvolved paraaortic nodes in a patient with carcinoma of the cervix.
A. Lymphogram taken at the time of diagnosis. The paraaortic nodes are generally slightly enlarged and foamy in appearance, which is probably a result of reactive hyperplasia secondary to inflammatory debris from the tumor. No metastases are seen.
B. Follow-up films taken 9 months later show obvious replacement of the high left paraaortic node (*arrow*). Note the generalized dilution of contrast agent in the remaining nodes due to the passage of time.

False-negative examinations are often due to nonfilling of regional nodes or to microscopic tumor deposits too small to be detected. False-positive findings may be due to fibrolipomatosis or to reactive hyperplasia.

Conditions other than metastases that can cause filling defects include:

1. The hilus of a normal node (recognized by reviewing the vascular phase of the injection)
2. Fibrolipomatosis (defects often are central, the node is usually flat, and there is no evidence for collateral formation or obstruction)
3. Abscesses
4. Lymphomas

Other common conditions causing obstruction are:

1. Surgery
2. Lymphangitis and chronic inflammation
3. Irradiation and chemotherapy of malignant tissues

Lymphomas: Role of Lymphography

The principal role of lymphography in lymphoma is to determine the full anatomic extent, or stage, of the disease [9, 10, 22, 28]. The initial diagnosis requires biopsy. In lymphoma, the lymphographic abnormalities are more pronounced in the lymph nodes than in the lymph vessels (Figs. 24-23, 24-24, 24-25, 24-26, 24-27, 24-28). It is possible to have massive lymph node involvement without lymphatic obstruction. When obstruction does occur in lymphoma, it occurs relatively late (see Fig. 24-11). Lymphoma may produce an increase in the number and also the size of the nodes. Unlike metastatic disease, which usually involves the margin of the node, lymphoma proliferates throughout the whole node. The characteristic appearance is an enlarged node that maintains its marginal sinus even when the disease process is extensive

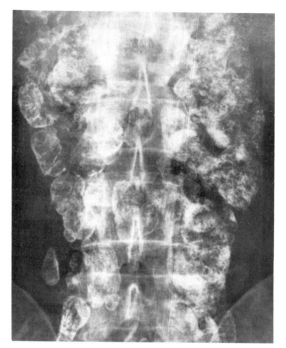

Fig. 24-23. Hodgkin's disease. This film shows ghost-like generalized enlargement of the paraaortic nodes.

(Fig. 24-23). Instead of the normal reticular pattern of the lymph node, one sees a somewhat foamy, loose architecture; this appearance is caused by the progressive separation and distortion of contrast-filled sinusoids and is characteristic of all lymphoproliferative disorders. Nodal replacement may also occur and may be so advanced as to leave a mere "ghost" of a node. The variability of involvement, both within the individual node and in the separate nodes in a chain, may help to differentiate lymphoma from nonmalignant lymphoproliferative disease. In the latter type of disease, there is more diffuse homogeneous involvement. With extensive involvement, a whole chain of nodes may be replaced. The contrast medium may stay in these pathologically involved nodes longer than in normal nodes.

The accuracy of lymphography in the staging of Hodgkin's disease has been correlated with the findings of staging by laparotomy [4, 5, 7, 17, 34, 37]. In such studies, biopsy of the paraaortic lymph nodes, liver biopsy, and splenectomy can be correlated with lymphographic findings. It has been found that the opacified nodes of a negative lymphogram rarely show evidence of disease on

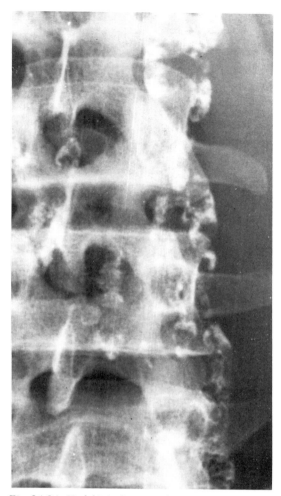

Fig. 24-24. Hodgkin's disease. The paraaortic nodes are of normal size with multiple filling defects.

biopsy. The diagnostic accuracy of lymphography in detecting abnormal retroperitoneal nodes has consistently exceeded 90 percent. In one large series, however, laparotomy has advanced the staging from that seen clinically and lymphographically in 30 percent of the patients. There is a correlation between the histologic type of lymphoma, the presence or absence of tumor demonstrated by lymphography, and disease in adjacent organs or nodes. Thus, even though liver, spleen, and mesenteric lymph nodes are not imaged, the presence or absence of lymphomatous involvement can be predicted by the presence or absence of tumor in the paraaortic lymph nodes [6]. Despite this ability to predict involvement in adjacent tissue, laparotomy is the most accurate method of

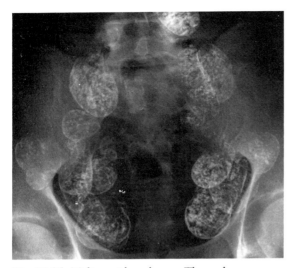

Fig. 24-25. Malignant lymphoma. The nodes are generally enlarged and foamy in appearance.

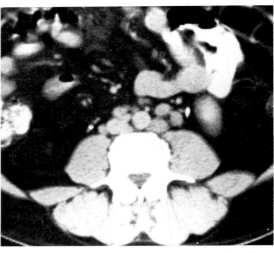

Fig. 24-26. Multiple enlarged paraaortic lymph nodes are clearly depicted by computed tomography and indicate involvement by underlying malignant lymphoma.

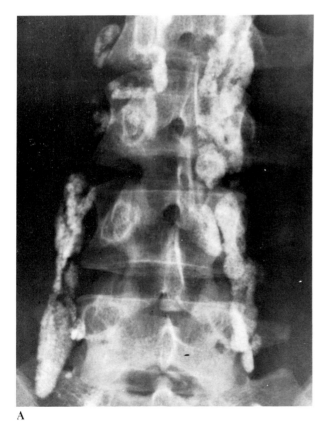

A

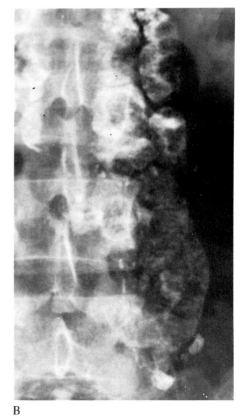

B

Fig. 24-27. Hodgkin's disease: progression over a 2-year period.
A. Normal paraaortic lymph nodes, stage I disease, confined to the supraclavicular area.

B. Repeat lymphogram shows enlargement and partial replacement of all the paraaortic nodes on the left.

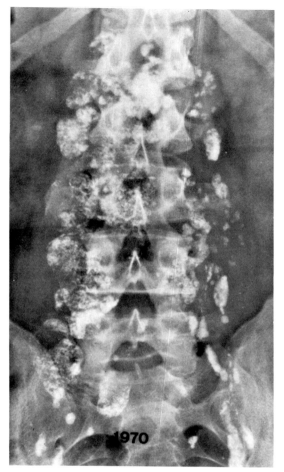

A

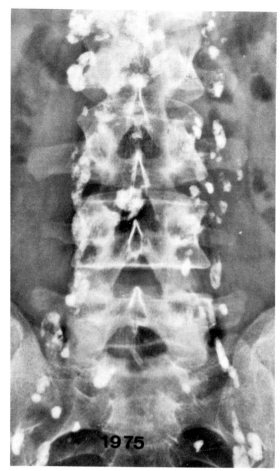

B

Fig. 24-28. Films of Hodgkin's disease, showing excellent response to therapy.
A. Film taken in 1970. There is foamy enlargement of the paraaortic nodes, primarily on the right.
B. Five years later, a repeat lymphogram shows a normal study.

demonstrating tumor involvement in those areas that are not directly imaged with bipedal lymphography.

One of the problems of lymphography is that the high sensitivity is obtained at a cost of specificity. Although very few false-negative diagnoses are made, there is a significant rate of false-positive interpretations. This rate could be altered by being more rigorous in the criteria for a positive lymphogram. However, if the overall accuracy remains the same, a decrease in false-positive diagnoses would be accompanied by an increase in false-negative reports. The role of the lymphogram

in the treatment protocol will determine whether it is more important to minimize false-positive or false-negative interpretations.

The accuracy of lymphography can be further enhanced by the use of percutaneous fine-needle aspiration biopsy. This technique uses a 22-gauge needle directed under fluoroscopic guidance into the most abnormal portion of the lymph node (Fig. 24-30) [18, 32]. Although it is more easily applied to patients with a solid tumor, it can also be successfully employed in patients with malignant lymphomas.

Several additional imaging techniques are available to evaluate the retroperitoneal lymph nodes, including ultrasonography, nuclear scintigraphy using gallium 76 citrate, computed tomography, and nuclear magnetic resonance. Ultrasonography is an attractive technique that avoids ionizing radiation and is often used in pediatrics; however, the impedance of sound transmission by bowel gas has resulted in many inadequate studies. The potential use of nuclear magnetic resonance is exciting, but it is too early to determine its role relative to lymphography. Computed tomography is the most commonly utilized modality and in many situations has replaced lymphography (see Figs. 24-26 and 24-29).

Although CT technology is expensive, it has become widely available and is routinely used to detect and monitor retroperitoneal lymphoma and malignant solid tumor metastases [1, 16, 30]. CT

Fig. 24-29.
A. Computed tomography reveals retrocrural lymphoma that is outside the expected area of opacification with lymphography.
B. Parailiac adenopathy is present bilaterally but is more marked on the left side.

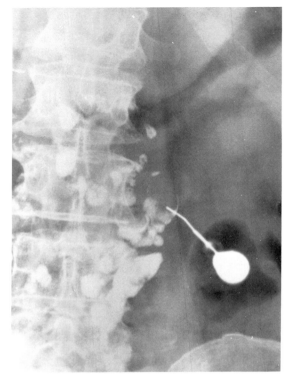

Fig. 24-30. Percutaneous biopsy of an abnormal lymph node confirms the presence of ovarian carcinoma.

has several advantages over lymphography, including the following:

1. CT is noninvasive, although intravenous and oral contrast agents are often needed, and requires little technical skill.
2. CT precisely defines the extent of abnormal

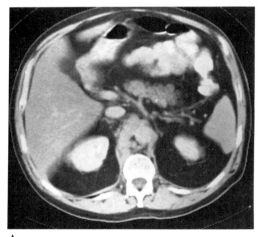

A

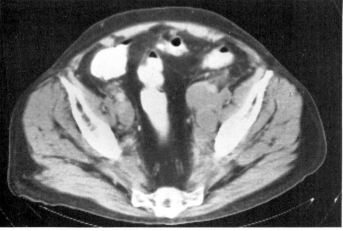

B

nodes, which provides a baseline for evaluating subsequent therapy, and aids in the delineation of treatment ports for radiation therapy.

3. CT detects disease outside the lymphatic drainage pathways of the injected contrast material. Involvement of internal iliac, mesenteric, and high paraaortic lymph nodes can be detected by CT but not lymphography (see Fig. 24-29).

4. Because the entire abdomen is imaged by CT, disease in abdominal organs is also identified by CT.

Despite the widespread use of CT, lymphography remains a valuable technique and continues to be used in patients with malignant lymphomas and selected solid tumors prone to retroperitoneal lymph node metastases. Lymphography has several advantages over CT, including the following:

1. Because internal lymph node architecture is imaged, tumor can be detected in normal size nodes.

2. The characteristic appearance of reactive hyperplasia allows the distinction between a benign and a malignant process in some enlarged nodes.

3. Disease monitoring may be done with an abdominal radiograph, which is far less expensive than a repeat CT examination [8, 19].

References

1. Aisen, A. M., et al. Distribution of abdominal and pelvic Hodgkin disease: Implications for CT scanning. *J. Comput. Assist. Tomogr.* 9:463, 1985.
2. Beetlestone, C. A., et al. The lymphogram in abdominal tuberculosis. *Clin. Radiol.* 28:653, 1977.
3. Cahn, E. L., and Steinfield, J. L. Conference on lymphography. *Cancer Chemother.* 52:119, 1968.
4. Castellino, R. A., Billingham, M., and Dorfman, R. F. Lymphographic accuracy in Hodgkin's disease and malignant lymphoma with a note on the "reactive" lymph node as a cause of most false-positive lymphograms. *Invest. Radiol.* 9:155, 1974.
5. Castellino, R. A., et al. Computed tomography, lymphography, and staging laparotomy: Correlations in initial staging of Hodgkin disease. *A.J.R.* 143:37, 1984.
6. Castellino, R. A., et al. Predictive value of lymphography for sites of subdiaphragmatic disease encountered at staging laparotomy in newly diagnosed Hodgkin's disease and non-Hodgkin's lymphoma. *J. Clin. Oncol.* 1:532, 1983.
7. Castellino, R. A., et al. Radiographic findings in

8. Castellino, R. A., et al. Roentgenologic aspects of Hodgkin's disease: Repeat lymphangiography. *Radiology* 109:53, 1973.
9. Castellino, R. A., et al. Roentgenologic aspects of Hodgkin's disease. II. Role of routine radiographs in detecting initial relapse. *Cancer* 31:316, 1973.
10. Castellino, R. A., et al. The role of radiography in the staging of non-Hodgkin's lymphoma with laparotomy correlation. *Radiology* 119:329, 1974.
11. Clouse, M. E., Grimsson, J. H., and Wendhind, D. E. Complications following lymphography with particular reference to pulmonary oil embolization. *Am. J. Roentgenol.* 96:972, 1966.
12. Cunningham, J. J. Lymphographic appearance of nodal extramedullary hematopoiesis simulating lymphoma. *Lymphology* 10:216, 1977.
13. Davidson, J. W. Lipid embolism to the brain following lymphography: Case report and experimental studies. *Am. J. Roentgenol.* 105:763, 1969.
14. Dolan, P. A. Lymphography: Complications encountered in 522 examinations. *Radiology* 86:76, 1966.
15. Dunnick, N.R., and Castellino, R. A. Lymphography in patients with suspected malignancy or fever of unexplained origin. *Radiology* 125:107, 1977.
16. Dunnick, N. R., and Javadpour, N. Value of CT and lymphography: Distinguishing retroperitoneal metastases from nonseminomatous testicular tumors. *A.J.R.* 136:1093, 1982.
17. Dunnick, N. R., Parker, B. R., and Castellino, R. A. Pediatric lymphography: Performance, interpretation, and accuracy in 193 consecutive children. *Am. J. Roentgenol.* 129:639, 1977.
18. Dunnick, N. R., et al. Percutaneous aspiration of retroperitoneal lymph nodes in ovarian cancer. *A.J.R.* 135:109, 1980.
19. Dunnick, N. R., et al. Repeat lymphography in non-Hodgkin's lymphoma. *Radiology* 115:349, 1975.
20. Elliott, G. G., and Elliott, K. A. The variable fate of oily contrast media after lymphography compared with residues in other sites. *Am. J. Roentgenol.* 104:851, 1968.
21. Frainow, W., et al. Changes in pulmonary function due to lymphangiography. *Radiology* 85:231, 1965.
22. Goffinet, D. R., et al. Clinical and surgical (laparotomy) evaluation of patients with non-Hodgkin's lymphomas. *Cancer Treat. Rep.* 61:981, 1977.
23. Jay, J. C., and Ludington, L. G. Neurologic complications following lymphangiography: Possible mechanisms and a case of blindness. *Arch. Surg.* 106:863, 1973.
24. Johnson, D. E., et al. Lymphangiography as an aid in staging bladder carcinoma. *South. Med. J.* 69:28, 1976.
25. Jonsson, K., Libshitz, H. I., and Osborne, B. M. Lymphangiographic changes after radiation therapy. *Am. J. Roentgenol.* 131:803, 1978.

26. Kademian, M. T., and Wirtanen, G. W. Accuracy of bipedal lymphography in Hodgkin's disease. *Am. J. Roentgenol.* 129:1041, 1977.

27. Kapdi, C. C. Lymphography without the use of vital dyes. *Radiology* 133:795, 1979.

28. Kaplan, H. S. Hodgkin's disease: Unfolding concepts concerning its nature, management and prognosis. *Cancer* 45:2439, 1980.

29. Kinmonth, J. G. *The Lymphatics: Diseases, Lymphography and Surgery.* Baltimore: Williams & Wilkins, 1972. P. 97.

30. Korobkin, M. Computed tomography of the retroperitoneal vasculature and lymph nodes. *Semin. Roentgenol.* 16:251, 1981.

31. Kuisk, H. *Technique of Lymphography and Principles of Interpretation.* St. Louis: Green, 1971.

32. Macintosh, P. K., Thomson, K. R., and Barvaric, Z. L. Percutaneous transperitoneal lymph-node biopsy as a means of improving lymphographic diagnosis. *Radiology* 131:647, 1979.

33. Maier, J., et al. Lymphangiography of testicular tumors. *Am. J. Roentgenol.*114:482, 1972.

34. Marglin, S., and Castellino, R. Lymphographic accuracy in 632 consecutive, previously untreated cases of Hodgkin disease and non-Hodgkin lymphoma. *Radiology* 140:351, 1981.

35. Miller, W., et al. Lymphangiomyomatosis. *Am. J. Roentgenol.*111:565, 1971.

36. Musumeci, R., et al. Lymphangiography in patients with ovarian epithelial cancer. *Cancer* 40:1444, 1977.

37. Musumeci, R., et al. Usefulness of lymphography in childhood neoplasia. *Cancer* 29:51, 1972.

38. Parker, B. R., Blank, N., and Castellino, R. A. Lymphographic appearance of benign conditions simulating lymphoma. *Radiology* 111:267, 1974.

39. Piver, M. S., Wallace, S., and Castro, J. R. The accuracy of lymphangiography in carcinoma of the uterine cervix. *Am. J. Roentgenol.* 76:278, 1971.

40. Prando, A. Lymphangiography in staging of carcinoma of the prostate. *Radiology* 131:641, 1979.

41. Ruttimann, A. *Progress in Lymphology.* Proceedings of the International Symposium on Lymphology. Stuttgart: Thieme, 1967.

42. Spellman, M. An evaluation of lymphography in localized carcinoma of the prostate. *Radiology* 125:637, 1977.

43. Strijk, S. P., Debruyne, F. M. J., and Herman, C. J. Lymphography in the management of urologic tumors. *Radiology* 146:39, 1983.

44. Tegtmeyer, C. A new lymph duct cannulator (Technical Note). *Br. J. Radiol.* 46:143, 1973.

45. Threefoot, S. A., et al. Gross and microscopic anatomy of the lymphatic vessels and lymphaticovenous communications. *Cancer Treat. Rep.* 52:1, 1968.

46. Wallace, S., and Jackson, L. Diagnostic criteria for lymphographic interpretation of malignant neoplasia. *Cancer Treat. Rep.* 52:125, 1968.

47. Wallace, S., et al. Lymphatic dynamics in certain abnormal states. *Am. J. Roentgenol.* 91:1187, 1964.

48. Wiljasalo, M. Lymphographic differential diagnosis of neoplastic diseases. *Acta Radiol.* [Suppl.] 247, 1965.

49. Wilkinson, D. J., and MacDonald, J. S. A review of the role of lymphography in the management of testicular tumors. *Clin. Radiol.* 26:89, 1975.

50. Yune, H. Y., and Klatte, E. C. Lymphography in lymphatic obstruction. *Radiology* 92:824, 1969.

VI

Cardiopulmonary Resuscitation

Cardiopulmonary Resuscitation

The eventual outcome of a cardiopulmonary arrest following an angiographic procedure depends on prompt and effective management. Since the same techniques are used in both primary respiratory and cardiac arrest, waste no time in trying to differentiate one from the other. Cerebral anoxia lasting more than 4 minutes is irreversible and often fatal.

The radiologist has two primary responsibilities:

1. Summon the aid of the advanced cardiopulmonary team. If possible, reserve for them those duties that require expertise and constant practice, i.e., endotracheal intubation, ventricular defibrillation, and drug therapy. As a rule, these procedures can await the arrival of the special team. The necessary equipment, however, must be immediately available (Table 25-1).
2. Promptly initiate basic cardiopulmonary resuscitation, namely, external cardiac massage and effective ventilation of the lungs.

Any patient at high risk undergoing intravascular or interventional studies, and any patient in whom intracardiac studies or pulmonary angiography are performed should be monitored by electrocardiogram (ECG). Intravascular pressures should also be available. These measures quickly detect life-threatening events.

Of all the resuscitative modalities available today, successful *early* cardioversion of ventricular fibrillation is most important in establishing a favorable outcome. High-risk patients should be provided with an intravenous drip as a precautionary measure before a study begins.

Recognition of Cardiopulmonary Arrest

Eye contact and verbal communication with the patient must be maintained at all times during angiographic procedures. The signs of cardiac arrest are as follows: there is cessation of the heart with an absent carotid pulse, breathing becomes inef-

fectual, the pupils begin to dilate, and the patient becomes unconscious (Table 25-2).

In primary respiratory arrest, the cessation or obstruction of ventilation is rapidly followed by cardiac arrest, and treatment is the same as for primary cardiac arrest. One should not be listening to the patient's heart or looking at his fundi when the patient's survival depends on vigorous cardiopulmonary resuscitation.

Treatment of Cardiopulmonary Arrest

The two essentials of treatment are adequate ventilation and effective external cardiac massage by manual chest compression. Either kind of therapy without the other is a waste of time. In the initial phase of resuscitation, physical action by the radiologist and his team is far more important than drugs, although an intravenous route for their administration should be established as soon as possible. Intracardiac administration of drugs is not usually required. Like the diagnosis of cardiopulmonary arrest, therapy can also be thought of under the headings ABCD (Table 25-3) [7].

ESTABLISHING AN AIRWAY
A major objective of establishing an airway is to elevate the posterior portion of the tongue away from the posterior pharyngeal wall, where obstruction usually occurs. An adequate airway is proved when the pectoral region of the chest rises with positive pressure ventilation. A proper airway may be achieved by one of three methods:

1. The operator tilts the patient's head, with one hand under the patient's neck and the other on the forehead. The neck is elevated while the head is tilted backward (Fig. 25-1A).
2. With the fingers of both hands behind the angles of the patient's jaw, the mandible is displaced forward and the head is tilted backward.
3. The patient's jaw is grasped with the thumb in the mouth and the fingers under the chin, and

Table 25-1. Emergency equipment needed
to treat cardiopulmonary arrest

Emergency equipment in the area
Oxygen
Defibrillator (portable)
ECG
Laryngoscope
Tracheostomy tray
Two 13- and two 15-gauge needles (for needle trache-
 ostomy)
Airways: Oropharyngeal, nasotracheal, and orotracheal
Portable resuscitator (anesthetic machine if possible)
Sphygmomanometer and stethoscopes
Intravenous stand, fluids, and equipment
Nasogastric tubes
Suction equipment

Emergency drugs
Diphenhydramine hydrochloride (Benadryl)
Epinephrine
Phenylephrine (Neo-Synephrine)
Aminophylline
Hydrocortisone sodium succinate (Solu-Cortef)
Levarterenol (Levophed)
Phentolamine (Regitine)
Nitroprusside
Reserpine
Atropine sulfate
Sodium bicarbonate (50-ml vials containing 50 mEq)
Lidocaine 1% (10 mg/ml) (do *not* use a mixture with
 epinephrine).
Phenytoin sodium (Dilantin)
Calcium chloride
Sodium amobarbital
Diazepam (Valium)
Nitroglycerine (dose tablets)
Lanatoside C (Cedilanid)
Digitoxin
Procainamide (Pronestyl; 100 mg/ml)
Isoproterenol (Isuprel; 1-mg ampules)
Dobutamine
Dopamine
Verapamil
Propranolol (Inderal)
Heparin
Dimenhydrinate (Dramamine)
50% glucose, 100 ml

Table 25-2. Signs of cardiac arrest

Diagnosis of cardiopulmonary arrest (*ABCD*)

Asystole—no heart sounds
Breathing—stopped
Carotid pulse—absent
Dilated pupils—present

Table 25-3. Treatment of cardiac arrest

Therapy for cardiopulmonary arrest (*ABCD*)

Airway	Establish and maintain
Breathing (artificial ventilation)	Initially mouth to mouth if necessary, but more effective with airway and bag plus oxygen. Start as soon as possible
Cardiac massage	Effective to produce a carotid pulse
Drugs	Epinephrine and sodium bicarbonate are the two vital drugs if the first three measures are not immediately effective

the mandible is drawn forward. The head is
extended by pressure downward on the forehead.

If respirations are weak or absent and chest
movement cannot be detected, artificial ventilation must be started at once, after establishment of
an adequate airway.

ARTIFICIAL VENTILATION
Mouth-to-Mouth Breathing
The operator positions himself at the side or above
the head of the patient. The mouth should be
explored quickly by hand to remove false teeth or
large particles of vomitus. One hand hyperextends
the neck and holds the jaw forward, while the
other pinches the nostrils shut (Fig. 25-1B). The
operator forcefully exhales directly into the patient's mouth at the rate of 15 times per minute. It
is important to monitor the first ventilation very
carefully; if there is no visible expansion of the
chest, the airway is probably obstructed despite the
previous maneuvers. A small plastic airway should
be inserted to hold the tongue forward and to
facilitate suctioning.

Bag-Valve-Mask Ventilation
Bag-mask ventilation should be substituted for
mouth-to-mouth breathing as soon as possible.
The mask is held firmly in place to form an airtight
seal around the patient's nose and mouth, and the
inlet valve on the end of the bag is connected to an
oxygen source at a flow rate of 15 liters per minute.
Room air has only 21% oxygen, but much higher

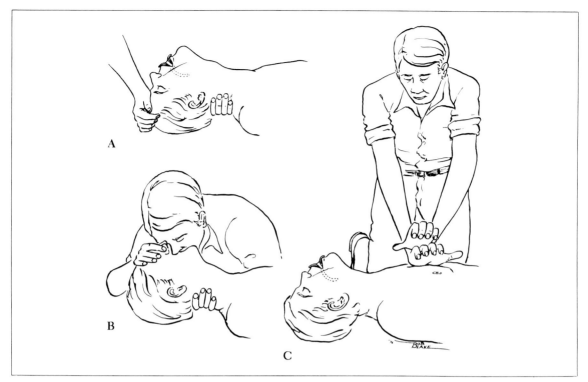

Fig. 25-1. Cardiopulmonary resuscitation.
A. Establishing an airway. Elevate the patient's neck with one hand and tilt the head back with the other. Introduce an airway after exploring the mouth for false teeth or large particles.
B. Mouth-to-mouth resuscitation. One hand hyperextends the patient's neck and holds the jaw forward; the other hand pinches the nostrils. Exhale forcefully directly into the patient's mouth 15 times per minute.
C. External cardiac compression. The operator exerts pressure over the lower third of the sternum by the heel of his hand, using the weight of his body rather than arm motion. Compress 60 times per minute, with a compression-ventilation ratio of 4:1.

concentrations (50 to 100%) can be provided by this oxygen source. The bag should be squeezed firmly, ventilating the patient approximately 15 times per minute. A patent airway may be confirmed by having another person listen for breath sounds, and the adequacy of ventilation can be monitored by observing the movement of the chest with each ventilation. A minimal tidal volume of 800 cc should be obtained with the bag-mask unit; this volume cannot be provided without adequate pressure on the bag.

Endotracheal Intubation
Endotracheal intubation should be performed whenever the patient's airway is threatened. Cardiac compression and indirect ventilation must not be suspended during unsuccessful attempts at endotracheal intubation. A maximum of 15 seconds should be allowed for endotracheal intubation if it is deemed necessary; this means that it must be performed by an experienced person. Endotracheal intubation is suggested when (1) an experienced person is present to intubate the patient; (2) an upper airway obstruction prevents adequate ventilation by the oropharyngeal route; (3) the patient has vomited, suction is ineffective, and there is considerable danger of fatal aspiration; (4) the patient has pulmonary disease, the cardiovascular collapse is primarily respiratory in origin, and indirect ventilation is probably not going to be effective; (5) there is an absent cough reflex; or (6) the situation has stabilized and assisted ventilation is likely to be necessary for a long period.

CARDIAC MASSAGE
External Cardiac Compression
External cardiac compression must be initiated immediately. It is performed by exerting pressure

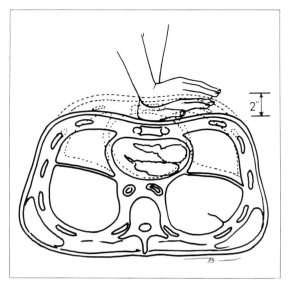

Fig. 25-2. Cardiac compression. The sternum can be depressed posteriorly directly over the heart for a distance of about 2 in. in adults.

over the lower third of the sternum. The only point of contact should be the heel of the operator's hand and the patient's midsternal line. By this means, the sternum can usually be depressed posteriorly for a distance of about 2 in. in adults (Fig. 25-2). To accomplish this, the operator must be in a position to exert pressure primarily by the weight of the body rather than by arm motion (see Fig. 25-1C), if necessary by standing on a stool.

The heart should be compressed at the rate of 60 times per minute. Practically, this implies a compression-ventilation ratio of 4:1. There should always be at least two people available in the angiocardiographic room, one for ventilation and the other for cardiac massage. If only one person is present to perform both functions, a more rapid rate of cardiac compression (i.e., 80 times per minute) must be accomplished to allow for the interspersed maneuvers of ventilation. In this case the compression-ventilation ratio would be 15:2. These ratios and rates are only guidelines. There is no scientific evidence to support efficacy of specific compression-ventilation ratios.

Palpation of the carotid or femoral pulses will provide a crude estimate of the effectiveness of cardiac compression. However, it is possible to produce a pressure wave without effective cardiac compression. A systolic pressure of 120 mm Hg

probably means that cardiac compression is effective. Cardiac massage may also restore and/or maintain the pupillary response to light.

External cardiac compression and ventilation should be continuous except for momentary interruptions to defibrillate. A continuous ECG recording should be instituted as soon as possible.

Internal Cardiac Compression

Physicians who perform thoracotomies must have training and experience in internal cardiac compression. The few indications for open cardiac massage in the angiographic setting include (1) cardiac arrest associated with penetrating chest trauma; (2) cardiac tamponade; (3) crushed chest injury; (4) unsuccessful use of closed chest compression. If tension pneumothorax is suspected, a large-bore needle may be inserted on the side of the pneumothorax through the second intercostal space 2 in. from the midline, and suction may be applied through a closed system. A catheter with multiple side holes may be quickly inserted percutaneously and, following suction, attached to a Heimlich valve.

Cardiac Monitoring

The radiologist in charge should be able to recognize arrhythmias and to provide effective treatment promptly. All high-risk investigations in patients should be accompanied by ECG monitoring throughout the procedure. The three types of arrhythmias that are seen with cardiac arrest are ventricular fibrillation, ventricular asystole, and electromechanical dissociation (profound cardiovascular collapse).

Ventricular defibrillation is the most valuable of the cardiopulmonary resuscitative methods that are available. The patients who survive ventricular fibrillation are most often those who are successfully defibrillated on the first or second attempt. Also, the incidence of successful defibrillation is higher if it is instituted early. The radiologist must take the initiative if ventricular fibrillation is suspected and an absent pulse does not respond to a precordial thump.

When ventricular fibrillation occurs in adults, the defibrillator should be promptly charged to 200 to 300 joules, or watt-sec. [3]. The manual compression is temporarily stopped, and the heart defibrillated. This is accomplished by applying the provided conducting gel to the paddles, firmly placing one paddle to the right of the upper sternum below the clavicle and the other just to the left of the left nipple in the left anterior axillary line. The countershock is delivered by depressing both paddle discharge buttons simultaneously. Skeletal muscle contractions should be observed. The operator should make sure that no one touches the patient at the moment of defibrillation and that the monitoring equipment is protected from the electrical burst. After the defibrillation attempt, cardiac compression must be resumed immediately; the effect of the defibrillation can be seen on the monitor while manual compression is continued. If the first shock is unsuccessful, shock the patient again immediately using the same energy. With subsequent efforts, increase the energy to 400 joules. If the defibrillation appears successful and the carotid pulse has returned, the external massage can be stopped. The use of the carotid pulse to diagnose the adequate return of the heartbeat is very helpful. One must not use the ECG monitor alone to determine when to discontinue external cardiac compression, because electromechanical dissociation may be present. In this condition, there is a normal ECG complex but little or no effective pulse or stroke volume. The prognosis is very grave if this condition occurs. Often the patient does not survive. Patients in asystole must be converted to ventricular fibrillation with epinephrine before one can expect to defibrillate the heart successfully (see the section on drugs). Since the diagnosis of asystole may be erroneous due to ECG monitor failure, an attempt should be made to defibrillate even if asystole is diagnosed. Basic arrhythmia problems occurring during cardiac catheterization are listed in Tables 17-3 and 18-2.

EMERGENCY TREATMENT WITH DRUGS

The major purpose of using drugs is to combat the hypoxemia (together with its side effects) that occurs during cardiorespiratory arrest. External cardiac compression alone cannot correct the problem of hypoxemia, because this treatment restores only one-third of the normal cardiac output. It is certain that prompt, expert tracheal intubation and early administration of high concentrations of oxygen go a long way toward correcting the problem. The correct choice of IV drugs may be life-saving. If an IV line has not previously been established, a

Table 25-4. Drugs used in the treatment of cardiac arrest

Essential drugs	Useful drugs
Oxygen	Vasoactive drugs
Sodium bicarbonate	Levarterenol
Epinephrine	(Levophed)
Atropine sulfate	Phenylephrine
Lidocaine	(Neo-Synephrine)
Calcium chloride	Isoproterenol (Isuprel)
	Propranolol (Inderal)
	Corticosteroids
	Morphine

long-term IV route should be obtained as quickly as possible. The superficial veins are often in a state of collapse. If rapid attempts at percutaneous venipuncture of the subclavian, femoral, or internal jugular veins are unsuccessful, a surgical exposure of the veins in the antecubital fossa or the external jugular or posterior tibial veins should be attempted. Intracardiac injections are usually limited to epinephrine early in the course of cardiac arrest if no intravenous routes are available.

Drugs used in treating cardiac arrest have been divided into two categories, essential and useful, by the American Heart Association (Table 25-4).

Essential Drugs

SODIUM BICARBONATE. Sodium bicarbonate combats metabolic acidosis that can occur rapidly in the presence of hypoxemia as a result of the accumulation of metabolites in the stagnant circulation. The bicarbonate (HCO_3^-) combines with the H^+ of acid to form carbonic acid (H_2CO_3), which rapidly breaks down to CO_2 and H_2O. The CO_2 is expired from the lungs, and acidosis is neutralized with the subsequent rise in pH. Removal of the CO_2 is necessary and requires adequate ventilation; if not, acidosis persists (reflected in a low pH), and the PCO_2 rises well above the normal limits of 35 to 40 mm Hg. This can lead to accentuation of intracellular acidosis and a depressant action on the myocardium.

In patients without initial acidosis who require resuscitation, severe acidosis can be prevented by good ventilation alone [2]; therefore, the bicarbonate need not be given if cardiopulmonary arrest has been of very short duration. Indeed, overenthusiastic use of bicarbonate can cause a very significant rise in PCO_2 to well above normal limits, with its depressant action on the myocardium and, in addition, hyperosmolarity that is potentially dangerous to brain function. Thus sodium bicarbonate should be used judiciously, and only if the duration of the arrest is over 1 or 2 minutes. At this point, the recommended dosage is 1 mEq per kilogram as an intravenous bolus or a continuous infusion over 10 minutes [2]. There should be repeated confirmation of the need for sodium bicarbonate by checking the pH (normal 7.36 to 7.44) and the PCO_2 (normal 34 to 46 mm Hg) level.

EPINEPHRINE. The use of epinephrine is based on the triple activities of restoring electrical activity in asystole, augmenting brain and heart perfusion during artificial cardiac compression, and facilitating defibrillation in cases of ventricular fibrillation. A 1-ml dose of 1:1000 solution (diluted to 10 ml in saline) should be administered intravenously every 5 minutes during cardiopulmonary resuscitation.

Sodium bicarbonate and epinephrine are the two most useful drugs for treating cardiopulmonary arrest. That should be kept in mind by all radiologists [4]. The combined use of both drugs will often convert asystole into ventricular fibrillation. Defibrillation may then be accomplished. When these drugs are used in patients with ventricular fibrillation, they may improve the state of the heart muscle and enhance the effectiveness of defibrillation.

ATROPINE SULFATE. Atropine sulfate is one of the most widely used drugs in our laboratory. Its parasympatholytic action rapidly counteracts the effects of the vasovagal reactions that are so commonly encountered. A dose of 0.5 to 1.0 mg is given intravenously as a bolus and repeated at 5-minute intervals until the pulse rate is greater than 60. A total dose of more than 2 mg should not be used in patients with third-degree atrioventricular block. If atropine sulfate fails to elevate pressures or pulse rate, one should resort to isoproterenol in an intravenous drip (see under Useful Drugs).

LIDOCAINE. Lidocaine (Xylocaine) is useful because of its action in depressing the irritability of the myocardium. It can be helpful when successful defibrillation repeatedly reverts to another episode of ventricular fibrillation. It is also useful for the treatment of multifocal premature ventricular contractions and ventricular tachycardia. A dose of 50 to 100 mg (a 1% solution contains 10 mg per milliliter) should be given as a bolus intravenously.

One should wait 5 to 10 minutes before repeating the dose; if after three doses there is no improvement in the ventricular tachycardia or premature ventricular contractions, 100 mg of phenytoin sodium (Dilantin) should be slowly given intravenously over a 2- to 3-minute interval. Although phenytoin sodium is used primarily as an anticonvulsant, it can also depress activity at the sinoatrial and atrioventricular nodes. The maximum recommended dosage of lidocaine is 300 mg (30 ml of 1% solution), or 4.3 mg per kilogram body weight. There is, however, a lower tolerance for this drug in the debilitated, the acutely ill, the elderly, or the very young.

CALCIUM CHLORIDE. Calcium chloride increases myocardial contractility and enhances ventricular excitability. It is useful in treating electromechanical dissociation. It also may restore an electrical rhythm in asystole, and it enhances electrical defibrillation. The usual dose is 5 ml of a 10% solution given as a bolus at intervals of 10 minutes.

Useful Drugs

VASOACTIVE DRUGS. The drugs levarterenol (Levophed) and phenylephrine (Neo-Synephrine) are potent peripheral vasoconstrictors and are used in the treatment of peripheral vascular collapse manifested by hypotension and absence of significant peripheral vasoconstriction. Levarterenol should be administered slowly and titrated against the blood pressure. One 4-ml ampule should be added to 500 ml of 5% dextrose. Neo-Synephrine should also be titrated with a minidrip of 10 mg of the drug added to 250 ml of 5% dextrose.

ISOPROTERENOL. Isoproterenol (Isuprel) is a sympathomimetic amine that acts almost exclusively on beta receptors. Its inotropic and chronotropic actions increase cardiac output sufficiently to maintain or increase the systemic systolic pressure. Peripheral resistance is decreased, however, and the diastolic pressure may fall. This drug is used in the treatment of profound bradycardia caused by complete heart block. The results are useful for severe sinus bradycardia that is refractory to atropine sulfate. It is also helpful in patients with systemic hypotension secondary to acute cor pulmonale. Isoproterenol should not be used in conjunction with epinephrine, which is also a sympathomimetic drug. A single 1-mg ampule is added to 500 ml of 5% dextrose; the dosage is approximately 1 ml (20 drops) per minute of this mixture administered intravenously, but it must be calibrated carefully with the pulse rate and blood pressure.

DOBUTAMINE. Dobutamine hydrochloride (a synthetic catecholamine) is a direct-acting inotropic agent with a short half-life (2 minutes) that stimulates the beta receptors of the heart to increase contractility while producing a relatively mild increase in heart rate, blood pressure, and arrhythmogenic and vasodilatory effect. Current literature suggests that dobutamine, although a less potent inotrope than Isuprel, is safer for patients with ischemic heart disease. The characteristics of dobutamine make it useful in the short-term treatment of the bradycardia and systemic hypotension that may occur secondary to acute cor pulmonale, or in treatment of adults with cardiac decompensation due to depressed contractility from other organic disease. The dosage is 2.5 to 10 μg/kg/minute, or 175 to 700 μg/minute in a 70-kg patient. Add a 250-mg ampule of dobutamine to 250 ml of 5% dextrose. Each milliliter contains 1000 μg dobutamine.

VERAPAMIL. Verapamil, a calcium channel blocker, has an antiarrhythmic function and is the drug of choice in treating supraventricular tachyarrhythmias such as atrial flutter and atrial fibrillation. In these conditions, it slows the ventricular response, and it is most helpful in the treatment of paroxysmal supraventricular tachycardia. These supraventricular arrhythmias are sometimes encountered during catheterization for pulmonary angiography. The dose in a 70-kg patient is 5 to 10 mg given intravenously over a period of 1 to 3 minutes while monitoring the heart rate. The peak therapeutic effects occur within 3 to 5 minutes. A repeat dose may be given 30 minutes later if an adequate response has not occurred.

PROPRANOLOL. The antiarrhythmic function of propranolol, a beta-adrenergic blocking agent, has been useful in cases of recurrent ventricular fibrillation that are refractory to lidocaine. The usual dose of propranolol is 1 mg given intravenously.

CORTICOSTEROIDS. A dose of 100 to 1000 mg of hydrocortisone sodium succinate (Solu-Cortef), given intravenously, may be used in cases of cardiac collapse occurring in anaphylaxis; this drug may also decrease the edema in conducting bundles in acute cardiac arrhythmias. The main use of corticosteroids is for prompt treatment of cardiogenic shock or shock lung occurring as a complication of cardiac arrest.

MORPHINE. Morphine, administered intramuscularly in a dose of 10 to 15 mg, may be used in the treatment of acute pulmonary edema complicating cardiac arrest. This drug should not be given if there is a history of asthma.

Basic life support and advanced cardiac life support systems are both important in cardiopulmonary resuscitation. The initial response of the radiologist must be to call for advanced assistance in cardiopulmonary resuscitation before initiating basic life support. Although the basic life support helps tide the patient over, it is limited in its efficacy. Early defibrillation in patients with ventricular fibrillation is essential for a successful outcome. Adequate facilities for advanced life support must therefore be immediately available at strategically placed, well advertised locations.

Treatment of Other Emergencies Occurring in the Cardiovascular Laboratory

ACUTE COR PULMONALE

The treatment of acute cor pulmonale is described on page 490.

CARDIAC TAMPONADE

The treatment of cardiac tamponade is discussed on page 490.

VASOVAGAL REACTION

Despite almost routine preangiographic preparation with atropine sulfate as an "on-call" drug, otherwise healthy patients may become dangerously hypotensive during an angiographic procedure. This reaction seems to occur most frequently at the onset of the study, sometimes even before the arterial puncture has been accomplished. Hypotension, bradycardia, pallor, sweating, nausea, and profound malaise may be singly or jointly present. Atropine sulfate is administered when the heart rate is less than 60 beats per minute in association with a systolic blood pressure below 90 mm Hg in an otherwise normotensive patient; it is given earlier in a patient who is otherwise hypertensive.

LARYNGEAL EDEMA
WITH OBSTRUCTION

Laryngeal obstruction usually accompanies an allergic anaphylactic reaction. Prior to the obstruction, other manifestations of an allergic response such as urticaria, bronchospasm, or convulsions may be seen [1]. The most useful drug is epinephrine, which may be given as 0.5 ml of 1:1000 solution subcutaneously in minor allergic reactions. A larger dose of 1 ml of 1:1000 epinephrine may be given intravenously in laryngeal edema with obstruction. It should be diluted in 10 ml of 5% dextrose or saline prior to administration. With severe obstruction, an emergency tracheostomy must be performed. An alternative treatment is the administration of oxygen through one or two 13-gauge needles rapidly inserted through the cricothyroid membrane or the upper trachea. Small endotracheal tubes may also be introduced through this membrane. In addition to epinephrine, an antihistamine (e.g., diphenhydramine, 100 mg) and corticosteroids (e.g., hydrocortisone sodium succinate, 100 mg) given intravenously may be effective. Tracheostomy is rarely required in these cases.

CENTRAL NERVOUS SYSTEM
EMERGENCIES

Convulsions

Convulsions may be secondary to the effects of the local anesthetic or, less often, the effects of contrast agents. They are treated with oxygen and also with slow intravenous administration of diazepam (Valium) to a dose of approximately 10 mg. The usual cause for toxic reactions to local anesthetics is overdosage or injection directly into the venous system. For this reason, it is important to aspirate the syringe before injecting any local anesthetic. There may be prodromal symptoms of paresthesias, tremors, tinnitus, slurred speech, or faintness before the convulsions.

Spinal Cord Damage

If spinal cord damage occurs, it is usually during aortography when a large dose of contrast agent is injected into a lumbar or intercostal artery, particularly one feeding the spinal cord. This type of injection is accompanied by an inordinate amount of back pain, clonic muscular contractions, and sometimes eventually paresthesias and paresis. Muscle spasm should be controlled with diaze-

pam, given intravenously in a dose of 10 mg. The same dose may also be administered directly into the intercostal or lumbar artery that was injected with contrast agent [5]. The most specific treatment is to perform a lumbar puncture and replace the cerebrospinal fluid with normal saline solution [6]. The rationale for this procedure is that there has been a breakdown in the natural barrier between the contrast-laden blood and the cerebrospinal fluid due to the high dose of contrast agent administered; the exchange reduces the concentration of the toxic material that has accumulated within the cerebrospinal fluid.

HYPERTENSIVE CRISES

Hypertensive crises usually complicate angiography in patients with pheochromocytomas or functioning paragangliomas. In the radiographic investigation of this condition, it is important that the patient be given phenoxybenzamine (Dibenzyline; a long-acting alpha-receptor blocking agent) for several days. An intravenous infusion must be started before the procedure is begun to allow rapid administration of drugs. Hypertensive crises may be treated by the administration of another alpha-adrenergic blocking agent, phentolamine (Regitine), given intravenously in a dose of 5 mg; this treatment rapidly brings the pressure down to preinjection levels. Diazoxide (Hyperstat) produces a prompt reduction in blood pressure by relaxing smooth muscle in peripheral arterioles. It is helpful in treating patients with an acute severe hypertensive episode when prompt and urgent decrease of systemic pressure is required. It is not effective against hypertension due to pheochromocytoma. Each ampule contains 300 mg of diazoxide. A 150-mg bolus (1 to 3 mg per kilogram) is given intravenously over a short period of time. This usually reduces the systemic pressure to an acceptable range. An additional 150 mg may be required over the next 15 minutes if an adequate response is not achieved. Sodium nitroprusside is a potent, rapid-acting antihypertensive agent when administered intravenously. It is also useful in these patients, but it must not be given unless there is continuous, beat-to-beat monitoring of intraarterial pressures. A rapid response in blood pressure results when the drug causes peripheral artery dilation and stops when the administration is terminated. The appropriate dose, carefully titrated with systemic intraarterial pressure readings, is 0.5 to 8 µg/kg/minute, or, in an average adult male, approximately 200 µg per minute. Fifty mg of sodium nitroprusside mixed with 250 ml of 5% dextrose and water (not saline) gives 200 µg per milliliter; therefore, approximately 1 ml per minute should be administered. Systemic cyanide toxicity and tachyphylaxis may occur if this dose is exceeded. Ideally the drug should be administered via an infusion pump. Since this medicine rapidly deteriorates on exposure to light, it must be protected by aluminum foil and should be discarded 4 hours after its preparation.

OTHER EMERGENCIES

Other emergencies resulting from angiography, such as loss of peripheral pulse, loss of the guidewire, knots in catheters, and clotted catheters, are dealt with in the appropriate sections of other chapters.

References

1. Barnhard, H. J., and Barnhard, F. M. The emergency treatment of reactions to contrast media: Updated 1968. *Radiology* 91:74, 1968.
2. Bishop, R., and Weisfeldt, M. Sodium bicarbonate administration during cardiac arrest: Effect on arterial pH, PCO_2 and osmolarity. *J.A.M.A.* 235:506, 1976.
3. Goldberg, A. H. Cardiopulmonary arrest. *N. Engl. J. Med.* 290:381, 1974.
4. Gordon, A. S. Standards for cardiopulmonary resuscitation and emergency cardiac care. *J.A.M.A.* 227(7) (Suppl.):833, 1974.
5. Gordon, D., and Levin, D. Treatment of angiographically produced cord seizures by intra-arterial diazepam. *Cathet. Cardiovasc. Diagn.* 2:297, 1976.
6. Miskin, M. M., Baum, S., and DiChiro, G. Emergency treatment of angiographically induced paraplegia and tetraplegia. *N. Engl. J. Med.* 288:1184, 1973.
7. McIntyre, K. N., and Lewis, J. A. *Textbook of Advanced Cardiac Life Support.* Dallas: American Heart Association, 1983.

Appendixes

Basic Drugs Used in Vascular Radiography

Indication	Drug and average dose	Remarks
Preangiographic medication	Atropine, 0.6 mg IM	Anticholinergic. Prevents vasovagal reactions.
	Meperidine (Demerol), 75 mg IM	Narcotic analgesic. Do not administer in cardiac or cerebral studies because of hypotensive effects of meperidine
	Diazepam (Valium), 10 mg PO or IV	Antianxiety. Respiratory depression in large IV doses
	Aspirin, 0.6 g PO	Decreases platelet adhesiveness. Give night before.
	Fluids IV	For dehydrated patients
	Hydroxyzine (Vistaril), 25–100 mg PO or IM	Antianxiety and antiemetic. May produce narcotic-enhanced respiratory depression
	Promethazine HCl (Phenergan)	
Narcotic antagonist	Naloxone HCl (Narcan), 0.4–2 mg IV; may repeat every 2–3 min to total of 10 mg	Used for overdose or exaggerated response to narcotics
Premedication of patient with previous allergic reaction to contrast medium	Prednisone, 20 mg q6h for 24 hr	Continue antihistamines for 24–48 hr after study
	Diphenhydramine (Benadryl), 50 mg IM 1 hr before study	
	Cimetidine, 300 mg IM or IV q6h for 2 hr	Histamine H_2 receptor antagonist.
Vasovagal reaction and brady-cardia	Atropine, 0.6–1.0 mg IV	Repeat at 5-min intervals until pulse rate is over 60. Maximum cumulative dose is 3 mg
Reactions to contrast medium (allergic), broncho-spasm, laryngeal edema	Diphenhydramine (Benadryl), 50 mg PO or 20 mg IV	Antihistamine
	Epinephrine 0.3–0.5 mg SQ or IM	Adrenergic. Give IV only in life-threatening situations
	Hydrocortisone sodium succinate (Solu-Cortef), 100–250 mg IV in 30 sec	May be repeated prn at increasing intervals (1, 3, 6, 12 hr)
	Cimetidine, * 300 mg in 20 ml 5% dextrose over 2–3 min	
Toxic convulsions	Diazepam (Valium), 10 mg IV	Tranquilizer and anticonvulsant
Hypertensive reaction to pheochromocytoma	Phentolamine (Regitine), 50 mg IV	Premedication with phenoxybenzamine (Dibenzyline), 10 mg qid for 1 week before arteriogram. Blocks hypertensive reaction
Acute hypertensive reaction (no pheochromocytoma)	Diazoxide (Hyperstat), 150-mg bolus IV; repeat in another 10–15 min if necessary	Peripheral arteriolar smooth muscle relaxant. Good for emergency reduction of BP
Gastrointestinal bleeding	Vasopressin, 0.2–0.4 units/ml/min	May also be used to reduce portal pressure (2.0-unit ampule in 100 ml saline = 0.2 units/ml)

(Continued on page 664)

* Use, together with Benadryl, if patient does not respond to epinephrine and steroids.
IM = intramuscularly; IV = intravenously; PTA = percutaneous transluminal angioplasty.

Indication	Drug and average dose	Remarks
Pharmacoangiography		
Vasoconstriction	Epinephrine, 5–10 μg	Preferential constriction of tumor vessels.
Vasodilatation	Tolazoline (Priscoline), 25–50 mg over 2 min	For better visualization of portal vein, peripheral tumors, and arteriovenous malformations. Also useful in treating arterial vasospasm
	Nitroglycerine (Nitrostat IV), 100 μg IA	Short half-life, 3–4 min. May be repeated with caution. Avoid hypotension. Use prophylactically during PTA below the diaphragm
	Nifedipine (Procardia), 10 mg PO or SL	Calcium channel blocker prevents smooth muscle spasm. Use prophylactically in PTA
	Verapamil, 5–10 mg IV over 2-min interval	
Acute cor pulmonale with left ventricular failure	Dobutamine, 2.5–10 μg/kg/min	Increases cardiac contractility with mild increase in heart rate and blood pressure. Half-life 2 min
Atrial fibrillation or flutter or supraventricular tachycardia	Verapamil, 5–10 mg IV over 1–3 min (in 70-kg patient)	Calcium channel blocker with an antiarrhythmic function
Cardiac arrest or ventricular fibrillation	Epinephrine, 0.5 mg IV	Ventricular fibrillation. Requires immediate defibrillation
	Sodium bicarbonate, 1 mg/kg IV bolus	Counters metabolic acidosis
	Oxygen	

Factors Influencing
Angiographic Quality

Factor	Poor quality study	Remedy
X-ray equipment and technique	Inadequate equipment with low power generator Low mA High kV Long exposure Large focal spot Low grid ratio (e.g., 5:1) Slow speed films and screens Poor film-screen contact Excessive object-film distance	Adequate generator of at least 100 kW output High mA Low kV (60–75) Short exposure Small focal spot* High grid ratio (e.g., 12:1) High speed film and screen combination Check film changers frequently Correct geometry
Coning	No coning, with primary x-ray beam beyond patient. Poor coning is the most frequent mistake contributing to a poor study	Tight coning to area of interest (e.g., kidney)
Film changer	Motion produced by cassette changer; inadequate maintenance of cut or roll film changer	Rigorous maintenance of equipment
Contrast medium and injector	Inadequate amount of contrast medium injected over a long time (e.g., hand injection through aortic catheter)	Power injection of adequate contrast medium in a brief time period
Catheter	Unsatisfactory use of catheter (e.g., aortic flush injection via selective catheter)	Correct size and shape of catheter
Improper technique	Absence of: Biplane studies Selective and superselective injection Magnification Digital subtraction Pharmacoangiography	These techniques are indicated in many special and difficult circumstances
Incorrect film timing	Capillary and venous phases of angiogram not recorded	Proper program selection

*Dual focal spot: 0.9–1.2 mm; 0.1–0.3 mm for magnification.

Characteristics of Different Ionic Angiographic Contrast Agents

Concentration	Trade name*	Anion	Cation	Remarks
Low				
Average iodine content	Conray-60	Iothalamate	NMG	Iothalamate is the best tolerated anion in
(mg/ml):280	Renografin-60	Diatrizoate	Na:NMG	the central nervous system, and Con-
Average viscosity	Reno-M-60	Diatrizoate	NMG	ray-60 is recommended
(37° centipoise):4	Hypaque-60	Diatrizoate	NMG	
	Angiovist 292	Diatrizoate	Na:NMG	
Medium				
Average iodine content	Renografin-76	Diatrizoate	Na:NMG	Renografin-76 is the ionic contrast agent
(mg/ml):370	Hypaque-M-75	Diatrizoate	Na:NMG	recommended for coronary arteriogra-
Average viscosity	Angiovist 370	Diatrizoate	Na:NMG	phy. Na$^+$ prevents ventricular
(37° centipoise):9	Vascoray	Iothalamate	Na:NMG	fibrillation. Do not use pure NMG
				salts in coronary arteries
High				
Average iodine content	Cardiografin	Diatrizoate	NMG	No advantage over medium concentra-
(mg/ml):400–460	Conray-400	Iothalamate	Na	tion group because of higher viscosity.
Average viscosity	Hypaque-M-90	Diatrizoate	Na:NMG	We do not recommend their use
(37° centipoise):13	Isopaque-440	Metrizoate	Na:NMG	

* Renografin and Cardiografin, Squibb Company; Hypaque and Isopaque, Winthrop Company; Conray and Vascoray, Mallinckrodt.
NMG is a cation of 1-deoxy-1-methylamino-D-glucitol 3.

Characteristics of Different Low Osmolarity Angiographic Contrast Agents

Concentration (Iodine mg/ml)	Viscosity (37° centipoise)	Trade name	Generic name	Remarks
Low				
300	4.7	Isovue	Iopamidol	Because of high cost, we recommend reserving for
300	6.8	Omnipaque	Iohexol	high-risk patients and possibly comfort reasons;
320	7.5	Hexabrix	Ioxaglate	history of allergies or previous contrast medium
				reactions; cardiac or renal disease or diabetes;
				suspicion of abnormal brain barrier; pulmonary
				hypertension or right heart failure; spinal or
				bronchial angiograms; external carotid and ex-
				tremity angiograms.*
Medium				
370	9.4	Isovue	Iopamidol	
350	11.15	Omnipaque	Iohexol	

*Fischer, H. W. Catalog of intravascular contrast media. *Radiology* 159:561, 1986.

Catheter Size and Approximate Maximum Injection Rates for Teflon Catheters*

Catheter	4.3 French	5 French	6 French	7 French	8 French
Outside diameter (mm)	1.4	1.6	2.0	2.3	2.6
65-cm catheter					
Standard		15–20 ml/sec	20 ml/sec	30 ml/sec	35 ml/sec
Thin-walled	22 ml/sec	25 ml/sec			
90–100-cm catheter					
Standard		10–15 ml/sec	15 ml/sec	20–25 ml/sec	25–30 ml/sec
Thin-walled	20 ml/sec	20–30 ml/sec	30 ml/sec		
Injection pressure (lb/sq in.)	1000	1000	600	300	200
Guidewire diameter (in.)	0.035	0.035–0.038	0.035–0.038	0.035–0.038	0.038–0.045

* With nonselective catheter position, one should use a catheter with end holes and side holes, a standard connecting tube, and medium-density contrast medium. Special high-pressure connecting tubes will permit delivery of 5 to 10 ml/sec more than with standard connecting tubes.

Film Timing to Cover
Arteriovenous Circulation

	Normal circulation time for:																		
	Heart and lungs ↓					Brain ↓					Renal ↓					Portal ↓				
Seconds	1	2	3	4	5	6	7	8	9	10	11	12	13	14	15	16	17	18	
Film exposure rate/second	2	2	2	1	1	1		1		1		1							Abdominal aorta
	2	2	2	2	1	1	1	1		1		1		1		1		1	Portal*
	2	2	2	2	1	1	1	1											Hepatic venous
	1	3	3	1	1	1	1												Aortic arch
	2	2	2	1	1		1		1										Selective carotid

* Portal hypertension may require extension to 30 seconds.

Amount of Contrast Medium and Rate of Injection

Time (seconds)	1	2	3	4	5	6	7	8	9	10	Total amount (ml)
Thoracic aorta	30	30									60
Abdominal aorta	25	25									50
Aortic bifurcation for peripheral vessels[a]	17	17	17	17	17	15					100
Translumbar	17	17	17	17	17						85
Main pulmonary artery	30	30									60
Right or left pulmonary artery selective	20	15									35
Celiac, superior mesenteric, and splenic	8	8	8	8	8	8	8				56
Hepatic	6	6	6	6	6	6	6				42
Inferior mesenteric and gastroduodenal	4	4	4	4	4						20
Carotid[b]	8	4									12
Renal[b]	6	4									10

[a] 60% ionic or low-osmolarity contrast agent (320 to 350 mg I/ml).
[b] 60% ionic contrast agent.
Note: As a general guide: Above the diaphragm, inject contrast medium over a 2-second period; below the diaphragm, inject contrast medium over at least 5 seconds (except selective renal and high abdominal aortic flush).

Risk Factors in
Angiography[*]

Complication	Complications of visceral and peripheral angiography (91,776 cases)[*] (Number of cases per 10,000 studies)			
	Femoral approach	Axillary approach	Translumbar arteriography	Remarks
Deaths	3	9	5	Femoral approach safer
Cardiac complications	29	26	36	Equal risk
Central nervous system complications	23	61	2	Axillary approach may embolize cerebral vessels
Local complications				
Arterial obstruction	14	76	2	Axillary approach indicated only
Hemorrhage	27	68	53	when femoral and translum-
Subintimal injection	44	37	175	bar approaches are not available

[*] After S. J. Hessel. Complications of Peripheral Angiography. Presented at the conference "Angiography, 1976—Interventional Radiology." Harvard Medical School, October, 1976.

Contraindications to Angiographic Procedures

General	A noninvasive procedure (e.g., ultrasonography) will give the same information.
	Information obtained will not influence management of patient.
	Risks of procedure outweigh the benefits that may be obtained.
	Patient's vital signs cannot be stabilized in an emergency situation.
Femoral approach	Severe aortoiliac occlusive disease.
	Severe blood dyscrasia.
	Femoral artery aneurysm.
	Prosthetic grafts in femoral region (relative contraindication).
Translumbar approach	High blood pressure (diastolic over 110 mm Hg).
	Bleeding diathesis or anticoagulant therapy.
	High aortic graft or infected aortic graft (relative contraindication).
	Suprarenal aortic aneurysm or dissecting aneurysm.
	Severe kyphoscoliosis.
Axillary approach	Subclavian artery occlusive disease or aneurysm.
	Subclavian artery bypass graft.
	Severe blood dyscrasia.

Radiologic Approach for Evaluating Renal Mass

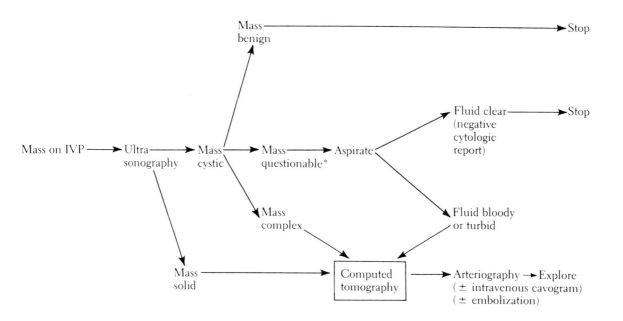

*Does not meet all three criteria of benign simple cyst: (1) anechoic, (2) smooth wall, (3) enhanced through transmission.

Management of Acute Gastrointestinal Bleeding

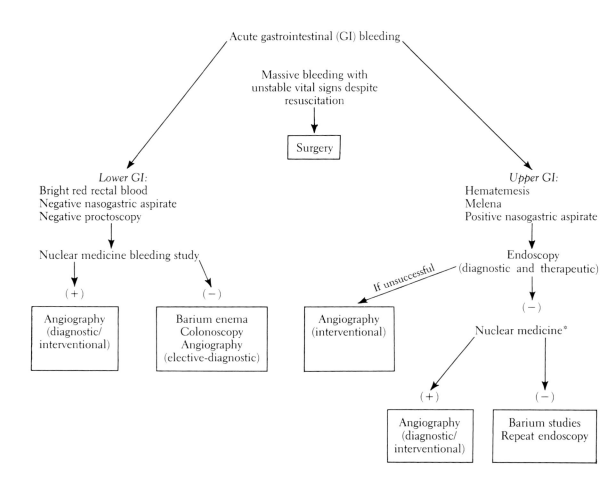

* The role of nuclear medicine in upper GI bleeding is controversial.

Essential Steps in Simple Subtraction

Subtraction is the removal of unwanted interfering images from an angiogram. The base film is the first film taken in the angiographic series, before any contrast agent has been injected. This base film is exposed, usually for 6 seconds, with a sheet of unexposed subtraction film with the emulsion side down to form a positive "mask." This film is then superimposed on a later film of the angiographic series together with a sheet of unexposed subtraction film for 30 to 60 seconds. The whole operation is most conveniently carried out using a commercial subtraction printer.* The directions for operation of the machine should be closely followed. Properly performed, simple subtraction leaves very little need for the more complicated second-order subtraction.

---

* Cronex printer, manufactured by E. I. duPont de Nemours & Co. (Inc.), Photo Products Dept., Wilmington, DE 19898.

The first step makes a positive mask of the base film (first film of angiographic series without contrast), thus:

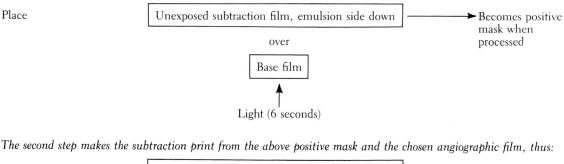

The second step makes the subtraction print from the above positive mask and the chosen angiographic film, thus:

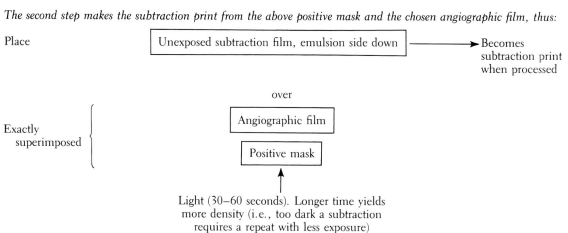

Catheter Diameters

Catheter (French size)	Outside diameter (mm)	Inside diameter (mm)	
		Standard	Thin-walled
3	1.00	0.50	
4	1.33	1.00	1.13
5	1.67	1.31	1.39
6	2.00	1.59	1.67
7	2.33	1.80	1.95
8	2.67		
9	3.00		
10	3.33		
12	4.00		
14	4.67		
16	5.33		
18	6.00		
20	6.67		
22	7.33		
24	8.00		
26	8.67		
28	9.33		
30	10.00		

Guidewire Conversions

Inches	Millimeters
0.015	0.39
0.018	0.46
0.021	0.53
0.025	0.64
0.028	0.71
0.032	0.81
0.035	0.89
0.038	0.97
0.045	1.14
0.047	1.19
0.052	1.32

Catheter Dimensions and Coaxial Systems

There should be a clearance of at least 0.10 to 0.13 mm (0.004 to 0.005 in.) between the outside diameter of the inner catheter and the inside diameter of the outer catheter. Generally, a difference of about three French sizes between the inner and outer catheter is required, maybe only two French sizes if a thin-walled outer catheter is used. Generally, a 3 French inner catheter (outside diameter 1.0 mm) will pass through a catheter that accepts a 0.097-mm (0.038-in.) guidewire. Check the inside and outside diameters before using, because there may be minor variations with different manufacturers.

In order to introduce a dilating balloon catheter through a sheath, select a sheath one French size larger than that of the catheter shaft.

Catheter Inside Diameter and Particulate Embolic Agents

There should be adequate clearance to prevent clogging the catheter lumen with small emboli. Powdered Gelfoam and smaller Ivalon particles (up to 250 μm) may be administered through a 3 French catheter (inside diameter 0.5 mm) but may occlude the catheter. Ivalon particles up to 400 μm may be passed through a 4 French thin-walled catheter (inside diameter 1.13 mm) but are best used through a 5 French thin-walled catheter; still larger particles (400–590 μm and 590–1000 μm) may be passed through thin-walled nontapered 6.5 and 7 French catheters, respectively. (1 mm = 1000 μm.)

Sterilization of Catheters

Most catheters are now commercially available in a sterilized form; those that cannot withstand autoclaving must be sterilized either by gas or by chemical means. Catheters made from Teflon are the only ones that can be autoclaved. The agent used in gas sterilization is ethylene dioxide, which requires a 24-hour washout period after sterilization.

The materials treated in the above manner remain sterilized for variable periods, but they probably should not have a shelf-life longer than 6 months. Quaternary ammonium salts, which were initially used for chemical sterilization, have been abandoned since the discovery that *Pseudomonas* can be freely grown in the solution. An agent currently available for sterilization is glutaraldehyde.* This toxic material can cause a contact dermatitis. It destroys bacteria, fungi, viruses, and tubercle bacilli in 20 minutes but requires 6 hours to eradicate spores. Catheters sterilized in this fashion must be thoroughly washed with normal saline solution prior to use in a patient.

---

*Available commercially as Sonacide (Ayerst Laboratories) and Cidex (Arbrook).

Preparation of FD&C Blue Dye No. 1 for Injection in Lymphangiography

Formula

1. FD&C Blue Dye No. 1 93%, 11 g.
2. Bacteriostatic water for injection, 100 ml.

Equipment

1. Magnetic mixer and spin bar.
2. Hot plate.
3. Beaker.
4. Erlenmeyer flask, 250 ml.
5. Cylindrical graduate, 100 ml.
6. 50-ml disposable syringe.
7. Millex filters,[1] 0.45 μm.
8. Alcohol swabs.
9. 16-gauge needle, 26-gauge needle.

Sterile Manufacturing Procedure[2]

1. Warm the bacteriostatic water for injection.
2. In a glass beaker with magnetic bar mixing, add the blue dye slowly to 90 ml of bacteriostatic water for injection.
3. When dye is dissolved, measure volume in 100-ml graduated cylinder and add water to 100 ml.
4. Mix in the original beaker.
5. Filter through 0.45-μm Millex filter directly into the vials, venting through 26-gauge needles.
6. Autoclave 15 minutes.

---

[1] Millipore Corporation, Bedford, MA 01730.

[2] Perform all operations under laminar flow hood.

Estimation of Percentage of Area of Stenosis*

The percentage of the area of stenosis can be estimated by comparing the diameter of the normal segment of vessel (D = abscissa) with that of the stenotic segment (d = curve) and reading the percentage of stenosis on the ordinate in Figures A1, A2, A3, and A4. Biplane studies are required to determine areas of stenosis accurately. Only percentage of area of stenosis is measured here, and not the length of stenosis, which is another important consideration in evaluating segmental narrowing.

Fig. A1. Concentric stenosis ($d_1 = d_2$).

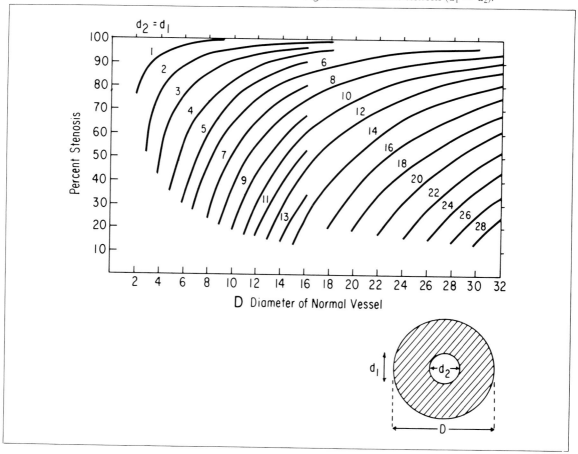

*Courtesy of Dr. Michael D. Miller, Elliot Hospital, 955 Auburn St., Manchester, NH 03103.

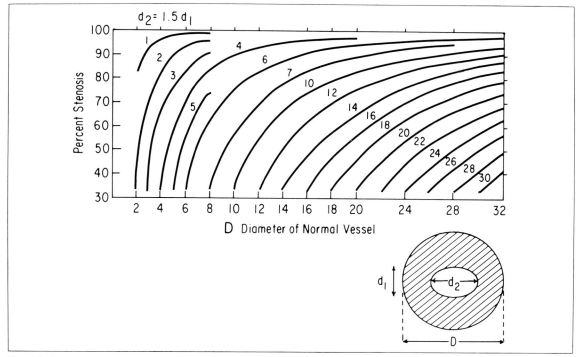

Fig. A2. Eccentric stenosis (area of an ellipse) with the large diameter 1.5 times that of the smaller. To find percent stenosis, locate the larger measured diameter (d_2) on the curve.

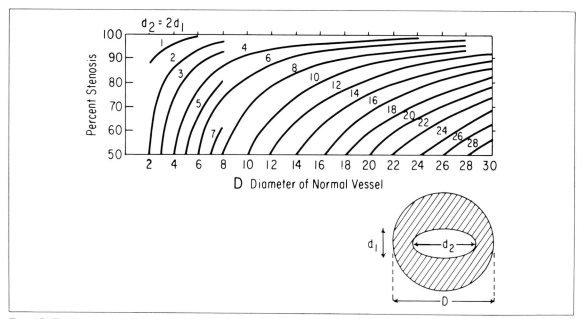

Fig. A3. Eccentric stenosis (area of an ellipse) with the larger diameter 2 times that of the smaller. To find percent stenosis, locate the larger measured diameter (d_2) on the curve.

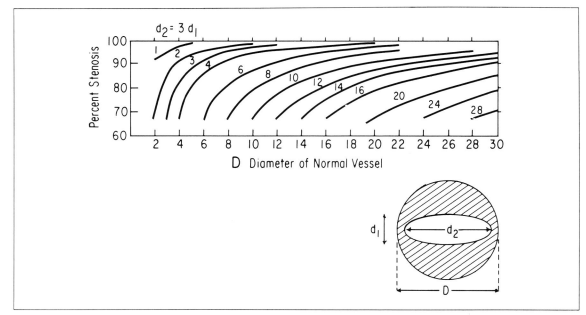

Fig. A4. Eccentric stenosis (area of an ellipse) with the larger diameter 3 times that of the smaller, as in an en face plaque. To find percent stenosis, locate the larger measured diameter (d_2) on the curve.

Less Commonly Used Embolic Agents and Their Delivery Systems

Calibrated-leak Miniballoon Catheter[1,2]

This catheter is used for delivering tissue adhesives or drugs selectively into a peripheral circulation (arteriovenous malformations, bleeding site, tumor bed) [5]. This is a 2.5 French single-lumen catheter with a small, nondetachable balloon at its tip that is calibrated to accept a given volume of fluid. If the volume is exceeded, the injectable substance (contrast agent, tissue adhesive) leaks out into the circulation. The small diameter of the catheter requires a coaxial delivery system. The tip of the larger diameter guiding catheter (7 French) is advanced as far as is practical into the parent vessel. The hub of the 2.5 French balloon catheter is fixed externally and attached to a tuberculin syringe while the body of the catheter is injected through the guiding catheter. The combined propulsion of the 2.5 French catheter and flow direction of the slightly inflated balloon advance the catheter to its final destination. For easier control, a propulsion chamber is attached to the hub of the guiding catheter in which the microcatheter is coiled while awaiting delivery. A series of Touhy-Borst adapters allows control of injections while controlling back-bleeding into the catheter system. The position of the flow-guided balloon tip is monitored fluoroscopically and may be readjusted by injecting contrast agent, which first fills the balloon and then spills over into the circulation. When in the correct position, the contrast medium (preferably nonionic) is first flushed with 5% glucose and then is replaced with accurately measured amounts (0.1–0.4 ml) of radiopaque tissue adhesive, which is flushed into the abnormal vascular bed with additional measured amounts of 5%

glucose. The tissue adhesive is made radiopaque by adding an equal volume of Pantopaque or 1 g tantalum to 1 ml of tissue adhesive. The balloon catheter tip and distal assembly should be lubricated with silicone. The balloon is deflated promptly following the injection, and both catheters rapidly withdrawn. This avoids trapping the balloon in the tissue adhesive. Carefully study the instructions provided by the manufacturer before use.

Detachable Balloons

Vessels feeding arteriovenous communications, bleeding sites, or lesions best treated by surgical ligation may be occluded by a detachable balloon. The balloon must be of sufficient size to occlude the vessel without migrating peripherally and remain inflated long enough to induce permanent occlusion. The balloon must be safely delivered into a peripheral circulation and accurately positioned before being detached.

There are two detachable balloon systems commercially available. Each has balloons of different size and materials. The two systems have different principles of delivery and balloon detachment.

LATEX MINIBALLOON (DEBRUN)

The Debrun latex miniballoon [2, 3][3] comes in a variety of sizes. Uninflated diameter ranges from 0.8 to 2.3 mm and length from 2 to 6 mm. Inflated diameter ranges from 4.5 to 14 mm and length from 10 to 25 mm. The sterile latex balloon must be manually attached to a 110-cm 2 French Teflon catheter immediately before use. The assembly also includes an overlying 3 French catheter, which engages and detaches the balloon when it is in final position. This 2 French/3 French coaxial system is advanced to its destination through

---

[1] Kerber balloon: Cook Inc., P.O. Box 489, Bloomington, IN 47401.
[2] Debrun's jet-controlled catheter system: Ingenor Medical Systems, 70 rue Orfila, 75020 Paris, France.

[3] Ingenor Medical Systems.

an overlying 80- or 90-cm 7.5 or 9 French non-tapered thin-walled guiding catheter previously shaped for selective placement in the parent vessel. The larger balloon requires the larger diameter guiding catheter. The guiding catheter is introduced into the femoral artery through an overlying catheter sheath. The assembly includes an appropriate adapter and hemostasis valves, which prevent back-bleeding, and side ports, which allow flushing with heparinized saline, both between the sheath and guiding catheter and between the guiding catheter and 2 French/3 French delivery systems.

Attaching the Balloon

Prior to attachment of the balloon to the 2 French catheter (Fig. A5), pull the distal few centimeters of the nonopaque 2 French Teflon catheter to attenuate it to make it more flexible and negotiable around difficult curves. Pass this 2 French Teflon through the 3 French dislodging catheter, which eventually will eject the balloon once in proper position. The balloon (with a small silver bead placed as a marker in its tip end) is next attached to the tapered-tip inner 2 French Teflon catheter. To do so, the 2 French Teflon delivery catheter is injected with 170 mg of metrizamide (through a Touhy-Borst adapter at its hub) as it is being introduced into the neck of the balloon. This allows easy passage of the catheter tip into the neck of the balloon and prevents air being injected into the balloon during subsequent dilation. Using a 1-ml tuberculin syringe, suction out bubbles within the balloon. Next, tie the neck of the balloon with at least 10 to 14 coils of latex thread, secure with three knots, and trim away excess latex sleeve. If nonsterile, the assembly is cold-sterilized. A newer model of balloon is now provided which has a mitered valve through which the 2 French catheter tip is simply advanced and firmly attached immediately prior to its use. The distance between the balloon and the tip of the 3 French dislodging catheter must be accurately measured. It is this measurement, together with the small silver bead marker in the balloon, that determines the balloon position prior to inflation with nonionic or isosmolar contrast agent.

Delivering the System (Fig. A6)

Once the sheath is introduced and sutured in place, the guiding catheter is advanced into the

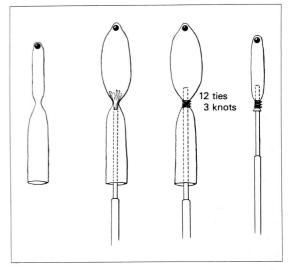

Fig. A5. The detachable latex miniballoon (Debrun) must be assembled manually prior to insertion (see text).

parent vessel. The vessel is first catheterized with a 5 French catheter, which is exchanged over a 220-cm long exchange guidewire for the 7.5 or 9 French guiding catheter. An inner coaxial catheter (5 or 7 French) facilitates this last maneuver. The 5 or 7 French catheter is next replaced by the 3 French/2 French coaxial balloon catheter assem-

Fig. A6. Delivering, inflating, and detaching the Debrun detachable balloon to occlude an arteriovenous fistula (see text). Large arrows indicate direction of blood flow.

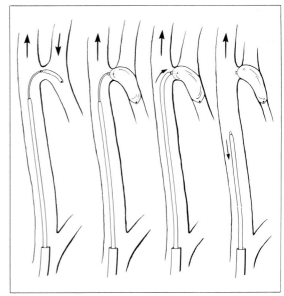

bly. During this maneuver, the deflated balloon is positioned a measured distance close to the 3 French tip. The 3 French/2 French combination is then advanced beyond the tip of the guiding catheter. The 2 French unit can be further advanced into the target vessel by inflating and deflating the balloon with small controlled injections of isosmolar contrast agent. Its progress is monitored by contrast injections into the outer guiding catheter. The partially inflated balloon is seen to change course and flutter as it enters the target fistula. At this point, the balloon is inflated and its correct position is monitored fluoroscopically with contrast injections through the outer guiding catheter. Optimally, the balloon should not impinge on the parent vessel but only occlude the fistula. When the inflated balloon position is correct, the 3 French dislodging catheter is advanced to engage and detach the balloon. To prevent leakage of contrast from the latex balloon, it is important to use the proper contrast agent for inflating the balloon. Metrizamide or other nonionic contrast agents (170 mg) may be expected to keep the balloon inflated long enough to induce thrombosis and permanent occlusion. The balloon may also be injected with silicone rubber which is allowed to harden and cause permanent inflation.

SILICONE RUBBER MINIBALLOON

The White silicone rubber miniballoon [8][4] is already attached by the manufacturer to a 2 French polyurethane catheter. The catheter material is sufficiently malleable to be injected at varying distances up tortuous arteries beyond the tip of the introducer catheter. The silicone rubber material of the balloon is semipermeable. When carefully inflated with precise amounts of isotonic or nonionic contrast media, it retains its inflated diameter for periods sufficiently long to permanently occlude vessels.

The balloon catheters come in two different dimensions and each has its own delivery system. The uninflated 1-mm (0.04-in.) diameter, 5-mm long balloon is inflated up to 5.3-mm diameter, 16-mm length and is used to occlude smaller vessels. It may be introduced through a standard non-tapered 6.5 French polyethylene catheter or through a 5 French thin-walled catheter (inside diameter must be greater than 0.044 in.). The 2-

[4] Becton-Dickinson Co., Rutherford, NJ 07070.

mm diameter and 7-mm long uninflated diameter balloon expands up to 8.7-mm diameter and 17-mm length, and is used to occlude larger vessels. This balloon requires a larger introducing catheter (8.8 French).

The introducing catheter should be inserted through an appropriate diameter thin-walled sheath with flushing sidearm and hemostasis valve; it may be introduced into the feeding vessel over a standard 220-cm-long, 0.038-inch guidewire previously positioned through a 5 French catheter as described for the Debrun system.

A special coiling chamber, similar to that described for controlling the calibrated-leak balloon catheter, facilitates injecting the balloon catheter through the introducing catheter (Fig. A7). A coaxial valve attached immediately in front of the chamber allows control of the length of the 2 French catheter injected and final manipulation of the balloon tip.

Prior to injection, air trapped in the 2 French catheter and its balloon is purged through its semipermeable membrane by injecting small amounts of isosmolar or nonionic contrast agent. The hub of the catheter is then passed through the coaxial valve and out through the back of the coiling chamber, where it is fixated with a Touhy-Borst adapter with attached contrast-filled tuberculin syringe. The body of the 2 French catheter is coiled within the sterile saline-filled chamber, and the protruding deflated balloon tip is inserted into the hub of the selectively placed introducing catheter. The balloon catheter is then propelled up the length of the introducer catheter and beyond by small controlled injections of saline through the sidearm of the coaxial valve. The course of the catheter is fluoroscopically visible and when the balloon tip is in proper position (monitored by contrast injections through the introducer catheter) it is gently inflated by injecting a small quantity of isosmotic contrast agent (0.15 ml in a 1-mm balloon and 0.6 ml in a 2-mm balloon) from a tuberculin syringe (Fig. A8). One should see a very small contrast-free gap between the tip of the catheter and the base of the inflated balloon. If this is not visible, the balloon may be coiled back on itself, and in that position it will not detach properly (Fig. A8). Deflate the balloon using a large 30-ml syringe and reposition the balloon if not properly located. When proper occlusion of the vessel is documented, open the coaxial valve of the

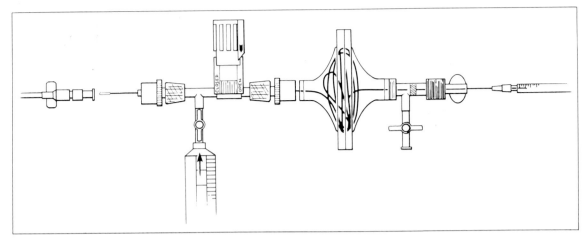

Fig. A7. The silicone rubber miniballoon (White) is attached by the manufacturer to a 2 French polyurethane catheter. It is delivered by injecting the polyurethane catheter beyond the tip of a previously positioned guiding catheter of larger diameter (see text). The coiling chamber facilitates the injection. A coaxial valve immediately in front of the chamber controls the length of 2 French catheter injected. The tuberculin syringe inflates the balloon with nonionic contrast agent when it is in optimal position.

coiling chamber and, while an additional small degree of inflation is applied, tug sharply on the 2 French catheter hub to dislodge the balloon.

PRECAUTIONS WITH DETACHABLE BALLOONS

Choose the correct concentration of contrast agent. If inadequately visualized, the balloon can be prematurely detached. If the contrast agent is hyperosmolar, the balloon will not remain inflated over the long term. If improperly placed, the balloon should be completely deflated before its withdrawal and repositioning. Occasionally, the balloon is difficult to detach once it is in proper position. It may displace during the detachment, and this insecure position may cause it to embolize elsewhere. Careful attention to detail and practice in an animal laboratory decrease the potential for complications.

Silicone Rubber[5]

This high-viscosity biocompatible liquid polymerizes to form an adhesive cast of the vascular bed, causing permanent occlusion [1, 4, 6].

[5] Ingenol: Ingenor Medical Systems.

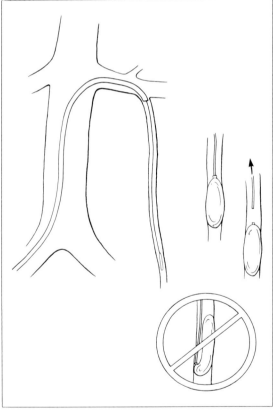

Fig. A8. Embolizing a testicular vein with the detachable silicone rubber balloon. The tip of the outer guiding catheter is in the testicular vein. The inner balloon catheter is injected peripherally to the desired site. The balloon is inflated with isosmolar contrast agent to firmly engage the walls of the vessel. A sharp tug disengages the catheter from the balloon. Be sure that the balloon is not coiled back on the catheter (see text for details).

The viscosity of this material (Silastic Elastomer 380R) can be reduced by adding and thoroughly mixing it with a diluent (Silicone Fluid 36 rs) in a ratio of one part Elastomer to two or three parts diluent. The time required to polymerize and solidify the material can be regulated. By adding one drop of catalyst (Stannous Octate-Catalyst M) per milliliter of silicone mixture, the mixture vulcanizes in 20 minutes. Adding another catalyst (one drop per milliliter) of Tetran Proxysilane, the mixture will vulcanize in 3 to 4 minutes; if one drop per 3 ml of mixture is added, it vulcanizes in 10 minutes. The material is made radiopaque by adding 1 g of tantalum powder[6] per milliliter of silicone mixture. Before the material is injected in vitro, vulcanizing time should be tested, and the necessary adjustments be made. Less-viscous materials with longer vulcanizing times are used to occlude smaller peripheral vessels, whereas more-viscous materials with rapid vulcanizing times are required to occlude larger, more central vessels. The material should be injected through a double-lumen balloon catheter (Berenstein) to more precisely control the location of the embolization.

Other Experimental Liquid Materials for Embolization

Polyurethane Bayer [7] is a solvent-free two-component vulcanizing polymer of urethane structures that requires a catalyst to form an elastic rubbery mass within the vascular system. It is made radiopaque by adding Pantopaque and changes from liquid to solid in approximately 10 minutes. It should be introduced through a coaxial occlusive balloon system. Results and precautions are similar to those for silicone rubber.

[6]Parke-Davis, Detroit, MI 48232.

Ethibloc [9] is a radiopaque viscous emulsion that, like bucrylate, precipitates when coming in contact with ionic substances. It takes 5 minutes to solidify, which allows a greater time for placing the material and removing the catheter tip. The catheter tip is less likely to stick to the vessel wall. The longer time interval allows greater penetration into the vascular system, possibly through the capillaries into the veins. It requires a coaxial system, and an occlusive balloon system allows greater control of the flow of the material.

References

1. Berenstein, A., and Kricheff, I. Catheter and materials selection for transarterial embolization: Technical considerations. 1. Catheters. 2. Materials. *Radiology* 132:631, 1979.
2. Debrun, G. Treatment of traumatic carotid, cavernous fistula using detachable balloon catheters. *A.J.N.R.* 4:355, 1983.
3. Debrun, G., et al. Endovascular occlusion of vertebral fistulae by detachable balloons with conservation of the vertebral blood flow. *Radiology* 130:141, 1979.
4. Doppman, J., Zapol, W., and Peirce, J. Transcatheter embolization with a silicone rubber preparation: Experimental observations. *Invest. Radiol.* 6:304, 1971.
5. Kerber, C. Balloon catheter with a calibrated leak: A new system for superselective angiography and occlusive catheter therapy. *Radiology* 120:547, 1976.
6. Kuntslinger, F., et al. Vascular occlusive agents. *Am. J. Roentgenol.* 136:151, 1981.
7. Novak, D., Wiener, S. H., and Ruekner, R. Applicability of liquid, radiopaque polyurethane for transcatheter embolization. *Cardiovasc. Intervent. Radiol.* 6(3):133, 1983.
8. White, R. I., Jr., et al. Therapeutic embolization with detachable balloons. *Cardiovasc. Intervent. Radiol.* 3:229, 1980.
9. Wright, K. C., et al. Experimental evaluation of ethibloc for nonsurgical nephrotomy. *Radiology* 145:339, 1982.

Index

Index